Being a Nursing Assistant

American Hospital Association

AHA

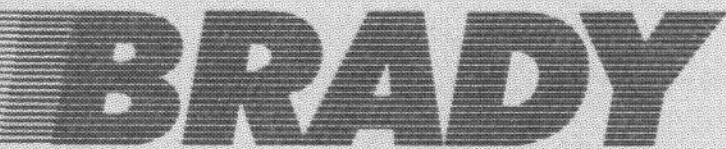

Being a Nursing Assistant

SIXTH EDITION, UPDATE

Rose B. Schniedman, R.N., B.S.N., M.S.Ed., C.N.A.
Susan S. Lambert, M.A.Ed.
Barbara R. Wander, B.S.N., R.N.

BRADY
REGENTS/PRENTICE HALL
Englewood Cliffs, New Jersey 07632

Library of Congress Cataloging-in-Publication Data

SCHNIEDMAN, ROSE B.
Being a nursing assistant / Rose B. Schniedman, Susan S. Lambert, Barbara R. Wander.—6th ed., update.

p. cm.
At head of title: American Hospital Association.
"Published for the Hospital Research and Educational Trust by Prentice-Hall, Inc."—T.p. verso.
Includes bibliographical references and index.
ISBN 0-8359-4902-8 (pbk.)
1. Nurses' aides. 2. Care of the sick.
I. Lambert, Susan M. II. Wander, Barbara R.
III. American Hospital Association. IV. Hospital Research and Educational Trust. V. Title.
[DNLM]: 1. Nurses' Aides. WY 193 S361b 1995]
RT84.S35 1995
610.73'069'8—dc20
DNLM/DLC 94–40683
for Library of Congress CIP

Acquisitions Editors: *Susan B. Willig, Natalie E. Anderson*
Cover design: *Richard Puder Design*
Cover illustration: *Mary Schmidt*
Interior design: *Lorraine Mullaney*
Photography: *Lightworks Studio/George Dodson*
Editorial/production supervision: *Patrick Walsh*
Prepress buyer: *Mary McCartney*
Manufacturing buyer: *Ed O'Dougherty*
Page layout: *Lorraine Mullaney, Charles Pelletreau, Karen Noferi*

Published for The Hospital Research and Educational Trust by Prentice-Hall Inc., A Simon & Schuster Company, Englewood Cliffs, New Jersey 07632

Printed in the United States of America
10 9 8 7 6 5 4 3 2 1

ISBN: 0-8359-4902-8

Prentice-Hall International (UK) Limited, *London*
Prentice-Hall of Australia Pty. Limited, *Sydney*
Prentice-Hall Canada Inc., *Toronto*
Prentice-Hall Hispanoamericana, S.A., *Mexico*
Prentice-Hall of India Private Limited, *New Delhi*
Prentice-Hall of Japan, Inc., *Tokyo*
Simon & Schuster Asia Pte. Ltd., *Singapore*
Editora Prentice-Hall do Brasil, Ltda., *Rio de Janeiro*

NOTICE

The procedures described in this textbook are based on consultation with nursing authorities. To the best of the authors' knowledge, these procedures reflect currently accepted clinical practice; however, they cannot be considered absolute recommendations. For individual application, the policies and procedures of the institution or agency where the Nursing Assistant is employed must be reviewed and followed. The authors of this textbook, and of the supplements written specifically to go with it, disclaim responsibility for any adverse effects resulting directly or indirectly from the suggested procedures and theory, from any undetected errors, or from the reader's misunderstanding of the text. It is the reader's responsibility to stay informed of any new changes or recommendations made by his or her employing health care institution or agency.

NOTE ON GENDER USAGE

Past attitudes have allowed our language to develop with the pronouns "he," "she," "his," or "her" used to signify persons of either gender. For example, when describing the care involved in turning a patient, most people will say "ask her to turn," or "ask him to turn," rather than "ask him or her to turn." Our editors tell us that the repeated use of "he or she" is not proper in long manuscript, and the use of "he or she" is incorrect in all cases.

Authorities in both professional journals and popular publications have stated that the "quick fix" approach should be discouraged. They recommend different sentence structures when appropriate and the traditional use of "he" and "she" when necessary. This is why you will find "he" and "she" used interchangeably when referring to the actions taken by a Nursing Assistant. It is not the intent of the authors or the publisher to imply that men should not be Nursing Assistants or that they are any less professional than women in carrying out Nursing Assistant level care.

TO THE STUDENT

A self-instructional workbook for this text is available through a college bookstore under the title, *Workbook for Being a Nursing Assistant.* If not in stock, ask the bookstore manager to order a copy for you. If your course is being offered off-campus, ask your instructor where to obtain a copy. The workbook can help you with course material by acting as a tutorial review and study aid.

A self-instructional pocket guide for this text is available through a college bookstore under the title, *Pocket Guide for the Nursing Assistant.* If not in stock, ask the bookstore manager to order a copy for you. If your course is being offered off-campus, ask your instructor where to obtain a copy. The *Pocket Guide* can help you in your clinical lab experience and on the job.

In loving memory of
Martin S. Schniedman

Contents

Preface

This sixth edition of Being A Nursing Assistant has been thoroughly redesigned and reorganized to increase its effectiveness as a superior teaching vehicle. Overall highlights of the sixth edition include:

- Total reorganization of content, blending theory with practice.
- Integrated presentation of material to facilitate student understanding.
- More comprehensive coverage to make teaching and learning easier.
- Numerous short chapters which organize the material into manageable lessons.
- Detailed lists of objectives, closely integrated with each chapter.
- Key Terms defined in the margin and a Glossary to clarify terminology.
- All units conclude with Key Questions that stimulate discussion and provide immediate reinforcement and maximum independence.
- Numerous new photographs and line drawings to clarify procedures and theoretical concepts.
- All procedures have been reviewed and updated to agree with current knowledge, standards, and practice.
- A completely new chapter on Emergency Care, including CPR.
- Expanded coverage of geriatric care, including the psychosocial and psychological aspects of geriatric care.
- New information on pediatrics, including children's common diseases/conditions.
- A completely new description of normal growth and development throughout the life span.
- Updated and expanded information on home health care.
- Revised explanations of intake and output.
- New discussions on current legal aspects, including responsibilities of the nursing assistant, invasion of privacy, slander, libel, assault, battery, informed consent, and false imprisonment.
- An entirely new presentation of sexuality.
- Revised and updated material on vital signs.
- Additional in-depth coverage of common diseases including Parkinson's, Hodgkin's, Alzheimer's and AIDS
- Psychological and psychosocial aspects of rehabilitative care.
- Updated job description.
- Current discussion of ethical behavior, including:
  - Ethics of accuracy
  - Ethics of dependability

- Human relations, including:
  - Transcultural nursing
  - Relating to people
  - Sympathy/empathy.
- Updated material on communication skills.
- Procedures reflecting the latest guidelines from the Center For Disease Control, Atlanta, Georgia (Universal Precautions).
- Reorganized material on medical terminology.

Acknowledgments

This sixth edition of *Being a Nursing Assistant* has been prepared by Rose B. Schniedman, R.N., B.S.N., M.S.Ed., C.N.A., Susan S. Lambert, M.A.Ed., and Barbara R. Wander, B.S.N., R.N.

Mrs. Schniedman

- Founded a School for Health Careers
- Directed the training of Nursing Assistants for Hospitals, Long Term Facilities, Home Health Agencies, and Rehabilitation Centers within the Miami, Florida area for many years
- Has been the Director of Nursing Education within an Acute Care Facility, and an Administrative and Educational Consultant for a Home Health Agency
- Pioneered the legislation of the Nursing Assistant Certification program in Florida, and has been a member of a special committee for the Certification of Nursing Assistants with the Florida State Board of Nursing
- Is currently Director of Professional Services for a nationwide Home Health Agency

Mrs. Lambert

- Is an Educational Curriculum Consultant specializing in Adult and Vocational Education, and an instructor of English as a Second Language in Charlotte, North Carolina

Mrs. Wander

- Has been a maternal and infant care patient educator in a teaching hospital in North-Central Florida, and a patient care supervisor for a Home Health Agency
- Is currently a Veterinary Hospital Administrator in Miami, Florida

The Trust gratefully acknowledges their wisdom, perseverance, and above all dedication as authors of this textbook.

The authors would like to acknowledge and thank the staff of the Prentice Hall College Book Division, who ensured that this edition maintained the quality and upheld the reputation of the previous editions. Special thanks go to

- Susan Willig, Publisher, Vocational Publishing, for sharing her professional expertise
- Natalie Anderson, Senior Editor, Vocational Publishing, for contributing immeasurably to this edition

- Louise Fullam, Editorial Assistant, who was always willing to help, for her hard work and high degree of professionalism
- Patrick Walsh, Senior Production Editor, for his guidance and help in maintaining the schedule
- The Design and Production Departments, for their efforts in developing and carrying out the production plan for this edition.

For providing the location, equipment, and personnel for many of the photographs taken for this edition, the assistance of the Division of Patient Care Services of Holy Cross Hospital of Silver Spring, Maryland is gratefully acknowledged.

Finally, the following individuals provided a careful and thorough review of the text and art for the sixth edition:

- Barbara A. Donaho, R.N., M.A.
Senior Vice President, Patient Services
St. Anthony's Hospital
St. Petersburg, Florida
- Julie Bell, R.N., M.S.
Nursing Support Staff/Student Affairs
Division of Nursing Research, Education and Program Development
Shands Hospital at the University of Florida
- Veronica Carr, R.N.
Inservice Program Director
Division of Nursing Research, Education and Program Development
Shands Hospital at the University of Florida

Their assistance in this manner is gratefully acknowledged.

Introduction

Welcome to *Being a Nursing Assistant* and to the beginning of a new career in the health care field. Delivering health care is a very special job, one you can take much pride in. You will be helping people and making your community a better place in which to live.

You are, or will be, working in a health care institution—hospitals, nursing homes, clinics, and the home where sick and injured people are treated and cared for. The most important people in these institutions are the patients. All health care personnel are there to meet their needs.

This book has been written to help you do well in your training and on the job. Your instructor will guide your training during class, lectures, practice sessions, and clinical experiences, and will teach you the procedures and policies that are required in your state and in the institution where you will be working. The reason for this is that methods and policies vary from state to state and from one health care institution to another. If your instructor demonstrates a procedure differently than it is explained in this book, follow that method.

Health care delivery is a field full of rapid changes and improvements. A textbook cannot be changed as quickly or as often as new insights, techniques, or equipment are adopted by modern health care institutions. Your instructor keeps informed of these changes and is your best source of current information. If this text, or any other source, takes one approach to a situation and your instructor takes a different one, follow your instructor. Your instructor is an expert in health care delivery and is the authority for your course.

On the job, you will be supervised by the head nurse, supervisor or team leader. They may not necessarily be the same person, although they might be. We use the term immediate supervisor throughout this book to refer to the person who supervises you and keeps a record of your performance. During your training, if you do not understand a procedure, ask your instructor for help. On the job, ask your head nurse or team leader. It is far better to get help if you are not sure than to do something wrong.

Use this book. Read through the procedures until you remember every step. Try to meet all objectives in each section of every chapter. Like a dictionary, this text is a learning tool and a reference book. Use it in class for taking notes. Look at it whenever you have a chance. *Study* this book at home, and *read* it before class. *Review* procedures you may not be sure of during your work. *Check* the illustrations, charts, and lists. They will help to make things clear. Work on your vocabulary. Use the Key Terms and the Glossary section in the back of the book to find the meaning of words you do not fully understand or that are unfamiliar to you.

How to Use This Manual Effectively

Contents

All of the chapters, key ideas in each chapter, and the procedures are listed in the Contents. Use it to find the page number of any concept or procedure you might want to review.

Chapters

The small chapters give you a smaller amount of material to learn at one time. This is designed to make it easier for you to study, understand the lesson, and learn the many nursing tasks that are involved in your job.

Objectives: What You Will Learn

Each chapter begins with a list of objectives. These objectives should serve as realistic goals for you to reach. Objectives tell you what you should be able to do by the end of each chapter. Objectives are things you are expected to accomplish.

Each objective gives you a specific goal or a particular action you need to be able to perform—actions or behaviors that can be observed by you and by others. For example, the best way for you and your instructor to see if you understand the procedure for making an occupied bed is for you to actually make an occupied bed.

Read each chapter and keep the list of objectives in mind. You can use the objectives as self-tests. When you finish reading a section, go back and reread the objectives. See if you are able to perform each objective in the list. Study the pages that deal with the objective you could not meet.

When you have completed each chapter you should be able to define, explain, apply, or demonstrate, the material covered in that section.

Key Ideas

Under the heading of *Key Ideas* you will find the reasons for each procedure. Knowing why you are doing something will help you to prepare for and to carry out the procedures in the best possible way. Pay careful attention to all the illustrations, charts, and lists, in every section. These are all designed to make it easier for you to remember the important information.

There are basic principles, ideas, and methods, that must be remembered for the overall total care of a patient. As an example, you will always treat the patient with courtesy, kindness, and empathy. Such a principle or rule does not make up a full procedure. In some situations, the order in which the tasks are done does not matter. For example, you will check the patient unit (the room) to make sure that everything needed is there. Tasks like this do not follow a definite numerical order. Therefore, they are not true procedures. They are called *Rules to Follow*.

Procedures

A task is an assigned duty, something you are expected to do. In this manual, each nursing task has been divided into a logical, orderly series

Sample Procedure

1. Assemble your equipment.
2. Wash your hands.
3. Identify the patient by checking the identification bracelet.
4. Ask visitors to step out of the room, if this is your hospital's policy.
5. Tell the patient what you are going to do. For example, "I am going to measure your vital signs."
6. Pull the curtain around the bed for privacy.
7. Do the procedure, each step of which is numbered in order of performance.
8. Discard disposable equipment in the proper containers.
9. Clean the standard reusable equipment and put it in its proper place.
10. Make the patient comfortable.
11. Lower the bed to a position of safety for the patient.
12. Pull the curtains back to the open position.
13. Raise the side rails where ordered, indicated, and appropriate, for patient safety.
14. Place the call light within easy reach of the patient.
15. Wash your hands.
16. Report to your immediate supervisor:
    - That you have completed the procedure.
    - The time and date the procedure was done.
    - The pertinent facts concerning the procedure.
    - The results of the procedure.
    - Area of the patient's body where the procedure was done, if appropriate.
    - The patient's reaction and tolerance to the procedure.
    - Your observations of anything unusual.

(sequence) of actions or steps. The entire set of steps is a procedure. In health care institutions, procedures are done according to a standard method. Nursing procedures will be somewhat different in different health care institutions. The underlying principles or ideas are always the same, but the wording, sequence, or style, for a task may be different. Be sure you know the methods, policies, and procedures, of the institution where you are working. Usually, the way things are done will be the same or similar to the series of steps given in this manual for a procedure.

There are several steps that are common to almost all of the procedures in this text. The numbers of those steps are printed in black. The steps that contain information unique to that procedure have numbers that print in color.

Words to Remember

New words are tools for communication. In your work as a nursing assistant, you will be introduced to medical terminology. You should increase your vocabulary as much as you can so you always understand what the head nurse or team leader tells you. Besides, learning new words can help to make you more confident.

When you are reporting to your supervisor, head nurse, or team leader, you must make yourself clearly understood. It is important that

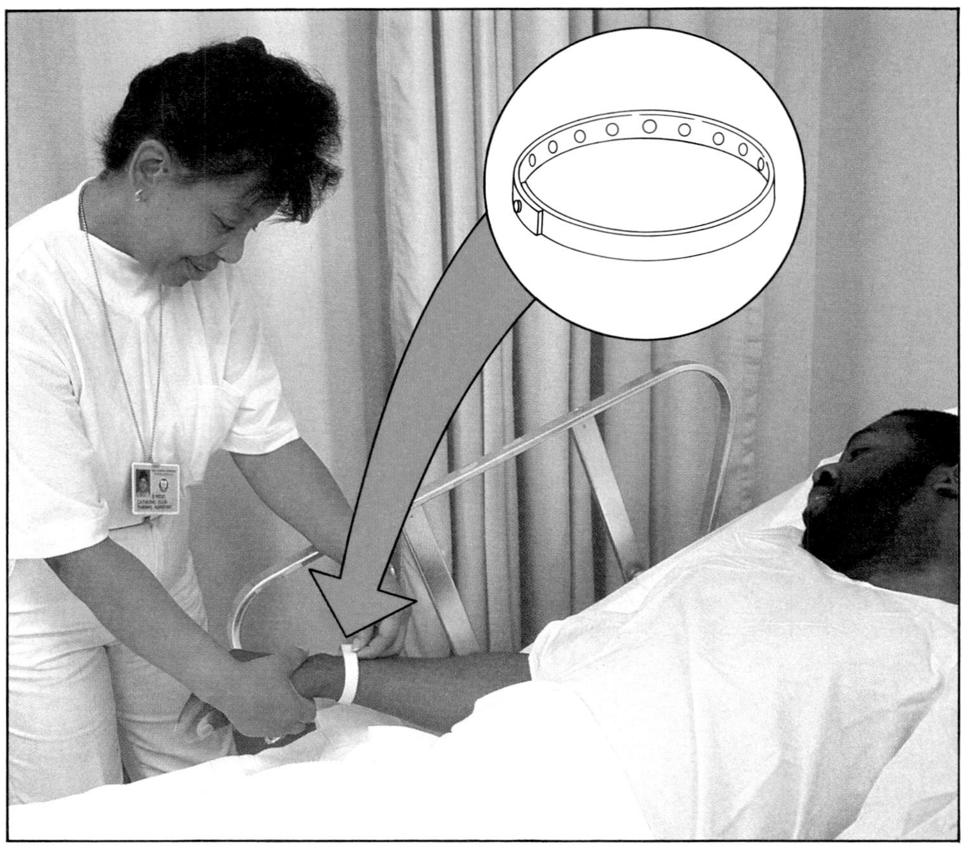

you accurately communicate information about patients and their situations or conditions. Chapter 3, Introduction to Medical Terminology, Key Terms in the margin and the Glossary will help you understand the meaning of many words used in the health care institution. Use the list throughout this course and on the job.

Notes Column

Use the blank space on each page to make notes, and underline the important information on each page. Writing things down will help you to remember them. Keep a pencil in hand as you study. Jot down key words and "thought clues." They will come back to you later when you need them. As your instructor goes over each procedure with you, he or she will explain things that may be done differently in your health care institution. Taking notes is a good way to record those differences.

Key Questions

These discussion questions will help you review the chapter's main ideas. They will remind you of the things you have learned and the objectives you have met. These questions are not intended to be a test quiz. Discussing the answers to these questions with classmates or your instructor can help you to remember what you have learned. Study any pages that deal with a question you could not answer.

WARNING

For all patient contact, adhere to Universal Precautions. Wear protective equipment, as indicated.

CHAPTER 1

The Health Care Institution

A NURSING ASSISTANT ALWAYS HAS WILLING HELPING HANDS FOR A PATIENT WHO NEEDS ASSISTANCE

- NURSING ASSISTANTS use their helping hands for the patient, the most important person in the hospital.
- NURSING ASSISTANTS understand that the patient is not an interruption to their work, but that the patient is their work.
- NURSING ASSISTANTS understand that the patient depends upon them and that their reputation and job depend on the patient.
- NURSING ASSISTANTS understand that the patient does them a favor when she or he calls; nursing assistants are not doing the patient a favor by answering the call.
- NURSING ASSISTANTS understand that the patient is someone to comfort and help, not someone to argue with.
- NURSING ASSISTANTS understand that the patient is not just a number but is flesh and blood and has feelings.
- NURSING ASSISTANTS understand that they must justify the trust the patient has in them.
- NURSING ASSISTANTS understand that the patient is a whole person, not just a disease.
- NURSING ASSISTANTS will use their helping hands to help the patient in a respectful, courteous, and attentive manner.

WARNING

For all patient contact, adhere to Universal Precautions (see page 91, 97, or the front cover flap). Wear protective equipment as indicated.

Objectives

What You Will Learn

When you have completed this chapter, you will be able to:

- Explain the purpose and organization of health care institutions and the purpose and role of the nursing assistant.
- Describe the effects of DRGs on the American health care system.
- Describe three ways of organizing the nursing health care team.
- Identify the nursing health care team.
- Explain the difference between the qualifications of the registered nurse and the licensed practical nurse, and between the jobs of the nursing assistant and the ward clerk.
- Explain the function of the in-service, staff development, and nursing education departments in your health care institution.
- Plan your career using the career ladder.
- Define: Diagnosis, DRGs, functional nursing, head nurse, team leader, or immediate supervisor, health care institution, patient oriented, primary nursing, task oriented, team nursing.

KEY IDEAS

The Health Care Institution

THE FIVE BASIC FUNCTIONS of a **health care institution** are as follows:

1. To provide care for ill and/or injured
2. To prevent disease
3. To promote individual and community health
4. To provide facilities for the education of health workers
5. To promote research in the sciences of medicine and nursing

Health Care Institution
Hospital, extended care facility, nursing home, convalescent home, or clinic where health care services are provided both on an inpatient and outpatient basis.

The Health Care Institution:

- Acute care facility
- Skilled nursing facility
- Long-term care nursing facility
- Rehabilitation facility
- Home health agency
- Outpatient clinic
- Mental health facility

KEY IDEAS

Diagnosis-Related Groups (DRGs)

Health care institutions and the people who work in them have always wanted to improve their roles and work. Change in the health care system is happening faster than ever. To give more people access to health care, to get the best possible results, and to keep costs down, health providers ask questions shown in Figure 1–1.

FIGURE 1-1
Questions Health Providers Ask.

- *What do they do*—thinking about the bigger issues of disease prevention and the health status of entire communities, not just about medical care for the sick and injured who come to an institution for help.
- *Where do they do it*—rethinking the roles of hospitals and the ways different institutions and providers can cooperate. People may go to walk-in or same-day surgery clinics rather than to hospitals, and many services may be provided in people's homes.
- *Who can do the work*—rethinking what must be handled by a doctor or a nurse and what can be done by others, including helping patients and their families assume an active role in self-care.
- *How can they get the best results at the lowest cost*—looking for the best ways to meet the goals of those who seek health services.

DRGs
Diagnosis-related groups of patients. A DRG classifies patients by diagnosis or surgical procedure to determine payment for hospital costs.

Diagnosis
Finding out what kind of disease or medical condition a patient has. A medical diagnosis is always made by a physician.

Many of these questions relate to insurance companies, managed care plans, and governmental legislation. For example, the federal Medicare program and others look at services used by patients who fall into **diagnosis-related groups (DRGs)**. A **diagnosis** is a physician's determination of what disease or condition a patient has. Researchers look at groups with related or similar diagnoses (a DRG) and develop statistics on the average length of hospital stay and average cost.

Medicare and others set their payments to health care institutions based on these statistics. Health care professionals also use DRGs to group patients and determine the best answers to the questions outlined above. These answers will change with advances in patient care techniques and technology.

You will learn new terms and see many changes as you enter the health care field. Don't look at change as a negative. Remember: the goal of all health care professionals is to improve patient care and the health of the community. If you stay focused on that important aim, you'll accept change as a necessary step to achieve that goal.

KEY IDEAS

The Nursing Assistant Is Part of the Health Care Team

Functional Nursing
A method of organizing the health care team in which the head nurse assigns and directs all patient care responsibilities for the nursing staff. This is sometimes called direct assignment.

Team Nursing
A task-oriented method of organizing the health care team in which the team leader gives patient care assignments to each team member.

As a nursing assistant, you are a member of a health care team (see Figure 1-2). Everyone on the team must understand teamwork and know what they are supposed to do and then to do it to the best of their abilities with a spirit of cooperation.

You will be working under the supervision of a professional nurse and cooperatively with other members of the nursing service staff. Remember that the nurse recognizes the nursing assistant as a valuable worker, as a member of the team. Look at your head nurse, team leader, or immediate supervisor as someone who will help you to learn and understand your job.

Organization of the Health Care Team

- **Functional nursing:** The head nurse assigns and directs all patient care responsibilities for the nursing staff. This system is sometimes called *direct assignment.*
- **Team nursing:** The **head nurse** is sometimes called the resource nurse. She or he divides the staff into teams. Each team has a leader.

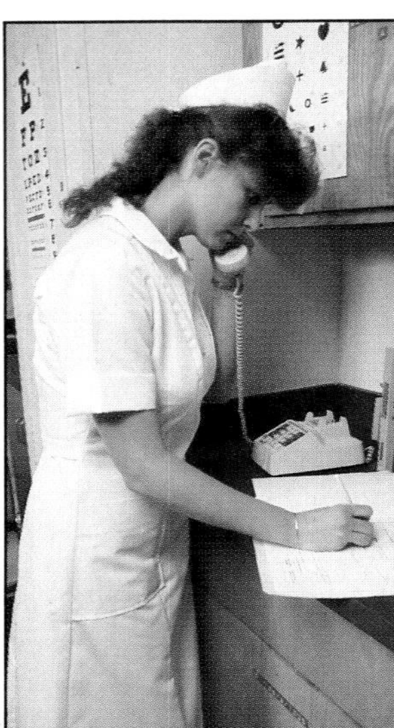

PROFESSIONAL REGISTERED NURSE

Four-year university education with a bachelor's degree
or
Two-year junior or community college education with an associate degree
or
Three-year diploma from a hospital nursing school
and
Passed state board examinations

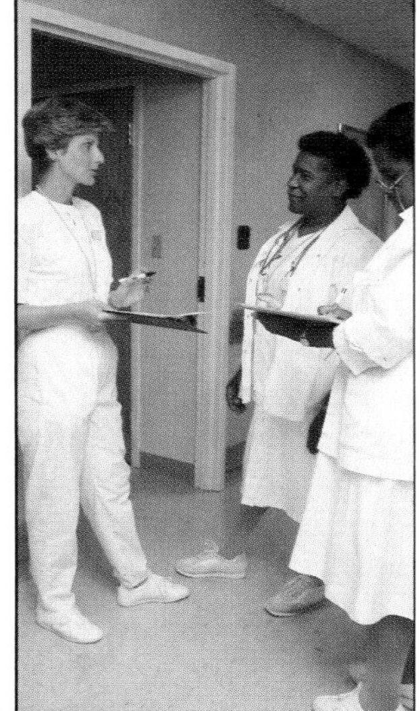

LICENSED PRACTICAL NURSE (LPN)
or
LICENSED VOCATIONAL NURSE (LVN)

One-year training program

Passed state board examinations

PLPN—Pharmaceutical Licensed Practical Nurse is one who administers drugs or medications after taking a special course and passing a special examination

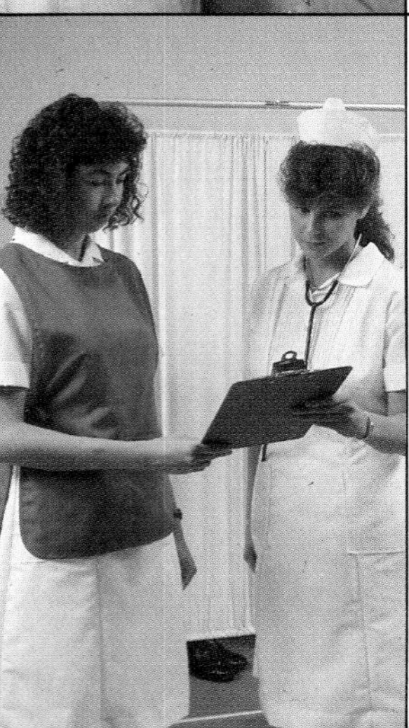

PERSONAL CARE ATTENDANT
PERSONAL CARE ASSISTANT
HOMEMAKER
NURSING ASSISTANT
NURSING AIDE
NURSE'S AIDE
NURSE'S ASSISTANT
HOME HEALTH AIDE
HOME HEALTH ASSISTANT
GERIATRIC AIDE
GERIATRIC ASSISTANT
ORDERLY
NURSING ATTENDANT

All are names used for the nonprofessional worker who, under the direction and supervision of the registered nurses, carries out basic bedside nursing functions

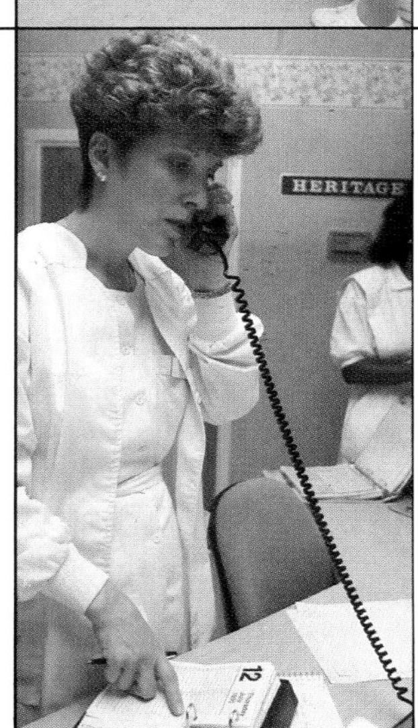

WARD CLERK
HEALTH UNIT SECRETARY
HEALTH UNIT CLERK
HEALTH UNIT COORDINATOR

Works at the desk of the nurses' station
- —Does clerical work
- —Answers the telephone at the nurses' station
- —Helps to direct traffic on the floor
- —Fills out requisition slips
- —Transcribes physician's orders

FIGURE 1-2 The nursing health care team.

Head Nurse or Team Leader The person who supervises the nursing health care team, including the nursing assistants. The head nurse or team leader will help you, the nursing assistant, keep track of your performance.

Task Oriented Nursing care that is arranged according to what must be done.

Primary Nursing A patient-oriented method of organizing the health care team in which the professional registered nurses are responsible for the total nursing care of the patient.

Patient Oriented Nursing care that is arranged according to the total needs of the individual patient.

The head nurse assigns a group of patients to each team. The team leader then makes outpatient care assignments for members of her or his team. Team members may be registered nurses (RN), licensed practical nurses (LPN), or nursing assistants (NA) (see Figure 1-2). The team leader is teacher, adviser, and helper to all the team members. This system is **task oriented**. This means that nursing care is arranged according to what must be done.

- **Primary nursing:** Primary nursing is a method of patient care delivery in which the professional nurse is responsible and accountable for the entire nursing care of the patient. She or he is responsible for assessing the patient's needs and for planning, implementing, and evaluating the patient's nursing care. The purpose is to ensure that the professional nurse works directly with the patient. In addition, responsibilities include family teaching, patient education, discharge planning, and recruiting community agencies to assist the patient after discharge. This system is **patient oriented**. This means that the nursing care is arranged according to the total needs of the individual patient; it is sometimes called *total nursing care.*

KEY IDEAS

Continuing to Learn

Continue your education! To keep up with new developments, all health care workers are expected to take refresher courses. As you continue to learn, your job will become more rewarding personally and professionally. You and your employer, the health care institution, will be happy and grateful that you decided to be a nursing assistant.

You can continue to learn while you are on the job. You can expand your knowledge of nursing care procedures, find better ways to do your work, and learn more about other aspects of health care. All this can make you a more effective nursing assistant, and you will become more secure in your job.

If you enjoy your work as a nursing assistant, you may be interested in advancement where you are employed. Maybe you would like to be a registered nurse or a licensed practical (vocational) nurse. The career ladder shown in Figure 1-3 can guide you in planning your advancement. The ladder can be changed to meet your needs and goals. Skills, time, hard work, and planning are needed to clmb to your level of desired work and educational satisfaction, or you may want to continue to climb to the top of the ladder.

If you do not have a high school diploma, that should be your first goal. Adult education programs at local high schools offer basic education programs that lead to a high school equivalency diploma. Community colleges offer the prerequisite courses necessary to move up to a program for the licensed practical nurse or registered nurse level. They have counselors to advise you along the way. The director of nursing education in your health care institution is the person to ask about planning your career ladder.

FIGURE 1-3 Career ladder for the nursing assistant.

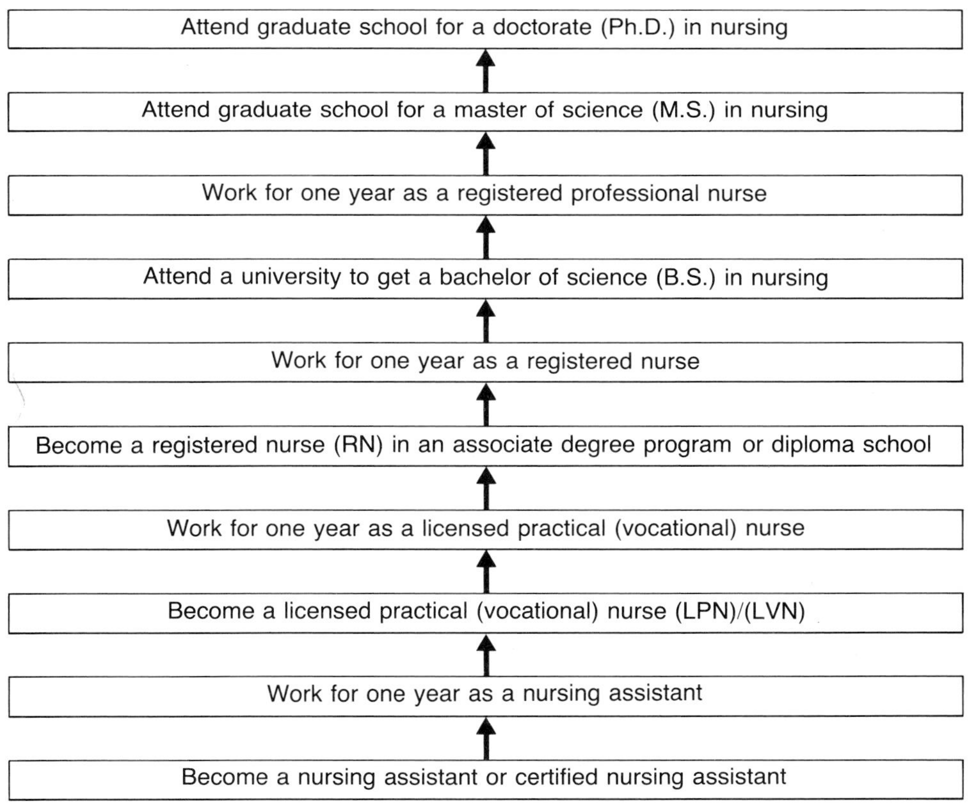
Attend graduate school for a doctorate (Ph.D.) in nursing
Attend graduate school for a master of science (M.S.) in nursing
Work for one year as a registered professional nurse
Attend a university to get a bachelor of science (B.S.) in nursing
Work for one year as a registered nurse
Become a registered nurse (RN) in an associate degree program or diploma school
Work for one year as a licensed practical (vocational) nurse
Become a licensed practical (vocational) nurse (LPN)/(LVN)
Work for one year as a nursing assistant
Become a nursing assistant or certified nursing assistant

KEY QUESTIONS

1. What are the purposes of health care institutions? How are they organized?
2. Describe three ways of organizing the nursing health care team.
3. Who are the members of the nursing health care team?
4. What are some differences between the qualifications of the registered nurse and the licensed practical nurse? What are some differences between the jobs of the nursing assistant and the ward clerk?
5. What are the functions of the in-service, staff development, and nursing education departments in your health care institution?
6. Write a career plan using the career ladder.
7. What effects are DRGs having on the American health care system?
8. Define: diagnosis, DRGs, functional nursing, head nurse, team leader, or immediate supervisor, health care institution, patient oriented, primary nursing, task oriented, team nursing.

KEY IDEAS

Legal Aspects of Being a Nursing Assistant

Negligence
The commission of an act or failure to perform an act, where the respective performance or nonperformance deviates from an act that should have been done by a reasonably prudent person under the same or similar conditions.

Malpractice
Negligence when applied to the performance of a professional.

Laws concerning patients and workers in health care institutions were written to protect both the patient and the worker. As a nursing assistant, you need to understand how the law affects you and the patients you care for. Patients are entitled to respect for their human rights. They must be kept safe and must be cared for properly.

The words negligence and malpractice are often used interchangeably, as if they were the same thing. Officially, **negligence** is the commission of an act or failure to perform an act where the respective performance or nonperformance deviates from the act that should have been done by a reasonably prudent person under the same or similar conditions. **Malpractice** is negligence when applied to the performance of a professional. If a nursing assistant does not follow the directions of her immediate supervisor and such failure causes or results in injury to the patient, then the nursing assistant has committed a negligent act. Examples are:

- If the nursing assistant fails to raise the siderails on a patient's bed and the patient falls, the nursing assistant has commited a negligent act.
- If the nursing assistant fails to open the bottom of the mechanical lift to its widest position before use and the patient falls, the nursing assistant has committed a negligent act.
- If the nursing assistant fails to follow instructions to turn the patient every two hours, and documents same, and the patient develops decubitus ulcers, the nursing assistant has committed a negligent act.
- If the nursing assistant fails to place the patient's feet on the provided footrests of the wheelchair and as a result the wheels of the wheelchair run over the patient's feet, the nursing assistant has committed a negligent act.

Standards of care are based on laws, administrative policy, and guidelines published for nursing assistants. The professional standards of care are usually defined with respect to community standards. These standards of care permit you to be judged based on what is expected of someone with your training and experience. All health care institutions and home health agencies have their standards of care, which you must follow.

Good Samaritan laws have been developed to protect individuals trying to give assistance to people requiring emergency care outside the health-care institution. In the states that have Good Samaritan laws, you will be granted immunity if you act in good faith to provide care to the level of your training, to the best of your ability, as a reasonable and prudent person.

Consent is the right to refuse your care when an adult is conscious and clear of mind. Whatever their reasons, they have this right. A parent or legal guardian can refuse to let you care for their child. You, the nursing assistant, must report to your immediate supervisor if any adult refuses to permit you to care for him or a significant other. **Informed consent** is a voluntary act by which a conscious and mentally competent person gives permission for someone else to do something for him.

Civil rights must be guaranteed to all citizens. This includes freedom from discrimination because of:

- Religion
- Ethnic origin
- Sex
- Race
- Physical handicap
- Age

For example:

- An employer cannot discriminate in hiring practices.
- A nursing assistant cannot discriminate in care for patients.

Defamation of character means making false or damaging statements or misrepresentations about another person that defame or injure his or her reputation. There are two types of defamation of character:

- *Slander:* A spoken statement (gossip)
- *Libel:* A written statement

Abandonment is the act of deserting or neglecting a patient. If the nursing assistant is unable to care for his patient, suitable and qualified substitutes must be made with consent of the patient; otherwise, a breach of duty could occur.

Criminal law applies to felonies against society. The elements of crime and punishment are usually part of each state's legislation and judicial opinions.

Restraining or detaining a person without proper consent is called **false imprisonment**. Restraints cannot be applied to any patient without a written order from the physician.

Incident
Any unusual event or occurrence such as an accident or a condition that is likely to cause an accident.

Accountable
To be answerable for one's behavior; legally or ethically responsible for the care of another.

Other legal terms include:

- *Accident/incident:* An unforeseen event that occurs without intent.
- *Accountability:* The act of being liable or legally responsible.
- *Advanced directive (living will):* A person giving instructions in advance that life-support systems shall not be used in the event that his or her death is imminent and a physician has determined that there can be no recovery and the application of life-support systems would only artificially prolong the dying process.
- *Assault:* An unsuccessful attempt or threat to commit bodily harm.
- *Battery:* An assault that is actually carried out where the person is injured.
- *Civil law:* Concerned with the legal rights and duties of private persons.
- *Crime:* A violation against a citizen or society.
- *Invasion of privacy:* Invasion of the right to live in seclusion without being subjected to undesired publicity.
- *Liability:* An obligation incurred or that might be incurred through any act or failure to act.
- *Wills:* A statement for the distribution of personal belongings and property following death.

KEY IDEAS

Incidents

Hazard
A source of danger, a possible cause of an accident.

An **incident** is an event that does not fit the routine operation of the health care institution or the routine care of the patients. It may be an accident or something that might cause one. For example, a staff person stumbles into a patient in a wheelchair because someone spilled liquid and failed to wipe it up. Such incidents can affect the patients, visitors, and members of the institution's staff.

FIGURE 2-6 Prevent accidents. Report hazards. Be alert for potential dangers, such as spilled liquids and trash.

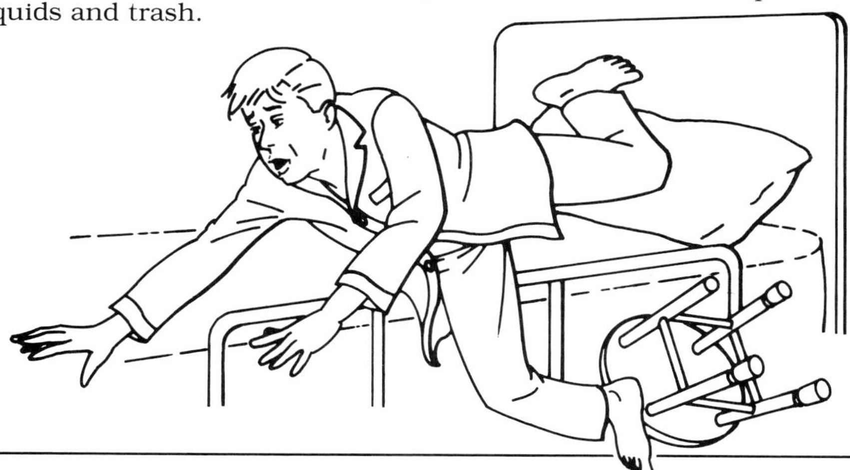

MEMORIAL HOSPITAL

ACCIDENT/INCIDENT REPORT

1. Patient ☒ Visitor ☐ Employee ☐ Other ☐
2. Date of this report 12/25 19xx Date of incident 12/25/xx
3. Name Johnson, Henry A. Age 43 Sex Male Marital Status ________
   Department ________ Position ________
4. Location incident occurred at Room 407 Time 1:00 a.m. p.m.
5. Reported to ________ Patient seen by Dr. Ralph A. Jones
   ________ Time ____ a.m. p.m. ________ Time 1:05 a.m. p.m.
6. Statement of doctor or resident (diagnosis, parts of body affected and treatment)
   Patient examined—no injuries sustained—left elbow slightly abraded.
   ________ Attending Physician ________ M.D.
7. Describe incident and how accident occurred. (Statement of nurse or person in charge.)
   Patient found on floor—stated he attempted to get out of bed, slipped off and fell to floor. Slight abrasion of left elbow. No hospital property damaged.
   Signed ________ Title ________
8. Witness's name Fred R. Smith Address 33 Yale St., New Brunswick, N.J.
   Witness's name ________ Address ________
9. Name of machine involved ________
10. Kind of work performed by machine ________
11. Part of machine causing injury ________
12. Any protective device on machine ________
13. Action taken to prevent recurrence ________
    ________ Signed ________ Title ________
14. Did employee lose time? Yes ☐ No ☐ If yes, give last day worked mo ☐ day ☐ yr ☐
    If unable to resume work, give probable date of return mo ☐ day ☐ yr ☐ if already returned mo ☐ day ☐ yr ☐
15. If patient accident, signed ________ Date ________
    Ass't. Adm. Nursing Service
    Reported to administration on ____ at ____ a.m p.m. Signed ________ Adm.

Department director must complete necessary information in duplicate. Duplicate must be forwarded immediately to chairman of the safety committee.

Reviewed by safety committee on ________ Signed ________ Chairman.

(FILL OUT IN DUPLICATE)

Types of incidents are:

- Patient, visitor, or employee accidents.
- Thefts from patients, visitors, or employees.
- Thefts of hospital property.
- Accidents occurring on outlying hospital property, such as sidewalks, parking lots, or entrances.

Whenever an incident occurs, a report must be made (see Figure 2-6). Report any incident you observe immediately. Also report any unsafe conditions you think might lead to an incident. Reporting is very important to the safety program of the health care institution and for the protection of all health care workers. For the institution to be prepared for possible liability suits or damage claims, all the facts related to the incidents must be known. Incident reports are filed with the hospital's administration and are not part of the patient's chart.

KEY QUESTIONS

1. Which qualities help to make a person a good nursing assistant?
2. What can you do to practice good personal hygiene?
3. Describe ethical behavior.
4. With whom should you not discuss patient information, if you want to respect confidences?
5. Why is it important for nursing assistants to be accurate in everything that they do?
6. In what ways can nursing assistants show they are dependable?
7. Why is it important to follow rules and instructions?
8. In what ways can you develop cooperative relationships with other staff members?
9. Discuss four examples of a nursing assistant's behavior that would be considered negligence.
10. What types of incidents should be reported?
11. Define: accountable, accuracy, cooperate, dependability, ethical behavior, hazard, hygiene, incident, malpractice, negligence.

CHAPTER 3

Communication and Human Relations

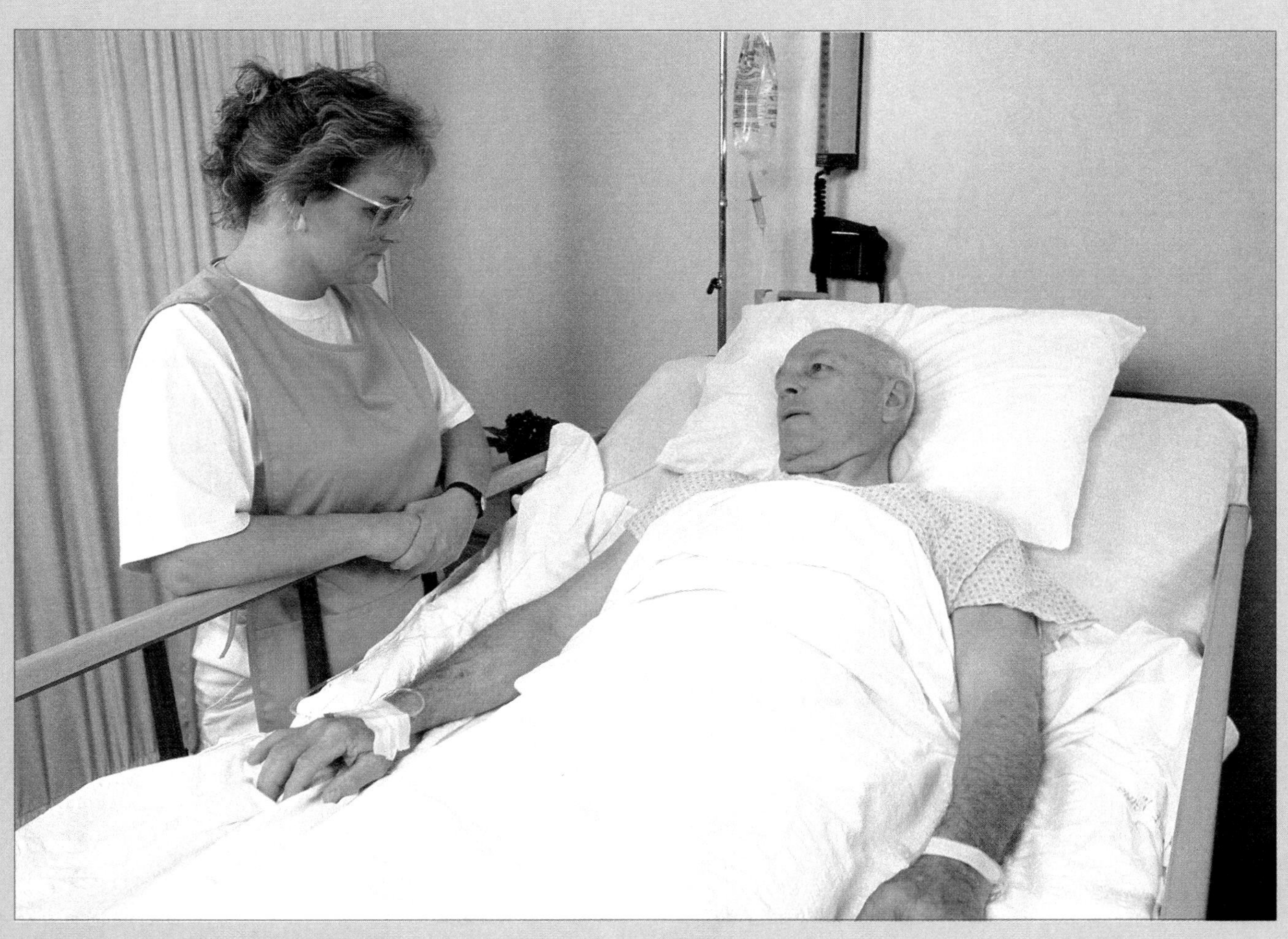

WARNING

For all patient contact, adhere to Universal Precautions (see page 91, 97, or the front cover flap). Wear protective equipment as indicated.

Objectives

What You Will Learn

When you have completed this chapter, you will be able to:

- Maintain a courteous and professional manner toward patients, visitors, and co-workers.
- Keep your emotions under control while on the job.
- Deal with patients and visitors in an empathetic and tactful manner.
- Show interest and concern about the patient's welfare.
- Communicate effectively with pediatric patients and their parents.
- Use communication skills effectively when relating to patients and their visitors.
- Answer the patient's signal promptly.
- Show respect for the patient's rights.
- Show respect for the patient's culture, language, customs, and beliefs.
- Meet the patient's physical and psychological needs.
- Teach a blind or deaf patient how to use the call signal.
- Take complete and accurate telephone messages.
- Define: body language, communication, courtesy, empathy, pediatric patient, tact.

KEY IDEAS

The Patient's Bill of Rights

THE AMERICAN HOSPITAL ASSOCIATION HAS WRITTEN a *Patient's Bill of Rights* to be used as a guide for doctors, hospitals, hospital employees, and patients. Patients are responsible for knowing and exercising their rights in accordance with the laws of their state. Twelve provisions are contained in the complete American Hospital Association's *Patient's Bill of Rights.* The following are the six major ones. Every patient has:

- The right to considerate and respectful care.
- The right to understandable, complete, and current information from the doctor about the diagnosis, the treatments that will be used, their risks and benefits, how long the sickness is likely to last, and the prognosis (the likelihood of recovery).
- The right to refuse to participate in experiments and the right to refuse treatment. This includes the right to leave a hospital against medical advice if the patient chooses.
- The right to be told which doctor is mainly in charge of the care, usually referred to as the primary physician.
- The right to privacy; records will be kept confidential, and permission is necessary if anyone who is not directly involved in the treatment is present during the treatment.
- The right to examine and receive an explanation of a bill regardless of the source of payment.

KEY IDEAS

Human Relations

Transcultural Nursing

Since you have chosen employment as a nursing assistant, you like working with and helping people. This is an important beginning because you will be dealing with people from all kinds of backgrounds. You must learn to treat all of them as individual human beings. To help sick people feel well, they must first be made to feel relaxed, comfortable, and safe.

As part of the nursing care team, you will assist with the delivery of nursing care to people from many different countries and backgrounds. These people may adhere to religious beliefs, values, traditions, practices, or rituals that are very different from your own. They may have very different food habits, manners, life-styles, social roles, family systems, birth and death practices, or perceptions of privacy, territoriality, and touch. They may use languages, customs, or behavior patterns completely foreign to your own. You must learn to be tolerant and understanding of these differences. Behave in ways that show respect for the patient's customs and beliefs. Each patient's culture is very important.

Different does not mean better or worse, only another way of doing things. Because your own ways are familiar to you, they seem like the right ways, and other languages, values, life-styles, traditions, or food habits may seem strange. Your customs may seem just as strange to the patient as his or her customs seem to you. This can lead to misunderstandings. There is no right or wrong in these matters.

Many patients are frightened by illness and the hospital environment. Part of your job is to show them that the health care institution is a friendly place and that your major concern is for their well-being. Patients born in other countries may be additionally fearful because of problems in understanding our language and culture. Be sure to discuss these problems with your immediate supervisor, who will suggest ways of dealing with these patients effectively.

For example:

- If the patient speaks and understands little or no English, your head nurse or team leader may suggest the use of flash cards, pictures, nonverbal communication, a translator, or materials written in the patient's language to communicate with the patient and thereby reduce stress and anxiety.
- Patients from another culture may answer yes to all questions asked because in their culture it is rude to say no. Your head nurse or team leader may suggest that you phrase your questions so that a yes or no answer is not required. For example, instead of asking, "Do you want the lights out now?" you could say, "What time would you like me to turn off the lights?"
- A patient may refuse to eat hospital food because of religious or cultural dietary laws or beliefs. Your head nurse or team leader may be able to make special arrangements for this patient's food.
- People from many cultures place more importance on modesty than most Americans. They may want to keep certain parts of the body such as the head, the face, arms, or legs covered at all times. Your head nurse or team leader may suggest ways of draping the patient so necessary care can be given without violating the patient's sense of modesty, dignity, and privacy.

- People have different ideas about death and the hereafter. Adherents of some religions believe that the body should not be touched or moved after death until the proper religious authority arrives. Your head nurse or team leader may suggest that you straighten the patient's limbs before death occurs.

KEY IDEAS

Basic Needs

Every person has basic needs that must be met. A need is a requirement for survival. Some people can satisfy their own needs; however, sometimes they need help. As a nursing assistant, you will help your patients meet some of their most basic needs until they no longer need your help. Your knowledge of these needs and your objective observations, when reported promptly, will help your supervisor, head nurse, or team leader to determine if all the patient's needs are being met by the plan of care.

Basic Physical and Psychological Needs

All human beings have basic physical needs that must be met in order to live. These needs do not all have to be met completely every day. But the more each person's needs are fulfilled, the better the quality of life.

Psychological needs must be satisfied to have a healthy emotional and social outlook. These, also, do not have to be met completely every day. However, the more completely each need is met, the better the emotional state of the individual.

Some psychologists divide human needs into five categories arranged into a hierarchy, or order of priority, developed by Abraham Maslow (see Figure 3-1). His idea is that human beings work on meeting their physical needs (food, water, shelter) first, then move on toward meeting their higher-level needs (security, belonging, and so on).

FIGURE 3-1 Maslow's Hierarchy of Needs.

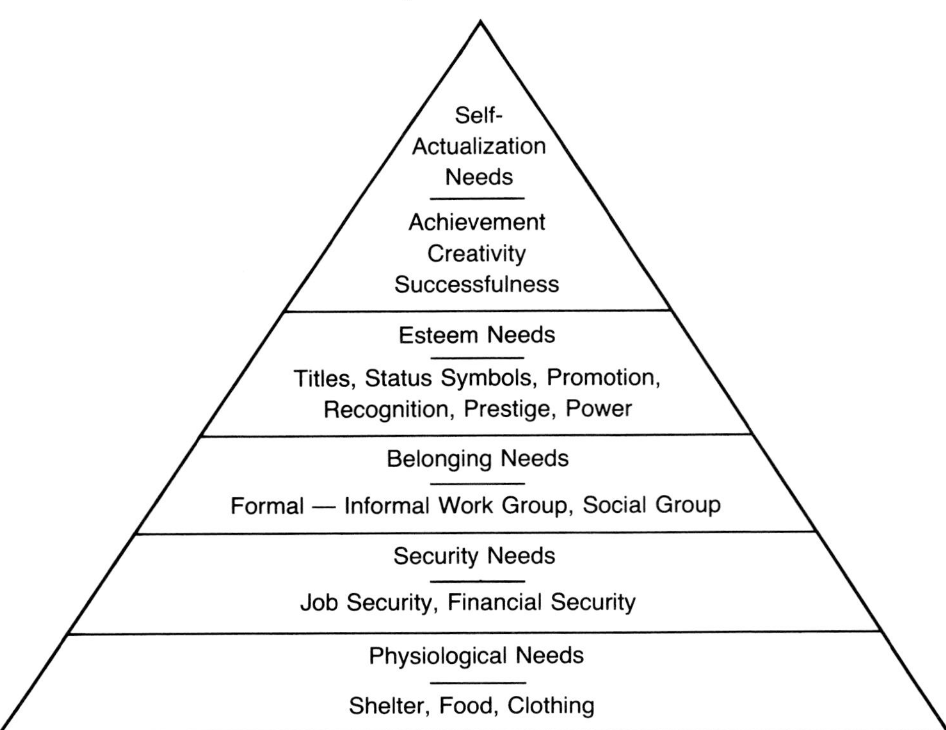

Unmet Needs

When basic needs are not met, most people show some reaction. If a physical need is not met, the person might become irritable or weak. When an emotional need is not met, the person's reactions may result in feelings of anxiety, depression, aggression, or anger or a physical ailment without apparent cause.

Report these reactions to your immediate supervisor. By reviewing a patient's actions, your supervisor will be able to determine if a need is unmet and evaluate the plan of care to attempt to fulfill the need and thus change the patient's behavior.

KEY IDEAS

Communication or Relating to People

Relating to people means making a connection between yourself and another person. The relations between yourself and patients, visitors, parents, and fellow workers depend on your approach to them. If you have a kind, courteous, tactful, empathetic, and open manner, you will find it easier to form positive connections (Figure 3-2). Relationships depend on receiving as well as giving information, so listening attentively is as important as what you say. Communication skills are necessary to be successful as a nursing assistant.

FIGURE 3-2 Helpful personal qualities include courtesy, emotional control, empathy, and tact.

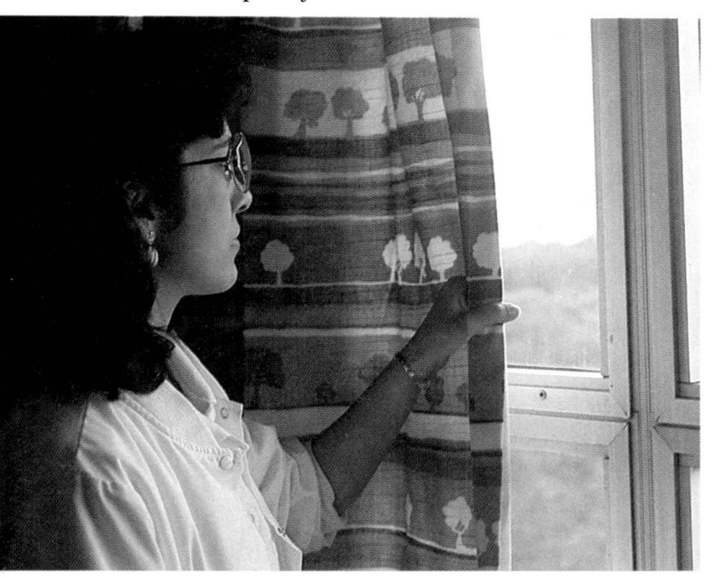

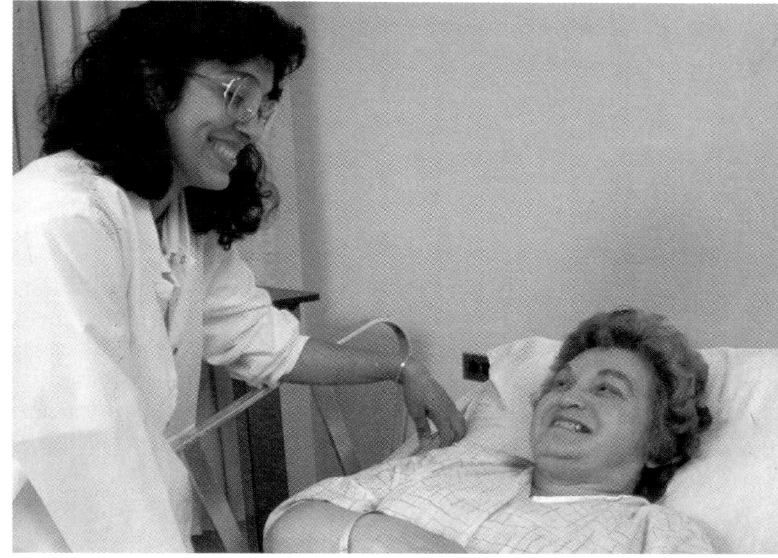

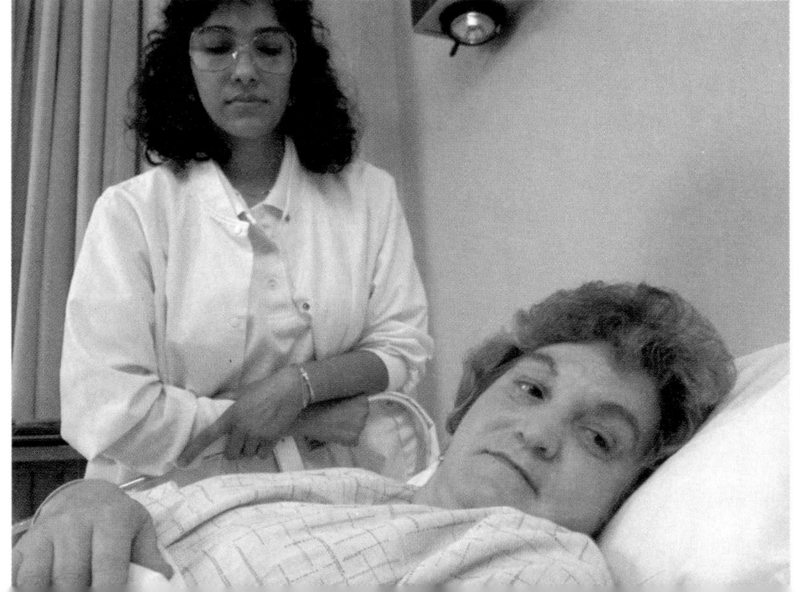

Courtesy
Being polite and considerate.

Courtesy

Behaving courteously means considering the needs of the other person as well as your own. It means cooperating, sharing, and giving. Being polite and considerate of others shows that you care about them. Think how you would feel if you were in their place and you will understand how far a cheerful word and a smile can go.

Emotional Control

Sometimes a patient, another staff member, or a visitor may upset and anger you. You may feel like making a rude or nasty remark. Don't do it. Stop and realize that the patient and his or her visitors may be worried, nervous, or tense. Fellow workers may be under stress because of a problem at home or on the job. Try to be understanding and learn to control anger and cope with all situations.

Learning to accept constructive criticism and suggestions without feeling you are being attacked is an essential part of your job. Try to avoid becoming defensive. If your supervisor criticizes you or tells you to do something, you may feel like saying, "That is not my job" or "Why do you pick on me?" Stop and examine your attitude. Calm down and then perform the right or correct action.

Empathy and Tact

Empathy
The ability to put yourself in another's place and to see things as they see them.

Tact
Doing and saying the right things at the right time.

- **Empathy:** feelings, thoughts, and motives of one person are understood and/or felt by another person without pity. A nursing assistant should use empathy or empathize with the patient, visitor, and coworkers.
- **Tact:** doing and saying the right things at the right time.

Relationships with Patients. Many things make a difference in a patient's behavior and attitude during an illness. The patient may become frightened, angry, or sad. Some factors or influences are the diagnosis, seriousness of the illness, age, previous illnesses, past experience in hospitals, and mental condition. Other things that might make a difference are the patient's personality, disposition, and financial condition.

Each patient's reaction to pain, treatment, annoyances, and even kindness is different. Always treat each patient as an individual, a person who needs your help.

Never talk to anyone except your immediate supervisor about a patient's condition. Discussing one patient's medical condition with another patient is an invasion of privacy.

Always try to give the patient confidence in the hospital, the doctors, and the nursing staff. Never discuss or criticize any of your fellow staff members in front of a patient.

Remember that the patient's behavior is the result of things that worry or bother her or him (Figure 3-3). The patient may be hostile, mean, and nasty. You may simply be the nearest person to talk to or to lash out against.

A patient's problems are very important to him or her. Try to be understanding. Be a good listener, even when you would rather leave.

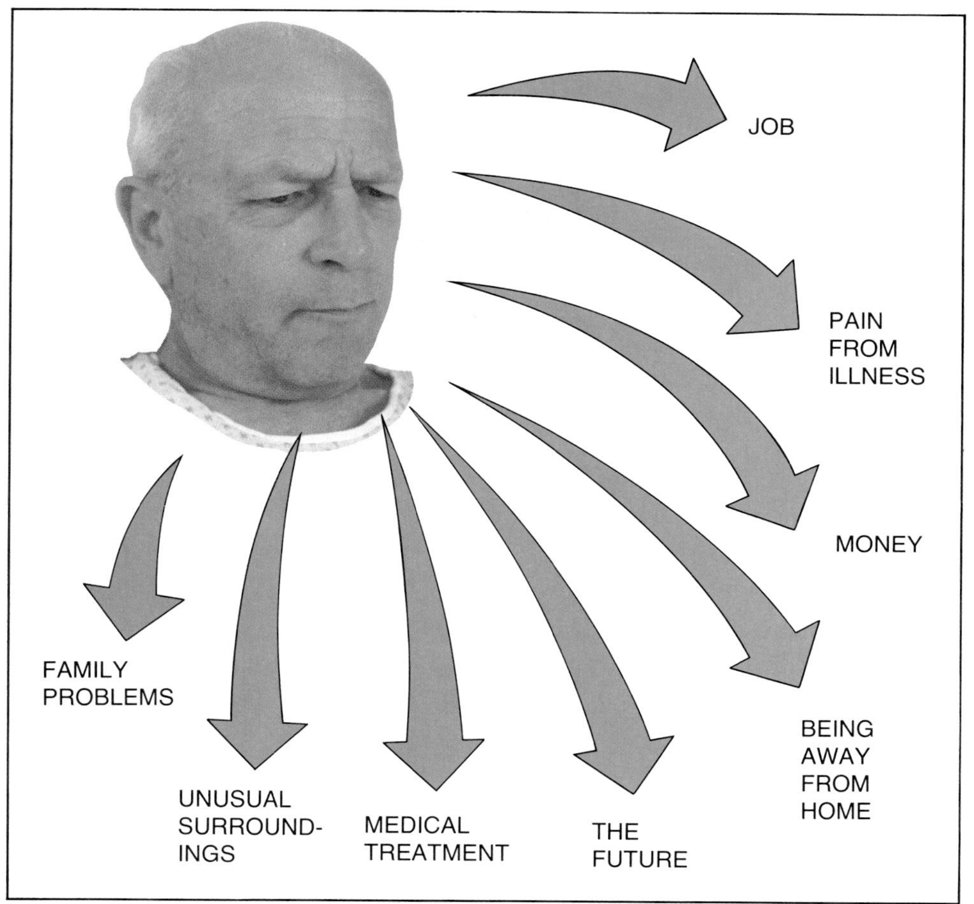

FIGURE 3-3 A patient worries about many things.

Patients and visitors often relieve their feelings of helplessness and hopelessness through words and behavior. They may try to take it out on you. Bear with them as much as possible. Remember that the patient may be suffering emotionally as well as physically; talking may relieve his or her emotional suffering.

Try to be as tactful as you can. When a patient begins to recover, give praise and encouragement.

Always listen when a patient makes a complaint or brings up a problem. The patient may ask you questions about the doctor or when she will be discharged. Refer such questions to your immediate supervisor.

Sometimes a child cries when his parents are getting ready to leave the hospital. You can show empathy to both the child and parents by making the separation easier for them. Pick up the child (if permitted) and pat and soothe him. Turn the child's attention to something other than the anxiety, fear, and pain of being separated from the parents.

Crying is the normal, natural way for children to express their feelings and fears. Try to understand why a child is crying excessively. Do not let it irritate you.

Never tell a child that you are going to *take* his temperature or blood pressure. The child may think you are going to take something away. Say you are going to *measure* his temperature or blood pressure instead. Explain the procedure; let the child examine the stethoscope or such to gain confidence and trust.

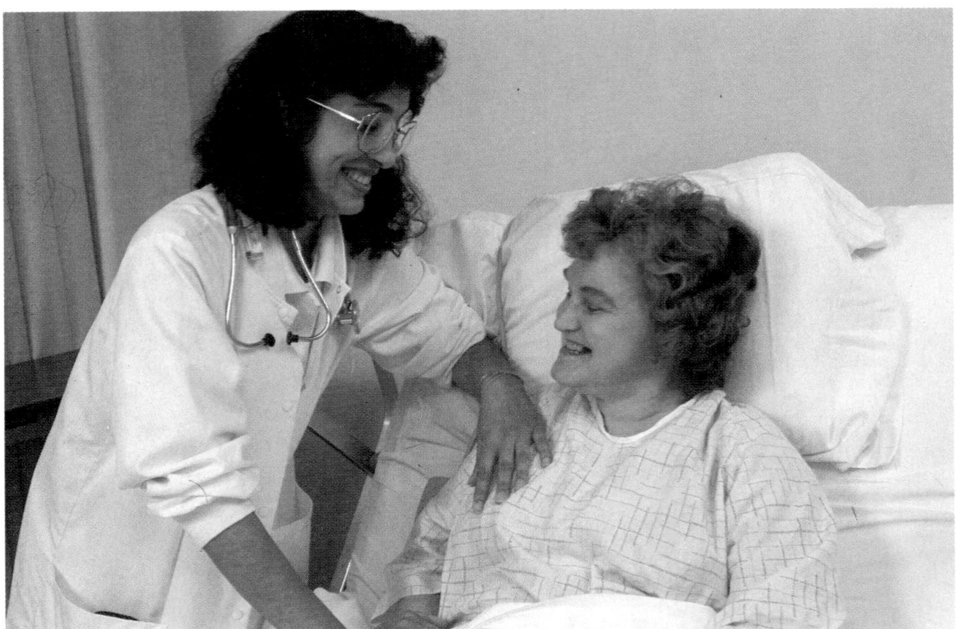

FIGURE 3-4 Communicating with patients is an important part of the nursing assistant's job.

Communication
The exchange of thoughts, messages, or ideas by speech, signals, gestures, or writing.

Body Language
Communication through hand movements (gestures), facial expressions, body movements, and touch.

Communicating with Patients

- Show an interest in what the patient is saying.
- Let your facial expressions show that you are interested (Figure 3-4).
- Use good manners.
- Speak clearly, distinctly, and slowly. Speak in a normal, pleasant tone.
- Use language that the patient can understand.
- Respect the patient's moods. Sometimes silence can help.
- Make your body movements look pleasing and energetic.
- When someone in need asks you for assistance, whether to bathe or turn him or her or to get something that is out of reach, you should give your assistance willingly and graciously, no matter whose assigned patient it is.

Nonverbal Communication and Body Language. Spoken and written words are used for most communications. But there are other ways that are sometimes more effective to get a message across. Hand movements (gestures), expressions on your face, and body movements may tell the story better than words.

As a nursing assistant, you are close to patients during their stay in the hospital. Often they tell you about their needs, pains, and worries. As you listen, you are both in close communication.

Every time you touch a person's body, whether you speak any words or not, you are communicating something. How you assist a person in any action that involves touching her body says something. If you are careful, firm, and gentle, it tells the person something far different than if you are rough.

Pay attention to your posture. The way you move when you enter a patient's room or how you stand by her bed are ways of communicating through body language. Try to make these movements communicate energy, a sense of interest, and a willingness to help. A frown, an impatient body movement, or a shrug may give the patient the message,

"Do not bother me." Also, a certain way of standing or walking may send the message "I am lazy" or "I don't want to be bothered."

Look at the patient when you speak to him. This tells the patient that he has your attention. If you are looking away when talking, the patient gets the impression that your attention is elsewhere. Speak clearly and distinctly in a normal tone of voice. Talk with the patient, not just to or at him. Ask the patient what he likes or dislikes, thinks, or wants. Listen to the responses in an interested manner.

Verbal Communication *(Communicating through Words).* Vulgar words are not appropriate or necessary. Also, do not use medical terms or abbreviations when talking to patients and their visitors. If you use medical language and the patient does not understand, you might give the patient the wrong idea about what is happening to him or her.

Keep your voice pleasant, not too loud or too high pitched. Speak clearly and slowly enough to be easily understood. Never whisper or mumble, even when you think the patient is asleep or cannot hear you. This is annoying to the patient.

Remember that, although some patients seem to be semicomatose, comatose, or unconscious, they may be fully aware of what is happening around them and can often hear what is happening. Therefore, always speak and behave as if the patient can hear every word. (They may hear more than you think.)

Be sensitive to those times when the patient does not want to talk. Respect his or her moods. Saying nothing may have more meaning than any words or facial expressions. Sometimes a pat on the shoulder or holding a hand means more to a patient than anything you might say. Simply being near the stretcher or bed at the moment of trouble may be the most comforting message of all.

Communicating with the Pediatric Patient

Pediatric Patient
Any patient under the age of 16 years.

Children or Pediatric Patients. **Pediatric patients** are children (Figure 3-5). In most hospitals, anyone under age 16 is called a pediatric patient. These patients may be grouped in several ways. For example, pediatric patients are sometimes grouped according to age because children of different ages need different kinds and amounts of care. Children also may be grouped according to their medical or surgical condition.

FIGURE 3-5 Pediatric patients have special needs.

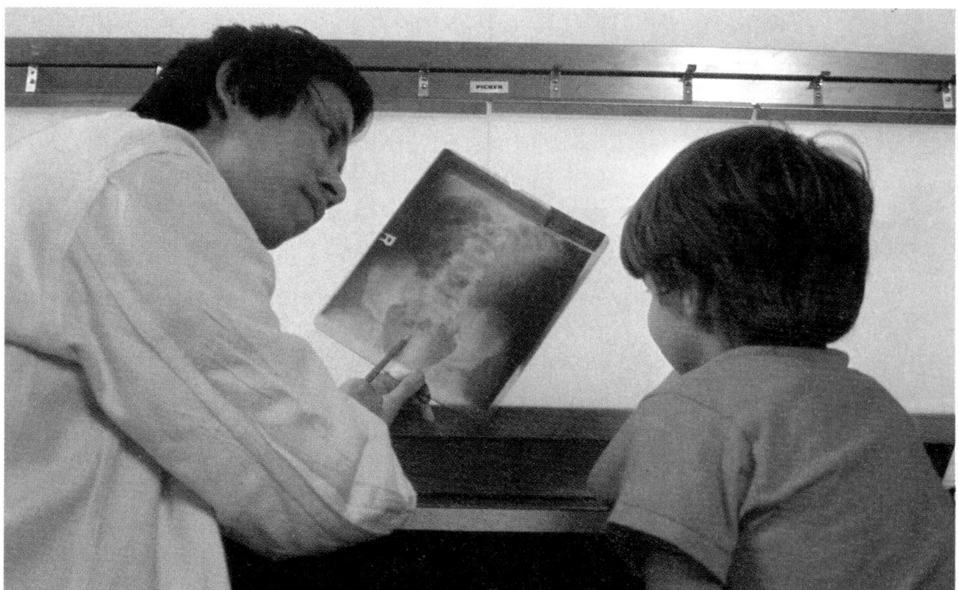

- *Premature* babies are born before the completion of 37 weeks of gestation (pregnancy) or 3 weeks less than full term (the normal gestation period is 40 weeks). Low birth weight babies are under 2500 grams or 5.5 pounds in weight.
- *Newborn* babies (neonates) are full-term babies from birth until 1 month of age.
- *Infants* are babies from 1 month to 1 year old.
- *Toddlers* are children from 1 to 3 years of age.
- *Preschoolers* are children from 3 to 5 years old.
- *School-age* children are from 6 to 12 years old.
- *Adolescents* are children from 12 to 19 years old.

Some Conditions for Which Children Are Admitted to the Health Care Institution

- Congenital defects (those a child is born with): cleft palate, club foot, hip dysplasia, skeletal limb deficiency
- Accidents: falls, poisoning, fractures, head trauma, burns
- Tumors
- Chronic conditions: diabetes, rheumatic heart disease
- Infectious or communicable diseases: meningitis, pneumonia, tuberculosis, chicken pox, AIDS
- Emotional disturbances: severe depression, acute anxiety
- Nutritional disorders: rickets, iron deficiency anemia, malnutrition
- Early childhood health problems: conjunctivitis, otitis media, urinary tract infections, child abuse
- Blood disorders: aplastic anemia, leukemias, lymphomas, sickle cell anemia
- Severe diarrhea and vomiting
- Acute or chronic renal failure
- Neuromuscular disorders: seizures, cerebral palsy

Communicating with Children. Call a child by his or her first name or nickname. Using his name tells the child that you know who he is. It shows respect for the child as a person and is a mark of courtesy.

Do not use commands (Figure 3-6). Do not call any child "stupid" or "dumb." Using such words can be very harmful to a child, because if they are repeated often enough children may begin to think of themselves as stupid or dumb. Then they may begin to behave as if they were stupid, because they think this is what is expected of them.

Very small children simply cannot tell you in words what they want. It is hard for them to communicate with you. Children will try to tell you things by the sounds they make and by the way they move. You should try to understand what their sounds and movements mean.

Try to learn the reason for their crying and then try to comfort them. Reasons for crying, of course, depend on how old the child is and perhaps on what happened before they started crying.

When you are giving children personal care, use every chance you have to show your interest in them and your affection for them. This is done in different ways with children of different ages. Although children may not complain or seem to feel sorry for themselves, they may be

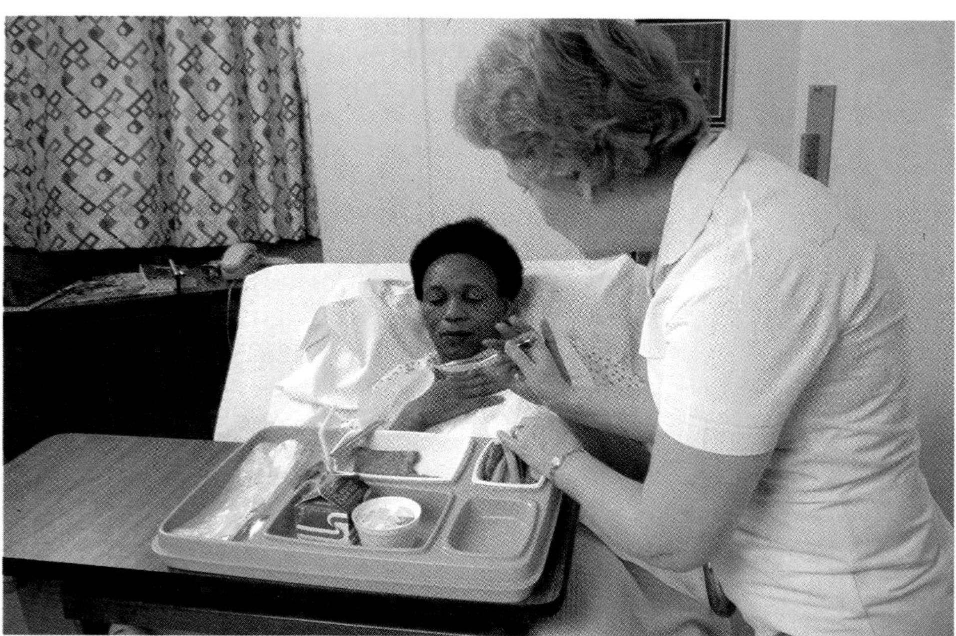

FIGURE 3-6 Do *not* say "Don't play with your food." You *could* say "Aren't you hungry?"

uncomfortable or unhappy. They need your kindness and empathy. Your smile, a tender touch, or affectionate words can tell the child that you are interested in and care about him or her.

Nursing Care of Pediatric Patients

The nursing care of children is based on what is normal in terms of growth and development for a child of a certain age. The parents of the child are also involved in various ways in the child's care. There are three categories of nursing care for children:

1. The things one normally does for a child at a certain age, such as giving a baby a bottle.
2. Nursing care related to the reason the child is in the health care institution, such as feeding a baby who has a cleft palate.
3. Regular nursing care procedures that have to be adapted to children, such as collecting a urine specimen from an infant.

Importance of the Family. A child is still a member of a family, even when in the hospital. The person or persons who care for the child at home represent the family. Many hospitals and pediatric patient care units have a policy of allowing a family member to stay with the child and even encourage them to do so.

This may be the first time the child has been away from home. The child may be frightened or may view hospitalization as punishment. Such a patient needs to be held, touched, and talked to in order to be comforted and reassured.

Communicating with Children (Pediatric Patients) and Their Families. Several important things need to be considered and remembered with the pediatric patient:

- Family members need to be with their children, and children need their families.
- Family members are normally concerned and often are worried and frightened.
- Most children first learn about the world from their families.
- The younger the child, the more the child needs his or her family to help ease his or her fears.

Things you can do to help are:

- Do the best possible jobs of caring for the child. This is usually reassuring to the family members.
- Show interest and concern about the family members' welfare. Ask, "Is there something we can do?"
- Do not make judgments about the family members' attitudes or behavior, even if they seem strange to you.
- Encourage and allow the family members to help take part in the child's care when possible and if permitted.
- Sometimes family members seem to be worried about something concerning their child in the hospital and are afraid to talk about it. If you suspect this, tell your immediate supervisor.

Relationships with Visitors. Visiting hours are often the highlight of the day for patients. Knowing that family and friends are interested and concerned can do a lot to relax a patient's tensions, ease feelings of loneliness or isolation, relieve fears, and cheer the spirit.

Visitors may be worried and upset over the illness of a member of the family. They need your kindness and patience. Pleasant comments about flowers or gifts brought by visitors for the patient may be helpful (Figure 3-7).

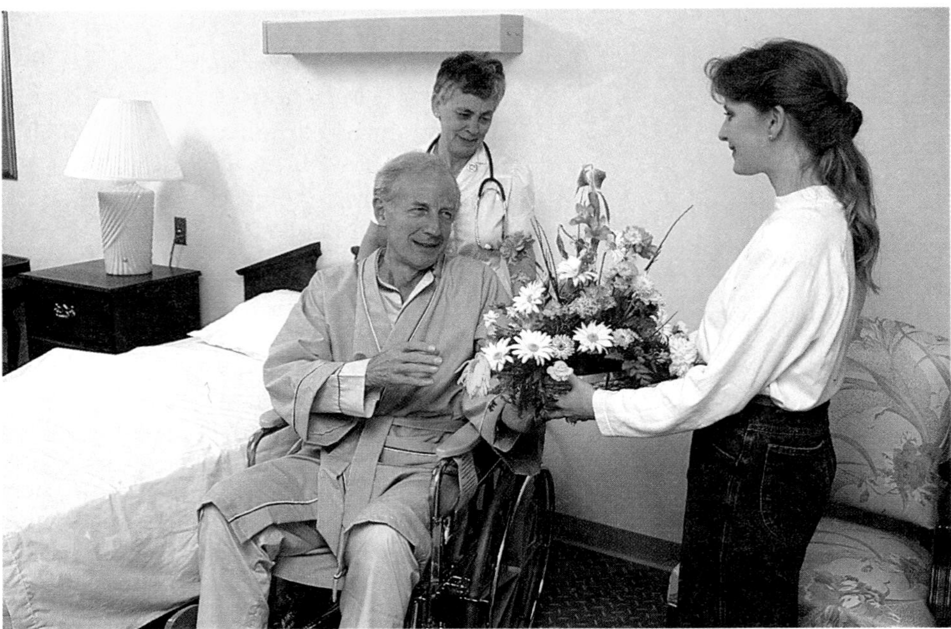

FIGURE 3-7 The nursing assistant should make visitors feel welcome.

If it appears that the visitors are upsetting the patient or making her or him tired, notify your immediate supervisor. He or she can caution visitors or ask them to leave.

In some situations, visiting hours may be longer or shorter. Your instructor will tell you about the visiting hours and any rules for visitors in your health care institution. These rules, of course, must be followed. Two main rules usually apply to visitors in any health care institutions:

- Visitors are not allowed to take institutional property away with them.
- Visitors cannot bring food or drink to the patient unless permission has been given by the nurse or doctor.

Communication with Visitors. Certain actions are helpful in your contacts with visitors:

- Listen to the visitor. Whether it is a suggestion, a complaint, or "passing the time of day," listen to the person. Some suggestions by visitors can be very helpful. Some complaints may be valid. When a complaint is presented, tell the person, "I will tell my supervisor about this," and then report it to your immediate supervisor.
- Do not get involved in the family's private affairs and feelings. Never take sides in family quarrels. Never give information or opinions to someone about other family members.
- Be prepared to give information regarding the hospital to visitors. Tell them what facilities are available for coffee, snacks, or meals, and the hours of operation. Tell them where a public telephone is. Direct them to other places in the institution, for example, the business office or the gift shop.

Answering the Patient Call Signal. Every patient has a way of sending a signal to the nursing staff when he or she wants something. It is important to answer the patient's call for service or help without delay (Figure 3-8).

All patients have a signal cord or call button. When the patient presses the button on the end of the cord, a light flashes near the nurses' station and over the patient's door. This device may be called a signal cord or call bell. You should always keep alert for such signals. Answer the signal as soon as it flashes. Every minute seems forever to the patient who is waiting. When the patient signals:

- Go to the patient at once, quietly and in a friendly way.
- Turn off the call signal, and address the patient by name.
- Say, "Mr. Jones, what can I do for you?"
- Do whatever the patient asks, but be sure it is correct and safe for this patient. If you are in doubt, ask your immediate supervisor. Tell him what the patient wants and then follow his directions.
- When necessary, use the emergency signal to get qualified personnel to assist you. Emergency signals are usually in one or more convenient locations: at the bedside, in the bathroom, shower, or tub room.
- Place the signal cord where the patient can reach it easily.
- *Caution:* A young child or an incapacitated adult may not be able to use the signal cord. Listen for calls for help from these patients and go quickly to see what they need. Check these patients often to see if

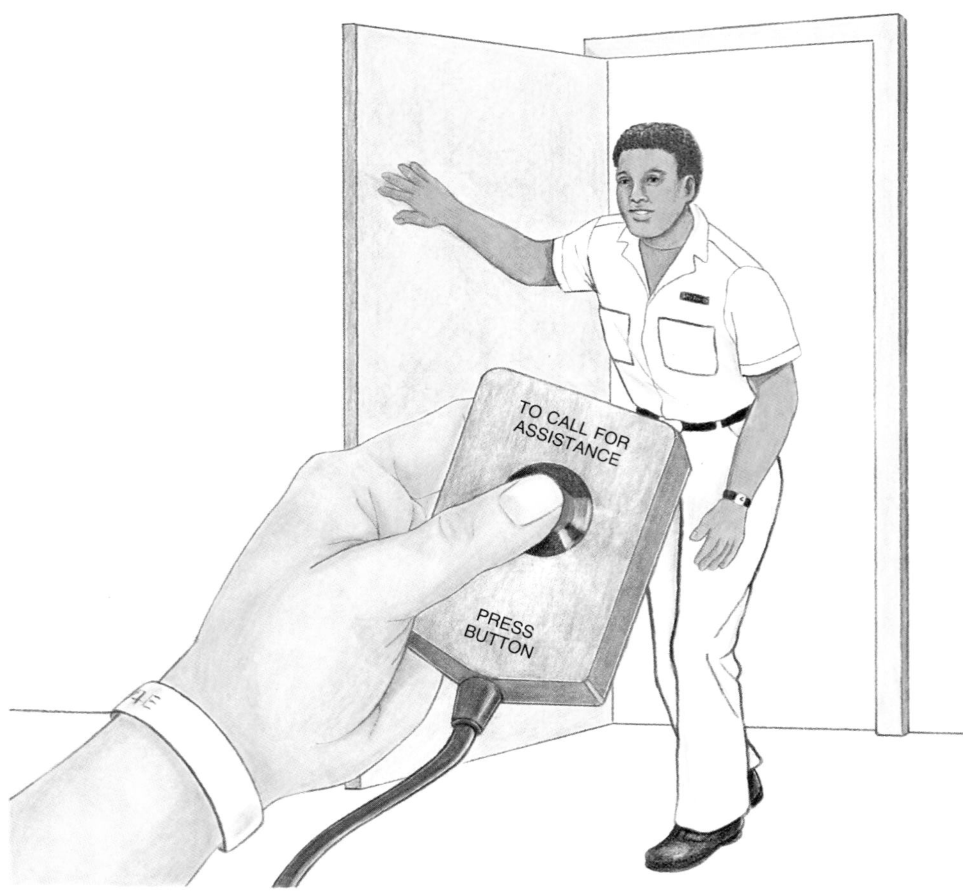

FIGURE 3-8 Answer the patient's call as quickly as possible.

they need something. Often special signal lights are available for patients with handicaps.

Communication with the Blind or Deaf Patient (Sensory Impaired). Patients with sensory loss present special challenges (Figure 3-9). For patients who have serious hearing and vision losses, the signal cord is used differently. *Blind or visually handicapped patients must be*

FIGURE 3-9 When working with patients who have a sensory loss (sight, hearing, speech, taste, or smell), be alert. Patients with impaired senses require special attention and help.

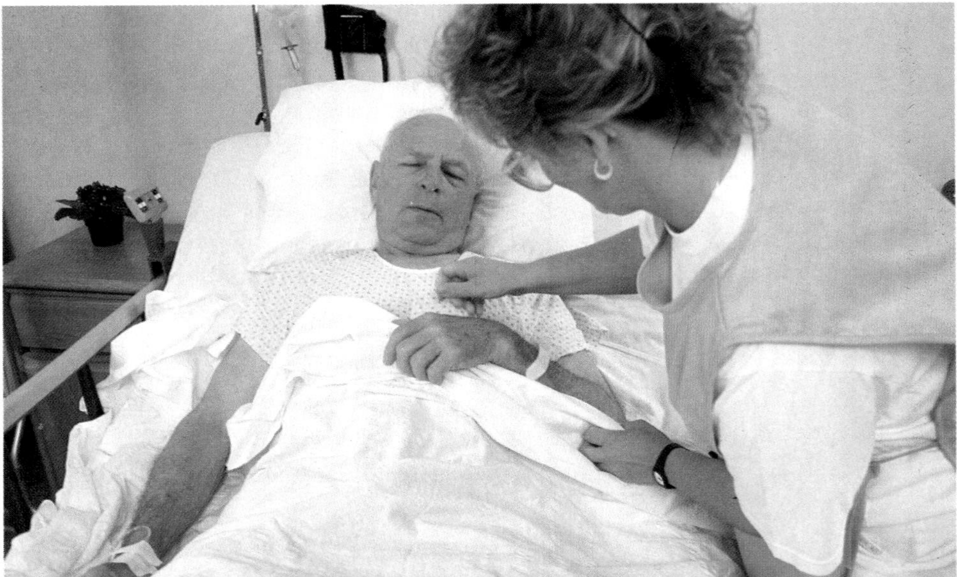

shown and taught how to use the signal. Have them feel around for the cord and practice using it while you are there.

If the signal is the kind that you push to turn on, you can call it a "push" button. If it works like a light switch, you can compare it to that. When working with patients who have serious visual losses, you should not expect them to turn off the signal. You can do that routinely when you respond to the signal call.

Patients with serious hearing losses can easily learn how to pull or push the signal cord on if you show them how to do it instead of telling them. Remember, they cannot hear you.

Communication When Using the Telephone. When you use the telephone or an intercommunication system (intercom), speak clearly and slowly. When you answer the telephone, for example, say, "Third floor, west. Mrs. Brown, nursing assistant, speaking." When you take a message for someone else, write it down immediately. Then, if possible, repeat it to the person calling to make sure it is correct. Ask the caller how to spell his or her name so you are sure you have it right. Record the following:

- The person being called
- The time the call was received
- The caller's name
- The message
- Your name and title

KEY QUESTIONS

1. Discuss the meaning of professional behavior toward patients, visitors, and co-workers. Give three examples.
2. Discuss situations in which it might be difficult for you to keep your emotions under control on the job and how you should behave.
3. How can you answer patient's and visitor's questions tactfully? Give examples.
4. What could you say to patients to communicate interest and concern? Give examples of conversations.
5. What should you take into consideration in order to communicate effectively with pediatric patients and their families?
6. What can you do to improve your communication skills?
7. What are the six things you should remember to do when answering the patient's call signal?
8. Explain five rights every patient has.
9. Discuss five ways you can show respect for the patient's culture, language, customs, and beliefs. Give examples.
10. Describe the role of the nursing assistant in meeting the patient's physical and psychological needs.
11. Demonstrate how you would teach a blind or deaf patient how to use the call signal.
12. List five items you should record when taking a telephone message.
13. Define: body language, communication, courtesy, empathy, pediatric patient, tact.

CHAPTER

4

Observing the Patient

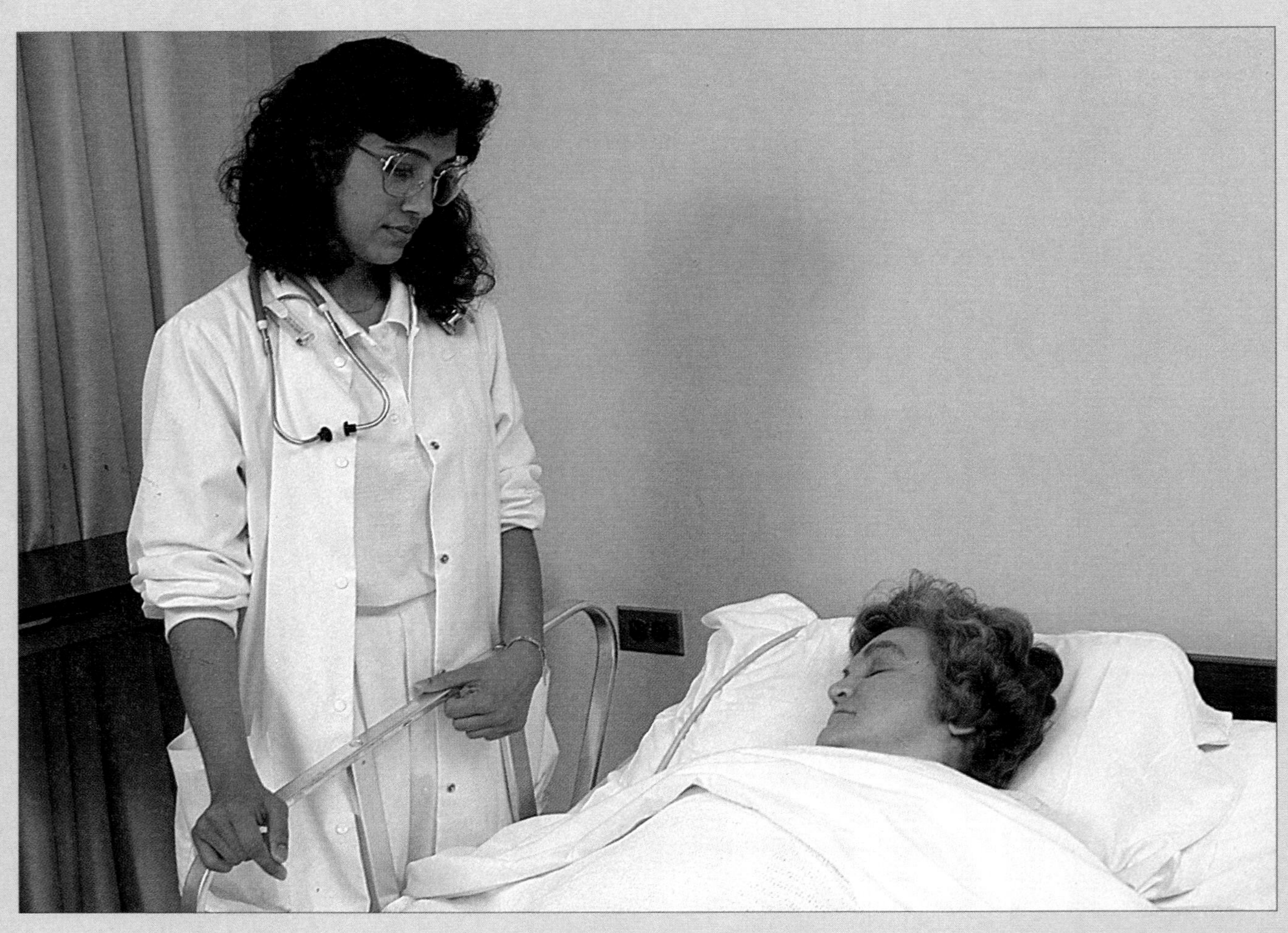

WARNING

For all patient contact, adhere to Universal Precautions (see page 91, 97, or the front cover flap). Wear protective equipment as indicated.

Objectives

What You Will Learn

When you have completed this chapter, you will be able to:

- Use your senses of sight, touch, hearing, and smell to observe the patients you care for.
- List the things to observe in a patient.
- List the things to report when they are observed in infants or children.
- Differentiate between objective and subjective reporting.
- Report observations promptly, accurately, and objectively.
- Define: cyanosis, edema, objective reporting, objective observations, observation, secretions, subjective reporting, subjective observations.

KEY IDEAS

Observing the Patient

Observation
Gathering information about the patient by noticing any change.

GET INTO THE HABIT OF OBSERVING the patient during all your contacts. These contacts include the bed bath, bed making, meal times, visiting hours, and any other time you are with him or her. **Observation** of the patient is a continuous process. Observing begins the first time you see a patient and ends when she or he is discharged from the hospital.

Observation means more than just careful watching. It includes listening and talking to the patient and asking questions. It means being aware of a situation and interpreting it. Be alert to changes in a patient's condition or anything unusual that occurs whenever you are with a patient. Report any changes in the patient's condition or appearance. Also watch for changes in the patient's attitude, moods, and emotional condition. Pay attention to any complaints. For example, report to your immediate supervisor if:

- A patient who had an abdominal operation two or three days ago says, "The calf of my leg is sore."
- A patient who is being given a blood transfusion says, "I feel itchy."

KEY IDEAS

Methods of Observation

Edema
Abnormal swelling of a part of the body caused by fluid collecting in that area. Usually the swelling is in the ankles, legs, hands, or abdomen.

Objective Observations: Signs and Symptoms

Use all your senses (looking, listening, touching, smelling) when making **objective observations**:

- You can see some signs of change in a patient's condition. By using your eyes, you can observe a skin rash, reddened areas, or swelling **(edema)**.
- You can feel some signs with your fingers: a change in the patient's pulse rate, puffiness in the skin, dampness (perspiration).

Objective Observations Symptoms that can be observed and reported exactly as they are seen.

- You can hear some signs, such as a cough or wheezing sounds, when the patient breathes.
- You can smell some signs, such as an odor on a patient's breath.
- Listen to the patient talking for other changes in his or her condition.

Subjective Observations Signs and symptoms that can be felt and described only by the patient, such as pain, nausea, dizziness, ringing in the ears, or headache.

Subjective Observations: Signs and Symptoms. **Subjective observations** are signs and symptoms that can be felt and described only by the patient. Examples are pain, nausea, dizziness, ringing in the ears, or headache.

Things to Observe in a Patient. Learning how to make useful observations is one of the most important things you will do in your work and will give you satisfaction and a feeling of achievement (Figure 4-1). The process of observation never ends, and you learn by doing. Because observations are so important in the total care of the patient, doctors and nurses never stop learning about a patient.

- *General appearance.* Has this changed? If so, in what way? Is there a noticeable odor (smell)?
- *Mental condition or mood.* Does the patient talk a lot? Very little? Does he talk about the future or the past? Does he talk about where he hurts? Is the patient anxious and worried? Is he calm? Or is he very excited? Is he talking sensibly? Or not making sense? Is he confused or disoriented? Is he speaking rapidly? Slowly? Is he cooperative? Uncooperative? Is he belligerent or aggravated?
- *Position.* Does the patient lie still or does she toss around? Does she like to lie in one position better than others? Does she prefer being on her back? Or on her side? Is she able to move easily?
- *Eating and drinking habits.* Does the patient complain that he has no appetite? Does he dislike his diet? How much does he eat? Does he eat some of each kind of food? Is he always thirsty or does he very seldom drink water? Does he eat all the food on his tray? Does he eat half the food on his tray? Does he refuse to eat?
- *Sleeping habits.* Is the patient able to sleep? Is he restless? Does he complain about not being able to sleep? Do these complaints agree

FIGURE 4-1 Be alert. You may be the first to notice a change in the patient's condition, attitude, or emotional behavior. For example, if a patient tells you that his family does not love him anymore and he is going to commit suicide, you should listen to his concerns and report the remark to your head nurse or team leader.

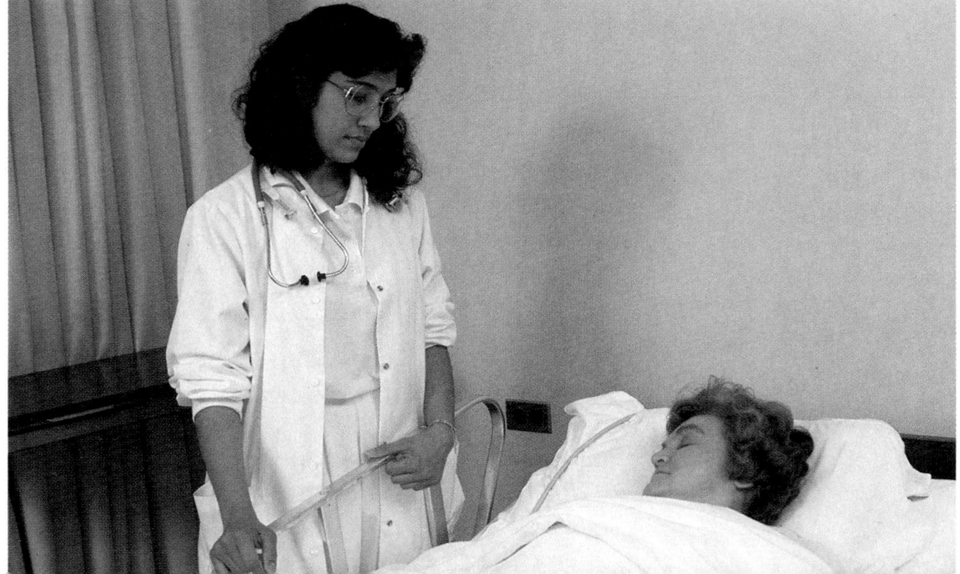

with your observations? Does he sleep more than is normal? Is he constantly asleep?

- *Skin.* Is the patient's skin unusually pale (pallor)? Is it flushed (red)? Is the skin dry or moist? Are her lips and fingernails turning blue (cyanotic)? Is any swelling (edema) noticeable? Are there reddened areas? Are these at the end of the spine, or on the heels, or at other pressure points? Is the skin shiny? Is there any puffiness? Is there puffiness in the legs and feet? Is her skin cold or clammy? Is it hot?
- *Eyes, ears, nose, and mouth.* Does the patient complain that he sees spots or flashes before his eyes? Does bright light bother him? Are his eyes red (inflamed)? Is it hard for him to breathe through his nose? Does he seem to have large amounts of mucous discharge from the nose? Does he complain that he has a bad taste in his mouth? Is there an odor on his breath? Is the patient able to hear you?
- *Breathing.* Does the patient wheeze? Does she make other noises when she breathes? Does she cough? Does she cough up sputum and how much? What is the color? Is it bloody? Does she have difficulty breathing (dyspnea) or shortness of breath?
- *Abdomen, bowels, and bladder.* Does the patient's stomach appear to be distended (puffed up)? Does he complain of gas, belching, or nausea? Is he vomiting (having emesis)? What is the appearance of the vomitus? Does it contain red blood? Does it look like coffee grounds? Is the patient constipated? How often does he have a bowel movement? What is the color and consistency (hard or soft) of feces (stool)? Is there any blood, or clumps of mucus, or pieces of white material in the feces? How often does the patient void (urinate)? How much does he void each time? Does he say that he has pain during urination, or that it is difficult to start to urinate? Is there sediment (cloudiness) or blood in the urine? Is it concentrated? Does the urine have a peculiar odor or color? Is the patient unable to control his bowels or urine (incontinent)?
- *Pain.* Where is the pain? How long does the patient say he has had it? How does he describe the pain? Is it constant? Does it come and go? Does he say that it is sharp, dull, aching, or knifelike? Has he had medicine for the pain? Does the patient say that the medicine relieved the pain?
- *Daily activities.* Does the patient dress herself? Does she walk without help? Does she walk with help? Does she avoid walking altogether?
- *Personal care.* Without help, does the patient brush her teeth? Comb her hair? Go to the bathroom? Wash her face? Does she ask for assistance?
- *Movements.* Is the patient shaking (having tremors or spasms)? Is he limp? Are his movements uncontrollable?

Secretions
The substances that flow out of or are produced by glandular organs; the process of producing this substance; for example, sweat, bile, lymph, saliva, or urine.

Observation of an Infant or Child. Observing an infant or a child means looking at his or her appearance and physical condition, bodily functions and **secretions**, movements, and behavior. When you observe changes in any of these, it is very important that you report them to your immediate supervisor right away. Report things that can be measured, such as a high temperature. Also report the things you see in a pattern of change, such as the child's behavior. Your careful observation and quick reporting could save a baby's life. The following are things to report when you observe them in infants or children:

Cyanosis
When the skin looks blue or has a gray color because there is not enough oxygen in the blood; often seen in the patient's lips and nailbeds and in the skin under the fingernails. In a black patient, it may appear as a darkening of color.

Appearance and Physical Condition

- The child's temperature is high or very low.
- The pulse is unusually fast, slow, or irregular.
- The child is breathing rapidly or is having trouble breathing.
- The abdomen seems to be swollen.
- The child's skin does not look normal. It may be yellow, show purplish patches, appear unusually pale, or have a blue cast.
- There may be blueness **(cyanosis)** in the fingernails or lips.
- There are secretions, bleeding, or odor coming from the baby's navel (umbilicus).

Bodily Functions and Secretions

- The child has not urinated during your hours of work or has voided very little.
- The child has diarrhea.
- A large amount of mucus is being secreted from the mouth or nose.
- The child is producing a large amount of saliva.
- The child is having trouble swallowing.
- The child is coughing or choking.
- The child is vomiting.

Movement and Behavior

- The child is lying in an abnormal position.
- The muscles are twitching.
- There is no movement in the legs or arms.
- The child is lying very quietly or seems unusually still.
- The child is crying or is excessively irritable.

KEY IDEAS

Subjective and Objective Reporting

Objective Reporting
Reporting exactly what you observe.

Subjective Reporting
Giving your opinion about what you have observed. The nursing assistant should never use subjective reporting.

It is very important for you to understand the difference between **objective reporting** and **subjective reporting**. Reporting subjective information must be done accurately by repeating what the patient tells you regarding himself or herself. Remember, only the patient can describe or make a judgment about what he or she feels.

Objective reporting means reporting exactly what you observe, that is, what you see, hear, feel, or smell. The nursing assistant must always use objective reporting (see Figure 4-2).

Here are some examples of objective reporting:

- Mrs. Barbary in Room 110, window bed, is perspiring profusely.
- Mr. Ellis in Room 432, door bed, had a bowel movement that was white. A specimen was collected.
- Mrs. Delcara, Room 510, A bed, has an area on her left heel that is hard, red, and the size of a quarter.
- Mrs. Walker in Room 330, A bed, lips are dark blue.

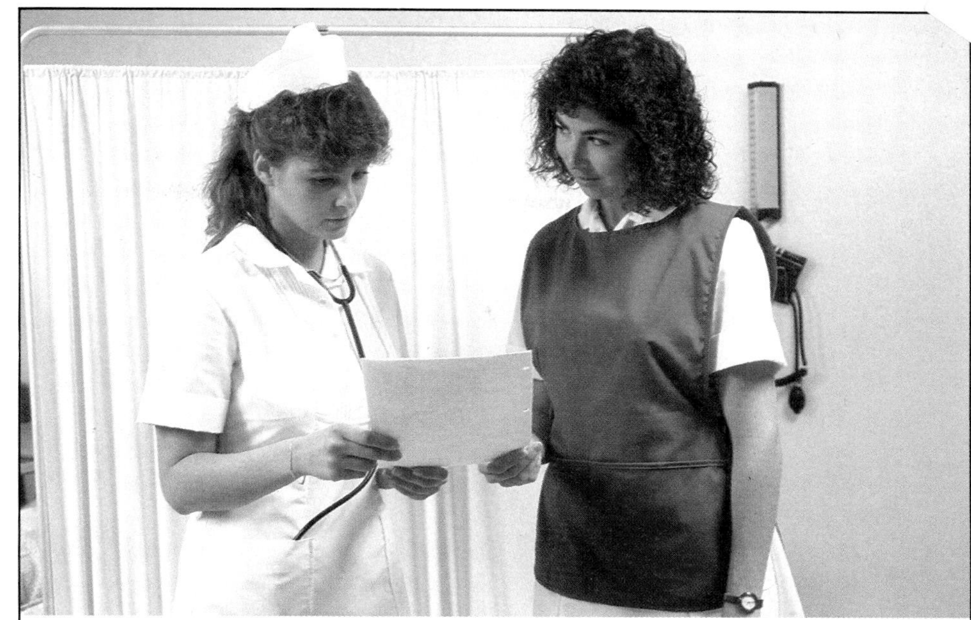

RULES TO FOLLOW WHEN REPORTING YOUR OBSERVATIONS

Write down the patient's name, room number, and bed number.
Write or report your observations to the head nurse or team leader as soon as possible.
Report the time you made the observation.
Report the location of the abnormal or unusual sign.
Report exactly, but report only what you observe, that is, report objectively.

FIGURE 4-2 Rules to follow when reporting your observations.

- Mrs. Carlin in Room 101, window bed, right ankle is much larger than her left ankle.
- Mr. Joseph in Room 404 is clenching his teeth together and is talking very differently than he was talking at breakfast.
- When Mr. Roberts in Room 581, B bed, breathes he makes loud wheezing sounds, which he was not doing when I made his bed an hour ago.
- Mrs. Smith, Room 404, B bed, is breathing rapidly and the breaths appear to be shallow.
- Mr. Williams, Room 204, B bed, urine looks red tinged. A urine specimen was collected.
- Cindy Jones, Room 107, A bed, has a red area the size of a dollar bill on her upper right back.
- Mr. Jones, Room 101, A bed, urine was bright red. Left in urinal in his bathroom for you to see.

Figure 4-3 gives examples of the right way and the wrong way of reporting.

FIGURE 4-3 Subjective versus objective reporting.

Right
Wrong
Objective Reporting: "Mr. Blike, 105, B bed, says his chest hurts on the left side. He says the pain started an hour ago."
Objective Reporting: "Mr. Jones, 402, B bed, the patient's lips are blue. They didn't look that way at 10 A.M."
Subjective Reporting: "There was a draft in the room. He was cold so his lips looked blue."

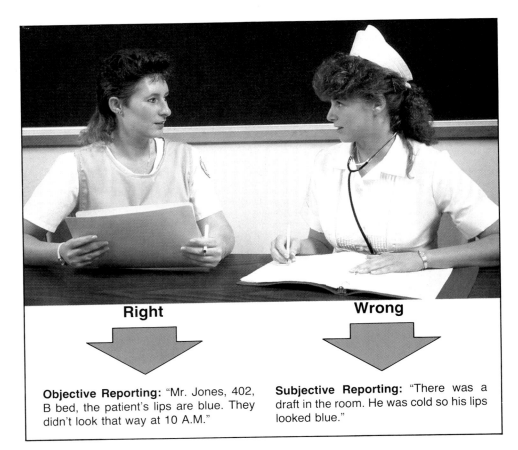

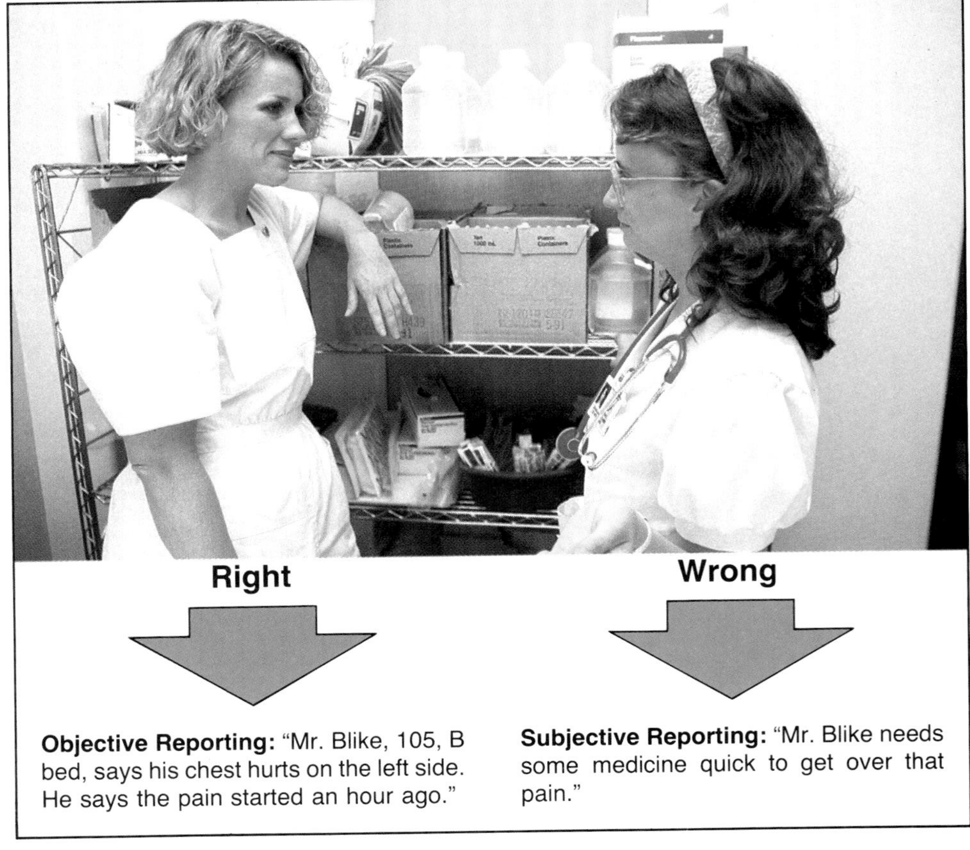

KEY QUESTIONS

1. List examples of observations of patients you can make by using your senses of sight, touch, hearing, and smell.
2. List ten categories of things to observe in a patient. Give examples for each group.
3. List 15 things to report when they are observed in infants or children.
4. What is the difference between objective and subjective reporting?
5. How should observations be reported?
6. Define: cyanosis, edema, objective reporting, objective observations, observation, secretions, subjective reporting, subjective observations.

CHAPTER

5

Medical Terms, Abbreviations, and Specialties

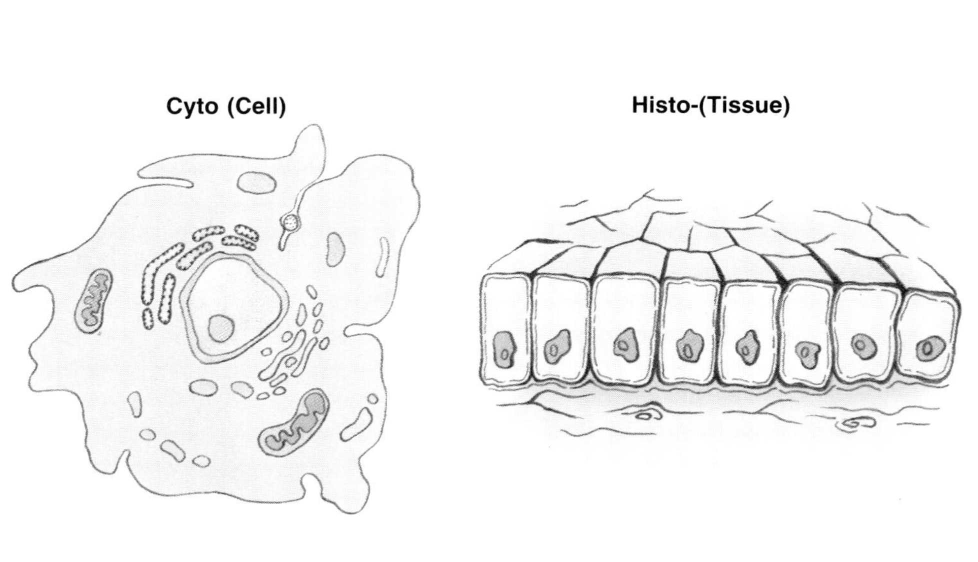

WARNING

For all patient contact, adhere to Universal Precautions. (see page 91, 97, or the front cover flap). Wear protective equipment as indicated.

Objectives

What You Will Learn

When you have completed this chapter, you will be able to:

- Define the list of abbreviations commonly used in health care institutions.
- Identify different physician's titles and describe their meanings.
- Name and describe medical specialties.
- Define: abbreviation, medical terminology, prefix, Roman numerals, root, and suffix.

KEY IDEAS

Abbreviations and Their Meanings

Abbreviation
A shortened form of a word or phrase used to represent the complete form.

ABBREVIATIONS ARE THE SHORTHAND OF THE health professions. They are clear and efficient tools for the nurse to tell you quickly what they want you to do. As a nursing assistant, you will use these abbreviations in your daily work. They will help you to understand instructions from your immediate supervisor. Abbreviations help you when you are receiving reports about your patients and in keeping your notes on your daily assignments.

Abbreviations Used in Keeping Notes

Abbreviation	Meaning
aa	Of each, equal parts
ABR	Absolute bed rest
abd.	Abdomen
ac	Before meals
AD	Admitting diagnosis
A&D	Admission and discharge
ad lib	As desired, if the patient so desires
ADL	Activities of daily living
Adm.	Admission
Adm. Spec.	Admission urine specimen
A.M. or a.m., AM or am	Morning
amb.	Ambulation, walking, ambulatory, able to walk
amt.	Amount
AP or A.P.	Appendectomy
aqua	Water or H_2O
@	At
Approx.	Approximately
B&B or b&b	Bowel and bladder training
bid or B.I.D. or b.i.d.	Twice a day
b.m. or B.M.	Bowel movement, feces
B.P. or BP	Blood pressure
BR or br or B.R. or b.r.	Bedrest

Abbreviations Used in Keeping Notes

Abbreviation	Meaning
BRP or B.R.P. or brp	Bathroom privileges
BSC or bsc	Bedside commode
°C	Celsius degree (or centigrade)
$\bar{c}$	With
Ca	Cancer
Cath.	Catheter
CBC or C.B.C.	Complete blood count
cc or c.c.	Cubic centimeter
CCU or C.C.U.	Cardiac care unit/coronary care unit
CBR or C.B.R. or cbr	Complete bed rest
C/O or c/o	Complaint of
CO_2	Carbon dioxide
CS or cs or C.S. or c.s.	Central supply
CSD or csd or C.S.D.	Central service department
CSR or csr and C.S.R.	Central supply room
CVA or C.V.A.	Cerebrovascular accident or stroke
CPR or C.P.R.	Cardiopulmonary resuscitation
dc or d/c	Discontinue
Del. Rm. or d.r., or DR	Delivery room
Disch. or dish or D/C	Discharge
D. & C. or D&C	Dilatation and curettage
drsg.	Dressing
DOA or D.O.A.	Dead on arrival
Dr. or Dr	Doctor
DX	Diagnosis
ECG or EKG	Electrocardiogram
ED or E.D.	Emergency department
EEG or E.E.G.	Electroencephalogram
EENT or E.E.N.T.	Eye, ears, nose, and throat
E. or E	Enema
ER or E.R.	Emergency room
°F	Fahrenheit degree
F. or Fe. or F or Fe	Female
FBS or F.B.S.	Fasting blood sugar
FF or F.F.	Forced feeding or forced fluids
ft	Foot
Fx	Fracture
Fx urine	Fractional urine
gal	Gallon
GI or G.I.	Gastrointestinal
gt	One drop
gtt	Two or more drops
Gtt or G.T.T.	Glucose tolerance test
GU or G.U.	Genitourinary
Gyn. or G.Y.N.	Gynecology
H_2O	Water or aqua
HOB	Head of bed
hr	Hour
HS or hs	Bedtime or hour of sleep
ht	Height
hyper	Above or high
hypo	Below or low
H.W.B. or hwb or HWB	Hot water bottle

Abbreviations Used in Keeping Notes

Abbreviation	Meaning
ICU or I.C.U.	Intensive care unit
I&O or I. & O.	Intake and output
Irr	Irregular
Isol. or isol	Isolation
IV or I.V.	Intravenous
L	Liter
Lab. or lab	Laboratory
lb	Pound
Liq or liq.	Liquid
LPN or L.P.N.	Licensed practical nurse
LVN or L.V.N.	Licensed vocational nurse
M	Male
Mat	Maternity
MD or M.D.	Medical doctor
Meas	Measure
mec	Meconium
med	Medicine
min	Minute
ml	Milliliter
Mn or mn or M/n	Midnight
N.A. or N/A	Nursing aide or nursing assistant
n/g tube or ng. tube or N.G.T.	Nasogastric tube
noct	At night
NP	Neuropsychiatric; or nursing procedure
NPO or N.P.O.	Nothing by mouth
nsy	Nursery
O_2	Oxygen
OB or O.B.	Obstetrics
Obt or obt.	Obtained
OJ or O.J.	Orange juice
Ord.	Orderly
OOB or O.O.B.	Out of bed
OPD or O.P.D.	Outpatient department
OR or O.R.	Operating room
Ortho	Orthopedics
OT or O.T.	Occupational therapy; or oral temperature
oz	Ounce
PAR or P.A.R.	Postanesthesia room
pc	After meals
Ped or Peds	Pediatrics
per	By, through
p.m. or P.M., pm or PM	Afternoon
PMC or P.M.C.	Postmortem care
PN or P.N.	Pneumonia
po	By mouth
post or $\overline{p}$	After
postop or post op	Postoperative
post op spec	After surgery urine specimen
PP	Postpartum (after delivery)
PPBS	Postprandial blood sugar
pre	Before

Abbreviations Used in Keeping Notes

Abbreviation	Meaning
prn or p.r.n.	Whenever necessary, when required
preop or pre op	Before surgery
pre op spec	Urine specimen before surgery
prep	Prepare the patient for surgery by shaving the skin
Pt or pt	Patient; pint
PT or P.T.	Physical therapy
q	Every
qd	Every day
qh	Every hour
q2h	Every 2 hours
q3h	Every 3 hours
q4h	Every 4 hours
QHS or qhs	Every night at bedtime/hour of sleep
qid or Q.I.D.	Four times a day
qam or q am or q.a.m.	Every morning
qod or Q.O.D.	Every other day
qs	Quantity sufficient; as much as required
qt	Quart
r or R	rectal or Rectal
Rm or rm	Room
RN or R.N.	Registered nurse
rom or R.O.M.	Range of motion
RR or R.Rm.	Recovery room
Rx	Prescription or treatment ordered by a physician
s or $\bar{s}$	Without
S&A	Sugar and acetone
S&A or S.&A. Test	Sugar and acetone test
S&K or S.&K. Test	Sugar and ketone test
SOB	Shortness of breath
sos	Whenever emergency arises; only if necessary
SPD	Special purchasing department
Spec or spec.	Specimen
ss or $\overline{ss}$	One-half
SSE or S.S.E.	Soapsuds enema
stat	At once, immediately
STD	sexually transmitted disease
Surg	Surgery
tid or T.I.D.	Three times a day
TLC or tlc	Tender loving care
TPR	Temperature, pulse, respiration
TWE	Tap water enema
U/a or U/A or u/a	Urinalysis
Ung.	Ointment, unguentine
VDRL	Test for syphilis
V.S. or VS	Vital signs
WBC or W.B.C.	White blood count
w/c	Wheelchair
wc or W.C.	Ward clerk
wt	Weight

Roman Numerals
The letters used to represent numbers in the ancient Roman system.

Roman Numerals. The dots or "eyes" are used to eliminate a margin of error:

$$1 = \text{I or } \dot{\overline{\text{I}}} \quad 2 = \text{II or } \ddot{\overline{\text{II}}} \quad 3 = \text{III or } \dddot{\overline{\text{III}}}$$

$$4 = \text{IV or } \overline{\text{IV}} \quad 5 = \text{V or } \overline{\text{V}}$$

$$10 = \text{X or } \overline{\text{X}}$$

KEY IDEAS

Word Elements

Many medical terms are composed of several smaller, simpler words or word elements. This discussion describes and shows how to use three primary word elements that are combined frequently to form medical terms. These three word elements are the prefix, the root, and the suffix.

Root
The body or main part of the word.

Prefix
A word element added to the beginning of a root.

Suffix
A word element used to change or add to the meaning of a root. It is always added to the end of a root.

- The **root** is the body or main part of the word. It denotes the primary meaning of the word as a whole.
- The **prefix** is a word element combined with the root. It changes or adds to the meaning of the words. A prefix is always added to the beginning of a root.
- The **suffix** is also a word element used to change or add to the meaning of a root. It is always added to the end of the root.

Examples of Similarity Between Terms

Word Element	Example	Meaning
ante	antefebrile	before onset of fever
anti	antifebrile	used against fever
cysto	cystogram	x-ray record of the bladder
cyto	cytogenesis	production (origin) of the cell
hyper	hypertension	high blood pressure
hypo	hypotension	low blood pressure
inter	interstitial	lying between spaces in tissue
intra	intracranial	within the skull
macro	macroscopy	seen large, as with the naked eye
micro	microscopy	seen small, as by microscope
per	percussion	striking through the body; use of fingertips to lightly tap the body
pre	preclinical	before the onset of disease

Word Element: Itis

Medical Terminology
The special vocabulary of words used in the health care professions.

The study of **medical terminology** can aid you in understanding the name of the specific disease for which the patient has been hospitalized. The suffix **itis** means inflammation. Almost every organ in the body is subject to infection by disease organisms that will cause an inflammatory reaction. The word to describe a diagnosis of this nature is formulated simply by adding the suffix itis to the word for the body organ affected.

appendicitis	inflammation of the appendix
dermatitis	inflammation of the skin
hepatitis	inflammation of liver tissue
rhinitis	inflammation of nasal mucosa
stomatitis	inflammation of the mouth

Word Element: Ectomy

The suffix **ectomy** means surgical removal. When used in combination with any word element denoting an organ or other body part, the term formed means that the organ or body part has been removed.

gastrectomy	surgical removal of the stomach
thyroidectomy	surgical removal of the thyroid gland
colectomy	surgical removal of the large intestine

In many cases, an organ may be removed only partially. To indicate this procedure, other words are used to modify the medical term, for example:

subtotal thyroidectomy	partial cystectomy

Other modifying words may precede the medical term. This identifies the surgery performed even more accurately.

left salpingo-oophorectomy	removal of the left ovary and Fallopian tube
vaginal hysterectomy	removal of the uterus through the vagina
transurethral prostatectomy	removal of the prostate through the urethra
total abdominal hysterectomy	removal of the entire uterus through abdomen

KEY IDEAS

Medical Specialties

Specialty	Physician's Title	Description
Allergy	Allergist	A subspecialty of internal medicine dealing with diagnosis and treatment of body reactions resulting from unusual sensitivity to foods, pollens, dust, medicines, or other substances.
Anesthesiology	Anesthesiologist	Administration of various forms of anesthesia in operations or procedures to cause loss of feeling or sensation.
Cardiology; cardiovascular diseases	Cardiologist	A subspecialty of internal medicine involving the diagnosis and treatment of diseases of the heart and blood vessels.
Dermatology	Dermatologist	The diagnosis and treatment of disorders of the skin.
Gastroenterology	Gastroenterologist	A subspecialty of internal medicine concerned with diagnosis and treatment of disorders of the digestive tract.
General practice	General practitioner	The diagnosis and treatment of disease by medical and surgical methods, without limitation to organ systems or body regions, and without restriction as to age of patients.

Specialty	Physician's Title	Description
General surgery	Surgeon	The diagnosis and treatment of disease by surgical means, without limitation to special organ systems or body regions.
Gynecology	Gynecologist	Diagnosis and treatment of diseases of the female reproductive system.
Internal medicine	Internist	The diagnosis and nonsurgical treatment of illnesses of adults.
Neurological	Neurosurgeon	Diagnosis and surgical treatment of brain, spinal cord, and nerve disorders.
	Neurologist	Diagnosis and treatment of disease of brain, spinal cord, and nerve disorders.
Obstetrics	Obstetrician	The care of women during pregnancy, childbirth, and immediately following.
Ophthalmology	Ophthalmologist	Diagnosis and treatment of diseases of the eye, including prescribing corrective lenses.
Orthopedics	Orthopedist	Diagnosis and treatment of disorders and diseases of muscular and skeletal systems.
Otolaryngology	Otolaryngologist	Diagnosis and treatment of diseases of the ear, nose, and throat.
Pathology	Pathologist	Study and interpretation of changes in organs, tissues, and cells and alterations in body chemistry to aid in diagnosing disease and determining treatment.
Pediatrics	Pediatrician	Prevention, diagnosis, and treatment of children's diseases.
Physical medicine and rehabilitation	Physiatrist	Diagnosis of disease or injury in the various systems and areas of the body and treatment by means of physical procedures, as well as treatment and restoration of the convalescent and physically handicapped patient.
Plastic surgery	Plastic surgeon	Cosmetic, corrective, or reparative surgery to restore deformed parts of the body.
Psychiatry	Psychiatrist	Medical branch concerned with diagnosis and treatment of mental disorders.
Radiology	Radiologist	Use of radiant energy, including x-rays, radioactive substances, and magnetic imagery in the diagnosis and treatment of diseases.
Thoracic surgery	Thoracic surgeon	Operative treatment of the lungs, heart, or the large blood vessels within the chest cavity.
Urology	Urologist	Diagnosis and treatment of diseases or disorders of the kidneys, bladder, ureters, urethra, and the male reproductive organs.

KEY QUESTIONS

1. Define the following commonly used abbreviations:

a) w/c
b) s
c) qs
d) QID
e) pre
f) per
g) O_2
h) hypo
i) hr
j) $\bar{c}$
k) @
l) Adm. Spec.
m) BID
n) Ca.
o) CCU
p) abd
q) CVA
r) Dx
s) gtt
t) po

2. Draw a line matching the physicians' titles with their descriptions.

a) Allergist	**1)** A doctor who treats patients with diseases of the heart and circulatory system
b) Cardiologist	**2)** A doctor who treats diseases and disorders of the muscular and skeletal systems
c) Gynecologist	**3)** A doctor who treats patients with allergies
d) Orthopedist	**4)** A doctor who treats patients with mental disorders
e) Psychiatrist	**5)** A doctor who treats patients with diseases of the female reproductive organs

3. Define the following: abbreviation, medical terminology, prefix, root, Roman numerals, and suffix.
4. Write the Roman numerals one to five.

CHAPTER

6

Safety

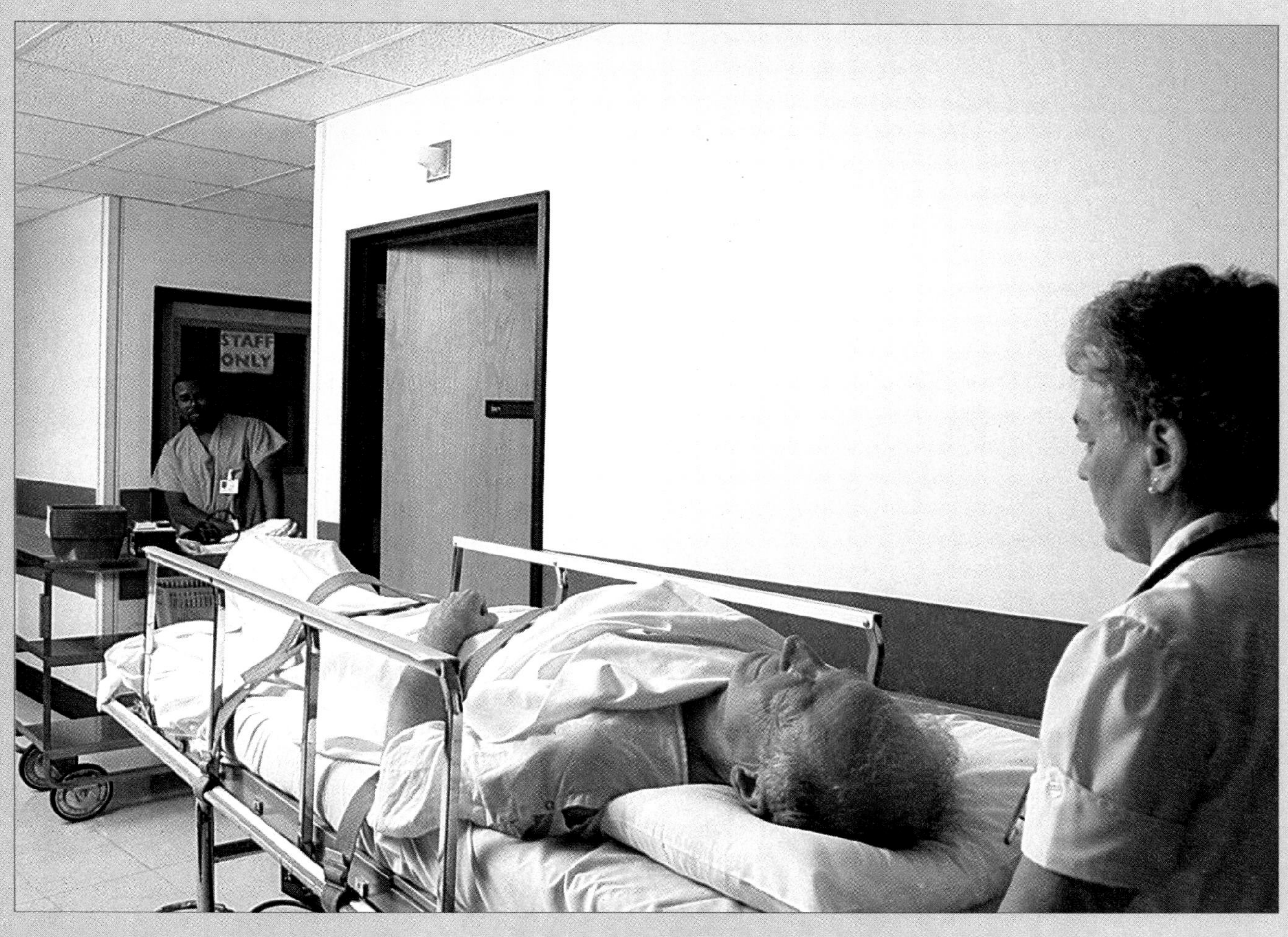

WARNING

For all patient contact, adhere to Universal Precautions (see page 91, 97, or the front cover flap). Wear protective equipment as indicated.

Objectives

What You Will Learn

When you have completed this chapter, you will be able to:

- List the general rules of institutional safety.
- List special safety precautions to take when caring for children.
- Describe the special safety precautions necessary when oxygen is being used.
- Explain what you can do to prevent fires and what to do in case of fire.
- Identify the safety precautions that should be taken when restraints are used.
- Deal with emergency situations.
- List the safety rules for patient ambulation.
- Define: ambulate, ambulation, cannula, gait training, nasal, oxygen, protective device, restraint.

KEY IDEAS

Safety

PATIENTS ARE CHALLENGED BY ILLNESS, DISABILITIES, worries, and medication. Many of them cannot take care of themselves in an emergency and must be protected. Therefore, health care personnel must be especially careful to guard against accidents, to prevent fires and other kinds of emergencies, and to know what to do if an emergency arises.

Rules to Follow

SAFETY MEASURES

- Walk, never run, especially in halls or on stairs. Keep to the right. Use the handrails on stairways (Figure 6-1) and avoid collisions. Take special care at intersections (Figure 6-2).

FIGURE 6-1 Be safety conscious at all times.

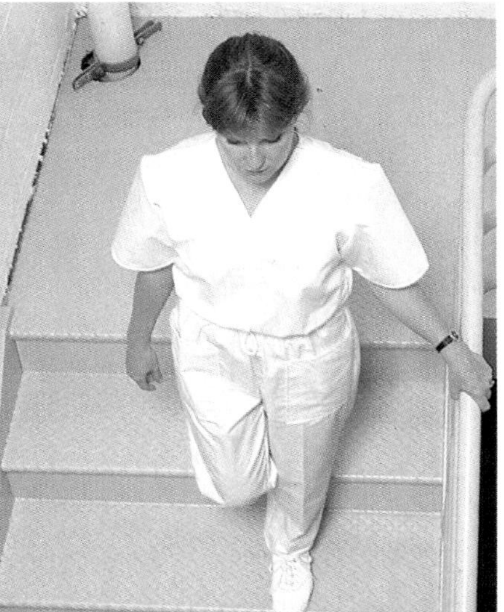

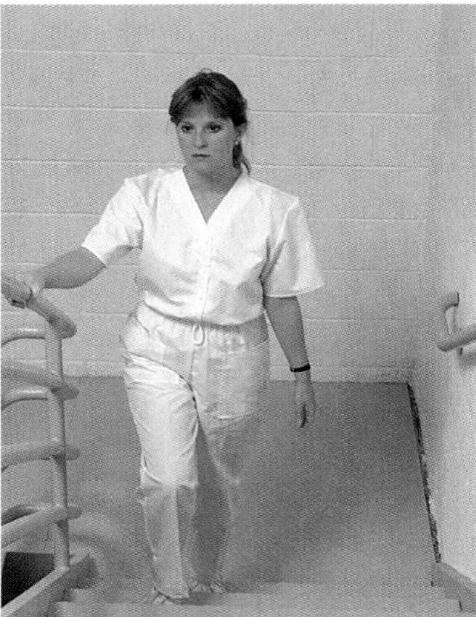

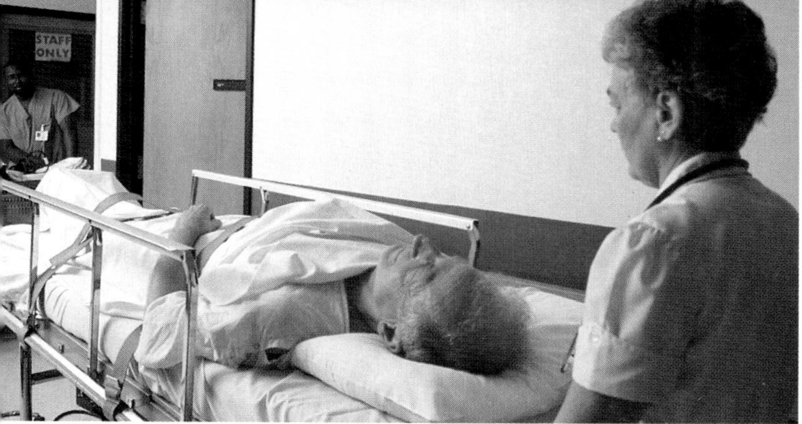

FIGURE 6-2 Use caution at intersections.

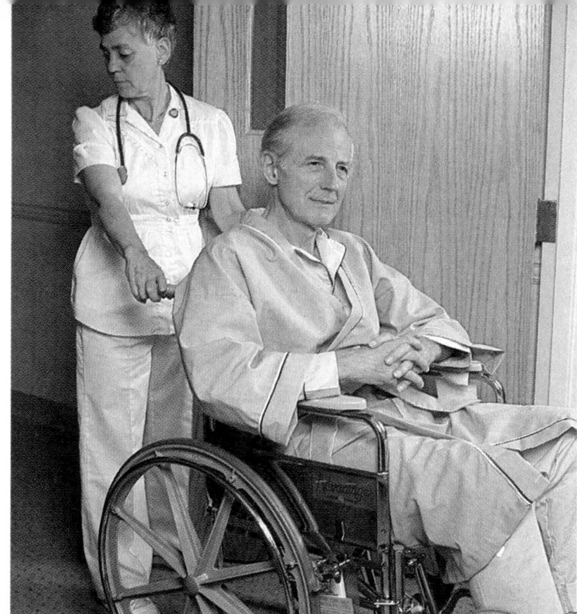

FIGURE 6-3 Watch out for swinging doors.

- Be sure to lock the brakes on the wheels of beds, stretchers, examining tables, or wheelchairs when moving patients on or off such equipment.
- Be very careful of the feet when transporting patients in wheelchairs or stretchers (Figure 6-3). Position feet on footrests so they are not in contact with the floor.
- When you see something on the floor that does not belong there, pick it up. If you see spilled liquid, wipe up the area (Figure 6-4).

FIGURE 6-4 Clean up spills immediately.

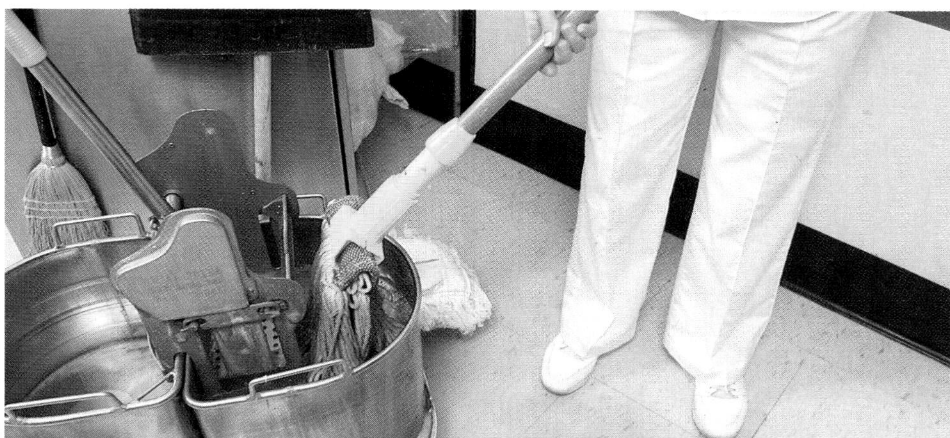

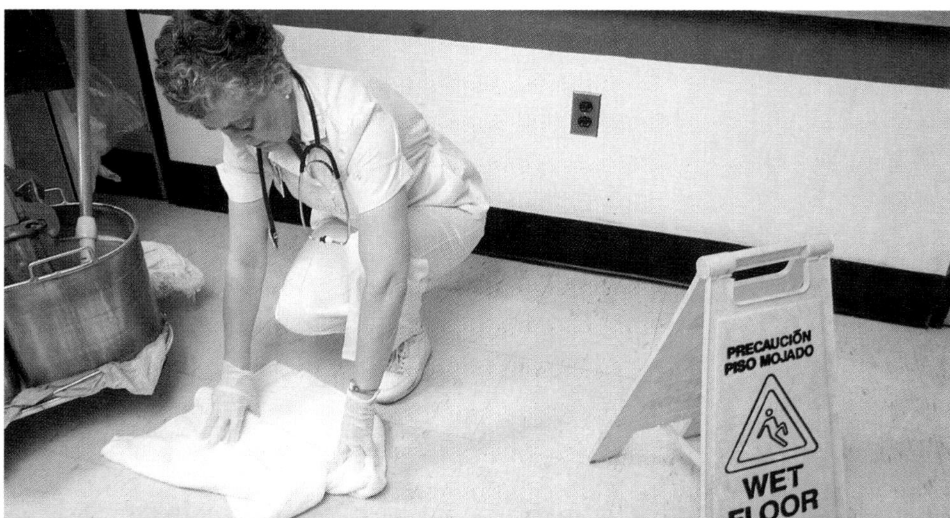

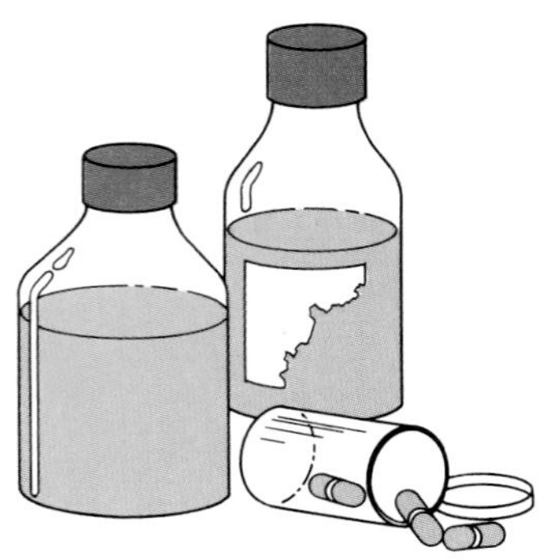

FIGURE 6-5 Never use the contents of an unlabeled container. Take the container to your immediate supervisor.

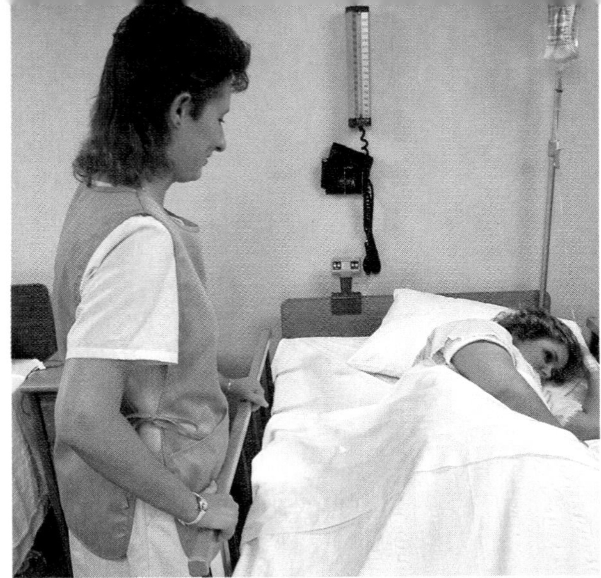

FIGURE 6-6 Keep the side rails in the up position for patients who are confused, elderly, restless, or coming out of anesthesia.

- Follow the instructions of your immediate supervisor when providing care. Many times the physician gives special orders, such as:
  - No weight bearing.
  - Keep head of bed elevated at all times.
  - Do not position patient on right side.
  - May be out of bed with assistance only.
- If you do not understand what is written on the label of a container, take it to your immediate supervisor and ask for an explanation.
- Check soiled linen for overlooked items before you send it to the laundry. Look for misplaced instruments, pins, needles, or other articles. Remove these and put them where they belong or dispose of them as instructed.
- Keep bed side rails in the up position for patients who are at risk (Figure 6-6).

Remove things that could be dangerous to children (Figure 6-7). Very small children must be watched continuously. They fall down, they

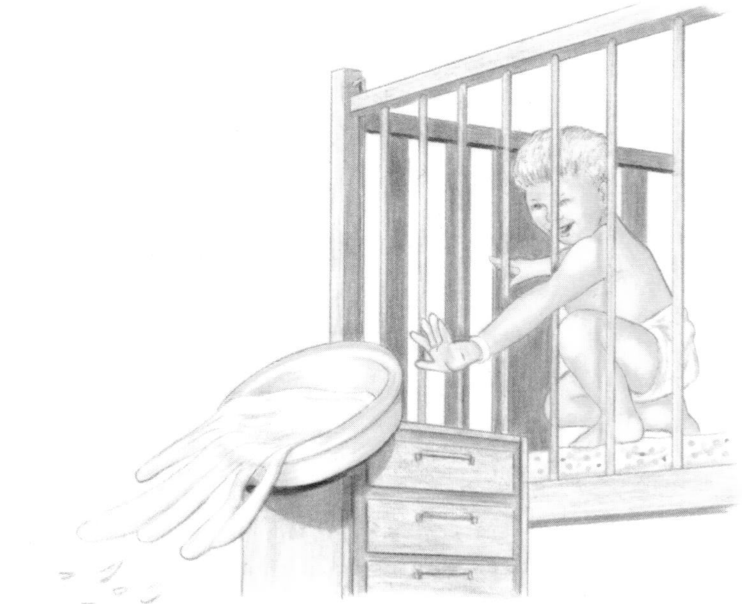

FIGURE 6-7 Keep items for child care out of reach. Remember, a child's reach is far and quick.

climb on things and fall from high places, they wander away, they find all sorts of things to try to do, and they can sometimes hurt themselves.

- People who work with children must always be alert to things that may cause accidents.
- Small children should never be left unattended when they are awake unless they are in a protected crib.
- Every child in a protective device should be checked frequently.
- Articles used in the child's care should be kept out of reach of a toddler when they are not being used. Watch especially for needles, water, safety pins, medication, matches, electrical equipment, syringes, or thermometers.
- Toys should never be left carelessly on the floor. Be especially alert to pick them up, as they could cause someone to fall.
- Clean up spills and messes, such as food, urine, and feces, right away.
- The sides of a child's crib should be up at all times except when someone is giving direct care to the child. For older children, bedside rails should be pulled up and locked in place.
- Doors to stairways, utility rooms, and the kitchen should always be closed immediately after use. They should be locked whenever possible.
- Linen chutes should be kept locked except when they are being used by hospital personnel.
- Venetian blind cords should be kept out of the reach of children.
- Be sure there are no small toys or objects in the crib or bed that can be swallowed. Examine all toys for small loose parts.
- Remove large objects that the child could stand on. The child might fall out of bed as a result. Also remove toys or objects with which the child could injure himself.
- Be sure all windows in the child's room are closed and locked.
- Lock the wheels on beds and cribs.

KEY IDEAS

Oxygen Safety

Oxygen
A colorless, odorless, tasteless gaseous element that is essential for respiration. Air is 21% oxygen.

A special device called a *regulator* or *flowmeter* (Figure 6-8) is necessary when **oxygen** is used. It controls or regulates the rate and flow of oxygen that is being given to the patient. Special procedures are to be followed in the care and use of portable oxygen tanks and regulators. Follow the instructions used in your facility. Pulmonary medicine or respiratory therapy departments often take care of this equipment in most health care institutions.

Respiratory therapy departments are responsible in most hospitals for the respiratory therapy treatments the patients might be receiving. This department takes care of the oxygen equipment and makes adjustments in the treatments by checking with the doctor or nurse. Special precautions must be observed when more than the normal amount of oxygen is present in a particular area, such as the patient's unit.

Extra oxygen supports combustion and can make things catch fire and burn much more rapidly than they would in normal air. To prevent fires when a patient is being given oxygen, the following rules of safety must be strictly observed.

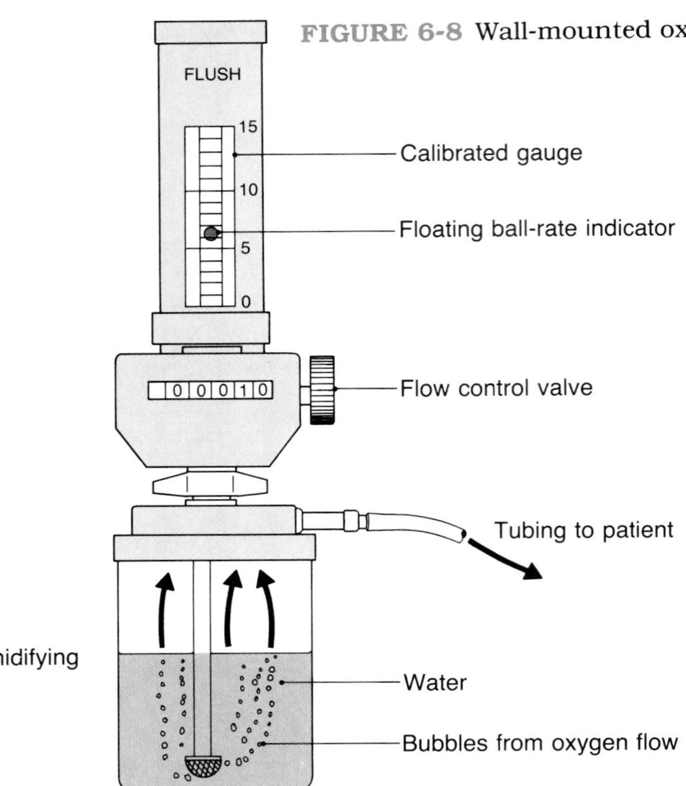

FIGURE 6-8 Wall-mounted oxygen flowmeter.

FIGURE 6-9 **No Smoking** sign used when oxygen is in use.

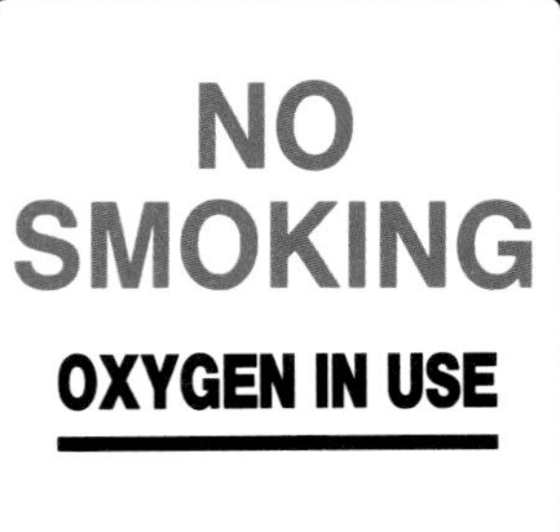

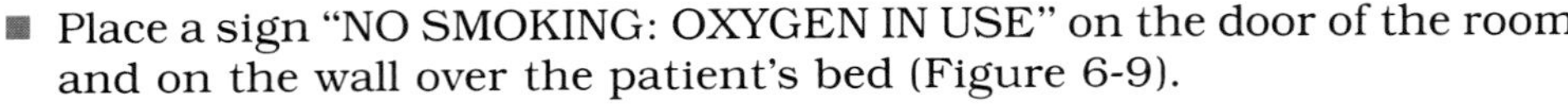

Rules to Follow

OXYGEN SAFETY

- Place a sign "NO SMOKING: OXYGEN IN USE" on the door of the room and on the wall over the patient's bed (Figure 6-9).
- The tubing connected to the source of oxygen should be free of kinks (Figure 6-10).
- Smoking is never permitted when oxygen is in use (Figure 6-11).

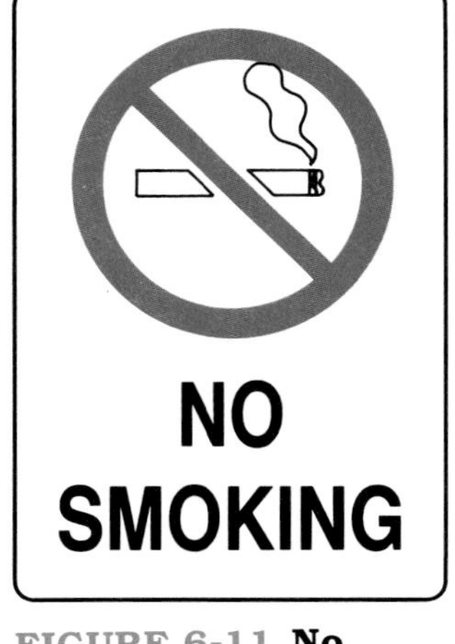

FIGURE 6-11 **No Smoking** sign.

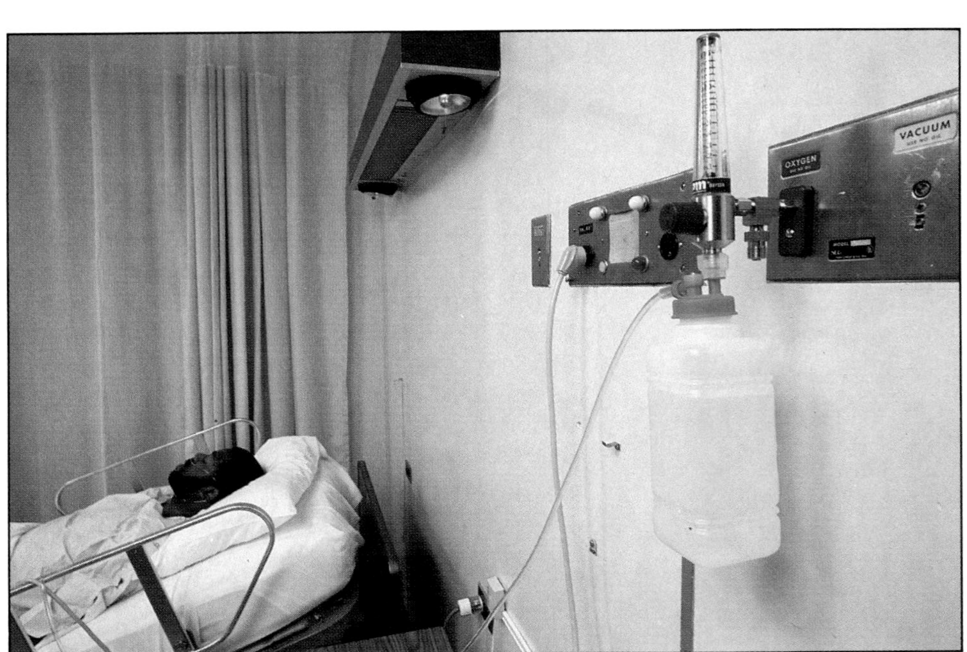

FIGURE 6-10 Safety precautions for oxygen include placing **No Smoking** signs inside and outside the room.

Nasal
Pertaining to the nose and the nasal cavity.

- A humidifying jar should be used with both the **nasal** oxygen cannula and the nasal oxygen catheter. The water level in the humidifying jar should be kept high enough so that it bubbles as the oxygen goes through it.
- Report cigarettes and matches belonging to the patient to your immediate supervisor.

KEY IDEAS

Oxygen Therapy

Invite a respiratory therapist to speak to the class.

Oxygen therapy is administered to the patient by a physician's order by way of:

- Mask (Figure 6-12)
- Cannula (Figure 6-13)

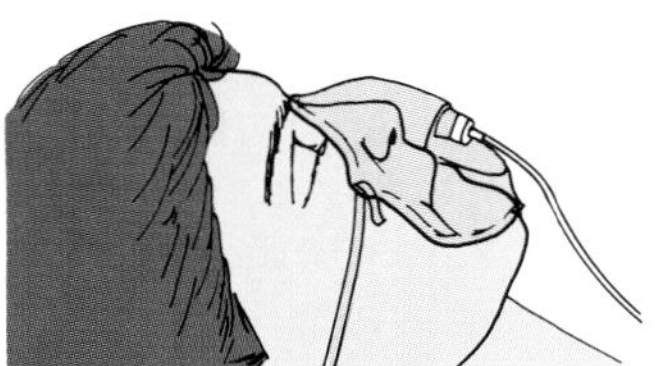

FIGURE 6-12 Face mask.

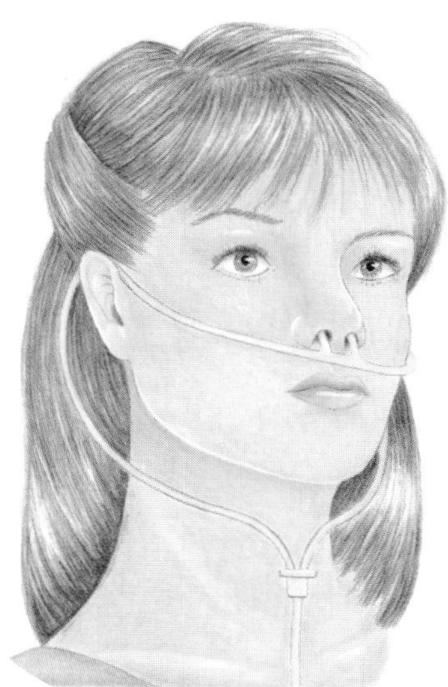

FIGURE 6-13 Nasal cannula.

Nasal Cannulas

Cannula
A flexible tube that can be inserted into one of the body cavities. A cannula may be used to draw fluids out or to give oxygen or fluids.

Nasal **cannulas**, or tubes, are used to give oxygen to a patient. The cannulas are inserted into the patient's nostrils. They are used when the patient needs extra oxygen. The cannula, which is made of plastic, is a circle of tubing with two openings in the center. The nose piece is inserted about $\frac{1}{2}$ inch into the patient's nostrils. The tubing can wrap around the patient's ears and is then connected to the source of oxygen by a length of plastic tubing. Check the skin frequently over the top of the patient's ears where the cannula sits. If there are red marks from pressure, alert the nurse.

KEY IDEAS

Misuses of Electricity

Be sure your hands are dry before using electrical equipment. Water should never come in contact with electrical equipment. For example, placing a container on top of a suction machine can create a hazard.

Always follow your institution's policies and procedures for the safe use of electrical equipment. For example, some institutions restrict the use of lightweight extension cords. Check equipment for defects such as frayed wires or broken plugs.

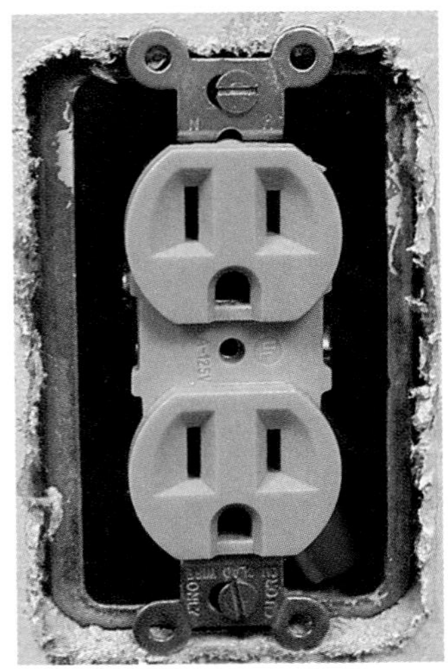

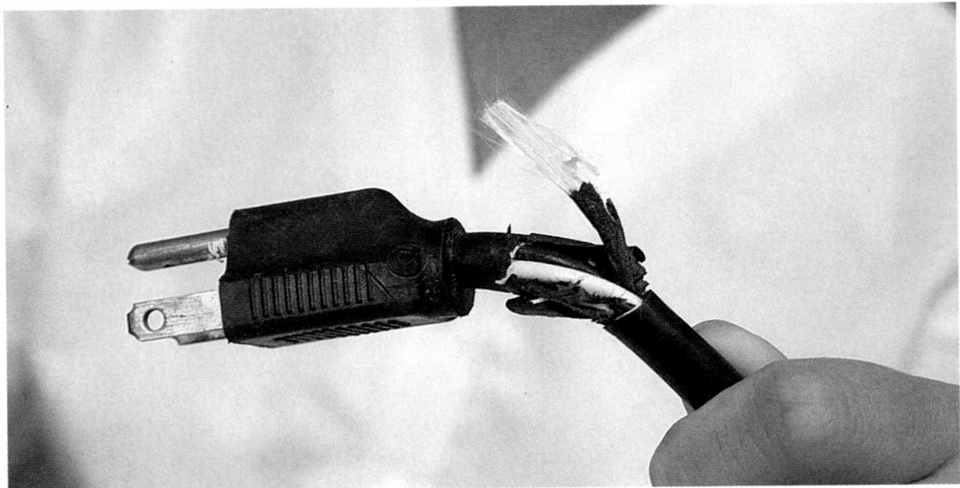

FIGURE 6-14 Defective outlets and frayed wires are electrical hazards.

Many electrical devices are equipped with three-pronged grounding plugs. Do not use any such device if the rounded middle pin on the plug has been broken or cut off. Do not use any piece of electrical equipment if you receive a shock when you touch it. Never touch a patient and an electrical device at the same time.

If you discover any electrical hazard report it to your immediate supervisor at once.

Figure 6-14, illustrates typical electrical hazards.

KEY IDEAS

Major Causes of Fire

- Smoking and matches
- Misuse of electricity
- Defects in heating systems
- Spontaneous ignition
- Improper rubbish disposal

Remember, it takes three things to start a fire (Figure 6-15).

FIGURE 6-15 It takes three things to start a fire: fuel, heat, and oxygen.

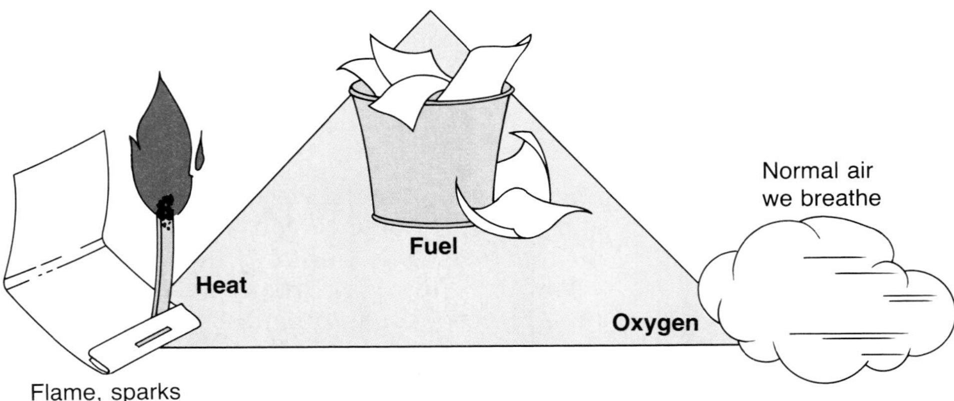

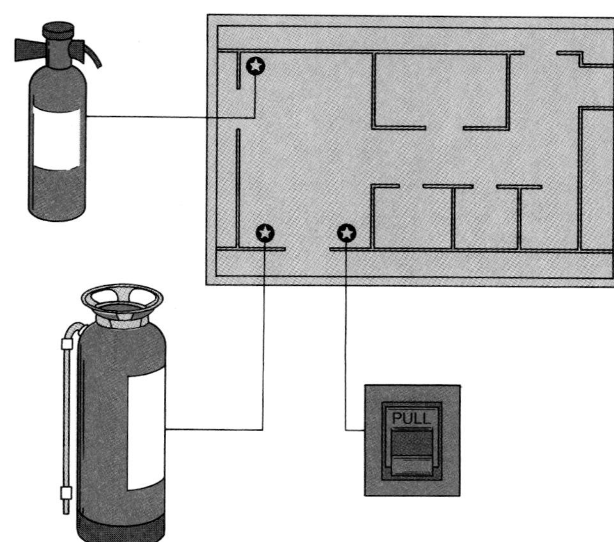

PULL
• Know the floor plan of your department and the hospital as a whole
• Pay particular attention to exit routes
• Know the exact location of fire alarms and fire extinguishing devices
• Know how to report a fire
• Know the emergency plan of your hospital and what you should do
• Know how to use fire extinguishers

FIGURE 6-16 Fire safety planning.

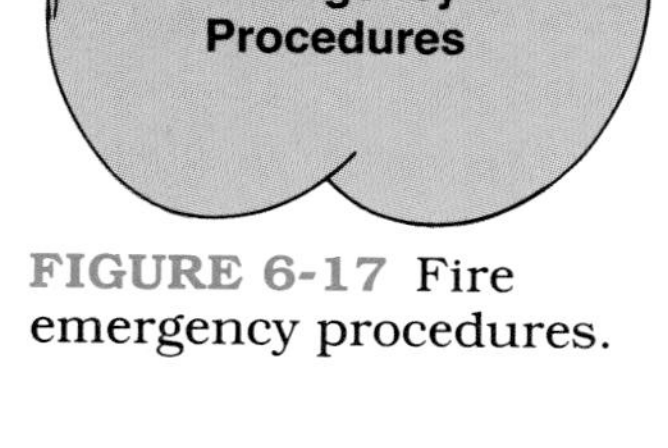

FIGURE 6-17 Fire emergency procedures.

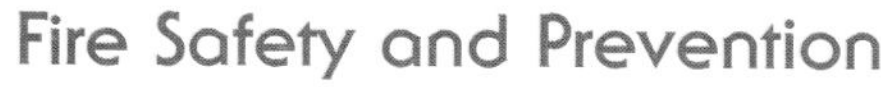

Fire Safety and Prevention

- Fire safety means two things:
  - Preventing fires
  - Knowing and doing the right things at the right time if a fire breaks out (see Figure 6-16)
- Be familiar with your institution's fire plan (Figure 6-17).

Fire extinguishers are rated A, B, or C, according to the type of fire they may be used on. Type A is for paper, wood, and trash; Type B is for liquids such as oil or grease; Type C is for electrical fires. Sometimes two or three ratings may be combined. For example, an extinguisher marked ABC may be used safely on all three types of fires. You should familiarize yourself with the fire extinguishers in your area: Where are they located? What type are they?

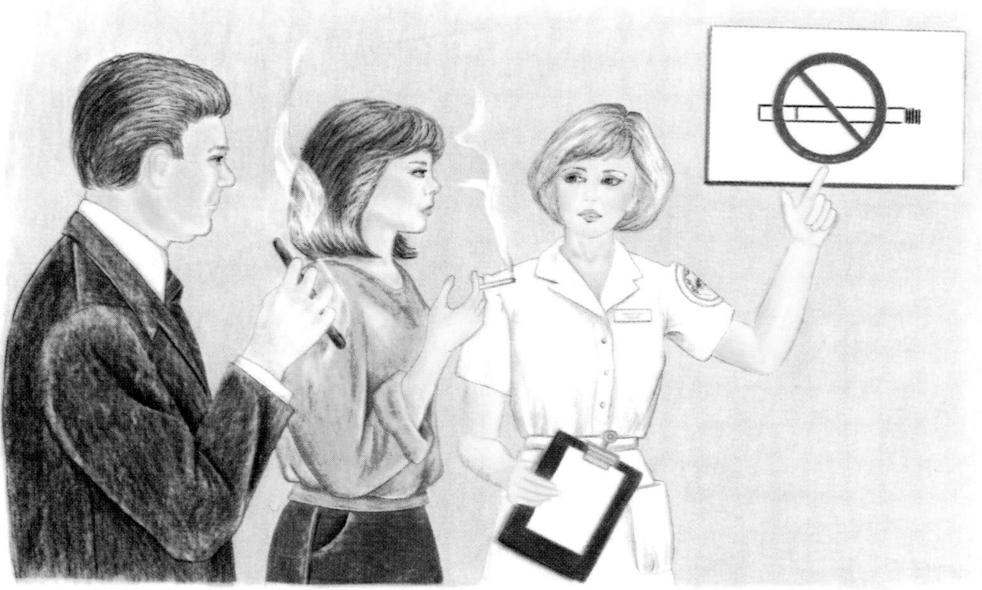

FIGURE 6-18 Be on the alert for smokers who disregard regulations. Smoking is the major cause of fires in health care institutions.

Smoking is the number one cause of fires in health care institutions. Observe the following rules:

- See that ashtrays are provided and that they are used.
- Empty ashtrays only after all smoking materials in them have been extinguished for a long time. Smoking materials should be collected in a separate metal container.
- Smoke only where it is permitted. Follow hospital policies regarding smoking.
- A patient who has been given a sedative should not be allowed to smoke or should have an attendant present.

FIGURE 6-19 In case of fire, use the RACE system.

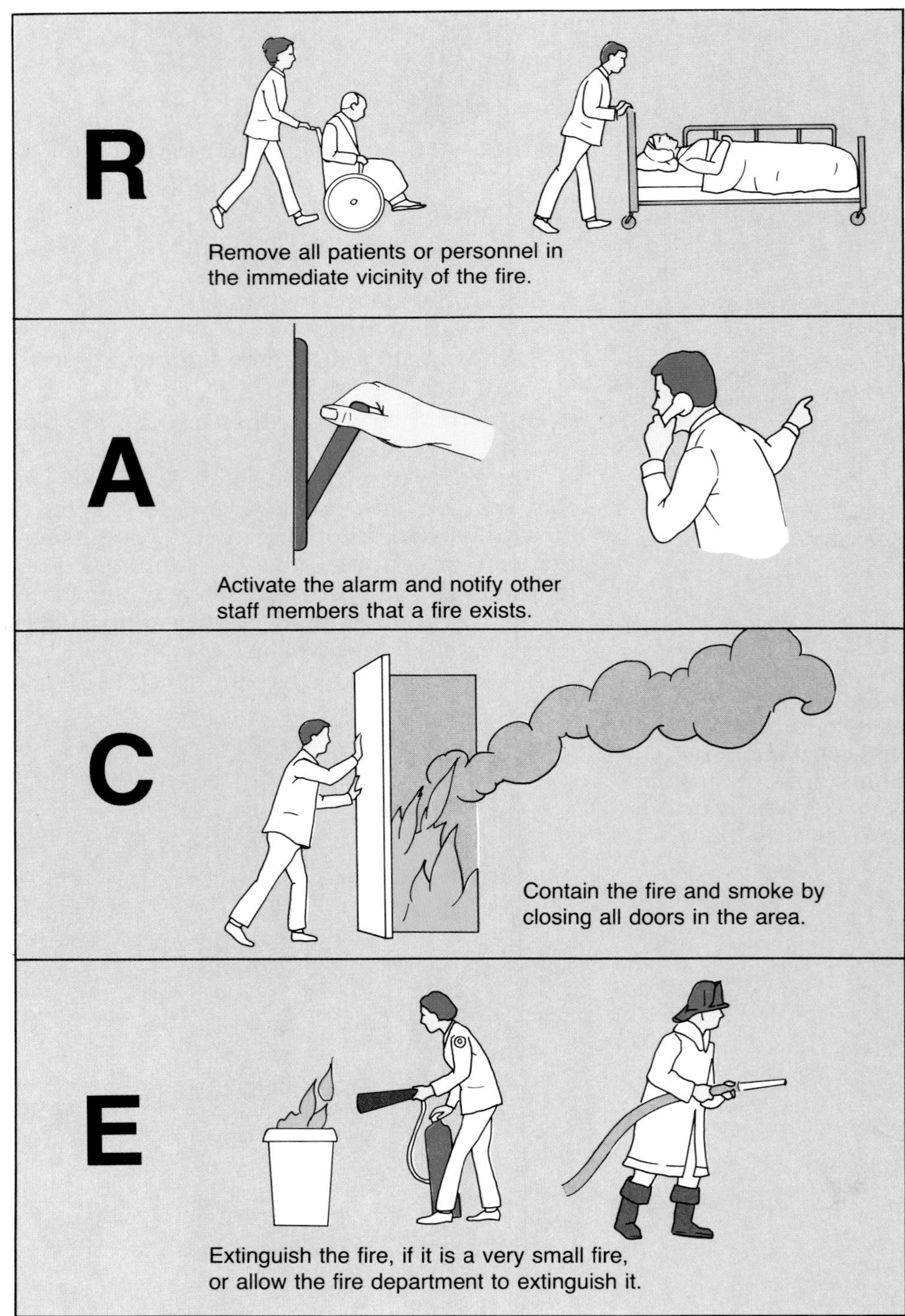

R
Remove all patients or personnel in the immediate vicinity of the fire.
A
Activate the alarm and notify other staff members that a fire exists.
C
Contain the fire and smoke by closing all doors in the area.
E
Extinguish the fire, if it is a very small fire, or allow the fire department to extinguish it.

- Constantly monitor patients, visitors, and employees to ensure safe smoking practices (Figure 6-18). Report any violation of smoking rules to your immediate supervisor at once. Remember, smoking is permitted only in designated smoking areas.

In Case of Fire

In case of fire, use the RACE System outlined in Figure 6-19, and observe the following guidelines:

- *If fire occurs in a patient area, move or assist the patients and visitors out of the danger zone by taking them to a safe area behind fire doors. Close the door after removing the patient from the danger area.*
- Most health care institutions have doorways that are large enough to move a bed through easily. However, if the building has to be evacuated, and since beds cannot be moved down stairs, many hospitals have evacuation policies that give directions on how to move many patients at one time. Follow the health care institution's policies.
- Pull the nearest fire alarm box.
- Notify the main switchboard as to the exact location and nature of the fire as soon as possible.
- Follow the fire emergency procedures for your department and health care institution.
- Do not panic. Many lives may depend on your actions in an emergency.

KEY IDEAS

Patient Safety

Falls in health care facilities account for almost 70% of all patient-related accidents! **You can help prevent falls by:**

- Properly positioning patients in beds and wheelchairs.
- Keeping frequently needed articles and the telephone within easy reach of patients.
- Answering the call light promptly so patients who require assistance do not attempt to get out of bed without your help.
- Reporting any lighting problems immediately.
- Reporting to your immediate supervisor your observations that a patient is unsteady, dizzy, slides out of the wheelchair, or climbs out of bed.
- Reporting hazards immediately, such as loose floor tiles or carpeting, loose or broken hand rails, leaks in bathrooms and shower areas.
- Reporting broken or malfunctioning equipment immediately.
- Maintaining a clear pathway between the bed and the bathroom.

Protective Device
A type of restraint that keeps the patient from harming himself and, therefore, creates a safe environment for the patient.

Restraint
Equipment used to protect, support, or hold a patient in a particular position.

Protective Devices: A Safety Measure

A **protective device** is a type of restraint that keeps the patient from harming himself or herself and provides a safer environment for the patient (Figure 6-20). Protective devices **(restraints)** are applied only on the instructions of a nurse, or team leader, or physician. They will determine the type of restraint to be used and the length of time it is to be left in place. Check your patient every 30 minutes, or according to

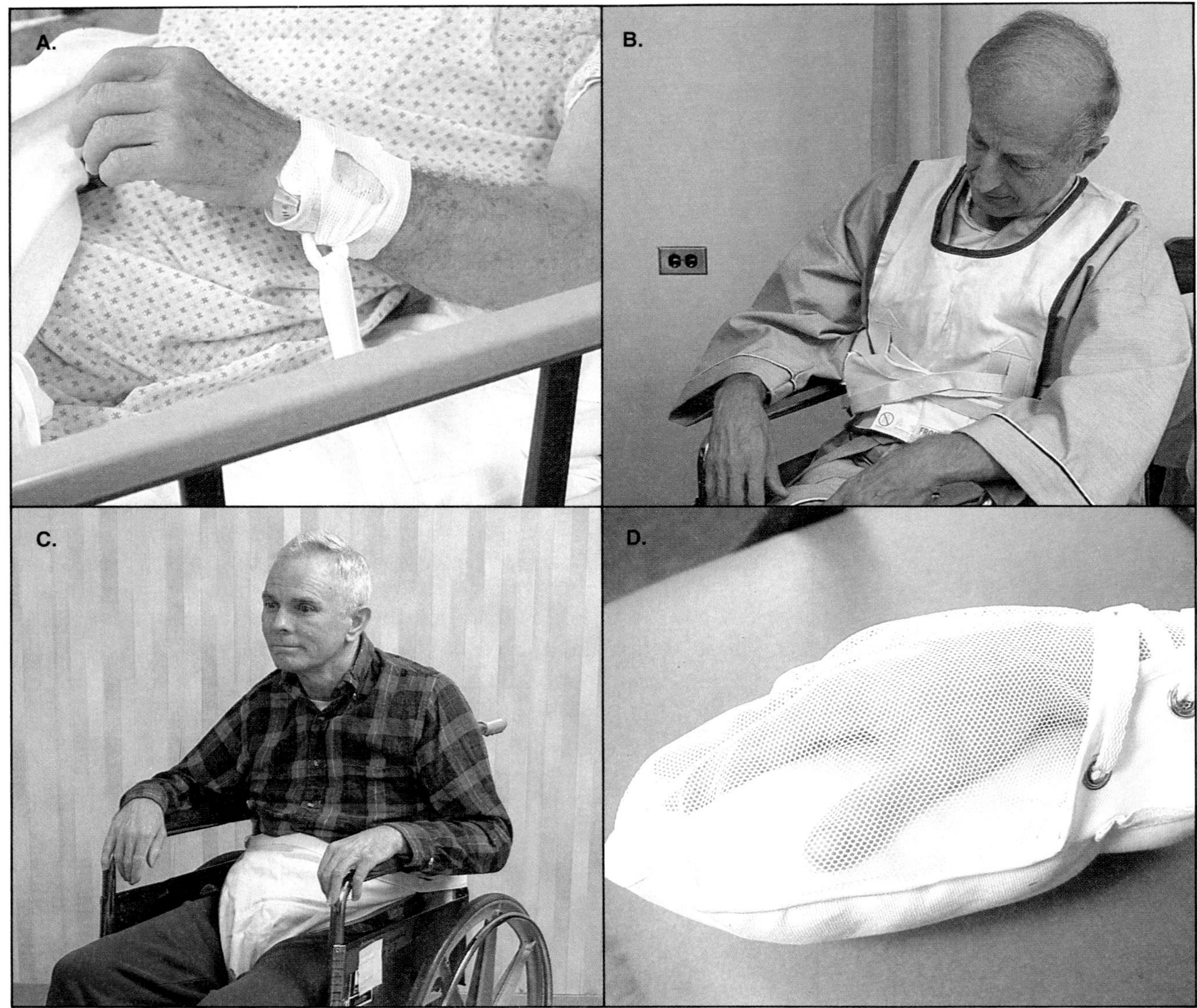

Report: Type of protective device used. Time you checked patient for safety, comfort, and any other unusual observations.

FIGURE 6-20 Soft protective devices. A. Soft limb tie. B. Safety vest. C. Pelvic support. D. Soft cloth mitten.

policy, for safety, pressure areas, circulation, and comfort when he or she is in a protective device.

If the patient is confined to a bed or chair, the restraint is to be removed every 2 hours, the patient repositioned, and the area restrained given special skin care before restraint is reapplied. Follow your hospital's policies; some states require that beds and chairs have wheels when the patient is in a restraint.

Rules to Follow

RESTRAINTS

- Restraining devices are to be used only to ensure the physical safety of the patient, upon a written order by a physician.

- Position a patient in a restraining device so as to allow as much movement as possible without injury.
- Before they are applied, all restraining devices must be explained to the patient and to the significant other even if the patient is confused, irrational, or in a coma.
- Devices must be applied correctly and appropriate care given in accordance with the policies and procedures of the employing health care institution or agency.
- Check the patient in a restraint every 30 (thirty) minutes for color, temperature, and the condition of the skin, to measure respirations, and to be sure that the restraint is not too tight.
- Follow your immediate supervisor's instructions to remove restraint, exercise the patient, offer toileting and drinking fluids, remake the bed, change the patient's clothing, and give extra skin care.
- Record all care, use of restraint, unusual skin problems, and emotional responses of the patient, type of restraint used, length of time it was applied, and every time the patient's condition was checked.
- Know the federal guidelines for the application and removal of restraints.
- Scissors should be taped to a wall near head nurse desk in case of a disaster or crisis to facilitate cutting a patient free of restraints.

Procedure Applying Limb Restraints

1. Obtain authorization from your immediate supervisor for the application of a limb restraint. *Note:* Know the Federal guidelines for application and removal of restraints.
2. Assemble your equipment:
   a) Adjustable limb restraint(s).
3. Wash your hands.
4. Identify the patient by checking the identification bracelet.
5. Ask visitors to step out of the room, if this is your hospital's policy.
6. Tell the patient and the significant other that you are going to apply a limb restraint. Explain the procedure even if the patient is irrational or confused.
7. Pull the curtains around the bed for privacy.
8. Raise the bed to a comfortable working position.
9. Lock the wheels on the bed.
10. Place the soft edge of the restraint against the patient's skin. Wrap the restraint smoothly around the limb. Make sure that no wrinkles are present.
11. Pull both ends of the straps through the tab or ring on the restraint. Then pull the restraint, secure but not too tight, against the patient's skin. *Caution!* If applied too tightly, the restraint could stop circulation or cause a pressure sore to form.
12. Test for fit and comfort by inserting two fingers between the restraint and the patient's skin.
13. Position the arm or leg in a comfortable position. Limit movement only as much as necessary.
14. Secure the straps to the bedframe or stretcher frame with a double-clove hitch. To make the double-clove hitch, bring the strap around the frame and then bring the strap up, over, and through the loop that has been made by the frame. Repeat the process for a double loop.
15. Recheck the patient before leaving the room. Make sure the patient is secure but not too tight.
16. Observe all checkpoints before leaving the patient. Position the patient in correct alignment.
17. Make the patient as comfortable as possible; offer adequate hydration.

18. Lower the bed to a position of safety for the patient.
19. Pull the curtains back to the open position.
20. Raise the side rails where ordered, indicated, and appropriate for patient safety.
21. Place the call light within easy reach of the patient.
22. Wash your hands.
23. Recheck the patient every 30 (thirty) minutes. Check color and temperature of the skin. Remove the restraint every two hours. Exercise the patient. Offer toileting and adequate hydration, make the bed and change the patient's clothing as needed, give extra skin care to the skin that is under the restraint.
24. Report to your immediate supervisor:
    - That you have applied the limb restraint.
    - The time it was applied.
    - The number of times when you rechecked the patient, including time of each recheck.
    - Your observations of anything unusual:

      Unusual skin problems

      The emotional response of the patient to the restraint.

Note: The restraint is removed when authorized by your immediate supervisor, when the danger of self-injury has passed.

Procedure Applying a Jacket Restraint

1. Obtain authorization from your immediate supervisor for the application of a jacket restraint. Note: Know the Federal guideline for application and removal of restraints.
2. Assemble your equipment:
   a) Jacket restraint, sleeveless.
3. Wash your hands.
4. Identify the patient by checking the identification bracelet.
5. Ask visitors to step out of the room, if this is your hospital's policy.
6. Tell the patient and the significant other that you are going to apply a jacket restraint. Explain the procedure even if the patient is irrational or confused.
7. Pull the curtains around the bed for privacy.
8. Raise the bed to a comfortable working position.
9. Lock the wheels on the bed.
10. Slip the armholes of the jacket restraint onto the patient's arms. Usually, the solid area is on the front for the most security. However, it can be placed in the back.
11. Crisscross the straps in the back. Check all of the material to make sure that it is free from wrinkles.
12. Bring the loose end of the strap through the hole provided in the jacket. The jacket should now completely encircle the patient.
13. Check the restraint to be sure that it is not too tight against the patient. *Caution!* Excessive tightness could interfere with breathing.
14. Position the patient in a comfortable position. Allow as much movement as possible without injury. Test for fit and comfort by inserting two fingers between the restraint and the patient's skin.
15. Secure the straps to each side of the bedframe or stretcher frame by bringing the straps down and secure on the frame with a double-clove hitch. To make a double-clove hitch, bring the strap around the frame and then bring the strap up, over, and through the loop that has been made by the frame. Repeat the process for a double loop.
16. In a wheelchair, the straps can be attached to the back frame. *Caution!* Never attach them to any part of the wheels.

17. Recheck the patient before leaving the room. Check the patient's respirations. Make sure the patient is secure but not too tightly restrained.
18. Observe all checkpoints before leaving the patient. Position the patient in correct alignment.
19. Make the patient as comfortable as possible; offer adequate hydration.
20. Lower the bed to a position of safety for the patient.
21. Pull the curtains back to the open position.
22. Raise the side rails where ordered, indicated, and appropriate for patient safety.
23. Place the call light within easy reach of the patient.
24. Wash your hands.
25. Recheck the patient every 30 (thirty) minutes. Check color and temperature of the skin. Check count and character of respirations. Remove the restraint every two hours. Exercise the patient. Offer toileting and adequate hydration, make the bed and change the patient's clothing as needed; give extra skin care to the skin that is under the restraint.
26. Report to your immediate supervisor:
    - That you have applied the jacket restraint.
    - The time it was applied.
    - The number of times when you rechecked the patient, including time of each recheck.
    - Your observations of anything unusual:
      Unusual skin problems
      Abnormal respirations
    - The emotional response of the patient to the restraint.

Note: The restraint is removed when authorized by your immediate supervisor, when the danger of self-injury has passed.

Patient Ambulation Safety with a Walker, Cane, or Crutches

Various pieces of equipment may be ordered by the physician to assist the patient to ambulate safely. These pieces of equipment include canes, crutches, and walkers (Figure 6-21). They support the patient while walking. Each of these pieces of equipment must be adjusted for each individual patient. The hand piece must be level with the patient's hip to accommodate a slight bend of the elbow while the patient is standing and holding the cane, crutches, or walker. The patient must never use these pieces of equipment to help get to a standing position. They are only something to assist the patient to walk.

- *Cane:* Usually used on the patient's stronger side to balance her or his weight between the cane and the weaker side.
- *Walker:* Ordered when the patient requires some support when walking due to imbalance or weakness. The walker is safe to push down upon only when all four legs of the walker are on the ground in a level position. When the walker is being moved the patient's feet should be stationary. When the walker is stationary, the patient can move his or her feet. The walker must be picked up and moved and never slid along the ground.
- Crutches: Ordered to decrease weight borne by one or both feet and legs or to provide stability. Instructions will permit full weight bearing, partial weight bearing, weight bearing to tolerance, or non-weight bearing. Make sure that all pads and grips are securely in

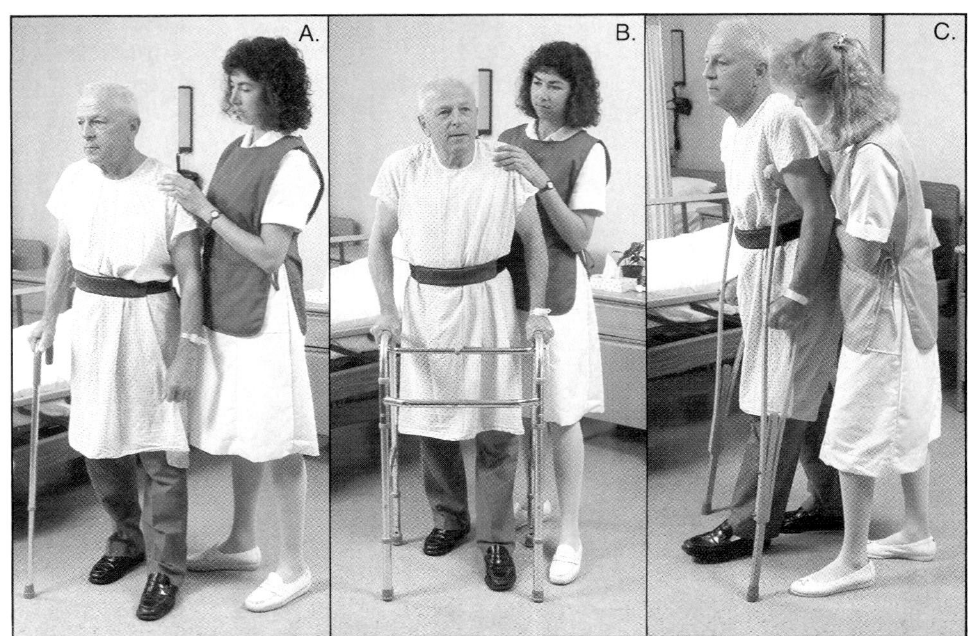

FIGURE 6-21 Walking aids. A. Cane. B. Walker. C. Crutches.

Ambulation
Walking or moving about in an upright position.

Gait Training
Rehabilitative exercise to help the patient improve his or her ability walking.

Ambulate
To walk or move about.

place. Check the screws to make sure all hardware is tight. Inspect the rubber tips for wear and make sure they are free of dirt and stones. If the patient is weak, unsteady or unable to maintain balance, help him or her to a position of safety and report this to your immediate supervisor.

Ambulation is the action of walking. Gait is the rhythm and movement of the feet and the speed of walking. **Gait training** is done by the physical therapist as the first step toward helping the patient to **ambulate** independently.

Rules to Follow

PATIENT AMBULATION SAFETY

- Apply good body mechanics at all times (see Chapter 16).
- Be sure of the patient's ability to ambulate before you attempt to assist him or her.
- If you need help or if you are in doubt, ask your immediate supervisor for assistance.
- Communicate with the patient by explaining the procedure and telling the patient what you expect of him or her.

KEY IDEAS

Restraining the Pediatric Patient

To restrain means to keep someone from doing something or to prevent an action from happening. All restraints are applied only on the instruction of the nurse or physician. The kind of restraint used for a child depends on why he or she is being restrained, age, and level of understanding.

- A toddler may be restrained by putting a cover over the top of his or her crib to prevent the child from climbing out (Figure 6-22).
- Elbow restraints (Figure 6-23) may be applied to a child who has eczema to keep him from scratching himself or to a child who has had surgery on his mouth or eyes, or has an IV, to keep his hands away from those areas. Elbow restraints prevent a child from bending his elbows and, therefore, from scratching or reaching his face.
- Mitten restraints are also used to prevent scratching.

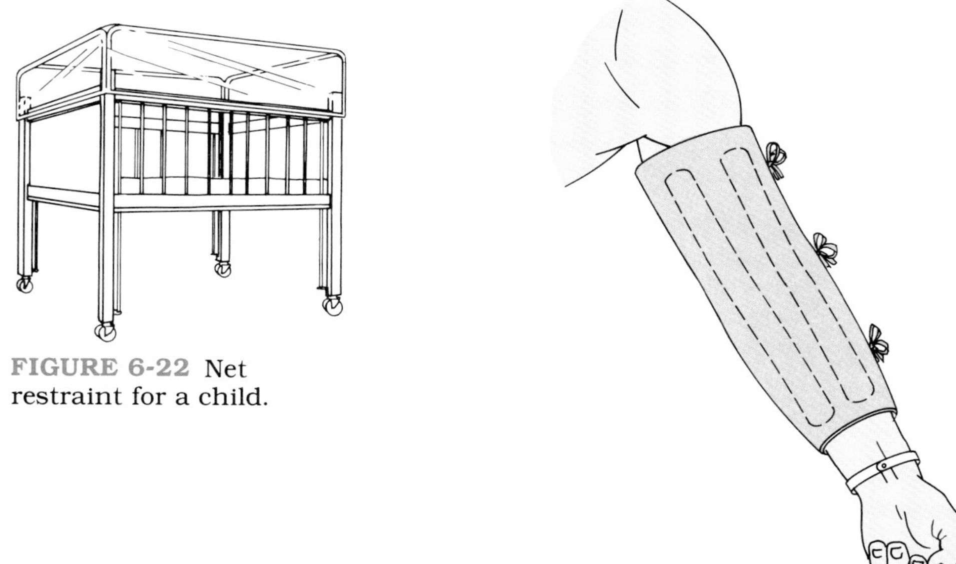

FIGURE 6-22 Net restraint for a child.

FIGURE 6-23 Elbow restraint.

Applying Elbow Restraints

Elbow restraints are made of canvas and tongue blades. They are tied firmly around the child's arm so that they will not slide below the elbow. The child can move the arm but cannot bend the elbow to reach his or her face.

Such restraints should be removed frequently to prevent muscle cramp and to assess the skin. One restraint should be removed at a time, and someone should be present to control the child's arm movements for the time it is off.

A child may often be frustrated emotionally because of the restraints. His or her satisfaction must be provided in new ways. Ask your immediate supervisor for guidance in caring for a restrained child.

KEY QUESTIONS

1. What are the rules that you as a nursing assistant can follow to make the health care institution a safe place for your patient, your co-workers, and yourself?
2. What special safety precautions should you take when caring for children?
3. Describe the special safety precautions when oxygen is being used.

4. What should you do in case of a fire?
5. What are the safety precautions that should be taken when restraints are being used?
6. List the safety rules for patient ambulation.
7. Define: ambulate, ambulation, cannula, gait training, nasal, oxygen, protective device, restraint.

CHAPTER

7

Emergency Care

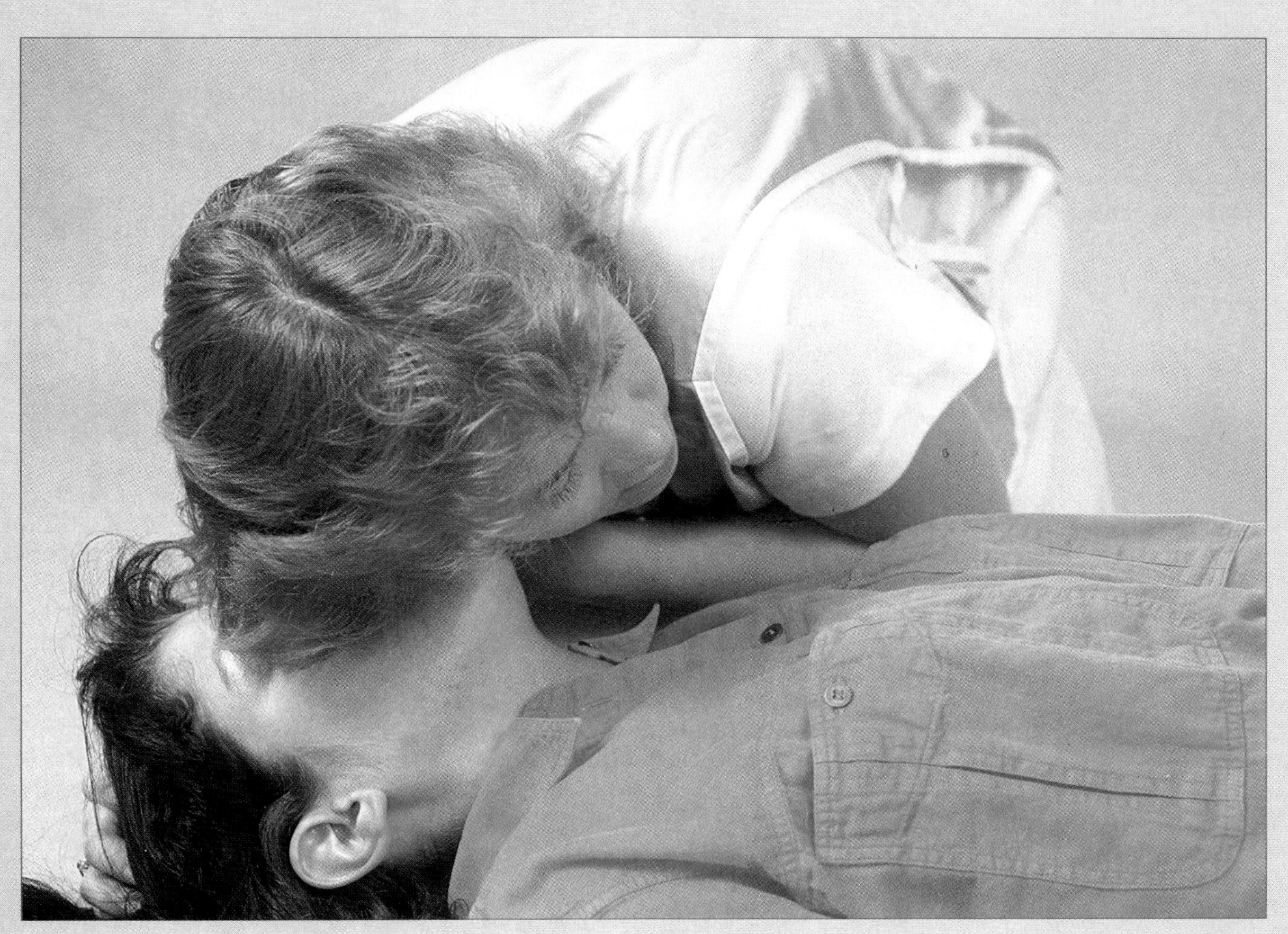

WARNING

For all patient contact, adhere to Universal Precautions (see page 91, 97, or the front cover flap). Wear protective equipment as indicated.

Objectives

What You Will Learn

When you have completed this chapter, you will be able to:

- List the rules to follow in an emergency.
- Describe the signs of shock and rules for care of a patient in shock.
- Explain the purpose of CPR and list its three basic elements.
- List the signs of heart attack, cardiac arrest, and stroke, and explain what should be done to help the person in crisis.
- Demonstrate the most effective way to control bleeding.
- Demonstrate first aid for a victim of a burn.
- Explain what to do for someone who has been poisoned.
- Define: cardiac arrest, cardiopulmonary resuscitation, cardiovascular system, emergency, first aid, heart attack, hemorrhage, poison, shock, stroke.

KEY IDEAS

Emergencies

Emergency
Events that call for immediate action.

First Aid
The first action taken to help a person who is in crisis.

EMERGENCIES ARE EVENTS THAT CALL FOR immediate action! **First aid** is the *first* action taken to help a person in crisis, which may range from a small cut to trauma due to an accident to a sudden illness. First aid is offered until outside help arrives. Every hospital, nursing home, ACLF (adult congregate living facility), extended care facility, clinic, senior citizen center, home health agency, and supplemental professional nursing service agency has written procedures for emergency and first aid care. Follow the procedures or policies of your employing health care institution. When caring for a person in the home, an emergency plan should be available to the care-giver (family member) or the employee of an agency. This plan should include phone numbers of the police (in many areas 911), fire rescue squads, emergency medical help, physicians, emergency rooms, the nearest hospital, telecommunication services for the deaf, and the regional poison control center. Follow the plan that is made available for you. Remember, if you are facing a situation where there is no one available to help you, take care of the person in crisis before you leave to call for help. If more than one person needs help, you will have to look over the entire situation and decide whom you will help first. Do not leave a person who needs immediate help. Have someone else call for additional assistance. If the person in crisis does not need immediate help to maintain life, your responsibility will be to prevent additional injury and to provide security and comfort until help arrives.

Rules to Follow
TO HELP A PERSON IN AN EMERGENCY

- Before you take any action, you must determine:
  - What is the problem or emergency.
  - What must be done immediately to maintain life for the person in crisis.
  - What you, the nursing assistant, are capable of doing.
  - If the person in crisis can be moved.
- Remove the person in crisis from immediate danger without endangering your own life.
- Restore or maintain breathing and heart function.
- Control bleeding.
- Treat poisoning.
- Call for medical help.
- Prevent shock.
- Be aware of the danger of electrical shock.
- Examine the entire body carefully for other injuries that may be life threatening.
- Keep the person in crisis as comfortable and safe as possible.
- Remain with the person in crisis until emergency medical help arrives.

KEY IDEAS
Shock

Shock
The failure of the cardiovascular system to provide sufficient blood circulation to every part of the body.

Cardiovascular System
Circulatory system.

Shock may accompany many emergency situations. **Shock** is the failure of the **cardiovascular system** to provide sufficient blood circulation to every part of the body. Diagnostic signs of shock are:

- Eyes are dull and lack luster.
- Pupils are dilated.
- Face is pale and cyanotic (blue).
- Respiration is shallow, irregular, or labored.
- Pulse is rapid and weak.
- Skin is cold and clammy.
- The patient may be:
  - Nauseated
  - Anxious
  - Thirsty
- The patient may:
  - Collapse
  - Vomit

Types of Shock

- Shock may be caused by many factors such as:
  - blood loss
  - insufficient oxygen
  - spinal cord damage
  - reaction of nervous system to fear, the sight of blood, and so on.

- inadequate heart function
- infection
- loss of body fluid or changes in body chemistry
- extreme allergic reaction

- *Hemorrhagic shock* is caused by blood loss. The reduction of blood volume means that circulation is impaired; this may occur for several reasons:
  - External bleeding
  - Internal bleeding
  - Loss of plasma due to burns or crushed tissues
- *Respiratory shock* is caused by insufficient oxygen in the blood. The inability to fill the lungs completely is the result of impaired breathing. This may happen because of:
  - A chest wound
  - Flail chest
  - Broken ribs
  - Pneumothorax
  - Airway obstruction
  - Spinal cord damage that has paralyzed the muscles of the chest and the patient must breathe with the diaphragm alone
- *Neurogenic shock* is caused by loss of control of the nervous system due to spinal cord damage.
- *Psychogenic shock* or fainting is caused by a reaction of the nervous system to fear, bad news, the sight of blood, or a minor injury. Sudden dilation of the blood vessels occurs, and the blood flow to the brain is interrupted. The person faints, and unless other problems are present, fainting is usually self-correcting. When the head is lowered, blood circulates to the brain and normal function is restored.
- *Cardiogenic shock* is caused by inadequate functioning of the heart. When the heart does not continuously operate, due to disorders that weaken the heart muscle, the heart can no longer develop the pressure required to move blood to all parts of the body.
- *Septic shock* is caused by infection. Toxins released into the bloodstream have a harmful effect on the blood vessels, causing them to dilate (get larger), which results in incomplete filling of the circulatory system.
- *Metabolic shock* is caused by loss of body fluids and changes in body chemistry. This happens because of:
  - Loss of body fluids through diarrhea, vomiting, or urination
  - Severe disturbance of body salts or the acid–base balance in diseases
- *Anaphylactic shock* or reaction occurs when a person contacts something to which he or she is extremely allergic. This may be caused by:
  - Insect stings (bees, yellow jackets, wasps, and hornets)
  - Inhaled substances (dust, pollen)
  - Injected substances (drugs such as penicillin)

Rules to Follow

TO GIVE ASSISTANCE TO THE PATIENT IN SHOCK

- Call for help.
- Maintain an open airway to assure breathing.

- Position the person in crisis with the head lower than the legs.
- If a broken bone is suspected, keep the person in crisis flat. Do not move.
- Control bleeding.
- Do not offer any food or drink.
- Talk to the person in crisis and reassure him.
- Stay with the person in crisis until emergency medical rescue help arrives.

KEY IDEAS

Heart Attack, Chest Pain, Myocardial Infarction, Cardiac Arrest

Heart Attack
Interruption or damage to the blood supply to the heart muscle; myocardial infarction.

The heart muscle has its own blood supply. Interruption or damage to this blood supply is a **heart attack** or myocardial infarction, which may cause damage to the heart muscle. Since it is difficult to determine if chest pain is really a heart attack, all chest pain is treated as if it is a heart attack.

Signs and Symptoms of a Heart Attack

- Shortness of breath
- Lowered blood pressure
- Shallow and difficult respirations
- Perfuse perspiration
- Wet clammy skin
- Rapid and weak pulse
- Pale color
- Nausea
- If there is chest pain it is severe and may radiate to the inner left arm, the jaw, or the neck; the person in crisis may refer to the chest pain as a belt around his chest

Rules to Follow

TO HELP THE PERSON HAVING A HEART ATTACK, CHEST PAIN, OR MYOCARDIAL INFARCTION

- Call for help.
- Help the person in crisis into a comfortable position.
- Loosen clothing if it is tight.
- Encourage the person in crisis to remain quiet.
- Measure respiration and pulse at frequent intervals.
- Talk to the person in crisis; reassure him.
- Do not offer any food or drink.
- Stay with the person in crisis until emergency medical rescue help arrives.

Cardiac Arrest
The unexpected stopping of the heartbeat and circulation.

Cardiac arrest is the unexpected stopping of the heartbeat and circulation.

Signs and Symptoms of Cardiac Arrest

- Loss of consciousness
- Absence of pulse
- Absence of heart sounds
- Absence of breath sounds
- Enlargement of the pupils of the eye
- Ashen gray color of the skin
- Lips and nailbeds may turn blue

KEY IDEAS

Cardiopulmonary Resuscitation (CPR)

Cardiopulmonary Resuscitation (CPR)
An emergency procedure used to reestablish effective circulation and respiration in order to prevent irreversible brain damage.

Cardiopulmonary resuscitation is a basic, life-saving procedure for sudden cardiac or respiratory arrest. The technique of CPR provides basic emergency life support until emergency medical help arrives. CPR keeps oxygenated blood flowing to the brain and other vital body organs until medical treatment can be given to restore normal heart function.

Note!

The following material is not intended to be a CPR course. An authorized CPR course includes practice on manikins supervised by a certified trained instructor to direct you in CPR with written and performance examinations. The American Heart Association and the American Red Cross, as well as other community service organizations, offer classes in CPR. Most health care institutions require all employees to be certified in CPR and to complete periodic recertification. *Remember*, only a person who has been trained in CPR can perform the rescue techniques. The only way of learning CPR is to enroll in an approved, supervised program.

There are three basic rescue skills to CPR. These are referred to as the ABC's of CPR:

- A, airway
- B, breathing
- C, circulation

Airway

The most important factor in successful resuscitation is the opening of the airway. There are many possible causes of an obstructed airway. The most common cause in an unconscious person is the back of the tongue.

There are several recommended methods for opening the airway that help to correct the position of the tongue. (a) The head-tilt maneuver is a simple repositioning of the head. This procedure is not recommended for use on any patient with possible injuries to the head, neck or spine. The trauma patient should be conscious. This procedure can be used on unconscious nontrauma patients. (b) The head-tilt, chin lift maneuver provides for the maximum opening of the airway. It is useful on conscious and unconscious patients and is one of the best methods for correcting obstruction caused by the tongue. This procedure is not recommended for use on any patient with possible neck or spinal injuries. (c) The jaw-thrust maneuver is the only widely recommended procedure for use on unconscious patients with possible neck or spinal injuries.

- *Look* to see if there is any chest movement.
- *Listen* for any breath sounds.
- *Feel* for the victim's breath on your cheek.

If the victim does not spontaneously begin breathing after you have opened the airway, then begin rescue breathing.

Breathing

Mouth-to-mouth rescue breathing is the most effective way of getting oxygen into the lungs of the victim. Pinch the nostrils shut using the hand that is on the victim's forehead. Open your mouth wide and place it tightly over the victim's mouth. Blow two breaths lasting 1–1½ seconds on inspiration, then remove your mouth. Turn your head to the side with your ear close to the victim's mouth and listen for a return of air. If there is no return of air, recheck the head and neck position. If the airway is obstructed, no air can flow to the lungs.

After you have given the victim two breaths, check to see if the heart is beating. To feel the carotid pulse, use your hand that has been lifting the chin. With the tips of your fingers find the groove next to the adam's apple and feel for a pulse. If the heart is beating you must breathe for the victim at a rate of 12 breaths per minute (one breath every 5 seconds) for an adult while maintaining the open airway. If the heart is not beating (no pulse) you will have to pump the heart and circulate the victim's blood using external chest compressions.

Note: To protect both the victim and yourself when performing CPR a protective device must be used as a barrier. The barrier will protect the victim and yourself from transferring any communicable diseases either individual may be carrying. There are many types of protective barrier devices; your instructor and the facility where you are working will determine which device you will use.

Circulation

External chest compression with mouth-to-mouth resuscitation will allow oxygenated blood to circulate to the brain and other organs. To perform external chest compression, kneel next to the victim's chest. Place the heel of one hand on the lower half of the sternum, place your other hand on top, and knit the fingers of the top hand through the fingers of your bottom hand to keep your fingers off the chest wall. As you compress downward your shoulders should be directly over the victim's midline and your arms straight. For an adult victim depress 1½–2 inches. When you release this pressure, do not remove your hands from the sternum. These compressions should be rhythmic so that compression and release are of equal duration. Deliver 15 compressions for every 2 breaths when you are providing mouth-to-mouth rescue breathing. Deliver a rate of 80–100 compressions per minute.

Emergency Medical Services

Most areas have emergency medical services systems, where you dial a given phone number and tell the operator the following information:

- Address of the emergency
- Phone number from which you are calling
- Cause of the emergency

- How many people need assistance
- What is being done for the victims

The operator will give you instructions as to when you can hang up.

By knowing your local emergency number and calling for help when an emergency arises, you can take responsibility for the rescue of the victims. CPR is provided until emergency medical rescue help arrives. All local emergency phone numbers should be written on or near your telephone.

KEY IDEAS

Stroke or Cerebrovascular Accident

Stroke
Interruption or damage to the blood supply to the brain; a cerebrovascular accident.

Stroke or cerebrovascular accident occurs when there is damage to a blood vessel in the brain. See Chapter 39, for details. If you suspect that someone is having a stroke, treat him until emergency medical help arrives.

Signs and Symptoms of a Stroke

- Seizures
- Difficulty breathing
- Headache
- Change in state of consciousness
- Difficulty with speech or vision
- Paralysis in an extremity

Rules to Follow

TO HELP A PERSON WHO IS SUSPECTED OF HAVING A STROKE

- Call for medical help.
- Maintain an open airway to assure breathing.
- Keep the person in crisis warm.
- Do not offer any food or drink.
- Stay with the person in crisis until emergency medical rescue help arrives.

KEY IDEAS

Seizures

See Chapter 39 for care of the petit mal and grand mal seizure and generalized tonic–clonic seizure patient. Remember:

- Turn the head of the person having a seizure to the side to promote the drainage of saliva or vomitus.
- Do not try to pry (force) the teeth apart.
- Pad any areas that may be dangerous to the patient (for example, the corners of furniture).
- Do not attempt to restrain the patient.

KEY IDEAS

Hemorrhage

Hemorrhage
The extreme or unexpected loss of blood; bleeding.

When **hemorrhage**, the extreme and unexpected loss of blood, occurs, there are several effects on the body:

- The loss of red blood cells, which carry oxygen to the body cells, causes lack of oxygen.
- The loss of blood volume results in lower blood pressure.
- The force of the heartbeat is reduced since there is less blood to pump.

If the bleeding or hemorrhage is not stopped, the body goes into shock. Death may occur in a matter of several minutes if the hemorrhage is due to arterial bleeding. The control of bleeding is secondary only to the maintenance of an airway and the restoration of breathing in first aid. Arterial blood, which is pumped away from the heart through arteries, can be bright red in color. The bright red color is due to the high oxygen concentration. The blood returning to the heart through the veins can be a different color because the oxygen has been exchanged for carbon dioxide and other waste materials. Bleeding may be classified according to its source:

- Arterial bleeding from an artery in spurts.
- Venous bleeding from a vein in a steady flow of blood.
- Bleeding from capillaries is characterized by the slow oozing of blood and is more easily controlled.

The most effective method of controlling external bleeding is direct pressure on the wound and elevation of the area if possible. Direct pressure should be applied with the palm of the hand. When the bleeding is in spurts, the application of pressure at a pressure point may control the bleeding. A *pressure point* is a site where a main artery lies near the surface of the body, directly over a bone. The use of pressure points requires skill on the part of the rescuer and should be used only after direct pressure and elevation have failed. If pressure on the pressure points does not effectively control the bleeding, then a tourniquet must be applied. The application of a tourniquet is very dangerous unless adequate measures are available to control shock. The loosening of the tourniquet may prove fatal or cause the loss of a limb. A tourniquet should be used only as a last resort to control life-threatening bleeding or hemorrhage that cannot be controlled by any other means. Follow the instructions of your immediate supervisor.

When the classic signs of shock are present but there is no obvious injury, internal bleeding may be suspected. The signs and symptoms of internal bleeding are:

- Rapid and weak pulse
- Pale, moist, and cold skin
- Shallow and rapid respirations
- Thirst
- Weak and helpless feeling
- Shaking and trembling
- Dilated pupils
- Coughing up bright red blood
- Vomiting blood that has the appearance of coffee grounds
- Blood in the urine or stool.

Rules to Follow

TO HELP THE PERSON WHO IS HEMORRHAGING

- Apply direct pressure.
- Elevate the limb.
- Call for medical help.
- Remain with person in crisis until emergency medical rescue help arrives.

KEY IDEAS

Burns

Tissue damage caused by excessive heat, regardless of the source, is a burn. Steam, electricity, sun, chemicals, or fire can all cause excessive heat and a burn. Burns are labeled from first degree to third degree. First degree is a minor or the least severe burn, and the third degree is the worst burn, where total destruction of the body part occurs. All first aid and treatment for burns are intended to prevent complication and further injury to the body part and to speed up the healing process. Complications of a burn may include infection, shock, pain, loss of body heat and fluid, swelling of breathing passages, and death.

Rules to Follow

TO HELP THE PERSON WHO HAS BEEN BURNED

For a minor first degree burn:

- Place the body part into cold water for 10 to 15 minutes.
- Cover area with clean or sterile pad.

For a large, deep burn:

- Call for medical help.
- Do not remove clothing stuck to the burned area.
- Keep the airway open to assure breathing.
- Cover the area with a clean or sterile cloth that is kept wet with sterile water and covered with an insulated cold pack or an ice pack.
- Stay with the person in crisis until medical help arrives.

KEY IDEAS

Poisoning

Poison
Any substance ingested, inhaled, injected, or absorbed into the body that will interfere with normal physiological functions.

Poison is any substance which is toxic to the body. Immediate action and good observation skills are necessary if poisoning or an overdose of medication is suspected. Poisons can enter the body by several means (Figure 7-1). Table 7-1 lists common poisons and the reactions they might cause.

FIGURE 7-1 How poisons enter the body.

INHALATION

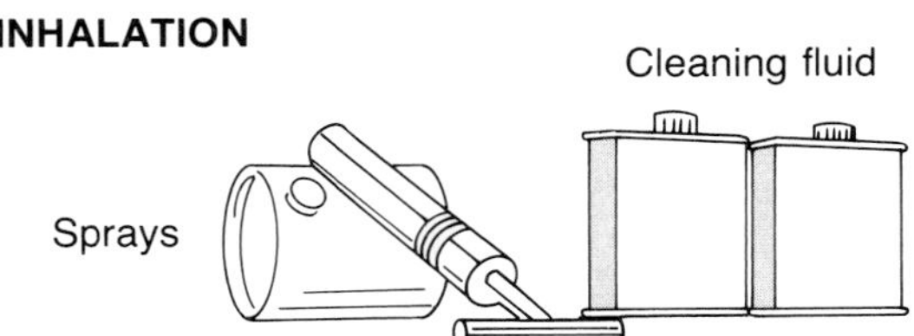

INJECTION

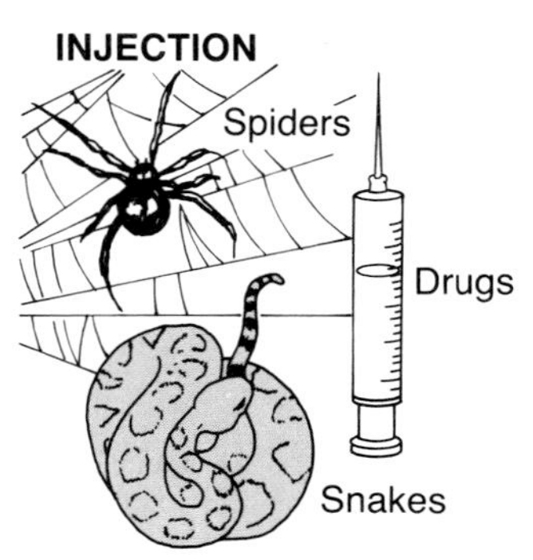

INGESTION

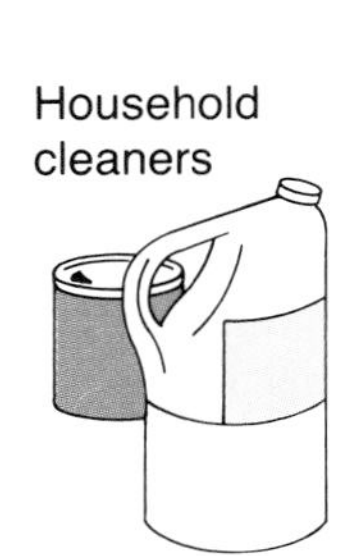

ABSORPTION

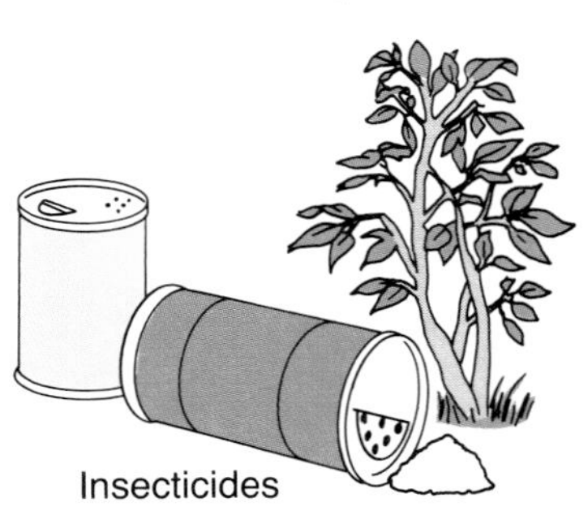

Table 7-1. Common Poisons

Poison	Helpful Symptoms and Signs	Poison	Helpful Symptoms and Signs
ACETAMINOPHEN	Nausea, vomiting, heavy perspiration. The victim is usually a child.	IODINE	Upset stomach and vomiting. If a starchy meal has been eaten, the vomitus may appear blue.
ACIDS	Burns on or around the lips. Burning in mouth, throat, and stomach, often followed by heavy vomiting.	METALS (copper, lead, mercury, zinc)	Metallic taste in mouth, with nausea and abdominal pains. Vomiting may occur. Stools may be bloody or dark.
ALKALIS (ammonia, bleaches, detergents, lye, washing soda, certain fertilizers)	Check to see if mouth membranes appear white and swollen. There may be a "soapy" appearance in the mouth. Abdominal pain is usually present. Vomiting may occur, often full of blood and mucus.	PETROLEUM PRODUCTS (some deodorizers, heating fuel, diesel fuels, gasoline, kerosene, lighter fluid, lubricating oil, naphtha, rust remover, transmission fluid)	Note characteristic odors on patient's breath, on clothing, or in vomitus.
ARSENIC (rat poisons)	"Garlic breath," with burning in the mouth, throat, and stomach. Abdominal pain can be severe. Vomiting is common.	PHOSPHORUS	Abdominal pain and vomiting. Vomitus may be phosphorescent.
ASPIRIN	Delayed reactions, including ringing in the ears, rapid and deep breathing, dry skin, and restlessness.	PLANTS—Contact (poison ivy, poison oak, poison sumac)	Swollen, itchy areas on the skin, with quickly forming "blister-like" lesions.
CHLOROFORM	Slow, shallow breathing with chloroform odor on breath. Pupils are dilated and fixed.	PLANTS—Ingested (azalea, castor bean, elderberry, foxglove, holly berries, lily of the valley, mistletoe berries, mountain laurel, mushrooms and toadstools, nightshade, oleander, rhododendron, rhubarb, rubber plant, some wild cherries)	Difficult to detect, ranging from nausea to coma. Always question in cases of apparent child poisoning.
CORROSIVE AGENTS (disinfectants, drain cleaners, household acids, iodine, pine oil, turpentine, toilet bowl cleaners, styptic pencil, water softeners, strong acids)	(See Acids)		
FOOD POISONING	Difficult to detect since symptoms and signs vary greatly. Usually, you will note abdominal pain, nausea and vomiting, gas and loud, frequent bowel sounds, and diarrhea.	STRYCHNINE (rat poisons)	The face, jaw, and neck will stiffen. Strong convulsions occur quickly after ingesting.

Rules to Follow

TO HELP THE PERSON WHO HAS BEEN POISONED

- Observe the person in crisis.
- Check the mouth for signs of burns.
- Check the breath for a significant odor.
- Ask questions of the person in crisis and other persons present to gather as many facts as possible before you act.
- Look for a medication container or bottle that may have been holding the poison.
- **Call the regional poison control center immediately.** The number is always found on the inside cover or on the first page of the telephone book. **Call for medical help also.**
- **Follow the directions given to you from the poison control center.**
- If you have been instructed to induce vomiting, save any vomitus from the person in crisis.
- If the person in crisis is unconscious:
  - Do not give anything by mouth.
  - Position the person on his or her back with the head facing you.
  - Maintain a clear airway.
  - If the person stops breathing, give mouth to mouth resuscitation. *Note:* This should be done only on the directions from the poison control center. There are times when you should *not* perform mouth to mouth resuscitation due to the type of poison ingested.
  - If it is necessary to move the person in crisis to a safe area, do so, but remember not to injure yourself while you are doing this.
  - Keep the person in crisis warm and comfortable.
  - Do not leave until emergency medical rescue help arrives.

KEY QUESTIONS

1. List the general rules to follow in an emergency.
2. What are the signs of shock and the rules for care of a patient in shock?
3. What is the purpose of CPR and what are the three basic elements of CPR?
4. What are the signs of heart attack, cardiac arrest, and stroke, and what should be done to help the person in crisis?
5. What is the most effective way to control bleeding?
6. What should be done to help a person who has been burned?
7. What should be done to help a person who has been poisoned?
8. Define: cardiac arrest, cardiopulmonary resuscitation, cardiovascular system, emergency, first aid, heart attack, hemorrhage, poison, shock, stroke.

CHAPTER

8

Infection Control

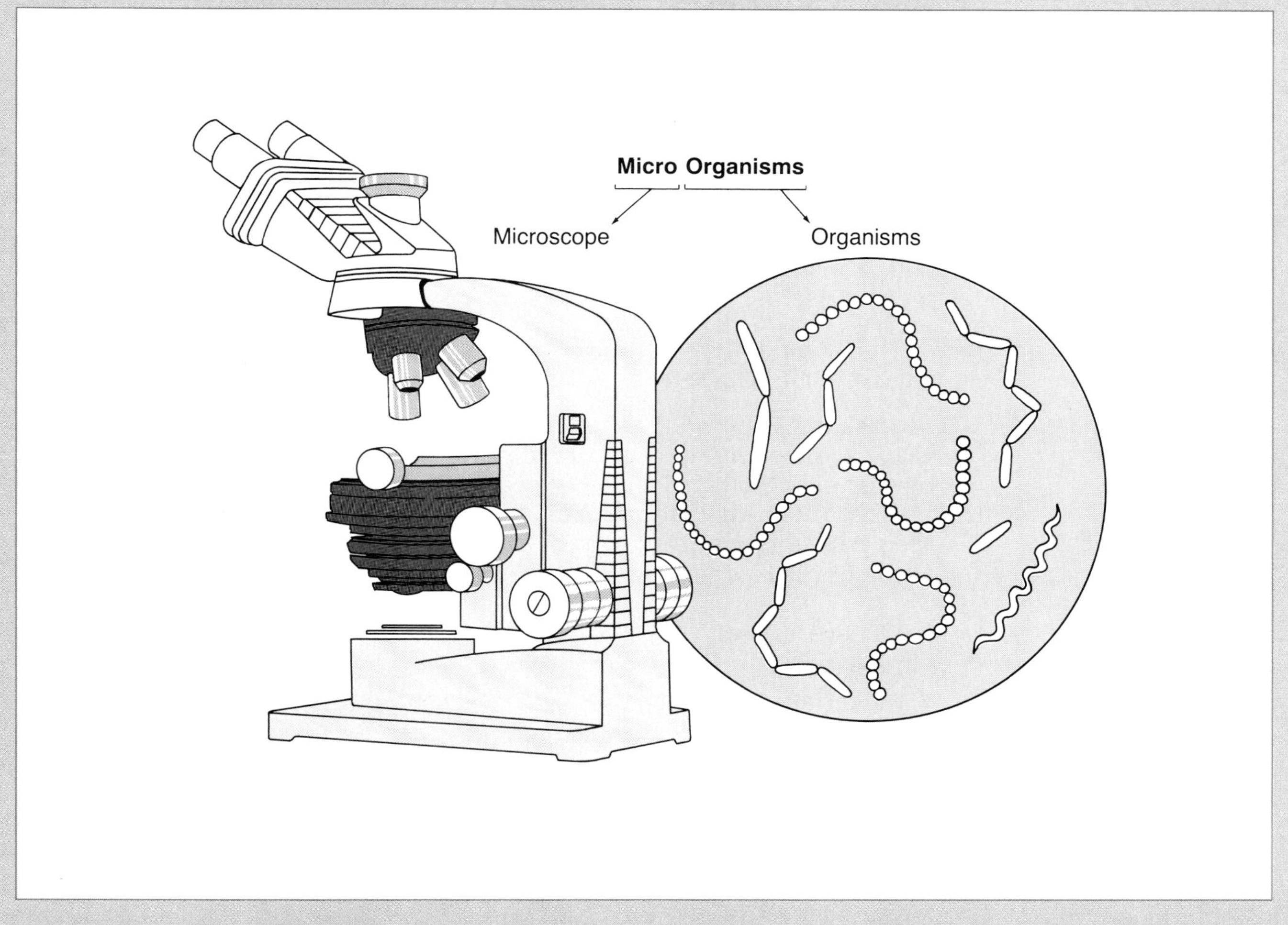

WARNING

For all patient contact, adhere to Universal Precautions (see page 91, 97, or the front cover flap). Wear protective equipment as indicated.

Objectives

What You Will Learn

When you have completed this chapter, you will be able to:

- Differentiate between helpful and harmful microorganisms.
- List six conditions affecting the growth of bacteria.
- Summarize the history of infection control.
- List five ways microorganisms are spread, giving examples of each.
- Explain how microorganisms are destroyed.
- Describe the five main purposes of medical asepsis.
- Demonstrate the procedure for handwashing.
- Define: aseptic, autoclave, bacteria, friction, hepatitis B, infection, medical asepsis, microorganism, nosocomial infections, pathogens, spores, sterilization, virus.

KEY IDEAS

Microorganisms

PEOPLE WHO WORK IN HEALTH CARE institutions must learn the importance of cleanliness. Everyone tries constantly in many ways to achieve ideal sanitary conditions. You, too, take part in this team effort to keep everything absolutely clean. Why? Because cleanliness is a part of every health care institution's effort to control disease and keep communicable diseases from spreading.

You will understand the importance of cleanliness in the health care institution if you know something about germs, the microorganisms that cause diseases. It may help to know what they are, how they spread, and how they can be destroyed.

Causes of Disease

People once believed that sickness was caused by evil spirits. About 500 years ago, scientists began to suspect that some diseases were caused by very small living things they called germs.

A germ is a **microorganism**. Micro means very small. Germs can be seen only under a microscope. Organism means a living thing. Different kinds of microorganisms (also called microbes) are:

Microorganism
A living thing so small it cannot be seen with the naked eye but only through a microscope.

Bacteria
Sometimes called germs; one kind of microorganism; many bacteria cause disease.

- Viruses
- **Bacteria**
- Rickettsiae
- Fungi, including molds and yeasts
- Protozoa

Diseases caused by microorganisms are shown in Figure 8-1.

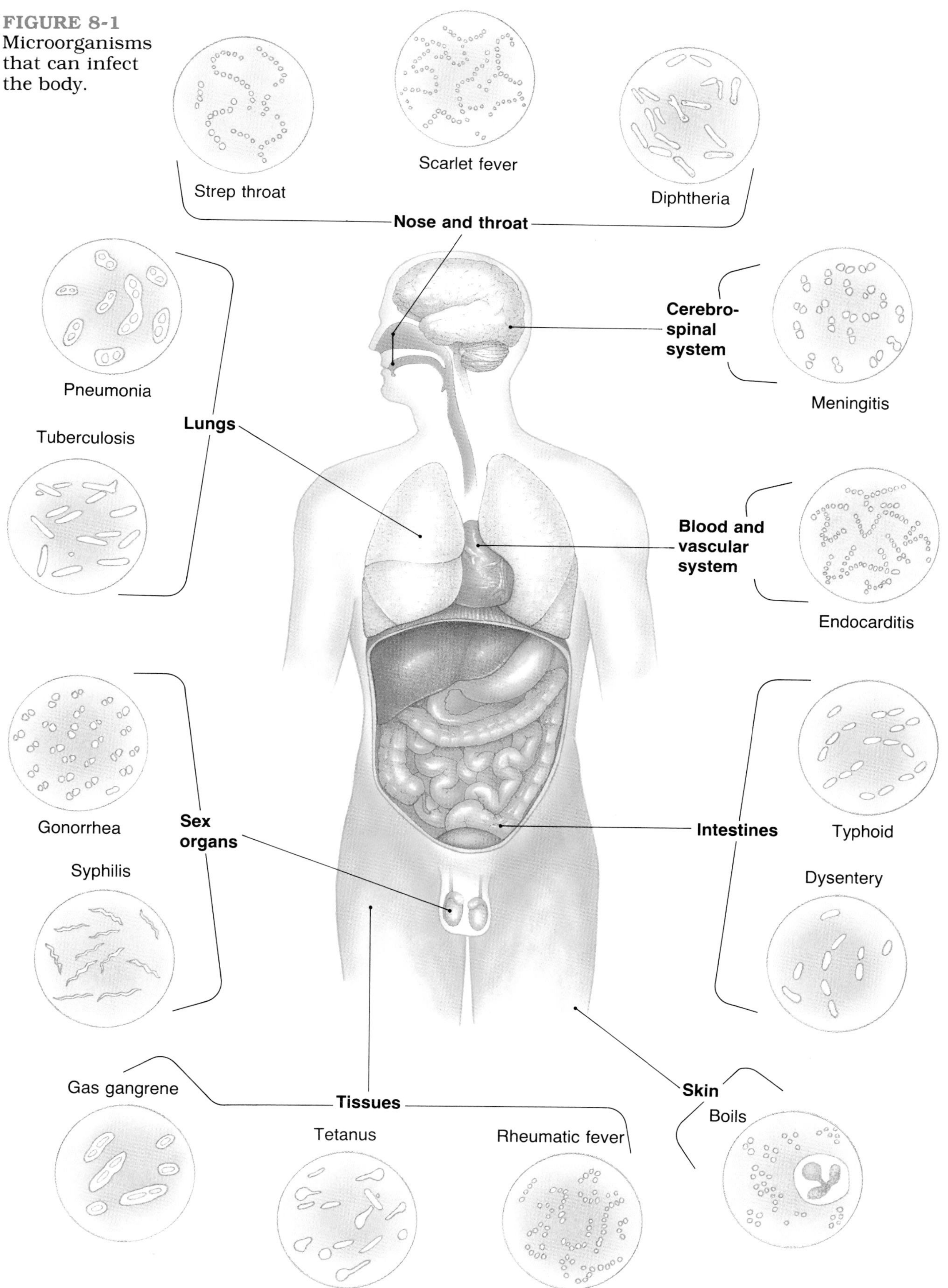

FIGURE 8-1 Microorganisms that can infect the body.

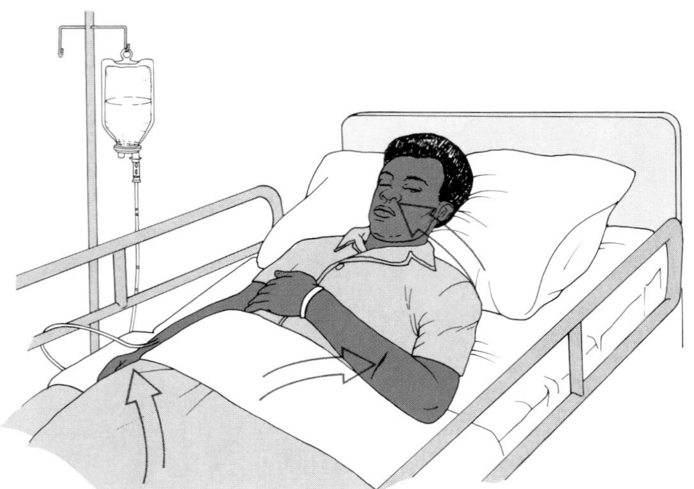

FIGURE 8-2 In the hospital bacteria enter the body through invasive points of entry such as IV sites, indwelling catheters, and surgical sites. Bacteria may also enter the body through cuts, or through the nose and mouth.

Nature of Microorganisms

Some microorganisms are helpful to people. For example, certain microbes cause a chemical change in food called fermentation. Fermentation is the change that produces cottage cheese from milk, beer from grains, cider from apples, and sauerkraut from cabbage. Other microorganisms in the human digestive system break down the foods not used by the body and turn them into waste products.

Pathogens
Disease-causing microorganisms.

Other kinds of microorganisms, however, are harmful to humans. These microbes cause disease and infection and are called **pathogens**. They grow best at body temperature, 98.6°F (37°C). Pathogens destroy human tissue by using it as food. They also give off waste products, called toxins, that are absorbed into and poison the body.

Microbes each have their own normal environment or home called their natural habitat. When organisms gain access to areas of the body in which they do not belong (see Figure 8-2) they become pathogens. For example, *Escherichia coli* belongs in the colon where it helps to digest our food. When it gets into the bladder or into the bloodstream, it can cause a urinary infection or a blood infection called bacteremia.

Figure 8-3 describes six conditions that affect the growth of bacteria.

In the hospital you will often hear the words staph or staphylococcus and strep or streptococcus. Staphylococcus and streptococcus are two types of bacteria. These organisms are found in all health care institutions. They are commonly found on the human skin and enter the body through a portal of entry. When staphylococci get inside the skin, they may produce a local infection. There may be soreness, tenderness, redness, and/or pus. Sometimes staphylococcus infections can affect the whole body.

Virus
A microscopic living parasitic agent that can cause infectious disease.

A **virus** is another type of microorganism. Viruses are much smaller than bacteria, and they cause many of our diseases. Examples are measles, AIDS, and influenza. Viruses can survive only in other living cells.

Table 8-1 lists a number of common communicable diseases.

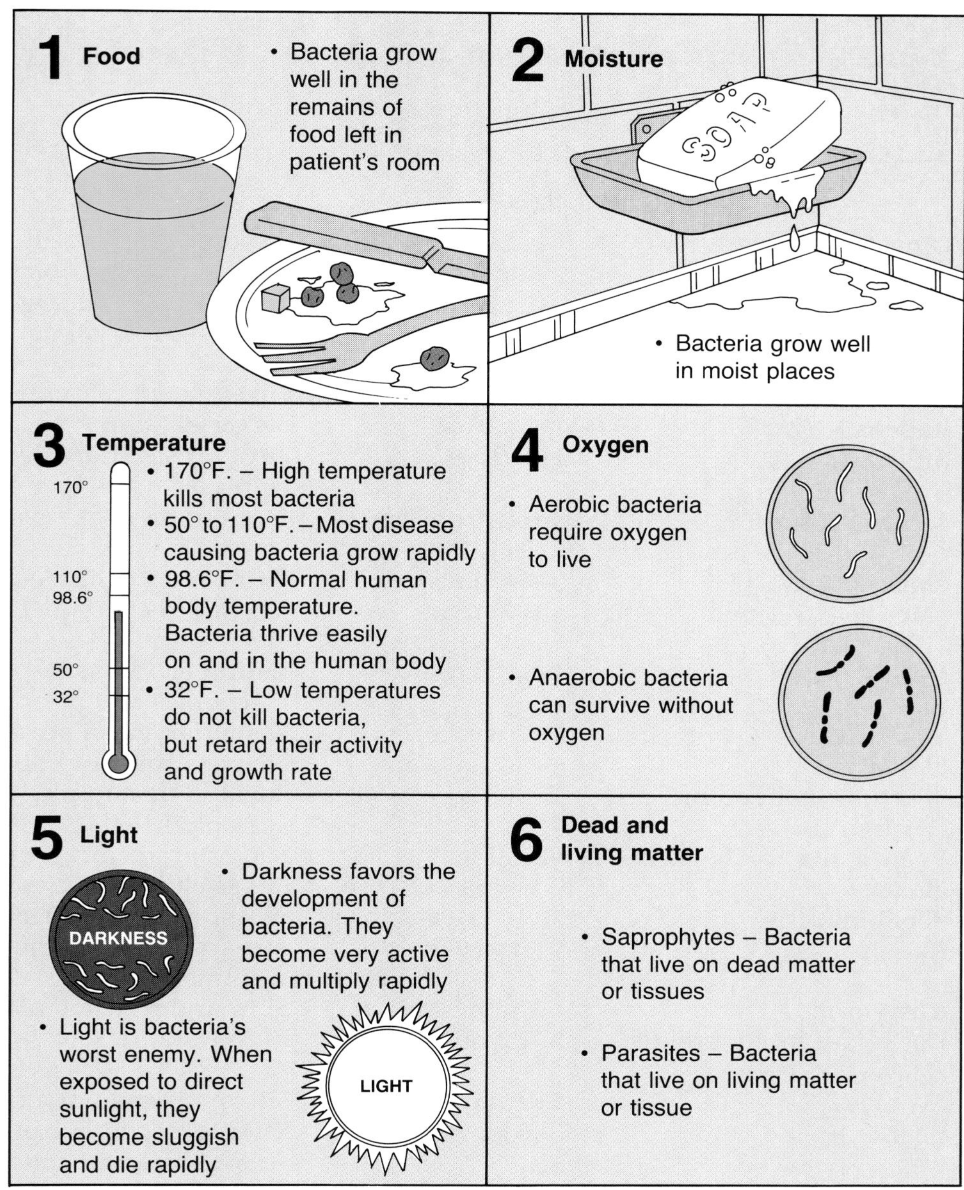

1 Food
• Bacteria grow well in the remains of food left in patient's room
2 Moisture
• Bacteria grow well in moist places
3 Temperature
170°
110°
98.6°
50°
32°
• 170°F. – High temperature kills most bacteria
• 50° to 110°F. – Most disease causing bacteria grow rapidly
• 98.6°F. – Normal human body temperature. Bacteria thrive easily on and in the human body
• 32°F. – Low temperatures do not kill bacteria, but retard their activity and growth rate
4 Oxygen
• Aerobic bacteria require oxygen to live
• Anaerobic bacteria can survive without oxygen
5 Light
DARKNESS
• Darkness favors the development of bacteria. They become very active and multiply rapidly
• Light is bacteria's worst enemy. When exposed to direct sunlight, they become sluggish and die rapidly
LIGHT
6 Dead and living matter
• Saprophytes – Bacteria that live on dead matter or tissues
• Parasites – Bacteria that live on living matter or tissue

FIGURE 8-3 Six conditions affecting the growth of bacteria.

History of Infection Control

The germ theory of disease was not actually proved until about 100 years ago. A French scientist named Louis Pasteur made two important discoveries about bacteria. First, he discovered that many diseases are caused by bacteria. Second, he discovered that bacteria could be killed by heat.

Pasteur's name has been used to refer to the heat method of killing germs. For example, *pasteurization* is the process of heating milk to 140°F (60°C) and keeping it at that temperature for one-half hour (Figure 8-4). Pasteurization kills harmful bacteria and makes milk safer for us to drink.

Table 8-1. Communicable or Infectious Diseases

Disease Name	Incubation	Transmission
A.I.D.S. (H.I.V.)	2 to 6 years	Sex, Blood, Needle Sticks, Hi-Risk Fluids: —Semen —Blood
Chicken pox (varicella)	14–21 days	Virus, respiratory droplets
Diphtheria	2–5 days	Nasopharyngeal secretions, respiratory droplets
Hepatitis (type A)	2–6 weeks	Virus, fecal–oral, parenteral injection
Hepatitis (type B)	6 weeks to 6 months	Virus, fecal–oral, parenteral injection, sexual
Hepatitis (Type C)	2–3 months	Virus, blood, parenteral injection, sexual
Impetigo	1–5 days	Bacterial (staph, or strep.), direct contact
Influenza	1–3 days	Virus, respiratory droplets, freshly soiled articles
Lyme Disease	3 to 21 days after Tick exposure	Presumably Tick-borne
*Measles (rubeola)	9–14 days	Virus, direct contact, respiratory droplets
*Measles, German (rubella)	14–21 days	Virus, direct contact, respiratory droplets
Meningitis	1–10 days	Meningococcus, respiratory droplets (could also be viral)
Mononucleosis, infectious	4–7 weeks	Nasopharyngeal secretions
*Mumps	8–30 days	Virus, respiratory droplets
*Pertusis (whooping cough)	7–20 days	Bacillus hemophilus, direct contact, respiratory droplets
Pneumonia	Variable	Bacterial, respiratory droplets, viral, rickettsial
Malaria	2 weeks	Anopheles mosquitoes
*Poliomyelitis	4–14 days	Feces, nasopharyngeal secretions
Rabies	2–6 weeks	Virus, saliva of rabid animals (usually dogs), animal bite
Ringworm	Variable	Skin and mucous membrane
Rocky mountain spotted fever	3–12 days	Rickettsia, tick bites, skin
Scabies	1–2 days	Mites, direct contact, skin
Scarlet fever	3–5 days	Streptococcus, nasopharyngeal secretions, contaminated articles
*Tetanus	4–21 days	Bacterial (clostridium tetani), penetrating wounds
Tuberculosis	Variable	Bacterial (mycobacterium tuberculosis), sputum, respiratory droplets
*Typhoid fever	5–14 days	Bacterial (salmonella typhi), infected urine and feces, contaminated food and water

*Today, immunization exists to prevent these diseases. Consult your local health departments for the schedules and availability of these immunizations.

A few years after Pasteur's discoveries, a British surgeon, Joseph Lister, found that germs could also be killed by carbolic acid. Lister recognized that many deaths in hospitals seemed to be connected with unclean conditions. He was the first to want surgical wounds kept clean and the air in the operating room kept pure.

Lister's theories led to changes in hospitals by introducing the principles and methods of aseptic surgery. **Aseptic** means germ free, without disease-producing organisms. Lister developed a technique to keep germs out of open wounds or to destroy them. His method was to spray

Aseptic
The condition of being free of disease-causing organisms.

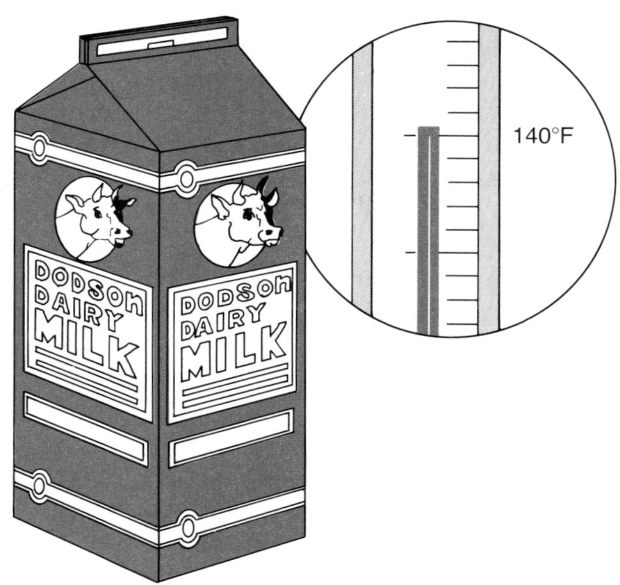

FIGURE 8-4 Heating milk at 140°F (60°C) for 30 minutes kills the germs in it and slows down the growth of other bacteria. This process is known as pasteurization.

the skin around the wound with carbolic acid. Also, surgical instruments were made aseptic by being dipped in a carbolic acid solution. This technique was a major advance in the battle against disease.

People working in hospitals began to realize that some disease-producing germs are everywhere (Figure 8-5). They are in the air, on the furniture, on and inside the patients' bodies, and on all the equipment.

FIGURE 8-5 Microorganisms are everywhere.

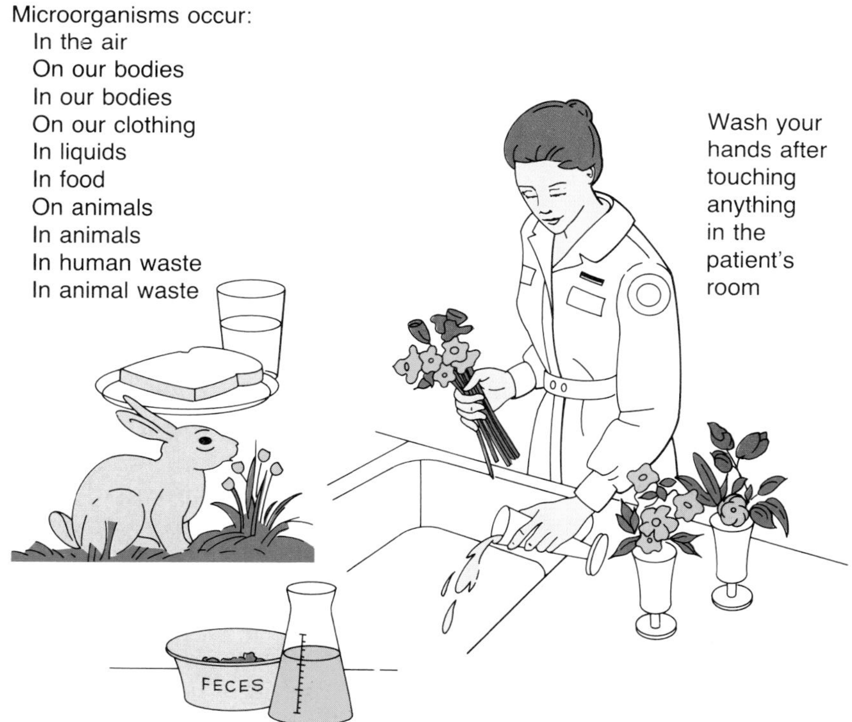

Microorganisms occur:
In the air
On our bodies
In our bodies
On our clothing
In liquids
In food
On animals
In animals
In human waste
In animal waste
Wash your hands after touching anything in the patient's room
FECES

Nosocomial infections
Hospital-acquired infections.

Scientists learned that germs multiply very rapidly. They also found that if germs are not killed, they spread infection and disease from one person to another. Therefore, it was necessary to apply the principles of asepsis to the entire health care institution in order to prevent **nosocomial infections** (hospital-acquired infections).

Figure 8-6 shows ways that microorganisms are spread.

Disinfection and Sterilization

A continuous battle goes on in health care institutions to prevent the spread of pathogens. This battle is called *medical asepsis*. In spite of the best efforts of health care personnel, there are always some harmful microorganisms around us. We can reduce the number of organisms, however, by maintaining simple cleanliness procedures. We can keep ourselves clean by bathing and frequent hand-washing. We can keep the institution and its equipment clean with soap, water, and special solutions that assist in keeping down bacterial growth. Two very important methods for killing microorganisms or keeping them under control are:

- **Disinfection:** the process of destroying as many harmful organisms as possible. It also means slowing down the growth and activity of the organisms that cannot be destroyed.
- **Sterilization:** the process of killing all microorganisms, including spores, in a certain area.

Sterilization
The process of destroying all microorganisms, including spores.

Spores
Bacteria that have formed hard shells around themselves for protection. Spores can be destroyed only by sterilization.

Autoclave
Equipment used to sterilize instruments and other articles in the health care institution.

Spores are bacteria that have formed hard shells around themselves as a defense. These shells are like a protective suit of armor. Spores are very difficult to kill. Some can even live in boiling water. Spores can be destroyed by being exposed to pressurized steam in a high temperature. Machines called **autoclaves** can produce this high-temperature, pressurized steam (Figure 8-7). Autoclaves are used to kill spores and other disease-producing bacteria. Another method of sterilization uses a chemical gas instead of heat to destroy microorganisms. This method can be used to sterilize equipment made of plastics without melting it. When an object is free of all microorganisms, it is called *sterile*. These are both effective ways of sterilizing objects used in a health care institution.

Sterilization is necessary if the article comes in direct contact with a wound, as in the case of surgical instruments. Most supplies and equipment used in the care of patients can be disinfected to prevent them from spreading disease or infection (Figure 8-8).

Medical Asepsis
Special practices and procedures for cleanliness to decrease the chances for disease-causing bacteria to live and spread.

Infection
A condition in body tissue in which germs or pathogens have multiplied.

Asepsis

Asepsis means preventing the conditions that allow pathogens to live, multiply, and spread. As a nursing assistant, you will share the responsibility for preventing the spread of disease and **infection** by using aseptic techniques. The main purposes for asepsis in caring for patients are:

- Protecting the patient against becoming infected a second time by the same microorganism. This is called *reinfection*.
- Protecting the patient against becoming infected by a new or different type of microorganism from another patient or a member of the hospital staff. This is called *cross infection*.

FIGURE 8-6 Ways by which microorganisms are spread. Use the Universal Precautions in any of the situations shown here.

Follow universal precautions in any of these situations

Direct Contact

Touching the patient
Rubbing the patient
Bathing the patient
Secretions from patient
Urine from the patient
Feces from the patient

Droplet Spread within Three Feet

Sneezing
Coughing
Talking

Indirect Contact

Touching objects:
- Dishes
- Bed linen
- Clothing
- Instruments
- Belongings

Airborne Transmission

Dust particles and moisture in the air

Vehicle

Contaminated:
- Food
- Drugs
- Water or blood

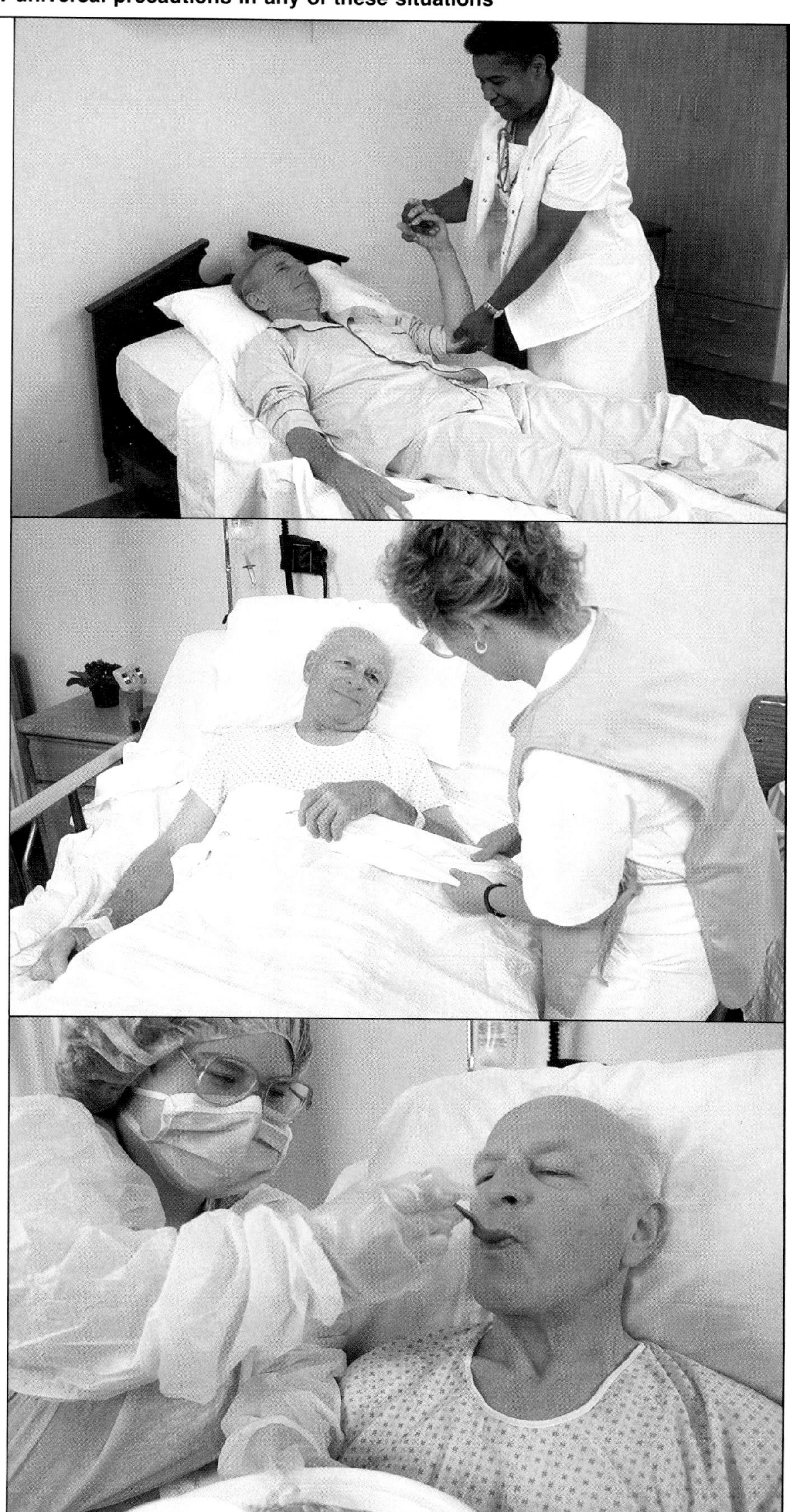

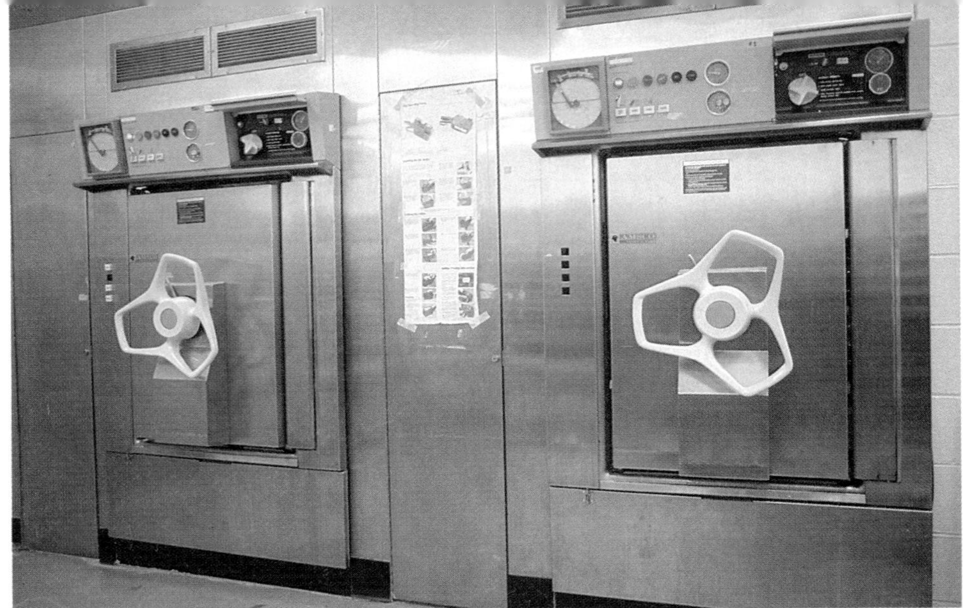

FIGURE 8-7 Autoclaving to achieve sterilization.

- Protecting all other patients and hospital staff against becoming infected by microorganisms passing from patient to patient, staff to patient, or patient to staff.
- Protecting the patient from becoming infected with his or her own organisms. This is called *self-inoculation.*

When the patient acquires an infection as a result of being hospitalized, it is called a nosocomial infection.

Universal Precautions

Nursing Assistants will adhere to the following precautions when delivering care to all patients. This will decrease the risk of transmission of disease when the infection status of the patient is unknown.

FIGURE 8-8 Intravenous poles should be wiped with antiseptic solution after each use.

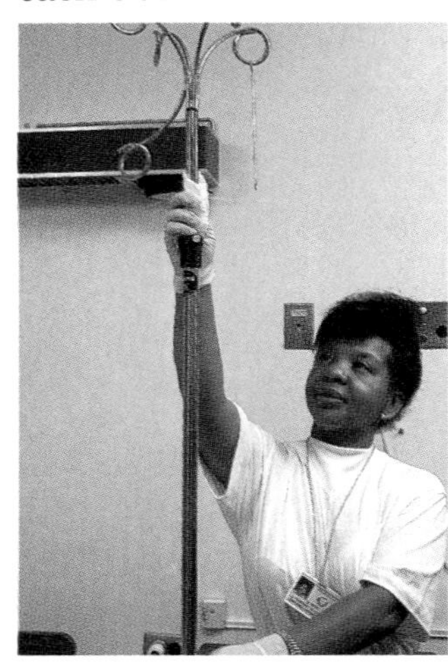

- Gloves must be worn when contact with blood or body fluids (urine, feces, emesis, etc.) is likely, for example, when taking a rectal temperature.
- Gowns or aprons must be worn during procedures or situations when there will be exposure to body fluids, blood, draining wounds, or mucous membranes.
- Mask and protective eyewear or face shield must be worn during procedures that are likely to generate droplets of body fluids or blood or when the patient is coughing excessively.
- Gloves are to be worn when collecting all specimens to prevent contamination from body specimen fluids or blood.
- Handwashing: Hands must be washed before gloving and after gloves are removed. (See Handwashing Procedures in the chapter on Infection Control.) Hands and other skin surfaces must be washed immediately and thoroughly if contaminated with body fluids or blood and after all patient care activities.
- Nursing Assistants who have open cuts, sores, or dermatitis on their hands must wear gloves for all patient contact.

KEY IDEAS

Handwashing

In your work you will be using your hands constantly. You will often be touching sick patients. You will handle supplies and equipment used in the treatment and care of patients. Germs will get on your hands (see Figure 8-9). They will come from the patient or from the things he or she has touched. Your hands could carry these germs to other persons and places or to your own face and mouth. Washing your hands frequently will help to prevent this transfer of germs.

Rules to Follow

HANDWASHING

- Handwashing must be done before and after each nursing task, before and after direct patient contact, and after handling any of a patient's belongings.
- The water faucet is always considered contaminated. This means there are germs on it. This is why you use paper towels to turn the faucet off (Figure 8-10).
- If your hands accidentally touch the inside of the sink, start over.
- Take soap from a dispenser, if possible, rather than using bar soap. Bar soap sits in a pool of soapy water in the soap dish, which is considered contaminated.
- Handwashing is effective only when:
  1. You use enough soap to produce lots of lather (Figure 8-11).
  2. You rub skin against skin to create **friction**, which helps to eliminate microorganisms.
  3. You rinse from the clean to the dirty parts of your hands. Rinse with running water from 2 inches above the wrists to the hands and then to the fingertips.
- Hold your hands lower than your elbows while washing. This is to prevent germs from contaminating your arms. Holding your hands down prevents backflow over unwashed skin.
- Add water to the soap while washing. This keeps the soap from becoming too dry.
- Never use the patient's soap for yourself.
- Rinse well. Soap left on the skin causes drying and can cause skin irritation.

Friction
The rubbing of one surface against another. Friction between the patient's body and his or her bedclothes often produces bedsores (pressure ulcers).

FIGURE 8-9 Washing your hands is important in preventing the spread of infection.

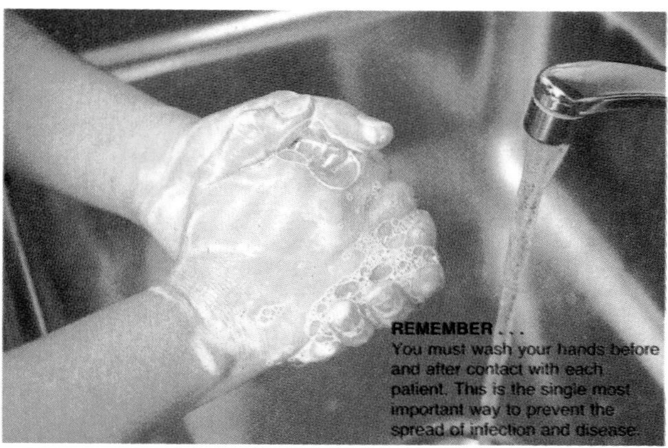

REMEMBER . . .
You must wash your hands before and after contact with each patient. This is the single most important way to prevent the spread of infection and disease.

FIGURE 8-10 Use a paper towel to turn the water faucet on and off.

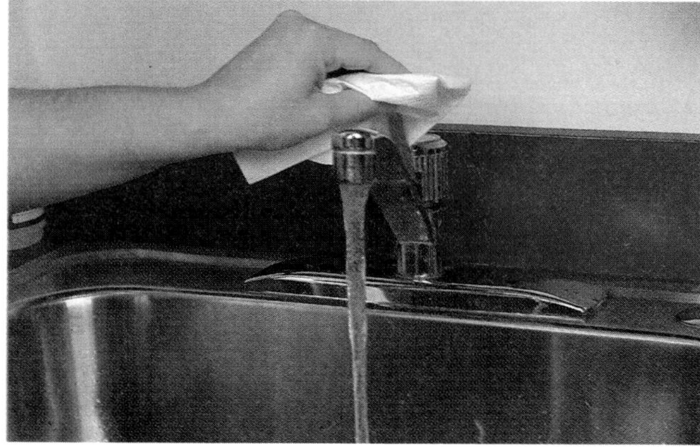

FIGURE 8-11 Use soap to work up a heavy lather on your hands.

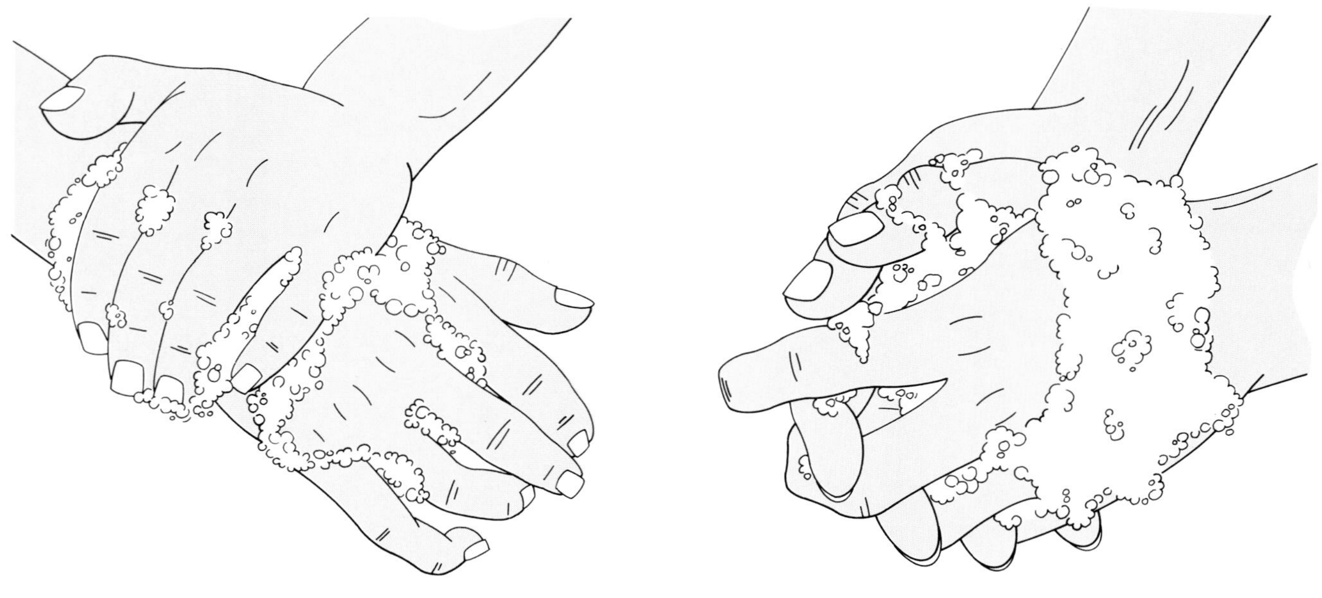

Procedure Handwashing

1. Assemble your equipment. The equipment used for handwashing is found at all times at every sink in all health care institutions.
   (a) Soap
   (b) Paper towels
   (c) Warm running water
   (d) Wastepaper basket
2. Completely wet your hands and wrists under the running water. Keep your fingertips pointed downward.
3. Apply soap.
4. Hold your hands lower than your elbows while washing.
5. Work up a good lather. Spread it over the

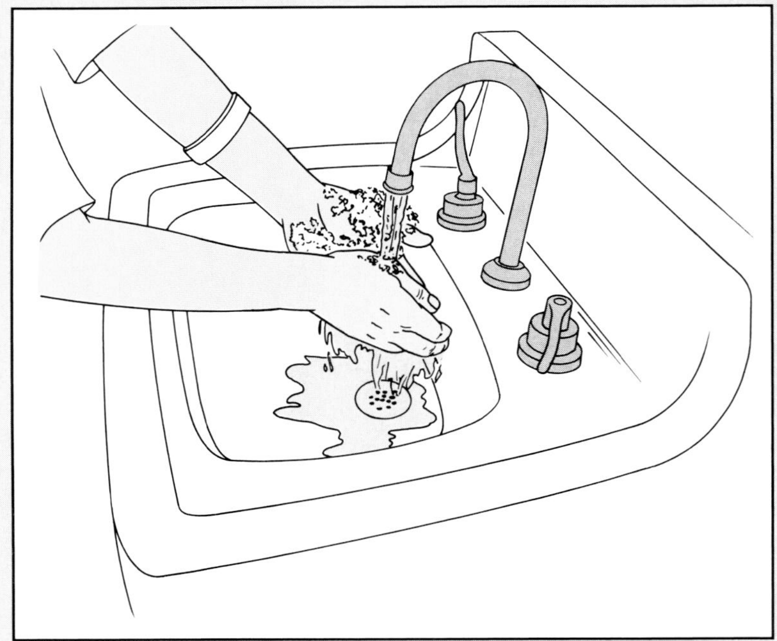

FIGURE 8-12 When rinsing, hold your hands and fingertips pointing down under the running water.

entire area of your hands and wrists. Get soap under your nails and between your fingers.

6. Clean under your nails by rubbing your nails across the palms of your hand.
7. Use a rotating and rubbing (frictional) motion for one full minute:
   a) Rub vigorously.
   b) Rub one hand against the other hand and wrist.
   c) Rub between your fingers by interlacing them.
   d) Rub up and down to reach all skin surfaces on your hands, between your fingers, and 2 inches above your wrists.
   e) Rub the tips of your fingers against your palms to clean with friction around the nail beds.
8. Rinse well. Rinse from 2 inches above your wrists to the hands. Hold your hands and fingertips down under running water (Figure 8-11).
9. Dry thoroughly with paper towels.
10. Turn off the faucet, using a paper towel. Never touch the faucet with your hands after washing.
11. Discard the paper towel into the wastepaper basket. Do not touch the basket.

KEY IDEAS

OSHA (Occupational Safety and Health Administration, U.S. Department of Labor) Standards for Occupational Exposure to Blood-Borne Pathogens

Hepatitis B
A blood-borne pathogen that can be life threatening. This infection is transmitted by exposure to blood and other infectious body fluids and tissues.

Who is at risk? All facilities where you are employed will identify all job classifications that have occupational exposure to blood and other potentially dangerous body fluids and materials.

Employers are required to provide a means of protecting their employees from potential exposure to **hepatitis B**. Employees must use universal precautions, protective clothing, and equipment to prevent exposure to potentially infectious materials. However, the best defense against infection by hepatitis B is vaccination.

Recombinant hepatitis B vaccine (grown on yeast) became available in 1987 and is now the only type produced in this country. There are minimal adverse reactions and no possibility of infection from this vaccine. Because the hepatitis B vaccine is recombinant it is contraindicated for individuals who are hypersensitive to yeast or any component of the vaccine. Employees with a history of cardiopulmonary disease should consult their physician prior to accepting this vaccination. Hepatitis B vaccination is **not** recommended for use by pregnant women or nursing mothers.

Immunization is accomplished in a three-injection series. Any employee with potential occupational exposure qualifies to receive the vaccine. All costs associated with this immunization must be provided by the employer.

Since July 6, 1992, OSHA standards mandate that training and immunization must be provided to all employees within 10 days of initial assignment to a job that puts that employee at occupational risk. This training must be updated annually. All employees must be given the choice to elect or refuse immunization. If refused the employee has the right to change his or her mind at a later date and receive immunization at no charge.

Another blood-borne pathogen that puts health care workers at potential risk is **human immunodeficiency virus (HIV)**. The **acquired immunodeficiency syndrome (AIDS)** caused by HIV is a severe viral disease that affects the immune system and is characterized by opportunistic infections. The risk is due to exposure by semen, vaginal secretions, cerebrospinal fluid, synovial fluid, pleural fluid, pericardial fluid, peritoneal fluid, amniotic fluid, saliva, blood, blood products, and other body fluids and waste. Annual reeducation and the enforced use of universal precautions is the best means of preventing exposure.

KEY QUESTIONS

1. What are the differences between helpful and harmful microorganisms?
2. What are the six conditions that affect the growth of bacteria?
3. What contributions did Pasteur and Lister make to the development of modern infection control practices?
4. How are microorganisms spread? Give examples in each category.
5. How are microorganisms destroyed?
6. What are the five main purposes of medical asepsis?
7. Discuss the ten rules to follow for proper handwashing technique.
8. What are the OSHA standards for occupational exposure to bloodborne pathogens?
9. Define: aseptic, autoclave, bacteria, friction, hepatitis B, infection, medical asepsis, microorganism, nosocomial infections, pathogens, spores, sterilization, virus.

CHAPTER

9

The Patient in Isolation

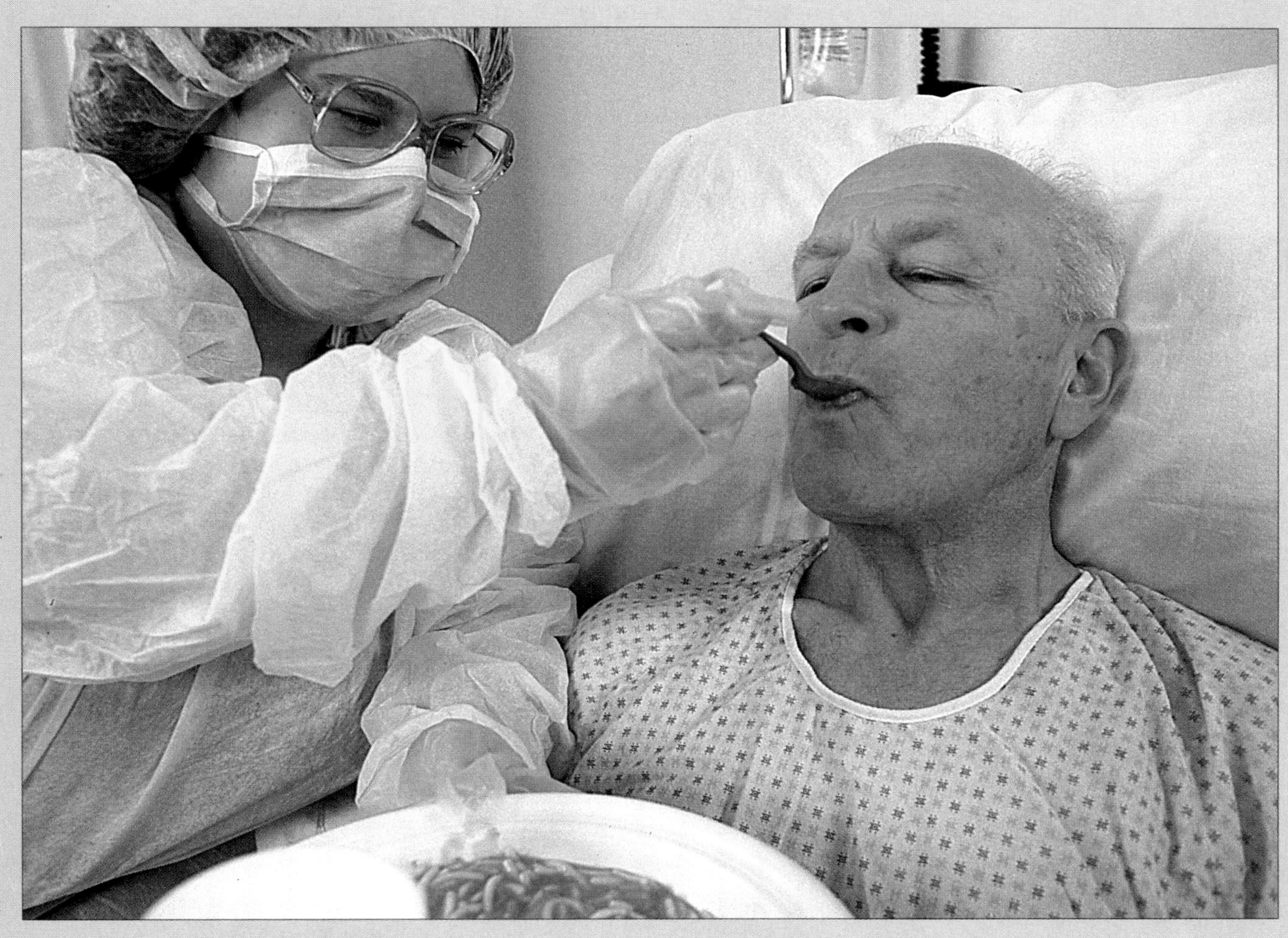

WARNING

For all patient contact, adhere to Universal Precautions (see page 91, 97, or the front cover flap). Wear protective equipment as indicated.

Objectives

What You Will Learn

When you have completed this chapter, you will be able to:

- Explain the purpose of isolation technique.
- Identify examples of items and areas considered to be clean and dirty.
- Differentiate between System A, Category-specific Isolation Precautions, and System B, Disease-specific Isolation Precautions.
- List the precautions to be taken for each system A category.
- Demonstrate mask and gown technique.
- Demonstrate double bagging.
- Describe good technique when caring for a patient in isolation.
- Demonstrate how to leave the isolation unit.
- Describe biohazardous waste materials and their proper disposal.
- Discuss the OSHA guidelines for preventing exposure to tuberculosis.
- Define: biohazardous waste, clean, communicable disease, dirty (contaminated), isolation gown, and isolation technique.

KEY IDEAS

Isolation Technique

ASIDE FROM HANDWASHING, SPECIAL METHODS ARE used to prevent infectious diseases from spreading. Isolation technique, including the use of masks and gowns, keeps disease germs away from equipment and personnel. Certain health care areas need extra precautions to prevent the spread of infection and disease (Figure 9-1).

Communicable Disease
A disease that is easily spread from one person to another; also called infectious disease.

Communicable Infectious Diseases. Infectious diseases spread very quickly and easily from one person to another. Examples are hepatitis and the common cold. Sometimes the more general term, communicable conditions, is used because it includes both diseases and infections. Ordinary cleanliness alone will not protect you and others from catching such diseases. When a patient has one of these diseases, special precautions are necessary. These safety measures are called **isolation technique**. The patient is separated (in isolation) from other people.

Isolation Technique or Protective Care
Special procedures used in caring for patients with infectious communicable diseases, to prevent infection or disease from spreading to other persons, as well as keeping other types of infections or diseases from coming in contact with the patient.

The purpose of isolation technique is to keep the germs that cause the disease inside the isolated patient's unit. As you know, these disease germs are everywhere in the sick room. They are on the floor, furniture, bedding, articles brought to the bedside, and on the patient himself. The area, the articles, and the patient are said to be contaminated. When you touch or brush your clothes against any of these, disease germs will contaminate your hands or clothing. Isolation technique is used to prevent the germs from leaving the unit on your hands, arms, and clothing or on articles used in the unit (cross contamination).

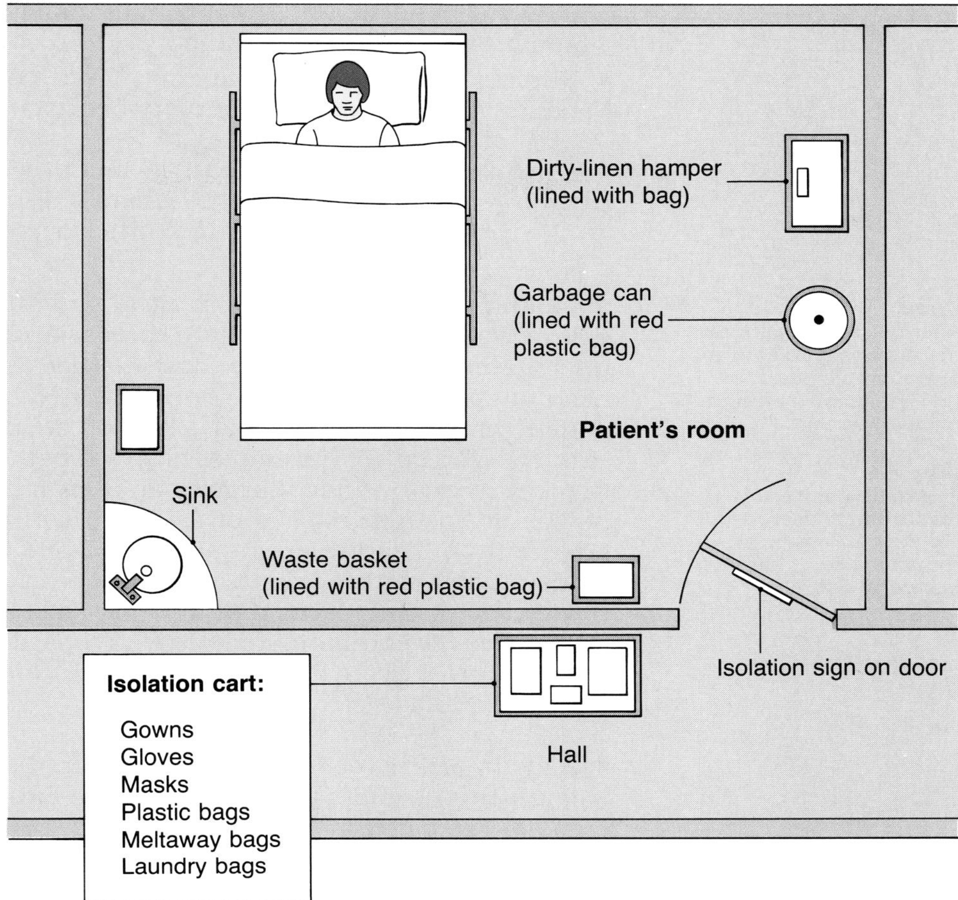

FIGURE 9-1 The isolation unit.

Universal Precautions

Nursing Assistants will adhere to the following precautions when delivering care to all patients. This will decrease the risk of transmission of disease when the infection status of the patient is unknown.

- Gloves must be worn when contact with blood or body fluids (urine, feces, emesis, etc.) is likely, for example, when taking a rectal temperature.
- Gowns or aprons must be worn during procedures or situations when there will be exposure to body fluids, blood, draining wounds, or mucous membranes.
- Mask and protective eyewear or face shields must be worn during procedures that are likely to generate droplets of body fluids on blood or when the patient is coughing excessively.
- Gloves are to be worn when collecting all specimens to prevent contamination from body specimen fluids or blood.
- Handwashing: Hands must be washed before gloving and after gloves are removed. (See Handwashing Procedures in the chapter on Infection Control.) Hands and other skin surfaces must be washed im-

mediately and thoroughly if contaminated with body fluids or blood and after all patient care activities.

- Nursing Assistants who have open cuts, sores, or dermatitis on their hands must wear gloves for all patient contact.

The following special precautions and procedures tell you how to protect yourself from catching the patient's disease and how to avoid carrying it outside her or his unit to other persons or areas.

Clean
A term used in health care institutions to refer to an object or area that is uncontaminated by harmful microorganisms.

Dirty
A term used in the health care institution to refer to an object or area as being contaminated by harmful microorganisms.

Clean and Dirty. The words clean and dirty have a special meaning when we are talking about health care isolation technique. **Clean** means uncontaminated. It refers to those articles and places to which disease has not spread. **Dirty** means contaminated. Articles or places near the patient who has an infectious condition are dirty areas from which disease can spread. For example, before a patient receives his meal tray, the tray is clean. After the tray has been in his room, no matter what he has or has not touched or eaten, it is dirty and can spread disease (Figure 9-2). Clean refers to all articles and places that have not been contaminated with or come in contact with pathogens. Dirty refers to those articles and places that a patient has been near or touched. The floor is heavily contaminated (dirty). Discard. Discard or put in a laundry bag any item if it falls to the floor. One good way to control the spread of disease is to have two areas:

- *A clean utility room.* Supplies are stored or prepared here that have never been near or had contact with a patient or any articles belonging to the patient.
- *A dirty utility room.* Supplies or articles are brought here after having been in contact with the patient or with the patient's belongings.

FIGURE 9-2 The words clean and dirty have a special meaning in isolation technique.

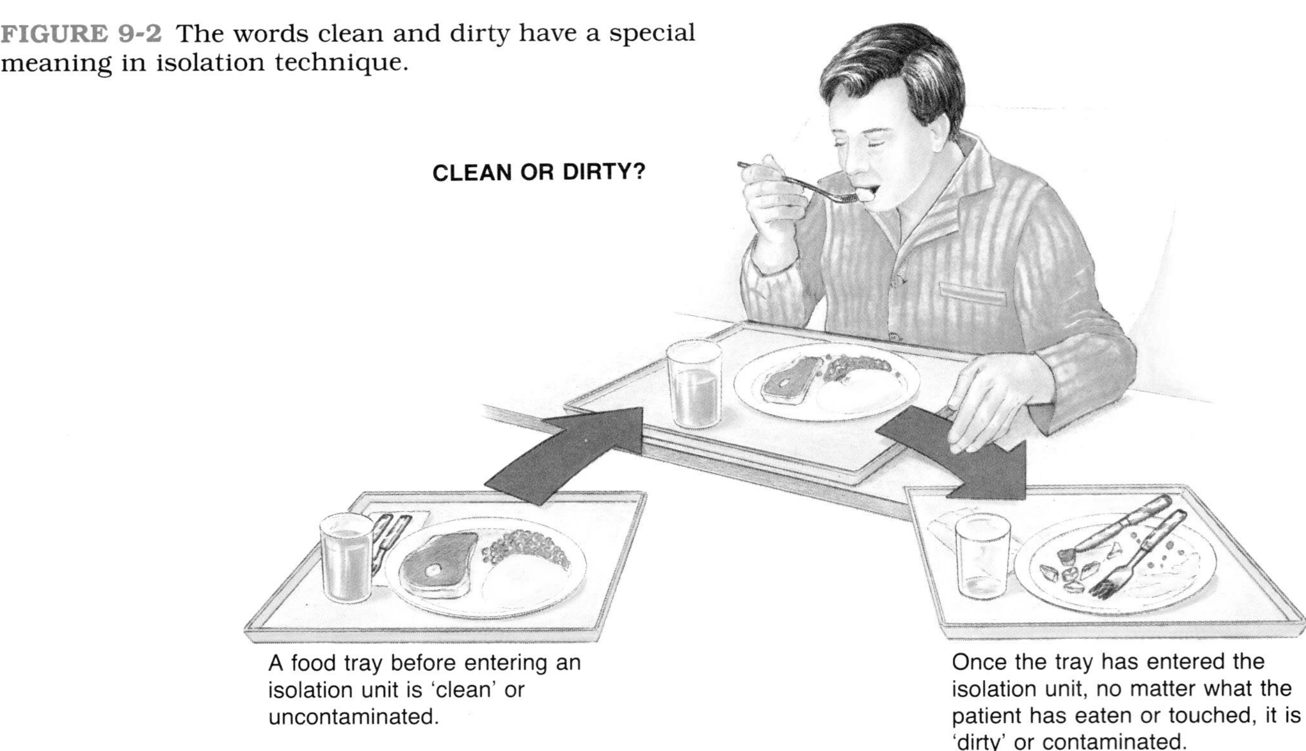
CLEAN OR DIRTY?
A food tray before entering an isolation unit is 'clean' or uncontaminated.
Once the tray has entered the isolation unit, no matter what the patient has eaten or touched, it is 'dirty' or contaminated.

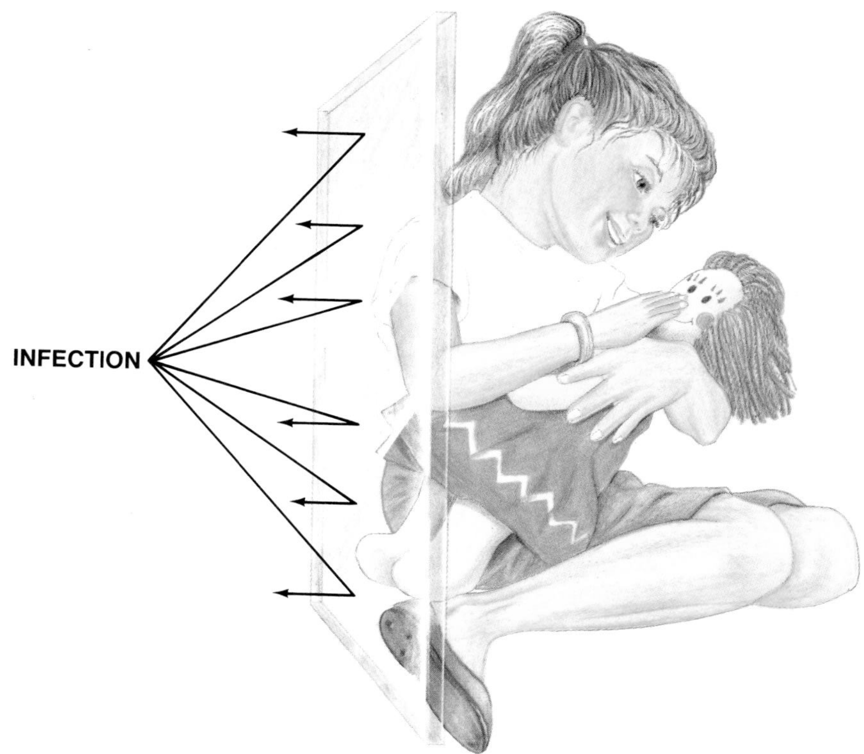

FIGURE 9-3 Compromised-host precautions (reverse isolation) prevent infection from reaching the patient.

Equipment kept in these utility rooms varies greatly from one institution to another. In most facilities there is a special area in the dirty utility room for items to be put that have to be returned to the central supply room after having been used for a patient. Dirty linen hampers should be stored in the areas designated at your institution.

Special Areas for Preventive Measures. Certain patient care areas in the health care institution need special attention to ensure cleanliness. Precautions to prevent infectious conditions from spreading are more strict because the patients in these areas may have a low resistance to disease (Figure 9-3). However, they may not have any communicable conditions. These areas include:

- Premature care nursery
- Surgical patient care unit (operating room)
- Burn unit
- Oncology (cancer) unit (certain rooms)
- Transplant unit (certain rooms)

Protective Care and Isolation Precautions

Each health care institution must follow policy and guidelines for isolation precautions (protective care). You, the nursing assistant, must follow the policies of your employing health care institution. These guidelines for isolation precautions in hospitals come from the Centers for Disease Control (CDC) in Atlanta, Georgia.

Some institutions utilize Universal Precautions plus category-specific isolation precautions. Others utilize Universal Precautions, with additional precautions utilized as necessary for specific disease states.

Category-specific Isolation Precautions

This system is used for grouping diseases for which similar isolation precautions are indicated. They utilize seven specific categories for which there are seven barrier cards with instructions for the group of diseases. The nurse posts the appropriate card on the patient's chart and door, and you follow the instructions on the cards before you enter the isolated area. These cards are shown in Figures 9-4 through 9-9.

FIGURE 9-4 Drainage/secretion isolation, system A.

SYSTEM A – CATEGORY SPECIFIC ISOLATION PRECAUTIONS

DRAINAGE/SECRETION PRECAUTIONS

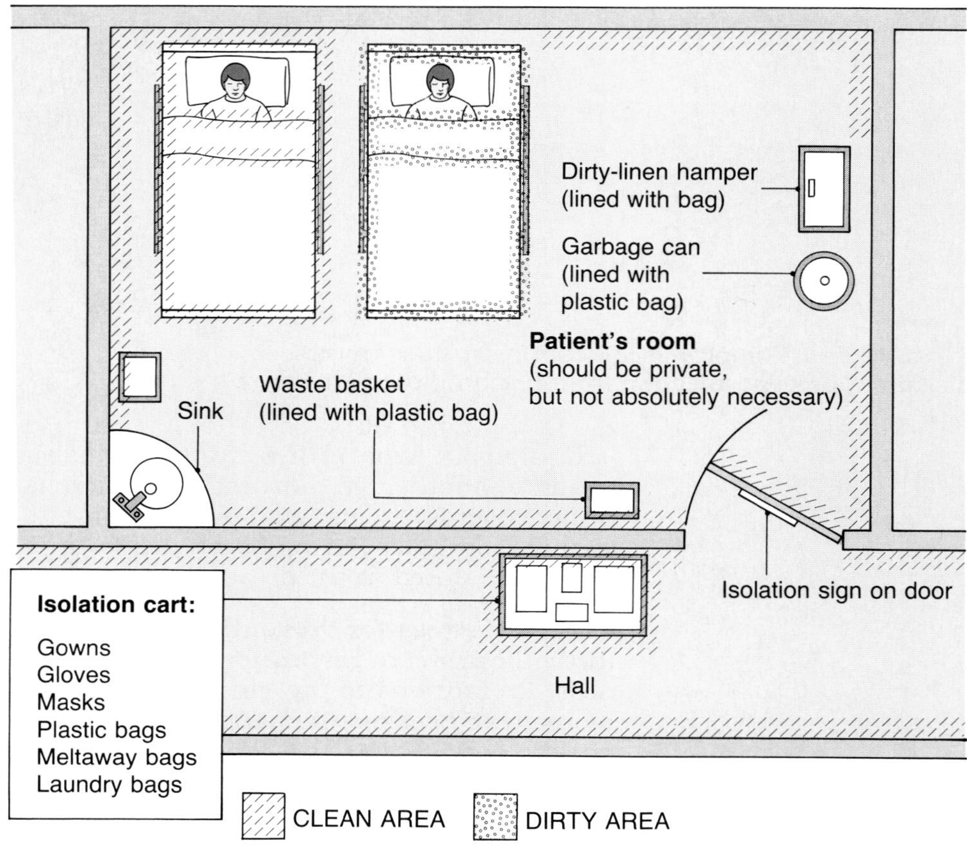

Drainage/Secretion Precautions

Visitors — Report to Nurses' Station
Before Entering Room

1. **Masks** are not indicated.
2. **Gowns** are indicated if soiling is likely.
3. **Gloves** are indicated for touching infective material.
4. **Hands must be washed after touching the patient or potentially contaminated articles and before taking care of another patient.**
5. **Articles** contaminated with infective material should be discarded or bagged and labeled before being sent for decontamination and reprocessing.

FIGURE 9-5 Respiratory isolation, system A.

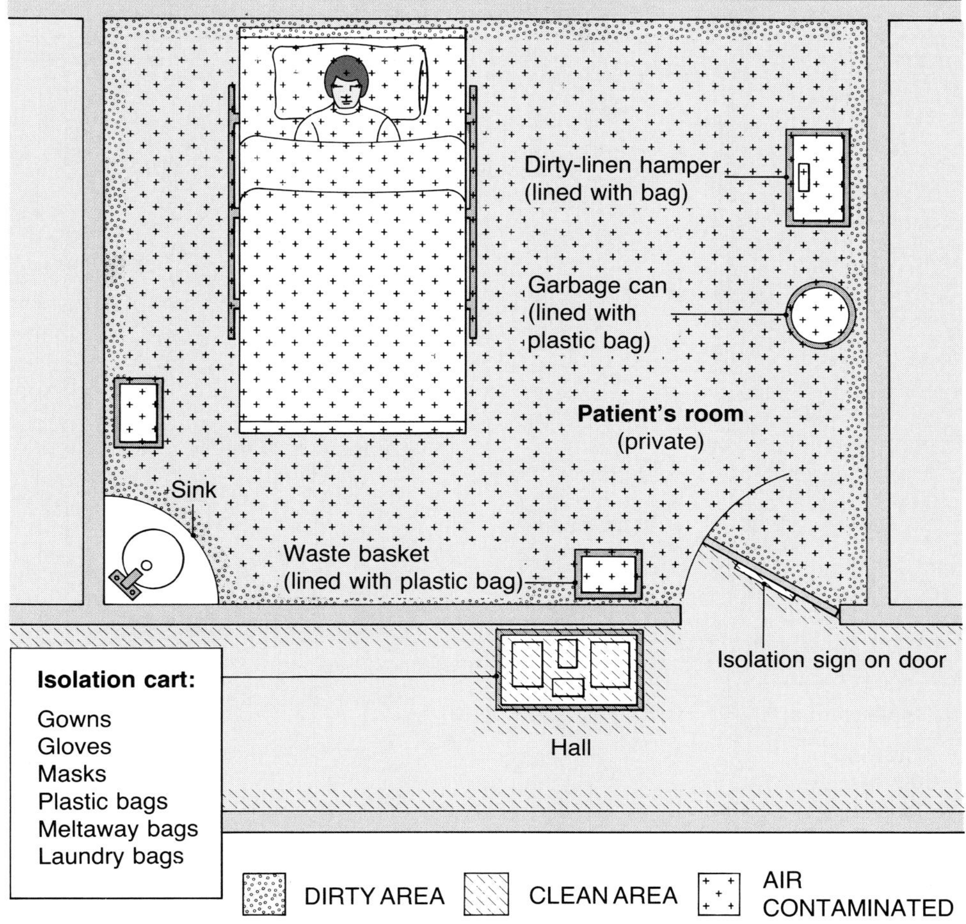

Respiratory Isolation

Visitors — Report to Nurses' Station Before Entering Room

1. **Masks** are indicated for those who come close to patient.
2. **Gowns** are not indicated.
3. **Gloves** are indicated per Universal Precautions (for contact with blood or body fluids).
4. **Hands must be washed after touching the patient or potentially contaminated articles and before taking care of another patient.**
5. **Articles** contaminated with infective material should be discarded or bagged and labeled before being sent for decontamination and reprocessing.

FIGURE 9-6 Strict isolation unit, system A.

SYSTEM A – CATEGORY SPECIFIC ISOLATION PRECAUTIONS

STRICT ISOLATION UNIT

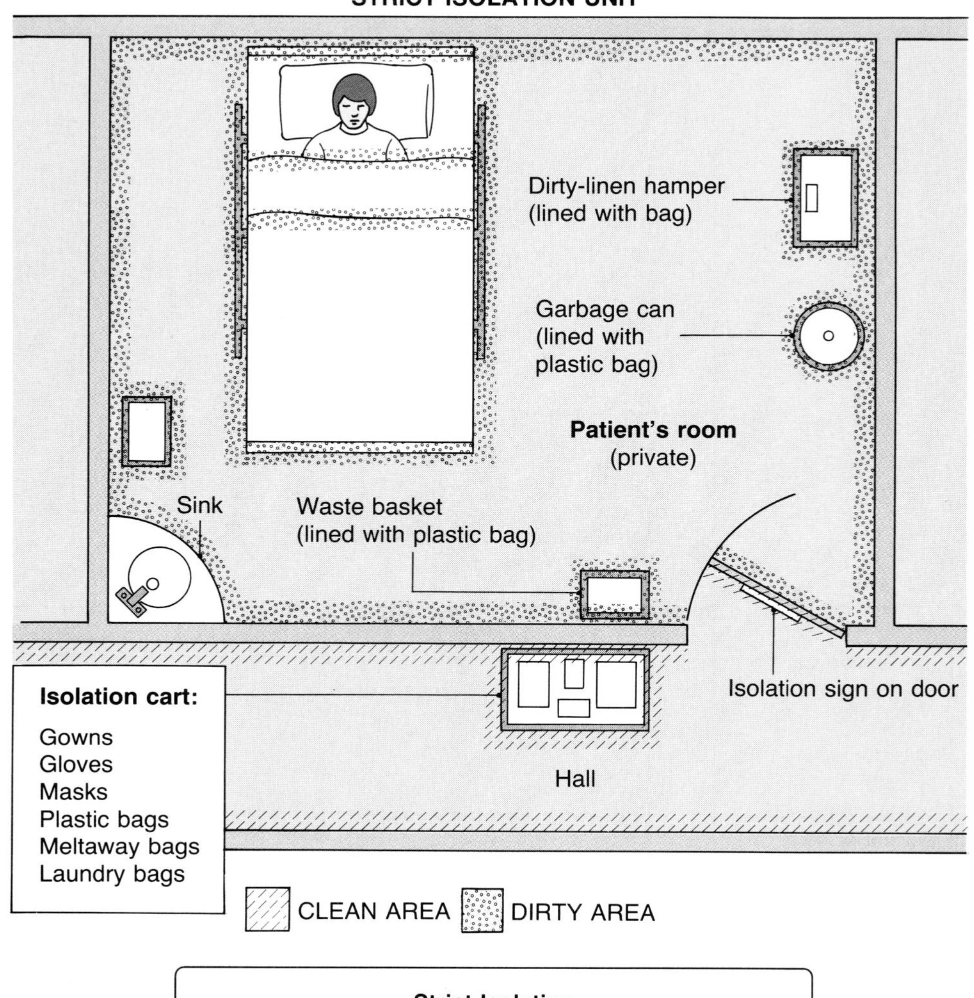

Strict Isolation

Visitors — Report to Nurses' Station
Before Entering Room

1. **Masks** are indicated.
2. **Gowns** are indicated.
3. **Gloves** are indicated.
4. **Hands must be washed after touching the patient or potentially contaminated articles and before taking care of another patient.**
5. **Articles** should be discarded, cleaned, or sent for decontamination and reprocessing.

FIGURE 9-7 Enteric precautions, system A.

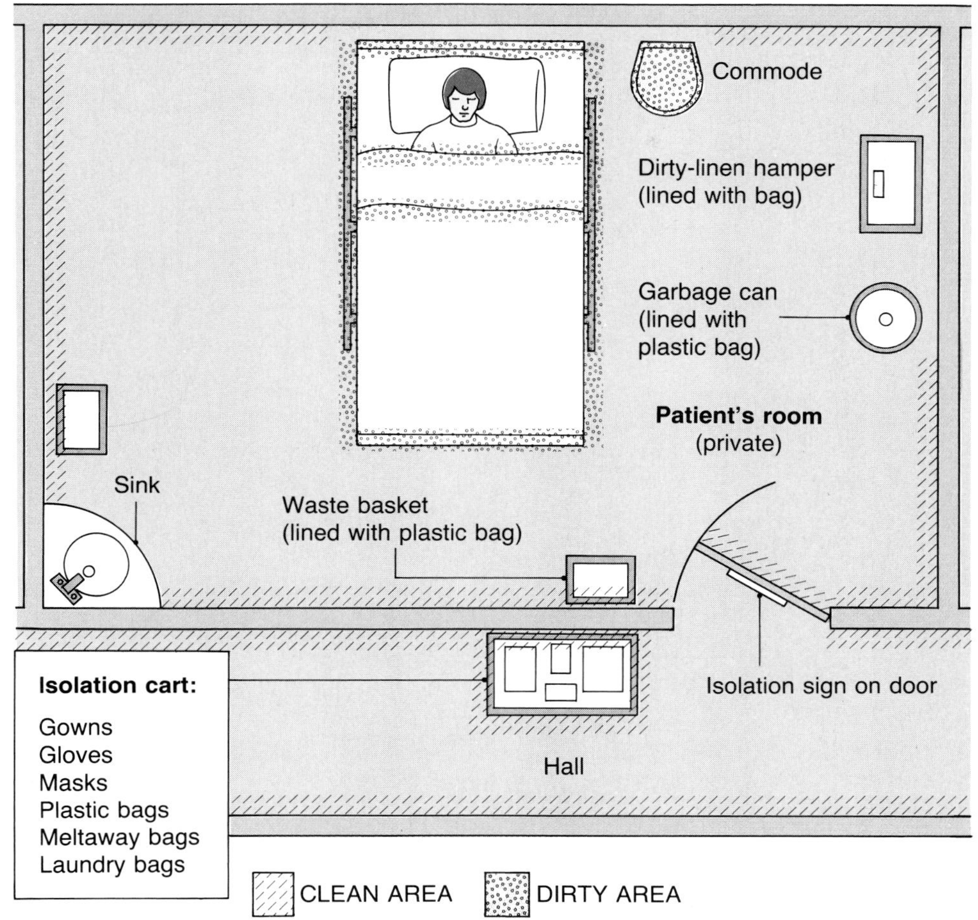

Enteric Precautions

Visitors — Report to Nurses' Station
Before Entering Room

1. **Masks** are not indicated.
2. **Gowns** are indicated if soiling is likely.
3. **Gloves** are indicated for touching infective material.
4. **Hands must be washed after touching the patient or potentially contaminated articles and before taking care of another patient.**
5. **Articles** contaminated with infective material should be discarded or bagged and labeled before being sent for decontamination and reprocessing.

A private room is indicated for Enteric Precautions if patient hygiene is poor. A patient with poor hygiene does not wash hands after touching infective material, contaminates the environment with infective material, or shares contaminated articles with other patients. In general, patients infected with the same organism may share a room.

FIGURE 9-8 AFB isolation unit, system A.

SYSTEM A – CATEGORY SPECIFIC ISOLATION PRECAUTIONS

AFB ISOLATION UNIT

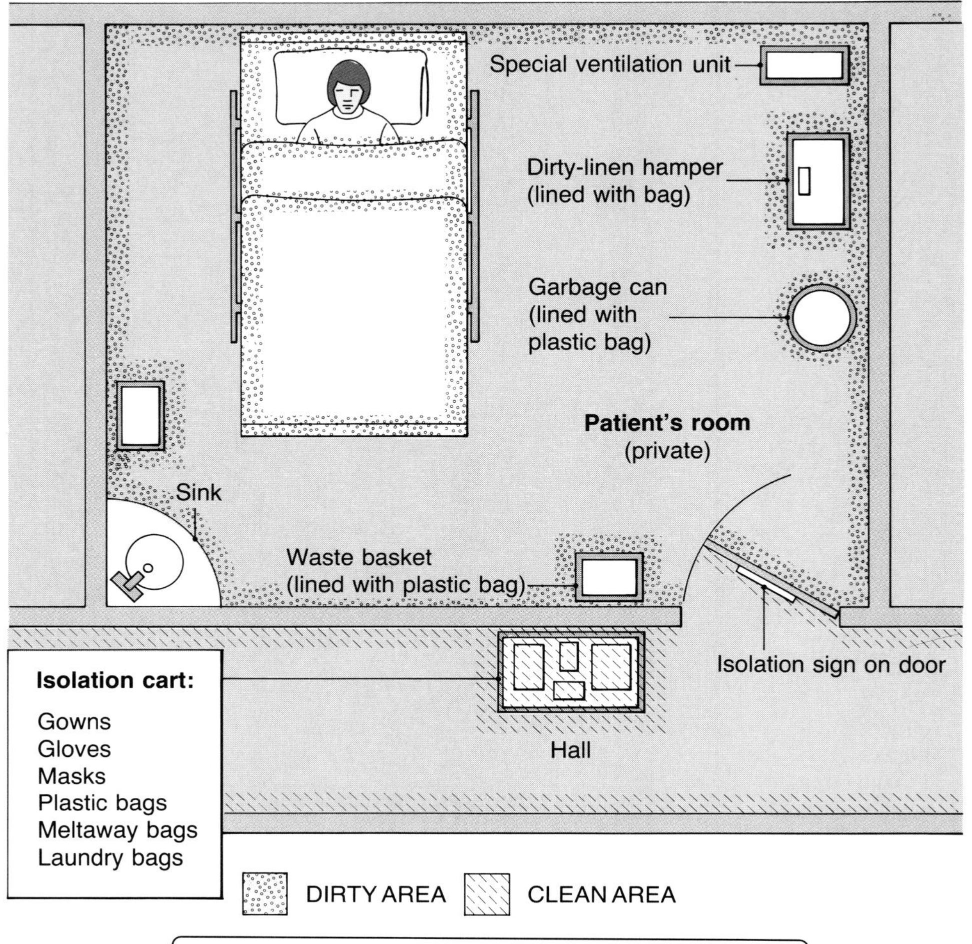

AFB (Acid Fast Bacillus) Isolation
Primarily for Tuberculosis

Visitors — Report to Nurses' Station
Before Entering Room

1. **Masks** are indicated.
2. **Gowns** are indicated only if needed to prevent gross contamination of clothing.
3. **Gloves** are indicated per Universal Precautions (for contact with blood or body fluids).
4. **Hands must be washed after touching the patient or potentially contaminated articles and before taking care of another patient.**
5. **Articles** should be discarded, cleaned, or sent for decontamination and reprocessing.

FIGURE 9-9 Blood and body fluid precaution unit, system A.

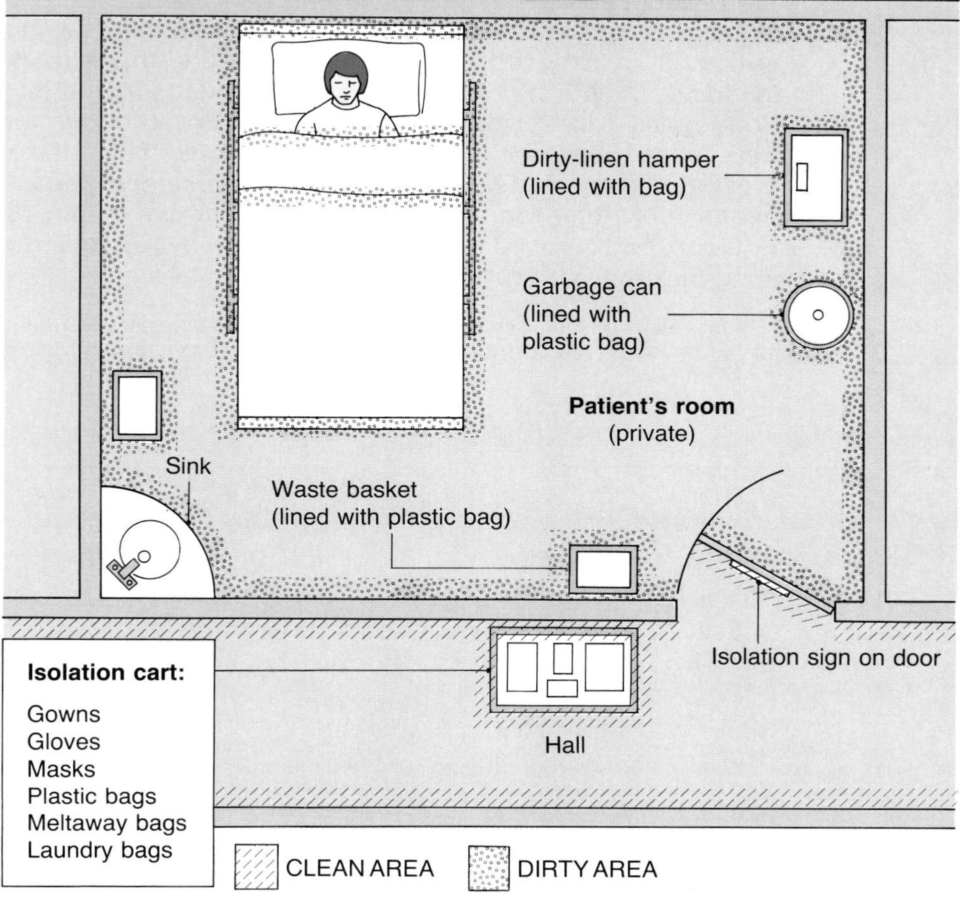

Blood/Body Fluid Precautions

1. **Masks** are not indicated unless aerosolization is likely.
2. **Gowns** are indicated if soiling with blood or body fluids is likely.
3. **Gloves** are indicated for touching blood or body fluids.
4. **Hands should be washed immediately if they are potentially contaminated with blood or body fluids and before taking care of another patient.**
5. **Articles** contaminated with blood or body fluids should be discarded or bagged and and labeled before being sent for decontamination and reprocessing.
6. **Care** should be taken to avoid needle-stick injuries. Used needles should not be recapped or bent; they should be placed in a prominently labeled, puncture-resistant container designed specifically for such disposal.
7. **Blood spills** should be cleaned up promptly with a solution of 5.25% sodium hypochlorite diluted 1:10 with water.

A private room is indicated for Blood/Body fluid Precautions if patient hygiene is poor. A patient with poor hygiene does not wash hands after touching infective material, contaminates the environment with infective material, or shares contaminated articles with other patients. In general, patients infected with the same organism may share a room.

Disease-specific Isolation Precautions*

This system is considered individually for each infectious disease so that only those precautions such as private room, mask, gloves, or gown indicated to interrupt the transmission for that disease are recommended. The nurse will follow a recommended list and fill in an instruction barrier card designed to give specific instructions regarding isolation precautions for a disease or syndrome. The instruction card is prepared by checking items and filling blanks and is posted on the patient's door, the head of the patient's bed, and/or on the patient's chart. This card will give you instructions to follow before you enter the isolated area. Figure 9-10 provides an example.

*This system is seldom used now. It is more likely that Universal Precautions will be enforced with attention drawn to specifics, as in the case of, for example, chicken pox, tuberculosis, or MRSA.

FIGURE 9-10 Sample instruction card, system B.

(Front of Card)

Visitors - Report to Nurses' Station Before Entering Room

1. Private room indicated? ______ No
   ______ Yes
2. Masks indicated? ______ No
   ______ Yes for those close to patient
   ______ Yes for all persons entering room
3. Gowns indicated? ______ No
   ______ Yes for all persons entering room
4. Gloves indicated? ______ No
   ______ Yes for touching infective material
   ______ Yes for all persons entering room
5. Special precautions indicated for handling blood? ______ No
   ______ Yes
6. Hands must be washed after touching the patient or potentially contaminated articles and before taking care of another patient.
7. Articles contaminated with ______________ (infected materials) should be discarded or bagged and labeled before being sent for decontamination and reprocessing.

(Back of Card)

Instruction for the Head Nurses or Team Leader

1. On Table B. Disease-Specific Precautions, locate the disease for which isolation precautions are indicated.
2. Write disease in blank space here: ______________
3. Determine if a private room is indicated. In general, patients infected with the same organism may share a room. For some diseases or conditions, a private room is indicated if patient hygiene is poor. A patient with poor hygiene does not wash hands after touching infective material (feces, purulent drainage, or secretions), contaminates the environment with infective material, or shares contaminated articles with other patients.
4. Place a check mark beside the indicated precautions on front of card.
5. Cross through precautions that are *not* indicated.
6. Write infective material in blank space in item 7 on front of card.

KEY IDEAS

Face Masks

When a patient's infectious condition can be spread by breathing, face masks are very important (see Figure 9-11). Before you put on or take off a face mask, be sure your hands are clean. Face masks are effective for 30 minutes only. If you stay in an isolated area longer, you must wash your hands and remove the old mask. Then wash your hands

FIGURE 9-11 If a patient's infectious condition can be spread by breathing, a face mask is an important piece of equipment. The mask must cover the mouth and nose.

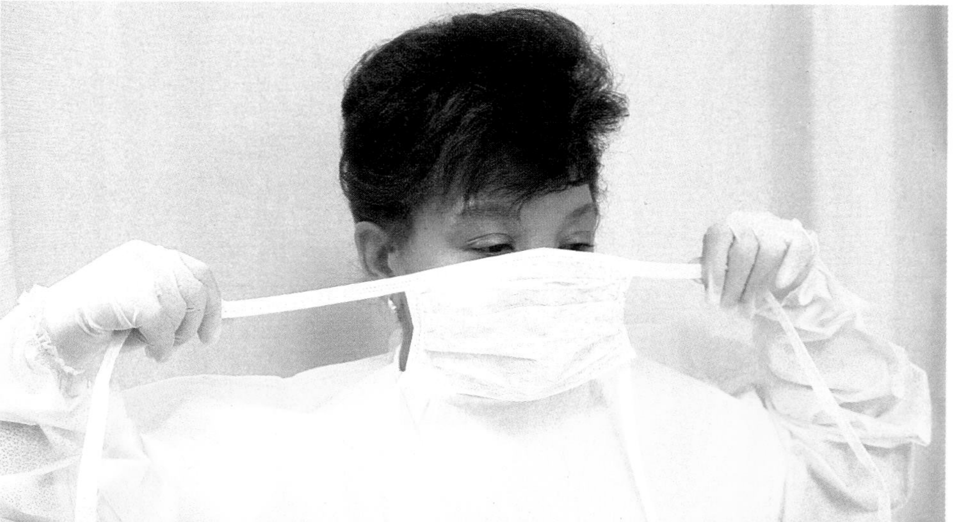

Procedure Mask Technique

1. Assemble your equipment: a disposable paper mask.
2. Wash your hands.
3. Remove a clean mask from its container.
4. Hold the mask firmly, avoiding unnecessary handling. Do not touch the part of the mask that will cover your face. Hold the mask by the strings or elastic only.
5. Place the mask over your nose and mouth. Tie the top strings over your ears first. Then tie the lower strings. Elastic loops are applied in similar fashion. If there is a nose piece, bend it to fit snugly.
6. Be sure the mask covers your nose and mouth during your task or procedure with the patient.
7. When you are ready to take off the mask, wash your hands.
8. Untie the bottom ties first, to avoid contamination. Hold the mask by the strings or loops only.
9. Untie the top strings. Remove the mask from your face. Discard it in the proper container inside the patient's room.
10. Wash your hands.

again and put on a clean mask. Masks are used only once and then discarded. If the mask gets wet, it must be changed. **Never let the face mask hang around your neck.**

KEY IDEAS

Isolation Gowns

Isolation Gown
A special gown worn over a uniform when coming in contact with a patient with a communicable infectious disease. The gown helps protect the uniform from being contaminated by harmful bacteria.

You will wear an **isolation gown** when indicated in caring for a patient in isolation. You will wear the gown if there is any possibility that your clothes could be contaminated with blood or body fluids or touch the patient or brush against any articles in the unit in strict isolation. Remember, everything in the unit is considered contaminated. There are three types of isolation gowns:

1. Cotton twill, which is reusable after proper washing.
2. A paper disposable gown, which is thrown away after one use.
3. A plastic disposable apron, which is worn once and thrown away.

Individual Gown Technique

A gown should be used only once. It is then discarded in the proper dirty linen container or trash can. This is done before you leave the isolation room.

To be effective, the isolation gown must cover your uniform completely. Therefore, it is made wide enough to overlap in the back.

Put on a clean gown in the hall before you enter the patient's room. Take off the dirty gown in the patient's room before leaving the unit.

KEY IDEAS

Double Bagging

***Note:* The Centers for Disease Control now indicate that all used linen is to be treated as contaminated. Follow the policy of your employing health care institution concerning bagging.** If double bagging is indicated, follow the steps shown in Figure 9-15.

Procedure Putting on an Isolation Gown in the Hall before Entering the Patient's Room

Refer to Figures 9-12 through 9-14.

1. If you are wearing a long-sleeve uniform, roll your sleeves above your elbows. Wash your hands.
2. Unfold the isolation gown so the opening is at the back.
3. Put your arms into the sleeves of the isolation gown.
4. Fit the gown at the neck, making sure your uniform is covered.
5. Reach behind and tie the neck band with a simple shoelace bow or fasten an adhesive strip.
6. Grasp the edges of the gown and pull to the back.
7. Overlap the edges of the gown; completely closing the opening and covering your uniform completely.
8. Tie the waist tapes in a bow or fasten the adhesive strip.

FIGURE 9-12

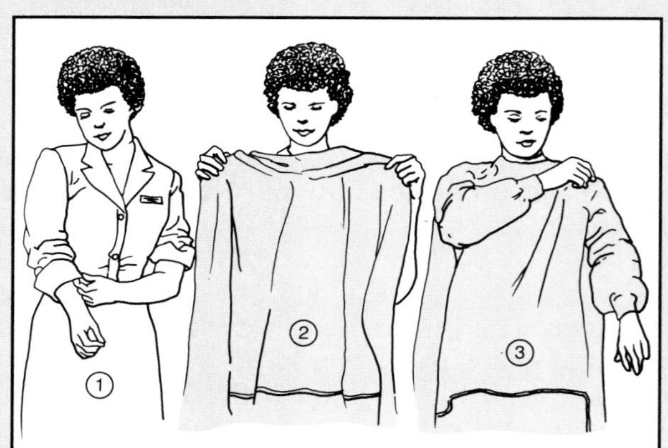

FIGURE 9-13

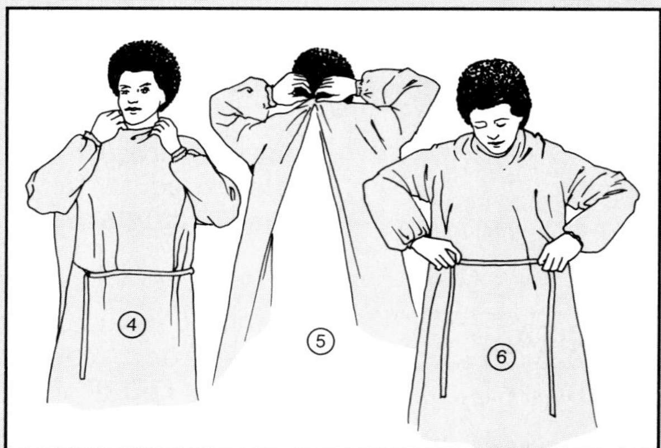

FIGURE 9-14

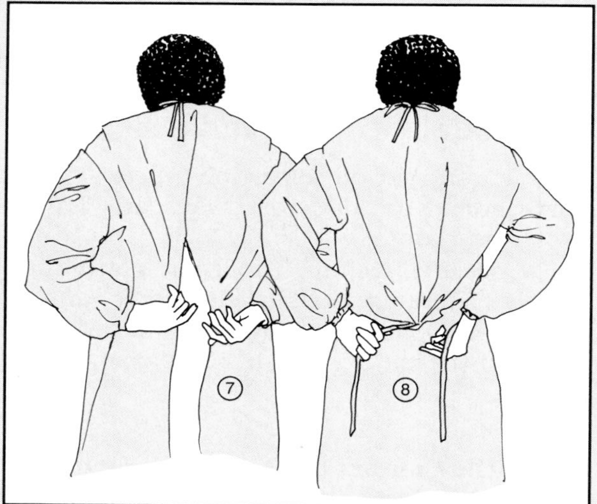

FIGURE 9-15 Double bagging technique. The double bag technique should be applied when removing linen, trash, and other contaminated articles from the isolation room.

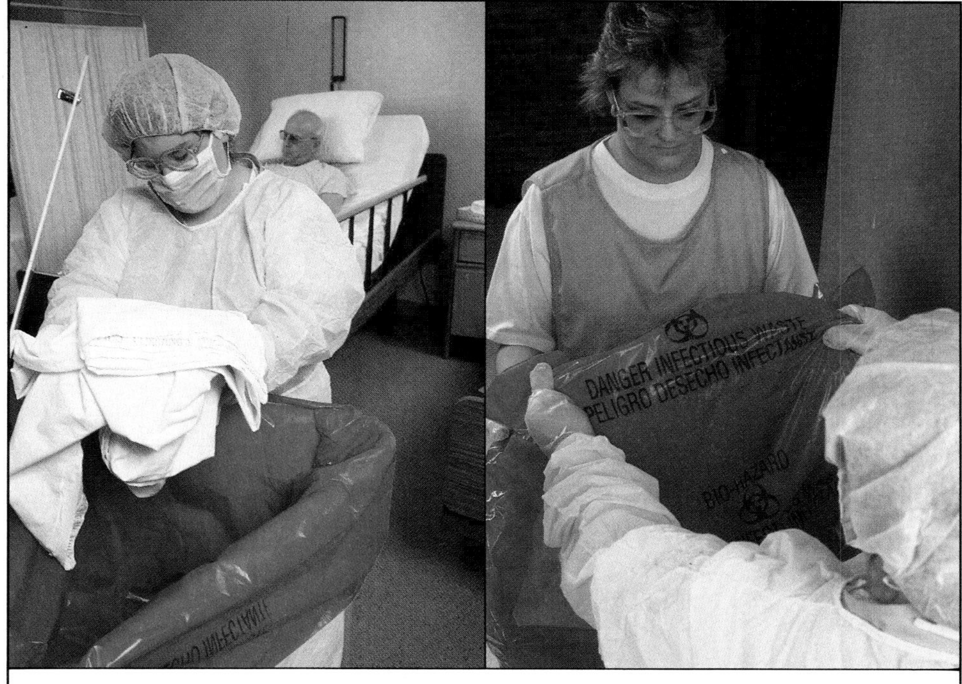

- Place linen in laundry bag inside isolation unit
- Seal bag

- Place sealed bag inside another bag outside the isolation unit

Procedure Removing an Isolation Gown inside the Patient's Room

1. If you are wearing disposable gloves, remove and discard them.
2. Untie the waist tapes and loosen the gown.
3. Open the neck band of the isolation gown by untying the strings. While still holding the strings, pull the gown off your shoulders.
4. Remove the gown by rolling it away from yourself into a ball.
5. Roll the gown with the contaminated portion inside.
6. If the gown is washable, put it in the dirty linen hamper inside the patient's room. If the gown is disposable, place it in the trash container inside the patient's room.
7. If also wearing a face mask, remove it at this time.
8. Wash your hands, using paper towels to turn the faucet on and off.

KEY IDEAS

Personal Care of the Patient on Isolation

The patient on isolation needs the same personal care as any other patient. It is very important to combine normal patient care with good isolation technique. These tasks should be performed in your usual pleasant and supportive style. Make it clear that it is the disease-causing microorganisms that are unwanted and not the patient. You will make continuous observations to note any pattern of change in the patient's appearance or behavior. Treat the patient as a complete and whole person (Figure 9-16).

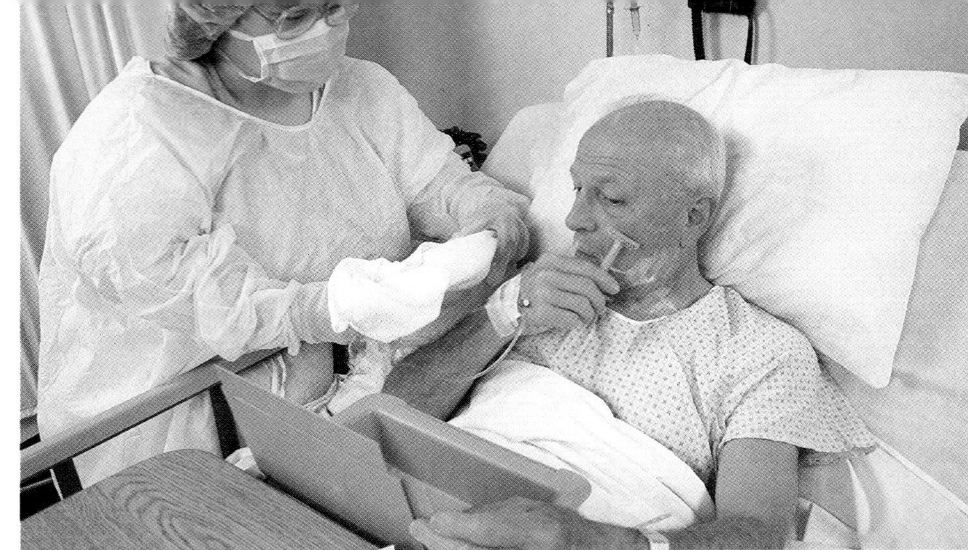

FIGURE 9-16 Disposable supplies are furnished to the isolation patient.

The Nursing Assistant's Watch

When a gown and gloves are to be worn, nursing assistants must be prepared to use a watch without contaminating it or themselves. Before entering the patient's room, the nursing assistant places the wristwatch on a clean piece of paper towel. The paper towel with the watch must be placed so that the assistant can read it easily without touching it. The nursing assistant must wash his hands before picking up the watch when leaving the isolated unit. The paper towel is picked up on the top surface only and then discarded. Some hospitals have a policy that central service provides a watch in a plastic covering, which stays inside the patient's room for the entire isolation period. Follow your institution's policy regarding a watch in an isolation unit.

Serving Food to the Patient in Isolation

Many health care institutions do not require you to wear a gown when serving meals to patients in isolation. If you are serving a patient, be careful that your uniform does not become contaminated. Wear a gown if you are required to provide patient care, for example, feed a patient or stay with him during his meal to help him eat (Figure 9-17). Food

FIGURE 9-17 Feeding an isolation patient requires the use of a gown. Head coverings are used if so instructed by the head nurse or team leader.

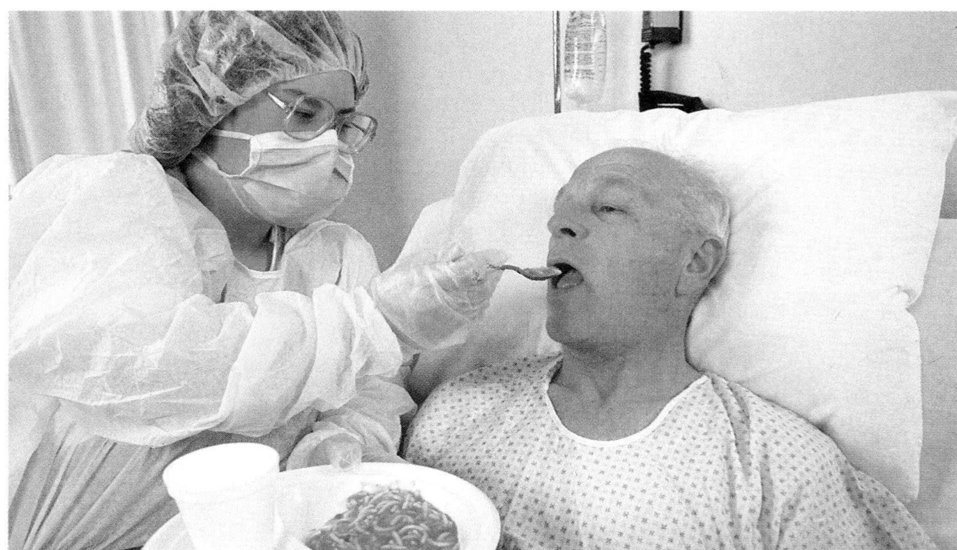

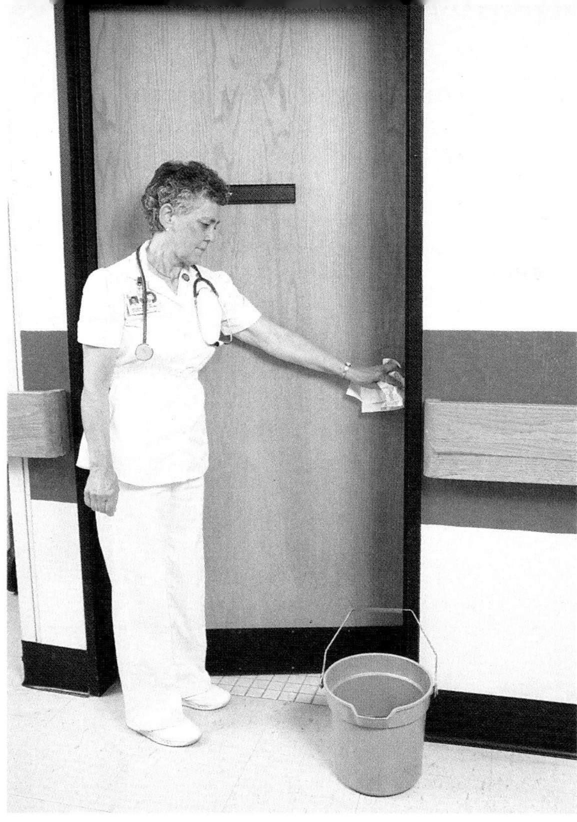

FIGURE 9-18 When leaving a patient's room after washing your hands, use a paper towel to open the room door. Then discard the paper towel in the waste paper basket inside the room as you leave the unit. Hold the door open on the outside, with your foot.

for the patient in isolation should be served in disposable dishes on a disposable tray. Uneaten food is considered to be contaminated. Scraps are disposed of in a trash container inside the patient's room. Liquids are poured down the toilet. Most institutions now treat all trays as contaminated (according to Universal Precautions). Therefore, patients in isolation often get regular trays.

Figure 9-18 shows the correct procedure for leaving the room of an isolated patient. Many institutions now have sinks in isolation-unit anterooms. Therefore paper towels are not necessary. Staff wash hands in anteroom before leaving isolation unit.

Biohazardous waste
Any solid or liquid waste that holds a potential threat of infection to humans. Examples include nonliquid tissue and body parts, laboratory waste, discarded sharps (needles, blades, etc.), blood and blood products, body fluids, and used absorbent materials (bandages, gauzes, and sponges) saturated with blood, body fluids (excretions or secretions), and/or solid waste materials.

Handling the Contaminated Articles of the Patient in Isolation

For some patients in isolation it is necessary to take special precautions with articles contaminated by urine or feces. For example, it may be necessary to disinfect (or discard) a bedpan and excreta. Follow your health care institution's procedure and the instructions of your immediate supervisor.

KEY IDEAS

Biohazardous Waste Disposal

Biohazardous waste collection containers must be clearly labeled. Sharps are collected in hard puncture-resistant and leakproof containers. Contaminated reusable linens are placed in separate collection containers and are disinfected when laundered.

Every facility must adhere to the standards set by its state regulating agency.

KEY IDEAS

OSHA (Occupational Safety and Health Administration, U.S. Department of Labor) Guidelines for Preventing Occupational Exposure to Tuberculosis

Since 1988 outbreaks of tuberculosis, which includes multidrug-resistant strains, have been identified nationwide. Tuberculosis bacillus is transmitted in the air by infectious droplet nuclei of 1 to 5 microns in size. These droplet nuclei may be generated when a person with infectious tuberculosis disease coughs, speaks, sings, or spits.

To protect the employee at occupational risk of exposure, universal precautions must be taken and a high-efficiency particulate air (H.E.P.A.) respirator mask that is NIOSH/MSHA (National Institute for Occupational Safety and Health/Mine Safety and Health Administration) approved must be worn when the employee comes in contact with suspected or active tuberculosis-infected patients. These respirators can filter particles of 0.3 microns with 99.97% efficiency. Prior to use these masks must be fit-tested.

KEY QUESTIONS

1. What is the purpose of isolation technique?
2. What is the difference between clean items or areas and dirty ones when referring to isolation technique? Give examples.
3. What is the difference between system A and system B isolation precautions?
4. Name the system A categories and list the precautions to be taken for each.
5. When, where, and how should masks and gowns be put on and taken off?
6. What is meant by double bagging technique, and when should it be used?
7. How should personal care be given to a patient in isolation?
8. How should you leave the isolation unit?
9. What is biohazardous waste and how do you dispose of it?
10. What does OSHA recommend to prevent the spread of tuberculosis?
11. Define: biohazardous waste, clean, communicable disease, dirty, isolation gown, and isolation technique.

CHAPTER

10

The Patient's Environment

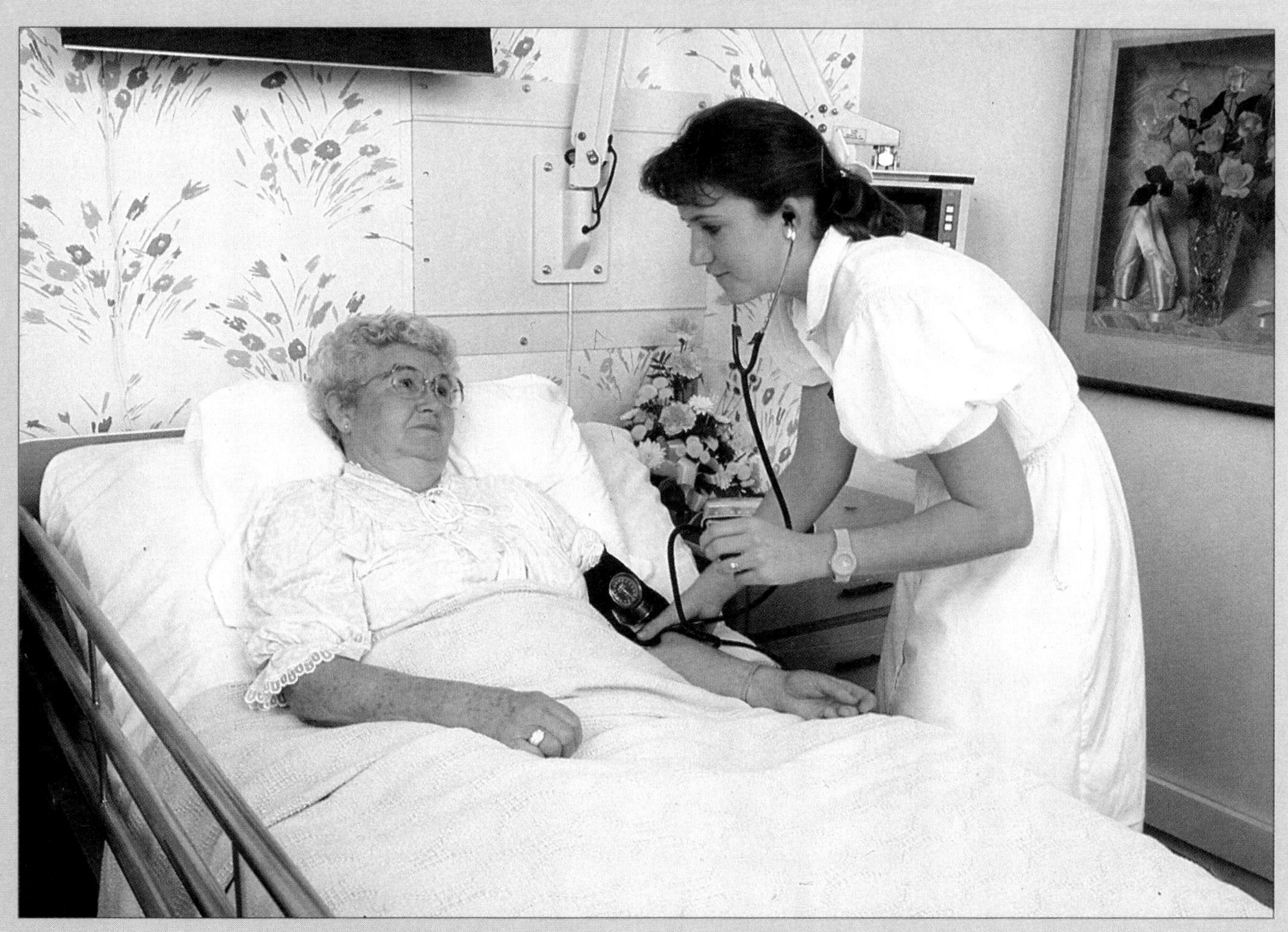

WARNING

For all patient contact, adhere to Universal Precautions. (see page 91, 97, or the front cover flap). Wear protective equipment as indicated.

Objectives

What You Will Learn

When you have completed this chapter, you will be able to:

- Describe the typical patient's unit and list the equipment it contains.
- Check the unit.
- Identify and describe the purpose of each piece of equipment.
- Define: alternating-pressure air mattress, bed cradle, bedpan, central supply room, disposable equipment, egg-crate mattress, emesis basin, equipment, heat cradle, intravenous pole, lamb's wool, patient lift, patient unit, specialty bed, stretcher, urinal, walker, wheelchair.

KEY IDEAS

The Patient's Unit

THE **PATIENT UNIT** CONSISTS OF ALL the room space, furniture, and **equipment** provided by the hospital for one patient. Each unit can be screened off for privacy by draw curtains (Figure 10-1).

Patient Unit
The space for one patient, including the hospital bed, bedside table, chair, and other equipment.

Equipment
Materials, tools, devices, supplies, furnishings, necessary things used to perform a task.

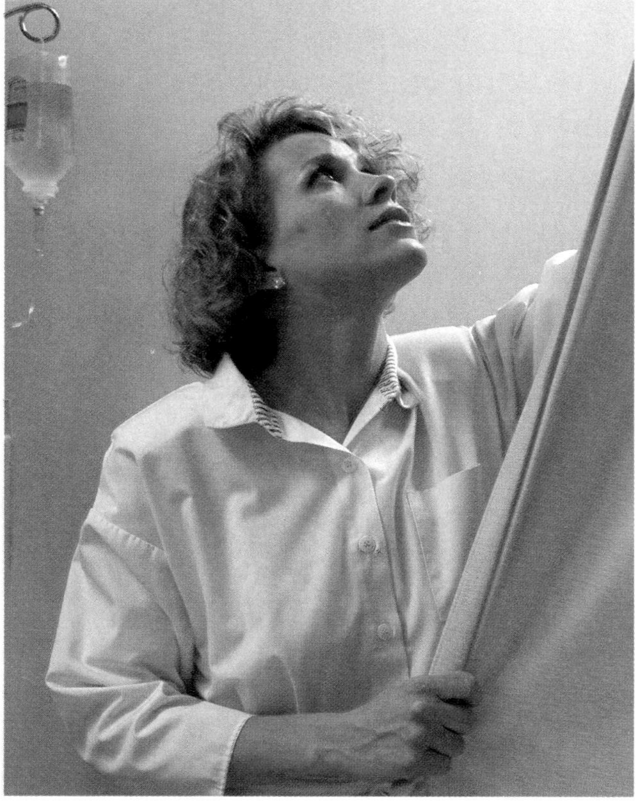

FIGURE 10-1 Adjust the curtain for the patient's privacy.

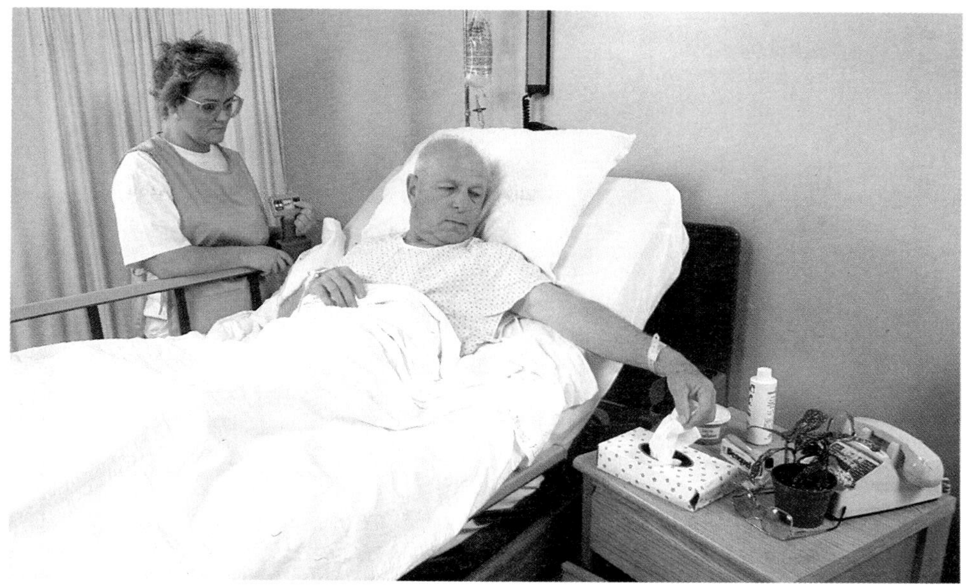

FIGURE 10-2 Check the patient's unit. Place the call signal where the patient can easily reach it. The patient should also be able to reach all articles on the table easily.

After a patient has been assigned to the unit for which you are responsible, make sure everything that belongs in the unit is there and in its proper place. If the patient is left handed, put the table and signal cord near the left hand; if the patient is right handed, place them near the right hand (Figure 10-2).

A hospital unit designed for children may be different from an adult unit (Figure 10-3). A child's age and the reason he or she is in the hospital will determine how the unit is arranged and the equipment that will be needed.

KEY IDEAS

Equipment

Alternating-pressure Air Mattress
A pad similar to an air mattress that can be placed beneath the patient to reduce pressure on the shoulders, back, heels, and elbows.

The modern health care institution has many pieces of large equipment needed for patient care and treatment. This equipment might include:

- **Alternating-pressure (A-P) mattress.** A device like an air mattress placed beneath the bedridden or elderly patient. It reduces pressure on the shoulders, back, heels, and elbows.
- **Bed board.** A large board placed beneth the mattress to provide additional support for patients with back muscle or bone problems.

FIGURE 10-3 The pediatric unit.

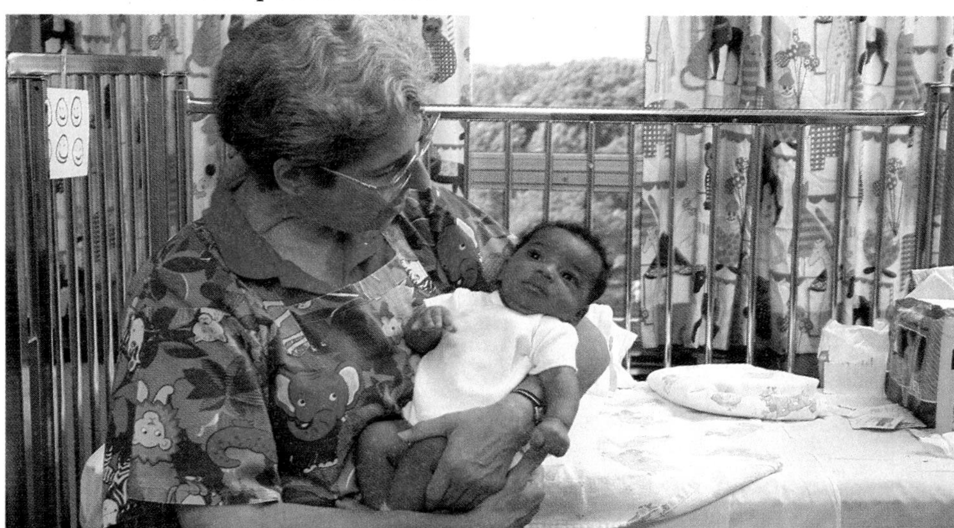

Bed Cradle
A frame shaped like a barrel cut in half lengthwise used to keep bed linens off a part of the patient's body.

Egg-crate Mattress
A foam pad shaped like an egg carton with many depressions and fingerlike projections used in addition to a mattress pad to reduce pressure on the back, shoulders, heels, elbows, and bony prominences.

Heat Cradle
A combination of a bed cradle and a heat lamp used for dry heat applications or to maintain the temperature of a warm compress.

Intravenous Pole
Also called IV pole. A tall pole on rollers or casters used to hold the containers or tubes needed, for example, during a blood transfusion.

Lamb's Wool
A wide strip of lamb's hide with the fleece attached or an imitation material used to relieve pressure in the treatment or prevention of bed sores.

Patient Lift
A mechanical device with a sling seat used for lifting a patient into and out of such equipment as the hospital bed, bathtub, or wheelchair.

Specialty Bed
A bed that constantly changes pressure under the patient. Used to minimize pressure points in the treatment or prevention of bed sores.

Stretcher
A narrow rolling table with or without a mattress or simply a canvas stretched over a frame used to transport patients. The latter may also be called a litter or a gurney.

Walker
A stable frame made of metal tubing using to support the unsteady patient while walking. The patient holds the walker while taking a step, moves it forward, and takes another step.

Wheelchair
A chair on wheels used to transport patients.

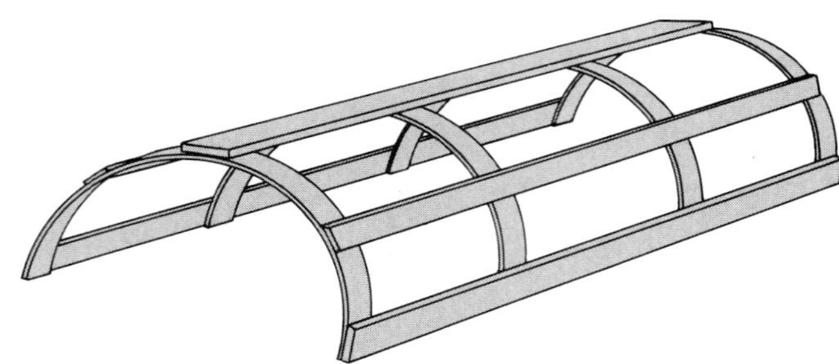

FIGURE 10-4 The bed cradle is used to keep bed linens off a part of the patient's body.

- **Bed cradle.** This cradle looks like a half-barrel cut the long way (Figure 10-4). It is used to cover a part of the patient's body where she or he is having great pain, to eliminate pressure and to support the weight of the top linen, to eliminate additional pain in the area, or when you do not want anything to touch that area.
- **Binders.** Strips of heavy cotton cloth with Velcro fasteners. Binders are wrapped securely around the patient's body over the abdomen to give support and comfort following abdominal surgery.
- **Egg-crate mattress** (sometimes called the egg-shell mattress). It reduces pressure on the back, shoulders, heels, elbows, and bony prominences.
- **Foot board.** A small board placed upright at the foot of the bed and used to keep the patient's feet aligned properly to prevent foot drop.
- **Heat cradle.** The heat cradle is the same as a regular bed cradle, but it has an electric light in it. It acts as a heat lamp. The heat cradle is sometimes ordered alone (dry). Sometimes it is ordered when the patient is having continuous warm compresses applied to an arm or leg. Here the purpose would be to keep the compress warm.
- **Intravenous poles.** These are often called IV poles. They support the containers or tubes used in various treatments. Some IV poles are on casters or rollers for easy movement. Other IV poles fit into the bed frame.
- **Lamb's wool.** Wide strips of lamb's wool cloth (or soft synthetic materials) used to relieve pressure in the treatment or prevention of bedsores.
- **Portable patient lift.** A mechanical device used to move the patient from bed to chair and back again, when the patient needs full assistance.
- **Protective devices.** Devices, usually of cotton, used to restrain a patient's arms, legs, or body to prevent him from injuring himself.
- **Specialty bed.** Used to eliminate pressure points and prevent bedsores.
- **Stretcher.** A narrow table on wheels used to transport patients. Also called a litter or gurney.
- **Walker.** The walker is a supportive device used by the patient for help in walking.
- **Wheelchair.** A chair with wheels used to transport patients.

A number of the preceding items are shown in Figure 10-5.

FIGURE 10-5 Health care equipment.

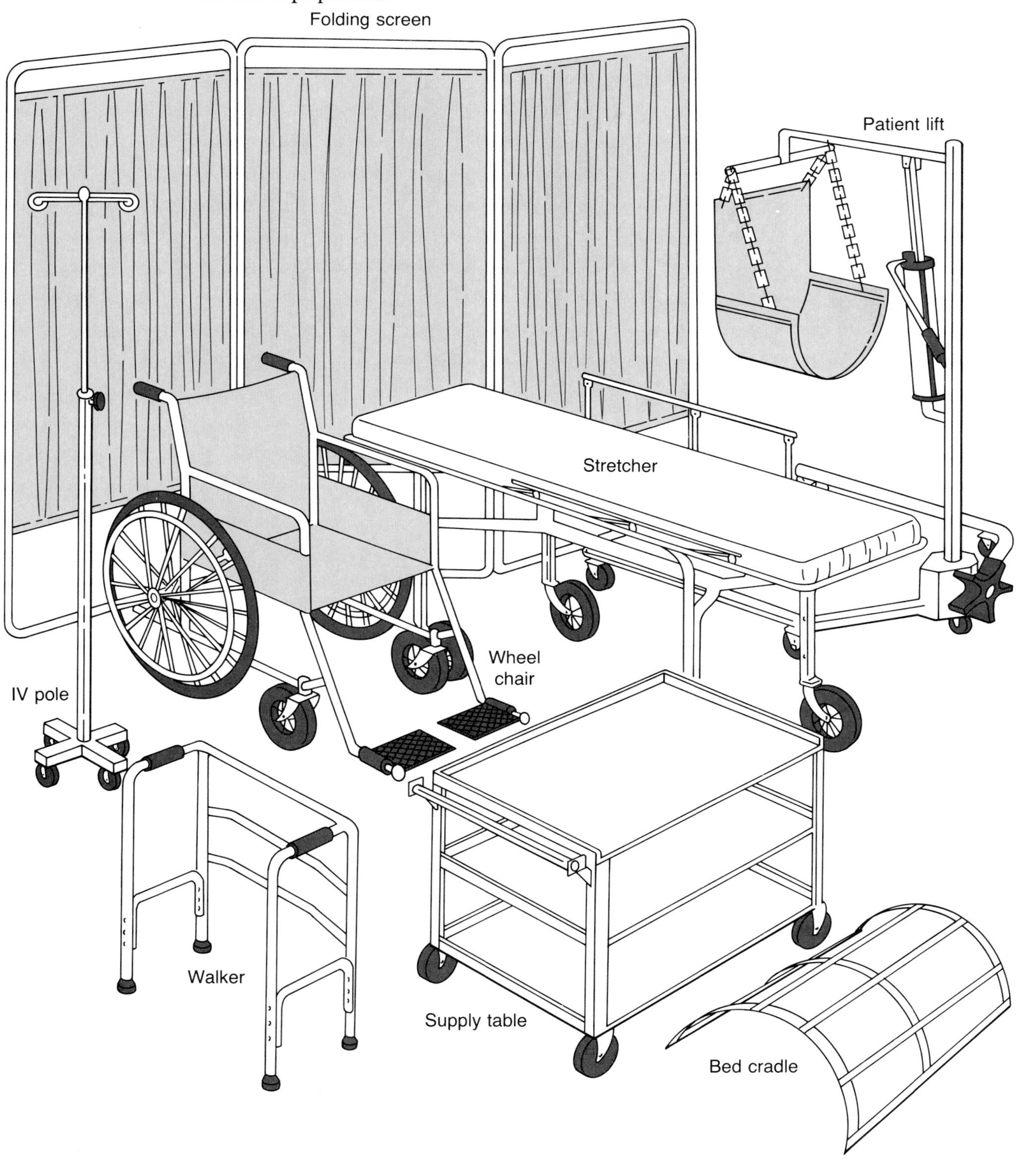

Disposable Equipment
Equipment that is used one time only or for one patient only and then thrown away.

Disposable Equipment

Today, in most health care institutions, standard equipment has been replaced by **disposable equipment** (Figure 10-6). Standard equipment requires washing, disinfecting, and sterilizing. Disposable equipment needs almost no care and is usually prepackaged. It may be made of

FIGURE 10-6 Disposable equipment.

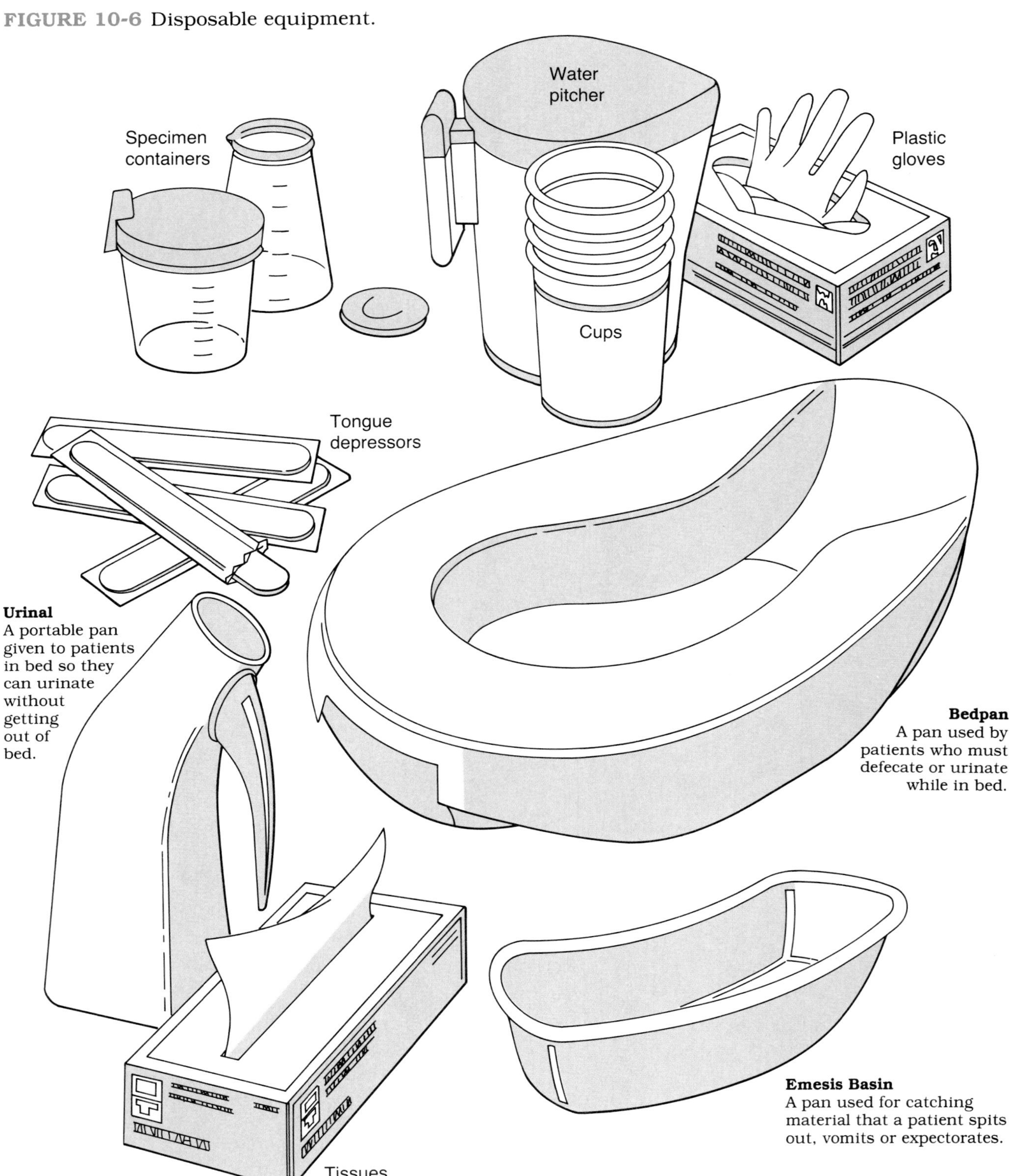

Urinal
A portable pan given to patients in bed so they can urinate without getting out of bed.

Bedpan
A pan used by patients who must defecate or urinate while in bed.

Emesis Basin
A pan used for catching material that a patient spits out, vomits or expectorates.

plastic, Styrofoam®, or paper. Some of this equipment is used only one time and then thrown away. Other disposable equipment may be used several times for one patient only, being cleaned between uses, and is thrown away when the patient is discharged.

Nursing assistants usually get disposable equipment from the **Central Supply Room** as needed. Central supply may also be called Special Purchasing Department or Central Supply Department. This is a central place for storing supplies and equipment. You will need a requisition slip to get equipment from Central Supply. In some institutions disposable equipment is stored in a clean utility room in each area, which is kept stocked by the central department.

Central Supply Room
A central place for storing supplies and equipment, also called special purchasing department or central supply department.

KEY QUESTIONS

1. What equipment does the typical patient unit contain?
2. What should you do to check the patient's unit?
3. Describe each piece of equipment and explain its purpose.
4. Define: alternating-pressure air mattress, bed cradle, bedpan, central supply room, disposable equipment, egg-crate mattress, emesis basin, heat cradle, intravenous pole, lamb's wool, patient lift, patient unit, specialty bed, stretcher, urinal, walker, wheelchair.

CHAPTER

11

Bedmaking

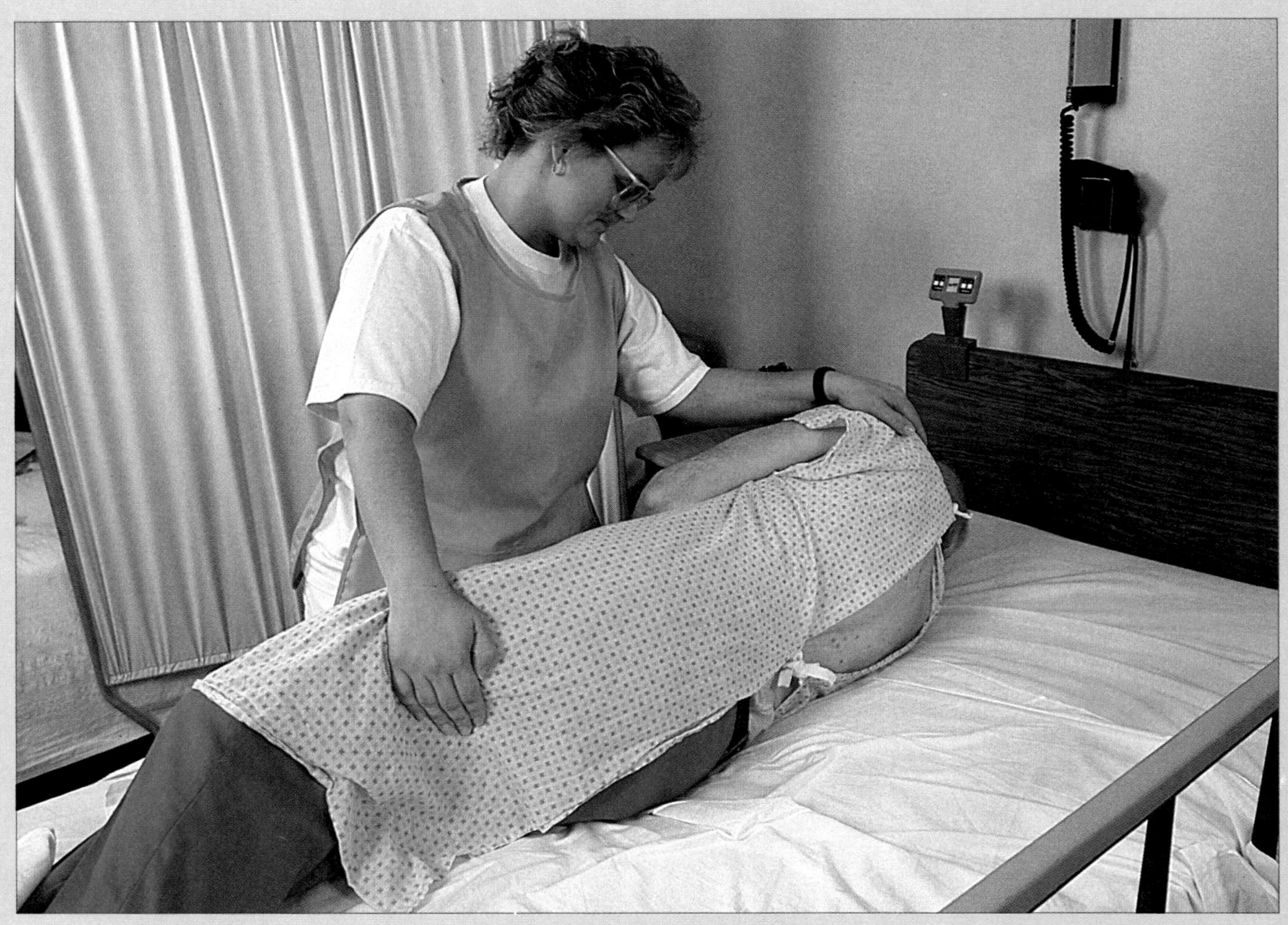

WARNING

For all patient contact, adhere to Universal Precautions (see pages 91, 97, or the front cover flap). Wear protective equipment as indicated.

Objectives

What You Will Learn

When you have completed this chapter, you will be able to:

- Explain the reason for making the patient's bed with great care.
- Identify and describe the four basic beds.
- List the rules to follow for bedmaking.
- Make the closed bed.
- Make the open, fan-folded bed.
- Make the occupied bed.
- Make the operating room bed (OR, stretcher, postoperative bed, surgical bed, recovery room bed).
- Define: bottom of the bed, closed bed, decubitus ulcers, draw sheet, fan-fold, occupied bed, open bed, postoperative bed, top of the bed.

KEY IDEAS

Bedmaking

Decubitus Ulcers
Now called skin breakdown or pressure ulcers. Once called "bedsores"; areas of the skin that become broken; often caused by continuous pressure on a body part.

PATIENTS SPEND MOST OF THEIR TIME in bed. Some patients are unable or are not permitted to get out of bed. As a result of this, many patients eat, bathe, and use a bedpan in bed. Therefore, it is important to make the patient's bed with great care.

Nursing assistants should make beds without any wrinkles in the sheets. Wrinkles are not only uncomfortable but restrict the patient's circulation and can cause skin breakdown **(decubitus ulcers)**. Making the bed carefully is very important to the patient's comfort and well-being.

Four Basic Beds

- **Closed bed** (Figure 11-1). This bed is made after environmental service personnel have cleaned the unit following a patient's discharge. The bed is made up *closed* so that it will stay clean until a new patient is assigned to it.
- **Open bed** (Figure 11-2). When a patient is assigned to a unit, the closed bed is made into an open bed by fan-folding the top sheets down to the foot of the bed.
- **Occupied bed** (Figure 11-3). Sometimes a patient is completely bedridden. The bed is made with the patient in the bed.
- **Postoperative bed** (Figure 11-4). This also may be called the OR (operating room), surgical, recovery, or stretcher bed. A special method is used to make this bed for a patient who is returning to the unit after surgery.

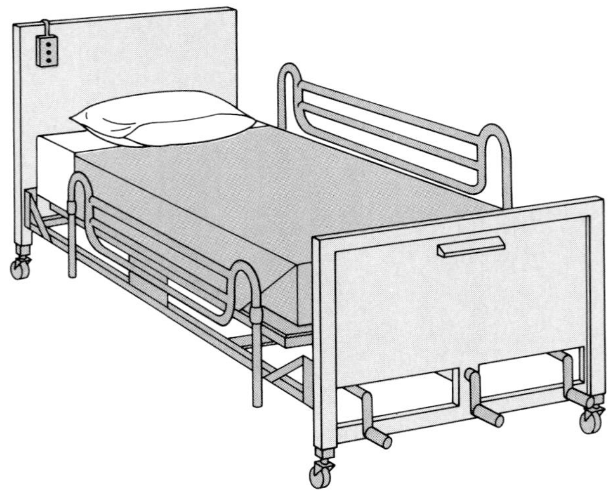

FIGURE 11-1 Closed bed.

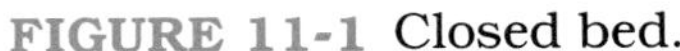

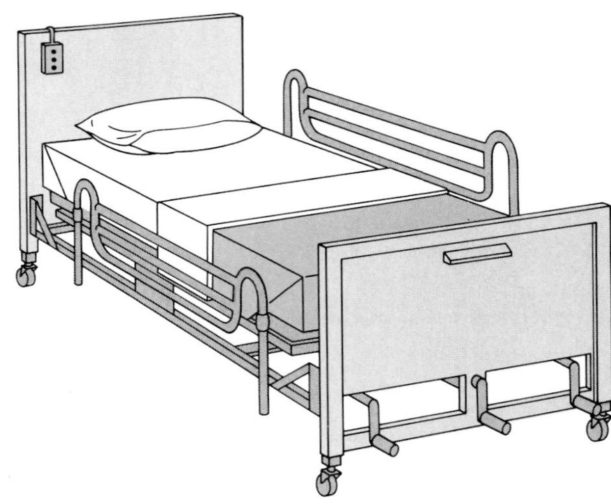

FIGURE 11-2 Open bed.

FIGURE 11-3 Occupied bed.

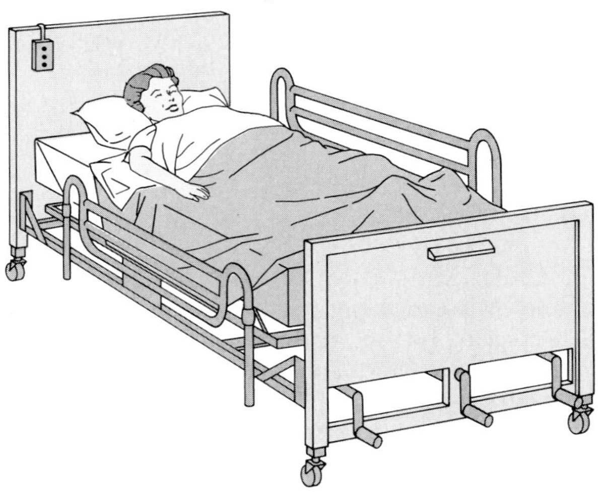

Closed Bed
A method of bedmaking where the top of the bed is closed so it will say clean until a new patient is assigned to it. This is also called an empty bed.

Open Bed
A method of bedmaking where the top of the bed is opened so that the patient can get into bed easily. This is also called a fan-folded or empty bed.

FIGURE 11-4 Postoperative bed.

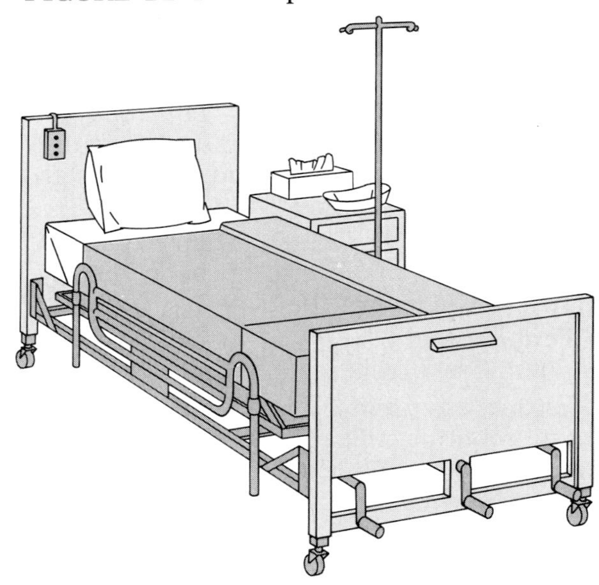

Occupied Bed
A method of making the bed with the patient in it. Used when the patient is not able or permitted to get out of bed.

Postoperative Bed
A standard hospital bed made up in a special way for a patient who is coming back to his or her unit after an operation. Sometimes called recovery bed, stretcher bed, or operating room bed.

Rules to Follow
BEDMAKING

- Return torn linen to a repair box in the linen closet for repair. Never use a torn piece of linen. It will probably tear even more.
- Never use a pin on any item of linen. Pins create holes in the linen.
- Never use bed linen for any purpose other than that for which it was intended.
- Report to your immediate supervisor if you see patients or visitors trying to remove articles of linen from the unit for any reason.
- Many health care institutions make the bed without the blanket or bedspread. However, the nursing assistant making the bed may leave a folded blanket at the foot of the bed to be used later, if needed.
- Do not shake the bed linen. Shaking spreads germs to everything and everyone in the room, including you.
- Never bring extra linen into a patient unit. It is considered contaminated (or dirty) and cannot be used elsewhere.
- Never allow any linen to touch your uniform.
- Dirty, used linen should never be put on the floor. Place in a laundry bag.
- In most health care institutions, the linen hamper is in the dirty utility room or on wheels in the corridor and is covered.
- Some health care institutions use melt-away plastic bags for laundry bags. These bags dissolve during the washing process. The dirty linen is put into these bags at the patient's bedside and then carried to the dirty laundry hamper or placed in a laundry chute.
- The bottom sheet must be firm, tight, and smooth under the patient. This is very important for the patient's comfort. Always make sure that the bottom sheet is tight and unwrinkled.
- By fan-folding the top of the bed, you make it easy for the patient to get back into the bed.
- The cotton **draw sheet** is about half the size of a regular sheet. When cotton draw sheets are not available, a large sheet can be folded in half widthwise (with small and large hems together). The fold must always be placed toward the head of the bed and the hems toward the foot of the bed.
- Plastic should never touch a patient's skin. If using a plastic draw sheet, be sure to cover it entirely with a cotton draw sheet.
- The plastic draw sheet and disposable bed protectors protect the mattress.
- Some health care institutions do not use a draw sheet at all. Instead, small disposable bed protectors are placed on the bed under the patient as necessary.
- **Bottom of the bed** refers to the mattress pad, if used, the bottom sheet, and the draw sheets.
- **Top of the bed** refers to the top sheet, blanket, if used, and bedspread.
- Remember that you save time and energy by first making as much of the bed as possible on one side before going to the other side.

Draw Sheet
A small sheet made of plastic or cotton placed crosswise on the middle of the bed over the bottom sheet to help protect the bedding from a patient's discharges and/or to lighten the foundation.

Bottom of the Bed
The bed linens used between the mattress and the patient, including the mattress pad, if used, the bottom sheet, and the draw sheets.

Top of the Bed
The bed linens used to cover the patient, including the top sheet, blanket, and bedspread.

Procedure Making the Closed, Empty Bed (Figure 11-5)

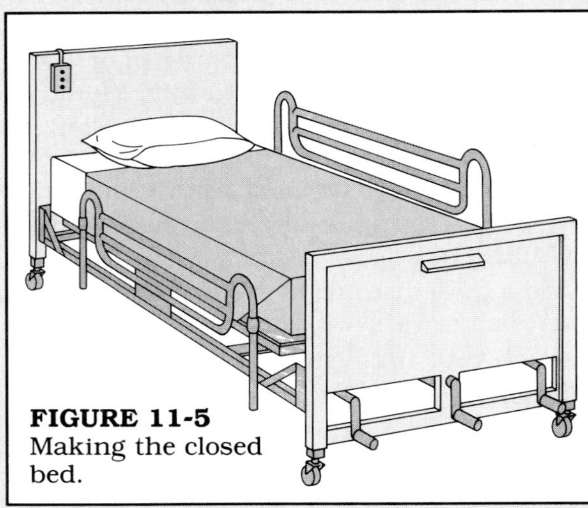

FIGURE 11-5 Making the closed bed.

1. Assemble your equipment—mattress cover (if used in your institution), bottom sheet, cotton and plastic draw sheet (or disposable bed protector), top sheet, blanket, bedspread, pillowcase, pillow, and pillow protector (if used in your institution).
2. Wash your hands.
3. Place a chair near the bed.
4. Put the pillow on the chair.
5. Stack the bedmaking linen items on the chair in the order that you will use them. First things to be used on top, last things to be used on the bottom.
6. Adjust the bed to the highest horizontal position that is comfortable for you to work at (Figure 11-6).

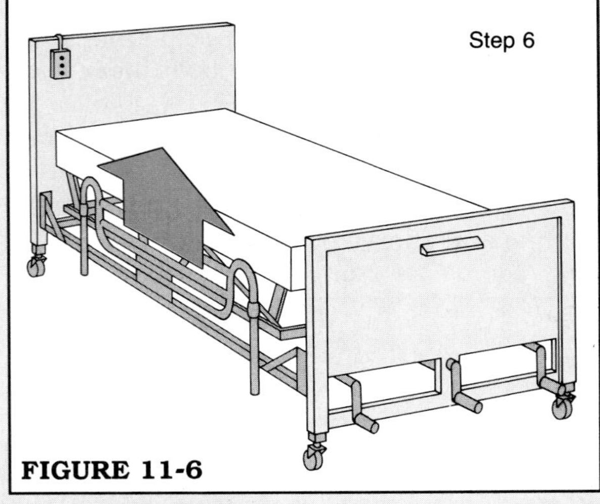

FIGURE 11-6

7. Pull the mattress to the head of the bed, until it touches the headboard.
8. Place the mattress pad on the mattress even with the head edge of the mattress, if used by your health care institution.
9. Fold the bottom sheet lengthwise and place it on the bed:
   a) Place the center fold of the sheet in the center of the mattress from head to foot (Figure 11-7).

FIGURE 11-7

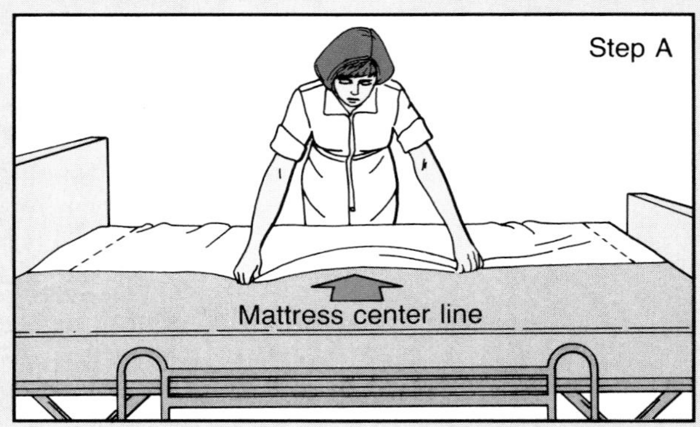

   b) Put the small hem at the foot of the bed, even with the edge of the mattress.
   c) Place the large hem to the head of the bed (Figures 11-8 and 11-9).

FIGURE 11-8

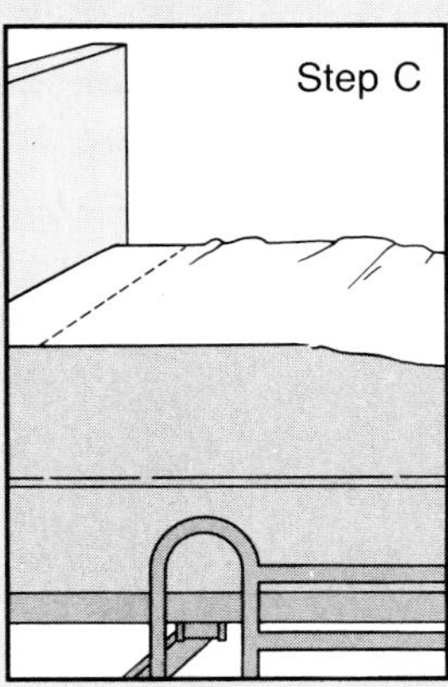

FIGURE 11-9

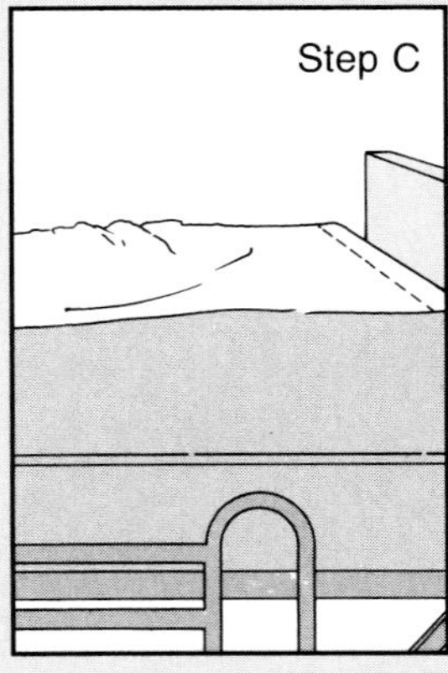

10. Open the sheet. It should now hang evenly the same distance over each side of the bed. The rough edges of the hem should now face down toward the mattress and away from the patient.
11. There should be 18 inches of the sheet to tuck smoothly and tightly under the head of the mattress.
12. To make a mitered corner:
    a) Pick up the edge of the sheet at the side of the bed 12 inches from the head of the mattress (Figure 11-10).

FIGURE 11-10

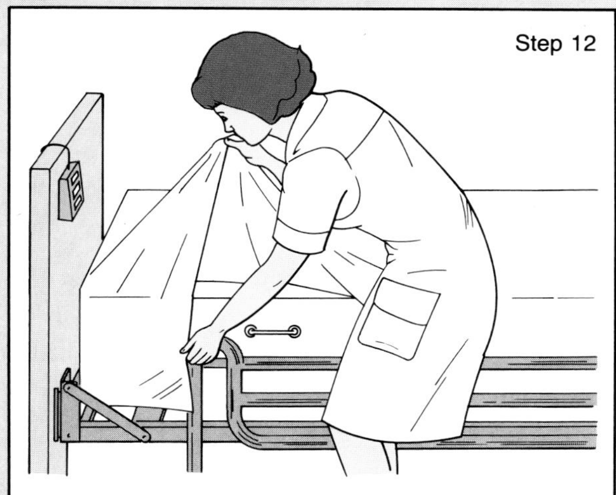

b) Place the triangle (the folded corner) on top of the mattress (Figure 11-11).

FIGURE 11-11

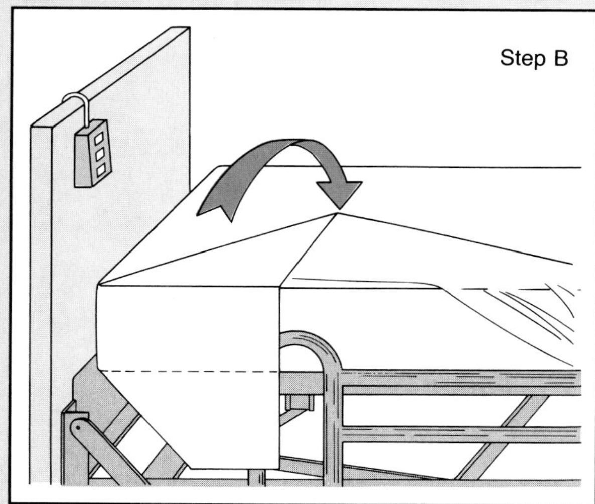

c) Tuck the hanging portion of the sheet under the mattress (Figure 11-12).

FIGURE 11-12

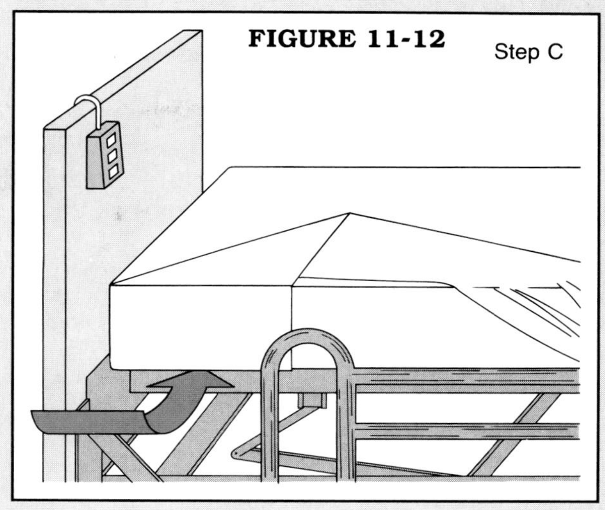

d) While you hold the fold at the edge of the mattress, bring the triangle down over the side of the mattress (Figure 11-13).

FIGURE 11-13

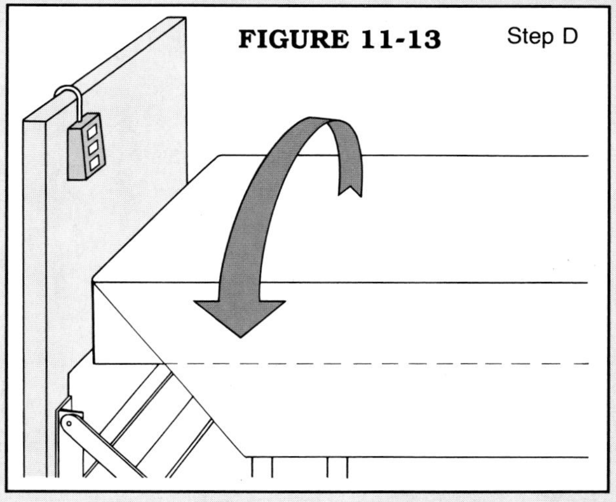

e) Tuck the sheet under the mattress from head to foot. Start at the head and pull toward the foot of the bed as you tuck (Figure 11-14).

FIGURE 11-14

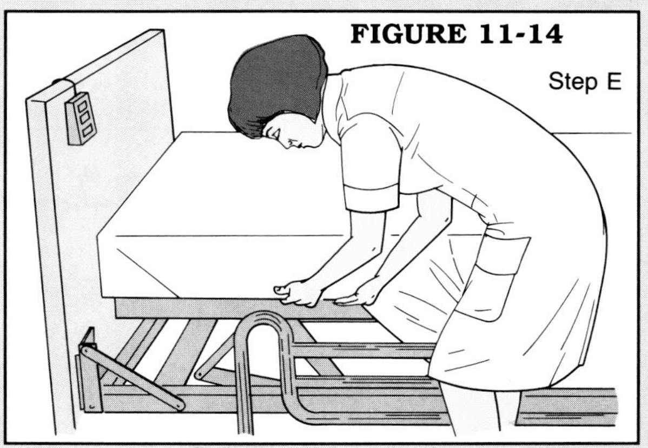

13. Stand and work entirely on one side of the bed until that side is finished.
14. Fold in half and place the plastic draw sheet 14 inches (two open-hand spans) down from the head of the bed. Tuck it in. Be sure each piece of linen is straight and even as you tuck it in (Figure 11-15).

FIGURE 11-15

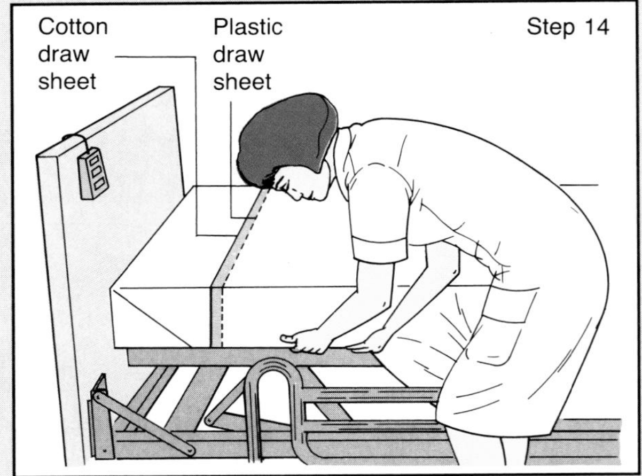

15. Cover the plastic draw sheet with the cotton draw sheet, and tuck it in.
16. Fold the top sheet lengthwise and place it on the bed:
    a) Place the center fold on the center of the bed from the head to foot (Figure 11-16).

FIGURE 11-16

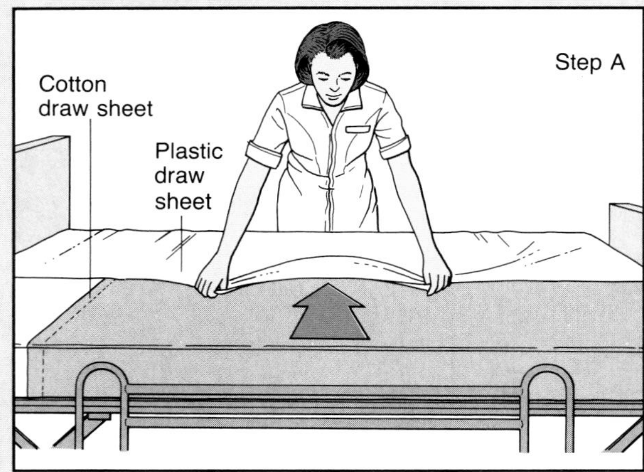

    b) Put the large hem at the head of the bed, even with the top edge of the mattress.
    c) Open the sheet, with the rough edge of the hem up, fan-folding half to the center of the bed.
    d) Tightly tuck the sheet under at the foot of the bed (Figure 11-17).

FIGURE 11-17

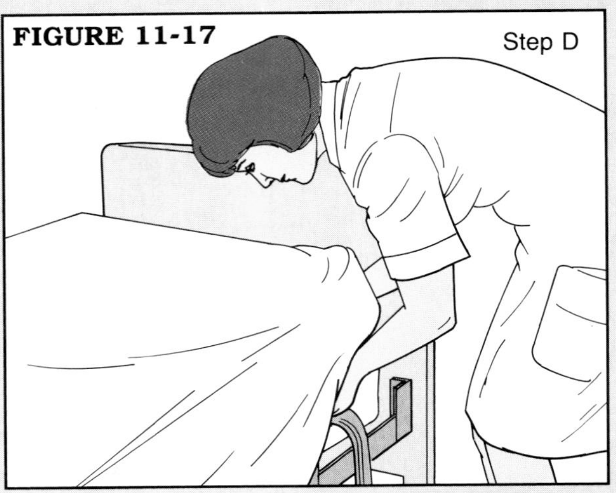

    e) Make a mitered corner at the foot of the bed (Figure 11-18).

FIGURE 11-18

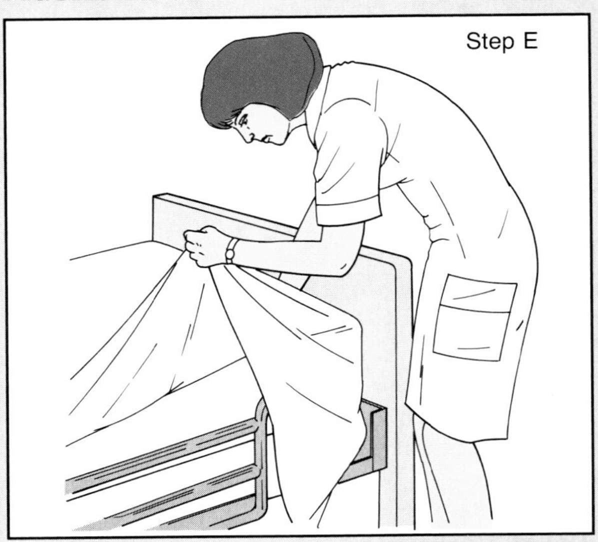

    f) Do not tuck in at the side of the bed.
17. Fold the blanket lengthwise and place on the bed.
    a) Place the center fold of the blanket in the center of the bed from head to foot.
    b) Place the upper hem 6 inches from the top edge of the mattress.
    c) Open the blanket.
    d) Tuck it under the foot tightly.
    e) Make a mitered corner at the foot of the bed.
    f) Do not tuck in at the sides of the bed.
18. Fold the bedspread lengthwise and place it on the bed.
    a) Place the center fold in the center of the bed from head to foot.
    b) Place the upper hem even with the head edge of the mattress.

c) Have the rough edge down.
d) Open the spread.
e) Tuck it under at the foot of the bed tightly.
f) Make a mitered corner at the foot of the bed.
g) Do not tuck in at the sides of the bed.

19. Now go to the other side of the bed. Start with the bottom sheet:
a) Pull the sheet tight to get rid of all wrinkles.
b) Miter the top corner.
c) Pull the plastic draw sheet tight and tuck it in.
d) Pull the cotton draw sheet tight and tuck it in (Figure 11-19).

FIGURE 11-19

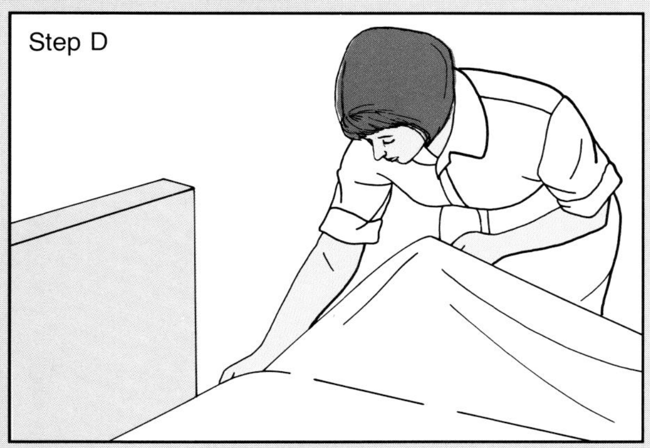

e) Straighten out the top sheet, making the mitered corner at the foot of the bed.
f) Miter the corner of the blanket.
g) Miter the corner of the bedspread.

20. To make the cuff:
a) Fold the top hem of the spread under the top hem of the blanket (Figure 11-20).

FIGURE 11-20

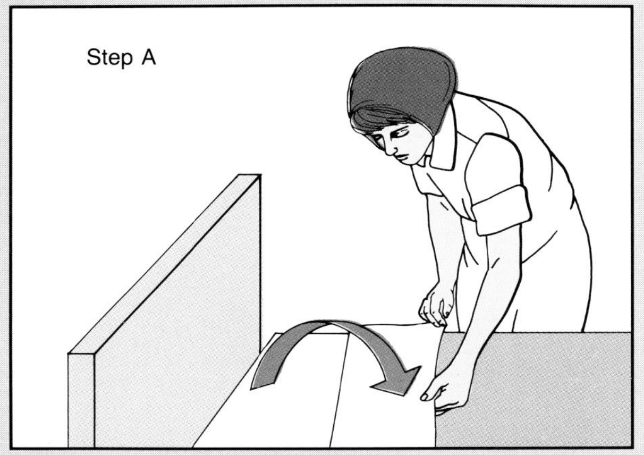

b) Fold the top hem of the sheet back over the edge of the spread and the blanket to form a cuff. The hemmed side of the sheet must be on the underside so that it does not come in contact with the patient.

21. To put the pillowcase on a pillow:
a) Hold the pillowcase at the center of the end seam.
b) With your hand outside the case, turn the case back over your hand (Figure 11-21).

FIGURE 11-21

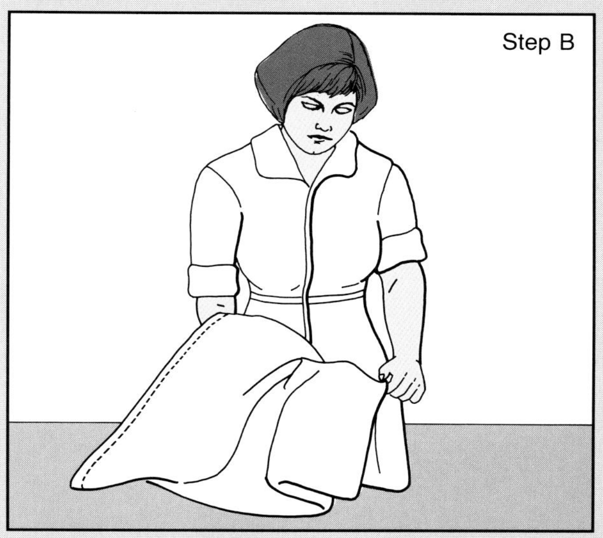

c) Grasp the pillow through the case at the center of one end of the pillow (Exhibit 11-22).

FIGURE 11-22

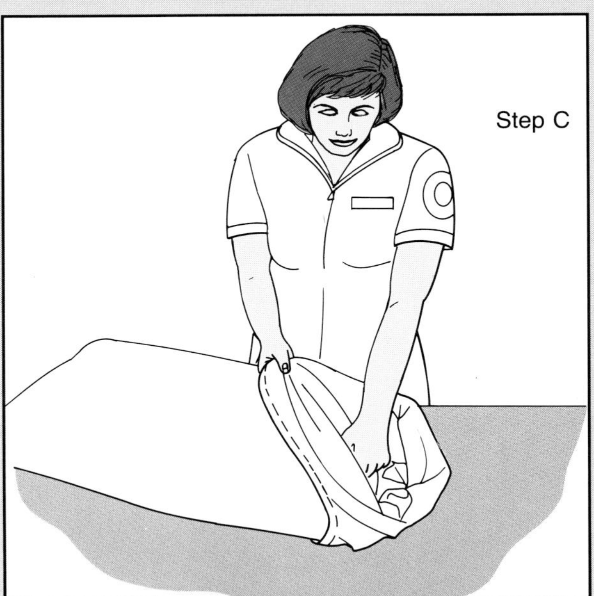

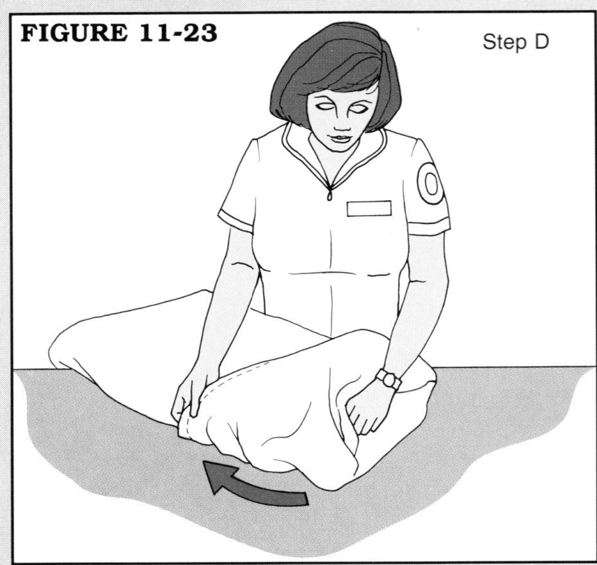

FIGURE 11-23

d) Bring the case down over the pillow (Figure 11-23).
e) Fit the corner of the pillow into the seamless corner of the case (Figure 11-24).
f) Fold the extra material from the side seam under the pillow.
g) Place the pillow on the bed with the open end away from the door.

22. Adjust bed to its lowest horizontal position (Figure 11-25).

FIGURE 11-24

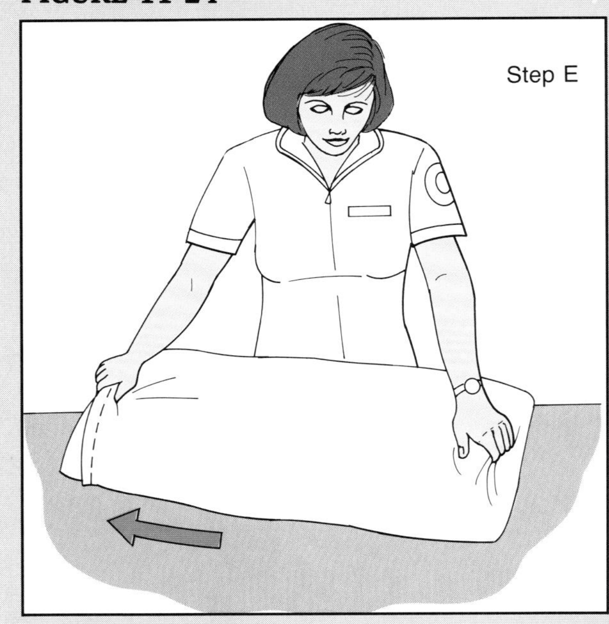

FIGURE 11-25

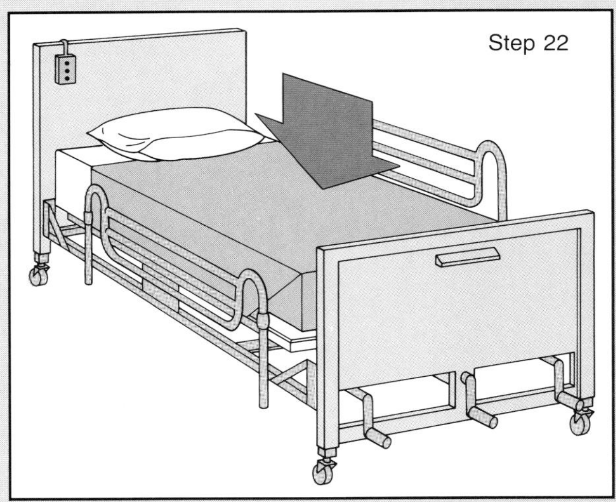

23. Wash your hands.
24. Report to your immediate supervisor that you have made the closed, empty bed.

KEY IDEAS

Open Bed, Fan-Folded Bed, and Empty Bed

Fan-fold
A method of arranging bed linens so that the covers and spread are folded back out of the way but still are on the bed and within easy reach.

The procedures for making the open bed, the **fan-folded** bed, and the empty bed are all the same. You will open the bed when a new patient has been assigned to a unit. You will be making an open bed when a unit is already occupied but the patient is able to get out of bed and move around while you arrange the unit.

The open bed is made exactly like the closed bed except for one thing. The top bedding is opened so that the patient can easily get into bed. This is done after you finish making the cuff at the head of the bed.

Procedure Making the Open, Fan-Folded, or Empty Bed

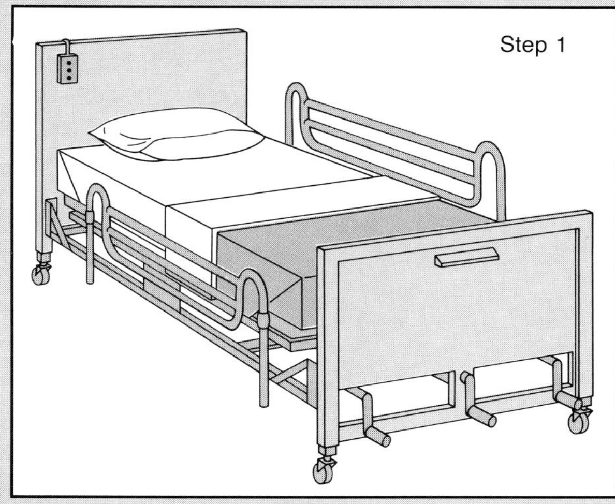

FIGURE 11-26

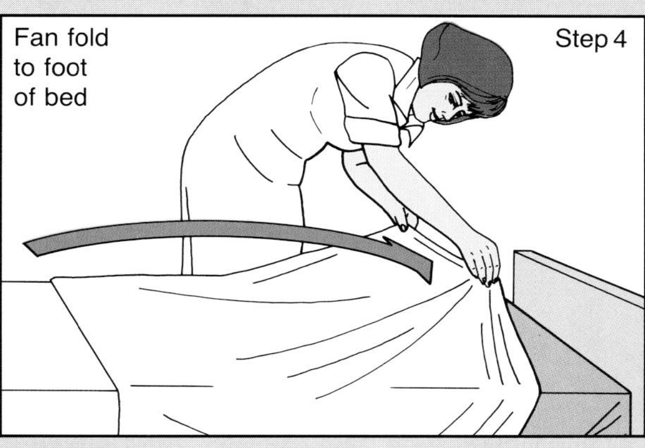

FIGURE 11-27

1. Assemble your equipment—a closed bed (Figure 11-26).
2. Wash your hands.
3. Grasp the cuff of the bedding in both hands.
4. Fan-fold to the foot of the bed (Figure 11-27).
5. Fold the bedding back on itself toward the head of the bed. The edge of the cuff must meet the fold (Figure 11-28).
6. Smooth the hanging sheets on each side neatly into the folds you have made.
7. Wash your hands.

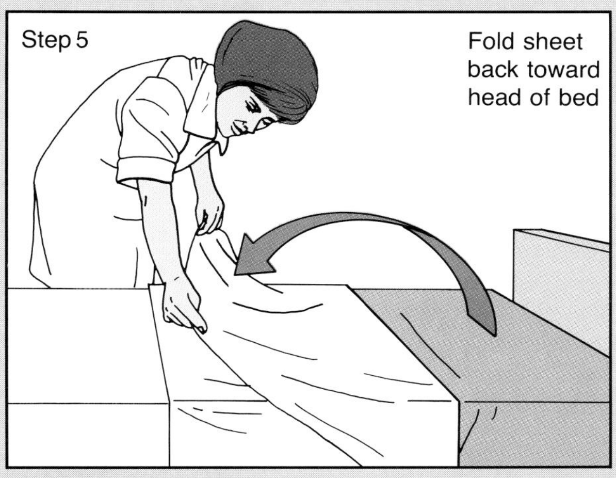

FIGURE 11-28

KEY IDEAS

Operating Room (OR) Bed

The operating room bed is also known as the postoperative bed, the OR bed, the stretcher bed, or sometimes the recovery bed. The operating room bed is used by patients returning from the postoperative recovery room or the postdelivery recovery room. The patient is brought in on a stretcher. The OR bed is positioned to match the stretcher height. The stretcher will be lined up alongside the bed to allow the transfer of the patient from the stretcher to the bed. Some institutions make this bed with bath blankets; others do not. Be sure you follow the policy of the institution that employs you. Bath blankets may be necessary due to the cold surgical environment, the probably lowered pulse and blood pressure, and the lack of patient mobility, resulting in poor circulation and poor production of body heat.

Procedure Making the Operating Room (OR) Bed or Stretcher Bed (Figure 11-29)

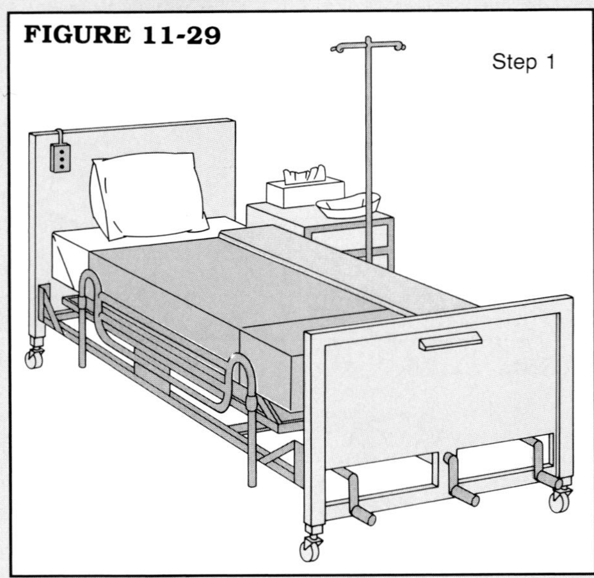

FIGURE 11-29

1. Assemble your equipment on a chair in the unit:
   a) Mattress cover, if used in your institution
   b) Bottom sheet
   c) Plastic draw sheet, if used in your facility
   d) Cotton draw sheet, if used in your facility
   e) Top sheet
   f) Blanket
   g) Pillowcase
   h) Pillow
   i) Bedspread
   j) Two cotton bath blankets. Follow the policy of your health care institution with regard to using bath blankets.
   k) Plastic laundry bag
   l) Pillow protector, if used in your institution
2. Wash your hands.
3. Adjust the bed to the highest horizontal, comfortable working position. Lock the bed in place. Strip all used linen from the bed and place in the plastic laundry bag.
4. Make the bottom part of the bed. Follow the instructions for making a closed bed.
5. Spread one bath blanket across the bed, on top of the draw sheet and bottom sheet. The bottom end of the bath blanket should be even with the foot of the mattress. Tuck the edge under the mattress on your side of the bed. Bath blankets are not used by every health care institution. Use only if applicable to your facility (Figure 11-30).

FIGURE 11-30

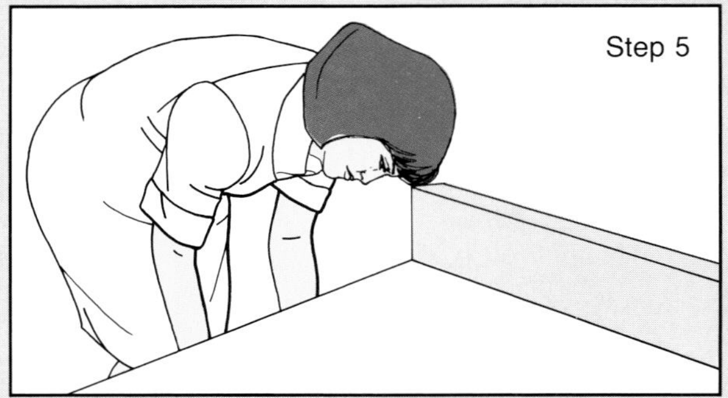

6. Go to the other side of the bed. Tuck the bath blanket under the mattress.
7. Spread the second bath blanket across the bed. The upper edge should be about 6 inches from the head of the bed. This blanket gives the patient extra warmth (Figure 11-31).

FIGURE 11-31

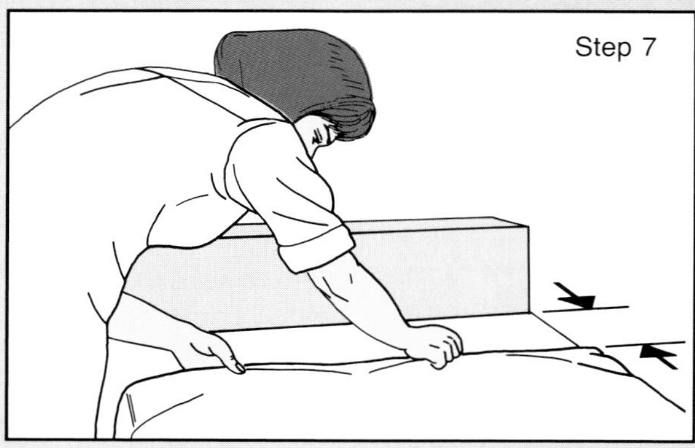

8. Put the top sheet, the regular blanket, and the spread on the bed. Do this the same way as when making the closed bed. But do not tuck them in at the foot of the bed. Instead, all the bedding at the foot end should be folded back on the bed so the folded edge is even with the foot of the mattress (Figure 11-32).

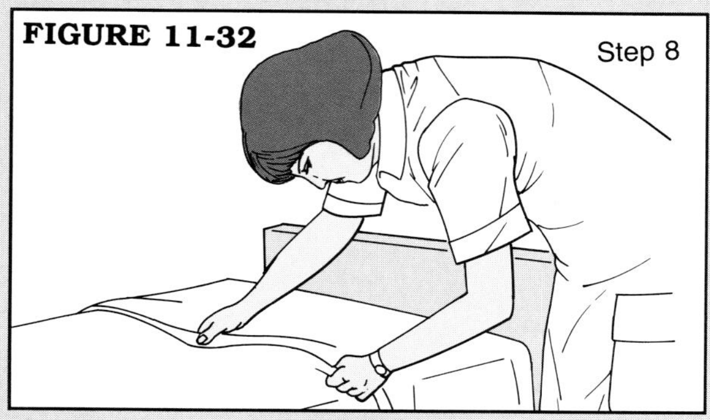

FIGURE 11-32

9. Make the cuff the same as for the open bed, except you fold the blanket over the cuff (Figure 11-33).

FIGURE 11-33

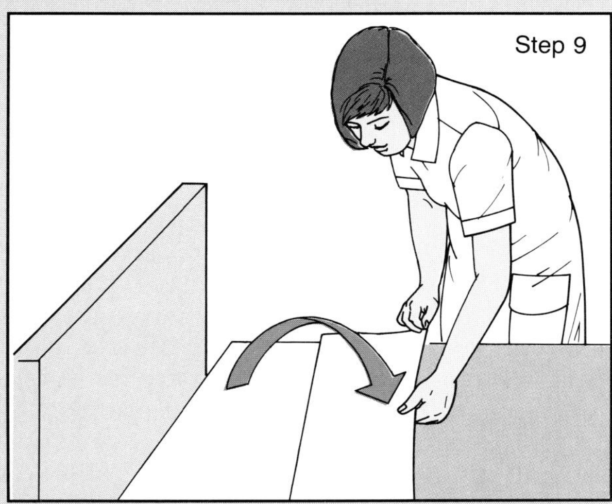

10. Go to the side of the bed where the stretcher will be in place.
11. Grasp the top bedding at the side with both hands. Fold the bedding across the bed so the folded edge is even with the far side of the mattress. Again, fold the bedding to the edge so it is twice folded onto itself (Figure 11-34).

FIGURE 11-34

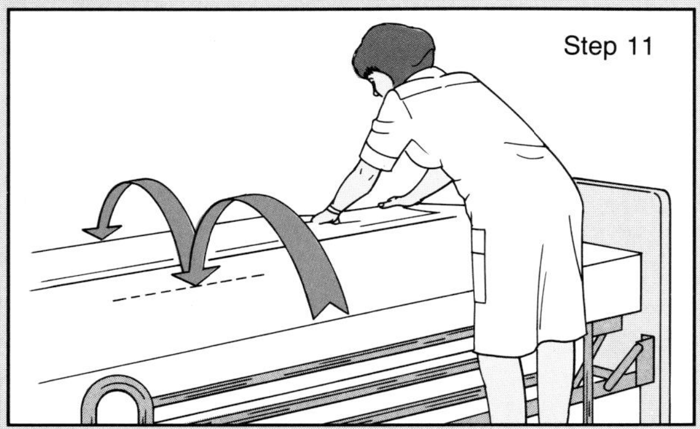

12. Put the pillow into the pillowcase. Put the pillow upright against the headboard. Place it so as to protect the patient from hitting his or her head on the headboard during the transfer procedure. When appropriate, you will place this pillow under the patient's head (Figure 11-35).

FIGURE 11-35

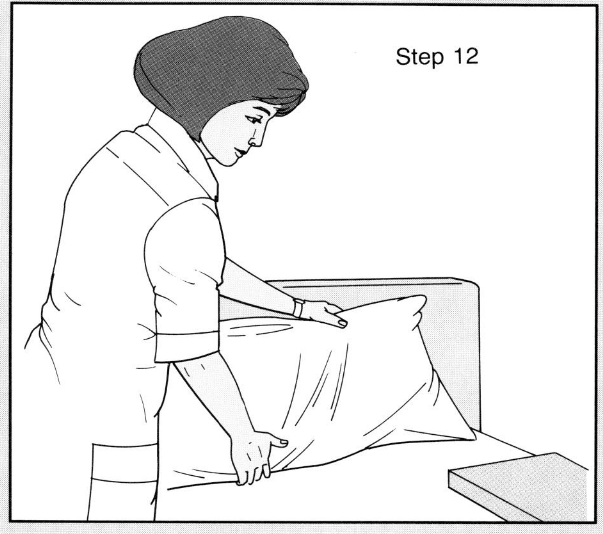

13. Move the bedside table, chair, and any other furniture out of the way to make room for the stretcher.
14. Remove everything from the bedside table except a box of tissues and an emesis basin (Figure 11-36).

FIGURE 11-36

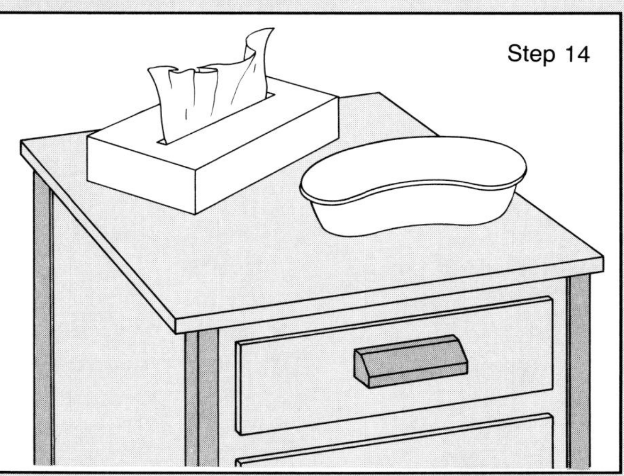

15. Bring an IV pole into the room and place near the head of the bed, out of the way (Figure 11-37).
16. Position the OR bed to match stretcher height.
17. Lower the bed to a position of safety for the patient after patient transfer from stretcher to bed. Raise the side rails.
18. Wash your hands.
19. Report to your immediate supervisor that the operating room bed has been made.

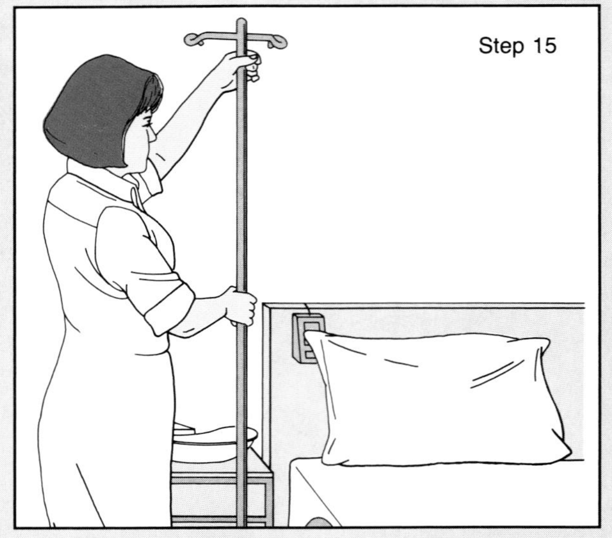

FIGURE 11-37

KEY IDEAS

Occupied Bed

The **occupied bed** is made when the patient is not able or not permitted to get out of bed. The most important part of making an occupied bed is to get the sheets smooth and tight under the patient so that there will be no wrinkles to rub against the patient's skin. When making the bottom of this bed, your job will be easier if you divide the bed in two parts—the side the patient is lying on and the side you are making, so the weight of the patient is never on the side where you are working. Always keep the side rail up on the patient's side. Usually, the occupied bed is made after giving the patient a bed bath. The patient should be covered with the bath blanket while you are making the bed. The sheets must be placed on the bed so that the rough seam edges are kept facing the mattress and away from the patient's skin.

Some institutions do not use plastic draw sheets covered by cotton sheets. Instead they use disposable bed protectors to protect the linen from getting dirty or wet. When the health care institution uses a plastic sheet covered with a draw sheet, the nursing assistant decides if the plastic sheet needs to be changed or if it can be used again according to institution policy. Usually, the plastic sheet is removed and replaced with a clean one if it is dirty or wet. If the plastic sheet does not need to be changed, follow steps 17, 18, 23, 24, 29, and 30. If you are removing the dirty sheets from the bed of an incontinent patient, simply protect the mattress by rolling the dirty wet sheets up toward the patient's back, and place a disposable bed protector around them to keep the wetness from coming through while you are making the bed. For institutions that do not use draw sheets, omit steps 17, 18, 23, 24, 29, and 30.

Some patients prefer the pillow to be moved with them from side to side as the bed is being made, and some patients ask you to remove the pillow while making the bed. Either way is acceptable for the average patient. However, there may be instances when your immediate supervisor instructs you to keep the patient flat in bed, elevated with a pillow, or in Fowler's position at all times. The nursing assistant must follow the instructions given by the immediate supervisor.

Procedure Making the Occupied Bed (Figure 11-38)

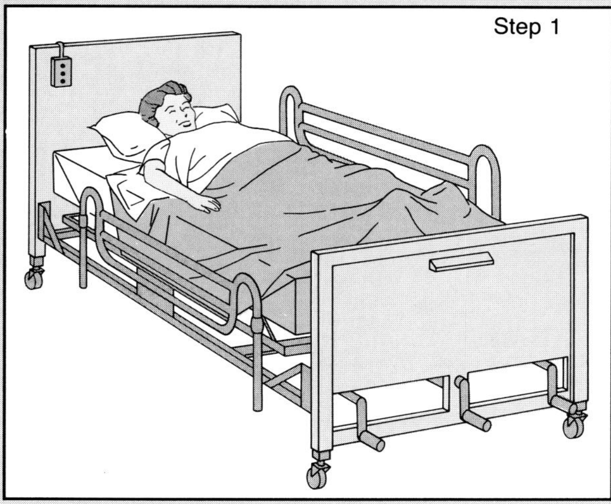

FIGURE 11-38

1. Assemble your equipment:
   a) Two large sheets
   b) One plastic draw sheet, if used
   c) One cotton draw sheet, if used
   d) Disposable bed protectors, if used
   e) One bath blanket
   f) Pillowcase
   g) One blanket (wool or thermal)
   h) One bedspread
   i) One plastic laundry bag (or whatever container is used in your institution for the dirty linen in the patient's room)
2. Wash your hands.
3. Identify the patient by checking the identification bracelet.
4. Ask all visitors to step out of the room, if this is your hospital's policy.
5. Tell the patient you are going to make the bed.
6. Pull the curtain around the bed for privacy.
7. Place a chair near the bed.
8. Place the clean linens on the chair in the order in which you will use them. That is, the last item to be put on the bed should be on the bottom of the stack.
9. Lower the backrest and knee rest until the bed is flat, if that is allowed. Raise the bed to a comfortable working height and lock in place.
10. Loosen all the sheets around the entire bed.
11. Take the bedspread and blanket off the bed and fold them over the back of the chair, leaving the patient covered only with the top sheet.
12. Cover the patient with the bath blanket by placing it over the top sheet. Ask the patient to hold the bath blanket. If the patient is unable to do this, tuck the top edges of the bath blanket under the patient's shoulders. Without exposing the patient, remove the top sheet from under the bath blanket. Fold the top sheet and place over the back of the chair (Figure 11-39).

FIGURE 11-39

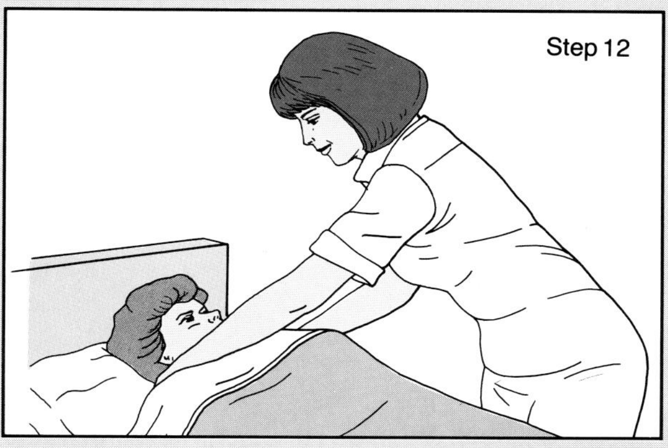

13. If the mattress has slipped out of place, move it to its proper position touching the headboard. Ask another nursing assistant to help, if necessary.
14. Raise the bedside rail on the opposite side from where you will be working and lock in place (Figure 11-40).

FIGURE 11-40

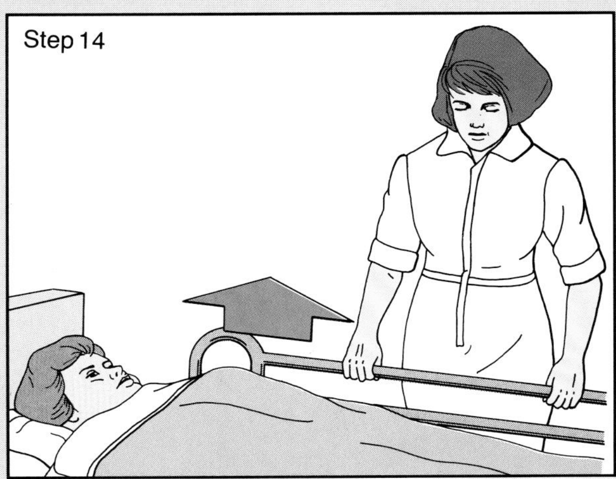

15. Ask the patient to turn onto his or her side toward the side rail. Help the patient to turn, if necessary. The patient is now on the far side of the bed (Figure 11-41).

FIGURE 11-41

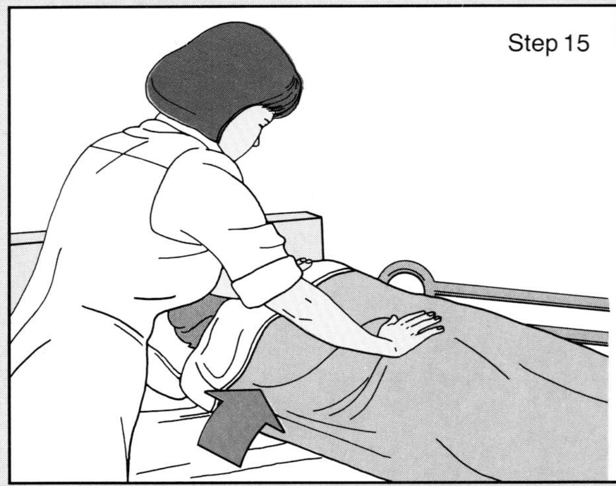

16. Adjust the pillow for the patient according to instructions. If the patient cannot sit up, lock arms with him and raise him to remove the pillow. If you are leaving the pillow under the patient's head, then move it over to the side of the bed, adjusting it so that it is comfortable.
17. Fold the cotton draw sheet toward the patient and tuck it against his or her back.
18. Raise the plastic draw sheet (if it is clean) over the bath blanket and the patient.
19. Fold the bottom sheet toward the patient and tuck it against his or her back. This strips your side of the bed down to the mattress (Figure 11-42).

FIGURE 11-42

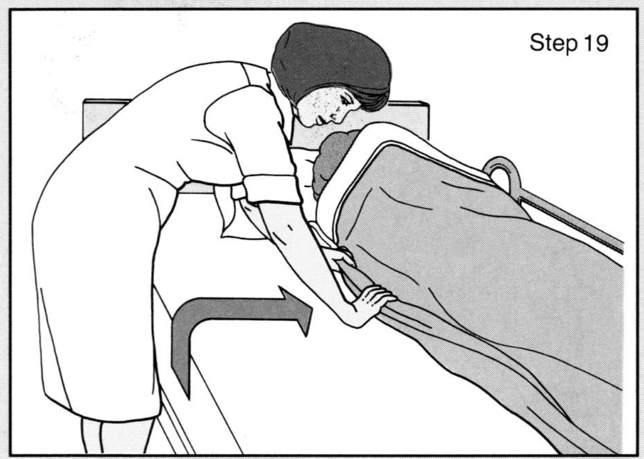

20. Take the large clean sheet and fold it in half lengthwise. Do not permit the sheet to touch the floor or your uniform.
21. Place it on the bed, still folded, with the fold running along the middle of the mattress. The small hem end of the sheet should be even with the foot edge of the mattress. Fold the top half of the sheet toward the patient. Tuck the folds against his or her back, below the plastic draw sheet (Figure 11-43).

FIGURE 11-43

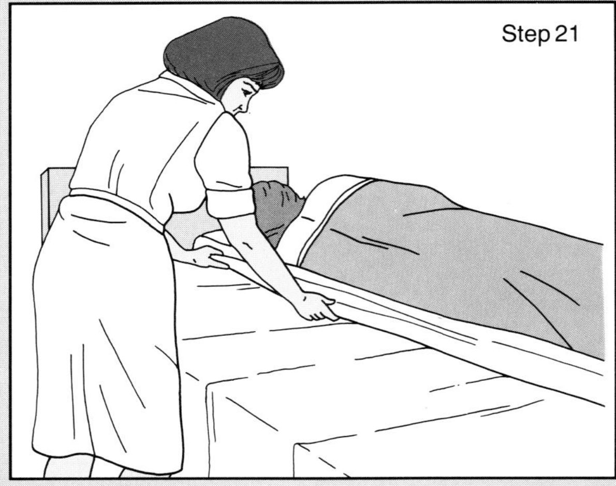

22. Miter the corner at the head of the mattress. Tuck in the clean bottom sheet on your side from head to foot of the mattress (Figure 11-44).

FIGURE 11-44

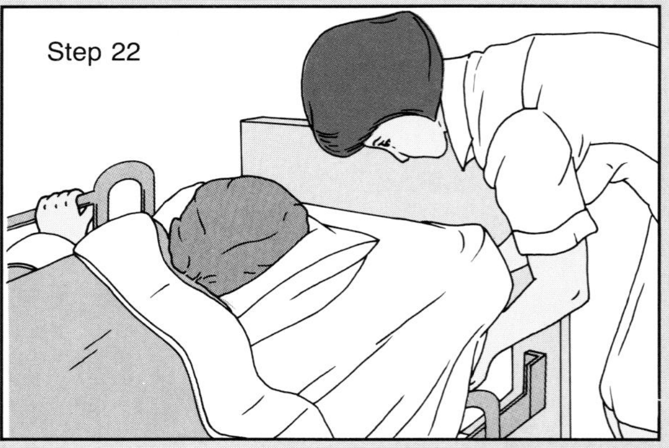

23. Pull the plastic draw sheet toward you, over the clean bottom sheet, and tuck in.
24. Place the clean cotton draw sheet over the plastic sheet, folded in half. Fold the

top half toward the patient, tucking the folds under his or her back, as you did with the bottom sheet. Tuck the draw sheet under the mattress.

25. Raise the bedside rail on your side of the bed and lock in place (Figure 11-45).

FIGURE 11-45

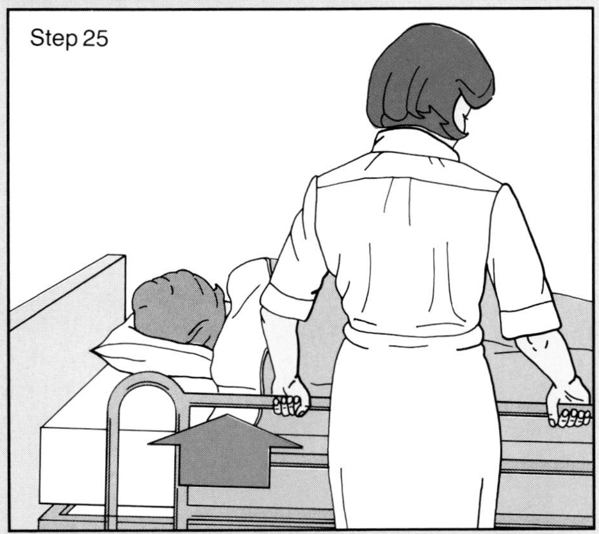

26. Go to the opposite side of the bed.
27. Lower the bedside rail. Ask the patient, or help him, to roll over the "hump" onto the clean sheets toward you. Be careful not to let the patient become wrapped up in the bath blanket whlie turning (Figure 11-46).

FIGURE 11-46

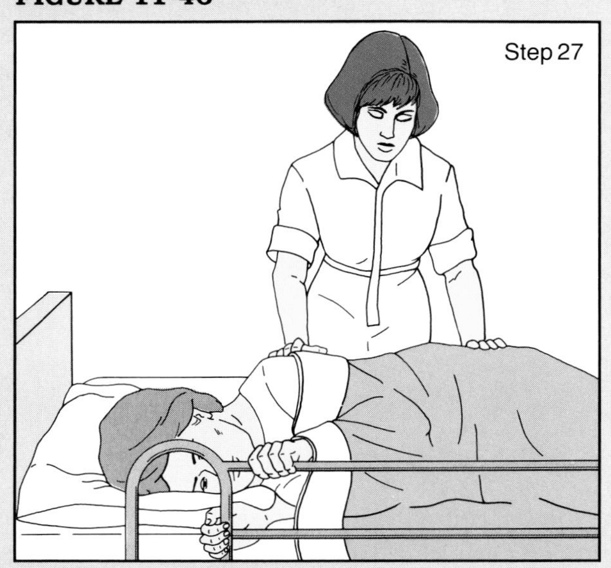

28. Remove the old bottom sheet and cotton draw sheet from the bed. Pull the fresh bottom sheet toward the edge of the bed. Tuck it under the mattress at the head of the bed and make a mitered corner. Then tuck the bottom sheet under the mattress from the head to the foot, pulling firmly to remove any wrinkles (Figure 11-47).

FIGURE 11-47

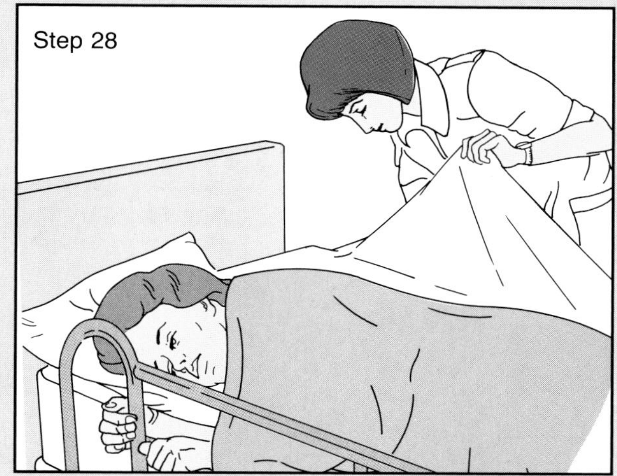

29. Pull the plastic draw sheet and clean cotton draw sheet toward you.
30. Then, one at a time, tuck the draw sheets under the mattress along the side.
31. Be sure to pull all the sheets tight as you tuck them in for a tight foundation.
32. Have the patient turn on his back, or turn him yourself, loosening the bath blanket as he turns (Figure 11-48).

FIGURE 11-48

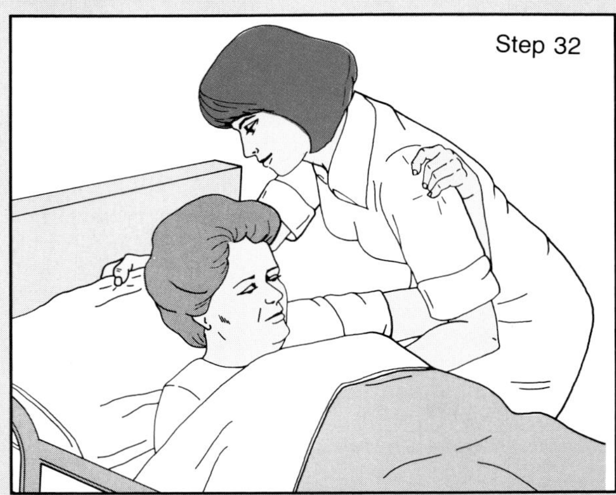

33. Change the pillowcase and place the pillow under the patient's head. If necessary, lock arms with the patient and raise him to place the pillow under his head.
34. Spread the clean top sheet over the bath blanket with the wide hem to the top. The middle of the sheet should run along the middle of the bed. The wide hem should be even with the head edge of the mattress. Remove the bath blanket, moving toward the foot of the bed, without exposing the patient (Figure 11-49).

FIGURE 11-49

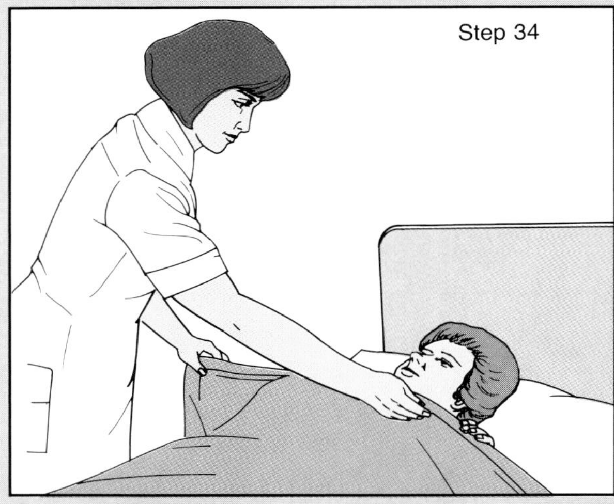

35. Tuck the clean top sheet under the mattress at the foot of the bed. Make sure you leave enough room for the patient to move his or her feet freely. Miter the corners of the sheet.
36. Spread the blanket over the top sheet. Be sure the middle of the blanket runs along the middle of the bed. The blanket should be high enough to cover the patient's shoulders.
37. Tuck the blanket in at the foot of the bed. Make a mitered corner with the blanket.
38. Place the spread on the bed in the same way. Make a mitered corner with the spread.
39. Go to the other side of the bed, turn the top covers back, and miter the top sheet; then miter the blanket, and then miter the spread. Be sure the top covers are loose enough for the patient to move his or her feet.
40. To make the cuff:
    a) Fold the top hem edge of the spread over and under the top hem of the blanket.
    b) Fold the top hem of the top sheet back over the edge of the spread and blanket to form a cuff. The rough edge of the hem of the sheet must be turned down so the patient does not come in contact with it.
41. Raise the backrest and knee rest to suit the patient, if this is allowed.
42. Make the patient comfortable.
43. Lower the bed to a position of safety for the patient.
44. Pull the curtains back to the open position.
45. Raise the side rails where ordered, indicated, and appropriate for patient safety.
46. Place the call light within easy reach of the patient.
47. Put used linen in the plastic laundry bag and place in hamper.
48. Wash your hands.
49. Report to your immediate supervisor:
    - That you have made the occupied bed
    - How the patient tolerated the procedure
    - Your observations of anything unusual

KEY QUESTIONS

1. Why is the patient's bed made with such great care?
2. Name the four basic beds and describe them.
3. Discuss the reason for each rule to follow for bedmaking.

4. How should the closed bed be made?
5. How should the open, fan-folded, or empty-bed be made?
6. Describe the process for making the occupied bed.
7. How should the operating room bed be made?
8. Define: bottom of the bed, closed bed, decubitus ulcers, draw sheet, fan-fold, occupied bed, open bed, postoperative bed, top of the bed.

CHAPTER

12

Personal Care of the Patient

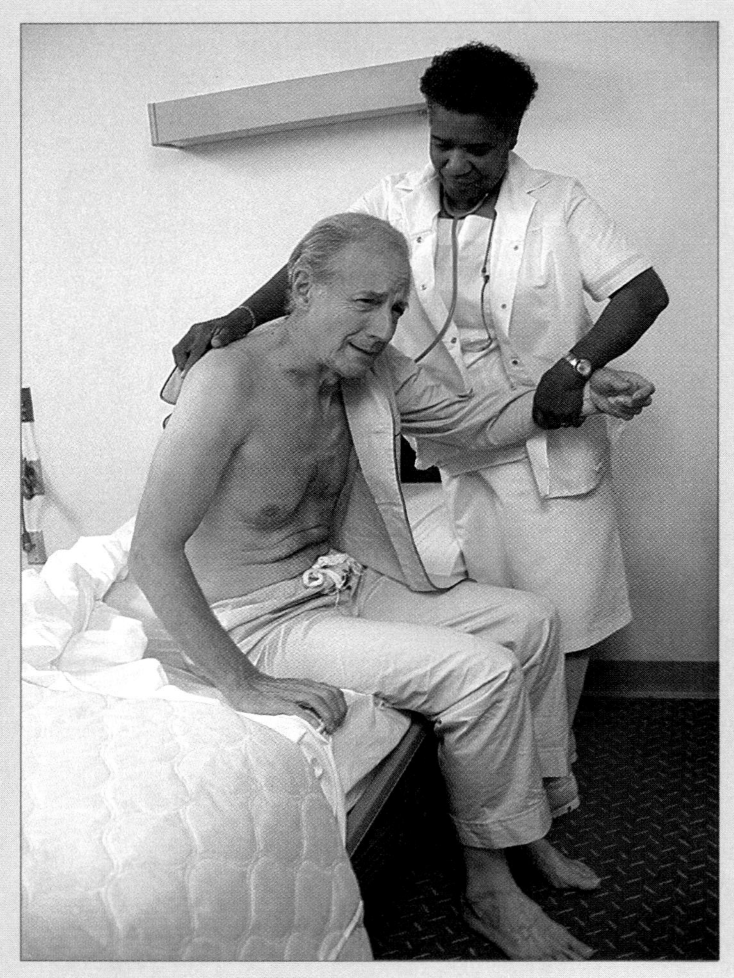

WARNING

For all patient contact, adhere to Universal Precautions (see page 91, 97, or the front cover flap). Wear protective equipment as indicated.

Objectives

What You Will Learn

When you have completed this chapter, you will be able to:

- Establish a schedule of daily care.
- Record what you have done for the patient on the activities of daily living (ADL) flow sheet (or other appropriate form).
- Care for the patient's mouth using good oral hygiene techniques.
- Bathe the patient.
- Give a back rub.
- Change the patient's gown.
- Care for the patient's hair.
- Shave the patient's beard.
- Define: activities of daily living, dentures, flow sheet, oral hygiene, self-care.

KEY IDEAS

Schedule of Daily Care; 24-Hour Needs of the Patient

Early Morning Care: Before Breakfast

(Sometimes called early A.M. care)

- Offer the bedpan or urinal.
- Wash the patient's hands and face.
- Help with oral hygiene.
- Pass fresh drinking water.
- Clean the overbed table and position to receive tray.
- Raise the head of the bed, if permitted.

Morning Care: After Breakfast

(Sometimes called A.M. care) Before giving personal care, pull the curtain around the bed for privacy (Figure 12-1).

- Offer the bedpan or urinal.
- Assist with oral hygiene.
- Help the patient to bathe. Follow instructions from your immediate supervisor. Give the patient a complete bed bath, partial bed bath, shower, or tub bath.
- Change the patient's gown.
- Help the male patient to shave his face, if allowed.
- Make the bed.
- Straighten the unit.

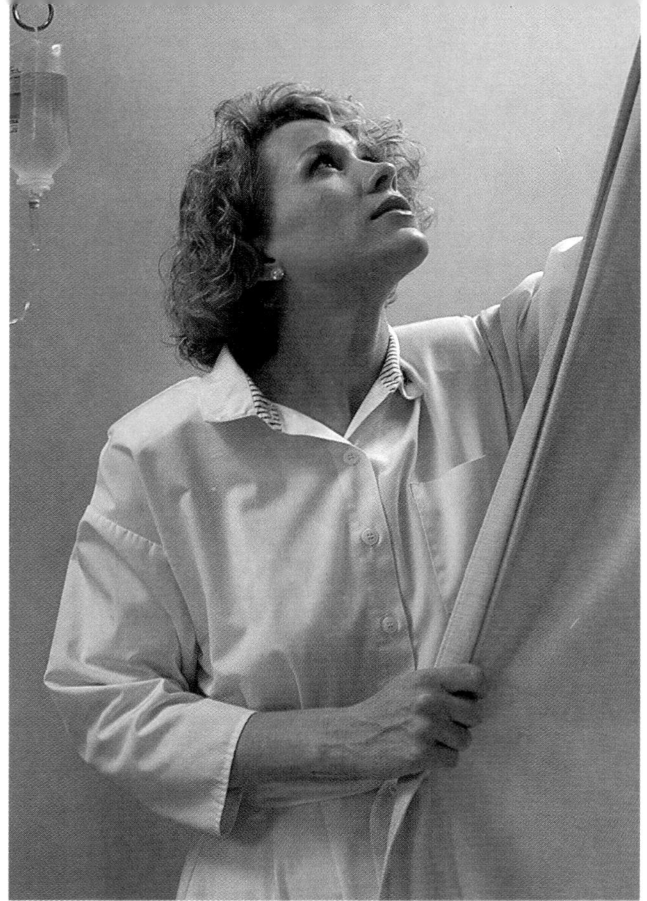

FIGURE 12-1 Before giving personal care, always pull the curtain around the bed for privacy.

Afternoon Care: After Lunch

- Change the patient's gown, if necessary.
- Straighten the unit.
- Pass fresh drinking water.
- Offer the bedpan or urinal.
- Assist with oral hygiene.
- Wash the patient's hands and face.

Evening Care: After Supper, Before Bedtime

(Sometimes called P.M. care)

- Offer the bedpan or urinal.
- Wash the patient's hands and face.
- Assist with oral hygiene.
- Give a back rub, if allowed.
- Change the draw sheet, if necessary.
- Smooth and tighten the sheets.
- Offer the patient an extra blanket.
- Pass fresh drinking water.

Activities of Daily Living
The activities or tasks usually performed every day, such as toileting, washing, eating, or dressing.

Flow Sheet
A checklist or chart for recording the activities of daily living.

Documentation of Activities of Daily Living: The Flow Sheet

In many hospitals, the nursing assistant is required to check off (√) or initial what she has done for the patient on an **activities of daily living** (ADL) **flow sheet** (Figure 12-2). Follow the nurse's instructions regarding this documentation.

FIGURE 12-2 The activities of daily living checklist.

ACTIVITIES OF DAILY LIVING CHECKLIST

SELF —Done by patient
ASSIST—Patient assisted by nursing staff
TOTAL —Done by nursing staff
✔ —Check procedure performed. Include time if appropriate.

DATE															
DIET	B'fast	Dinner	Supper	B'fast	Dinner	Supper	B'fast	Dinner	Supper	B'fast	Dinner	Supper	B'fast	Dinner	Supper
Ate all food served															
Ate approx. ½ food served															
Refused to eat															
PROCEDURE	11-7	7-3	3-11	11-7	7-3	3-11	11-7	7-3	3-11	11-7	7-3	3-11	11-7	7-3	3-11
A.M. or H.S. Care															
Oral Hygiene															
Bath–Bed bath complete															
Bed bath partial															
Shower															
Tub															
Self Care															
Back Care															
Bed Made															
ELIMINATION															
Bowel movement															
Involuntary B.M.															
Voided															
Incontinent															
Foley cath.															
Sitz Bath @															
ACTIVITY															
Bed rest complete															
Dangle															
Bed rest–B.R.P.															
Up in chair															
Up in room															
Walk in hall															
Ambulatory															
POSITION CHANGED															
Flat in bed															
Semi–Fowler's															
Deep breathe, cough															
Range of motion															
Turn from side to side															
Side Rails–Up															
Down															
Fresh Water @															
SIGNATURE & TITLE															

KEY IDEAS

Oral Hygiene

Oral Hygiene
Cleanliness of the mouth.

A person's mouth and teeth need as much care when a person is sick as when he or she is well. This care is called **oral hygiene**. A sick person's mouth often has a bad taste. Sometimes the mouth feels "fuzzy" because of medications or an illness. The tongue may be covered with a grayish coating that spoils the appetite. With good care, the patient's mouth will feel fresh and clean. Cleaning the patient's teeth and mouth, that is, giving oral hygiene, is an essential part of daily patient care (Figure 12-3). Teeth should be brushed every morning, every evening, and after each meal. In your work, you will be giving oral hygiene to conscious and unconscious patients. When necessary, you will be cleaning their false teeth (dentures).

Oral hygiene is given to unconscious patients and patients who are NPO (nothing by mouth) every 2 hours. The purpose is to keep the lips and oral tissues moist. Unless this is done, tissues tend to dry out, split, and bleed, and they develop a mucous coating much more rapidly.

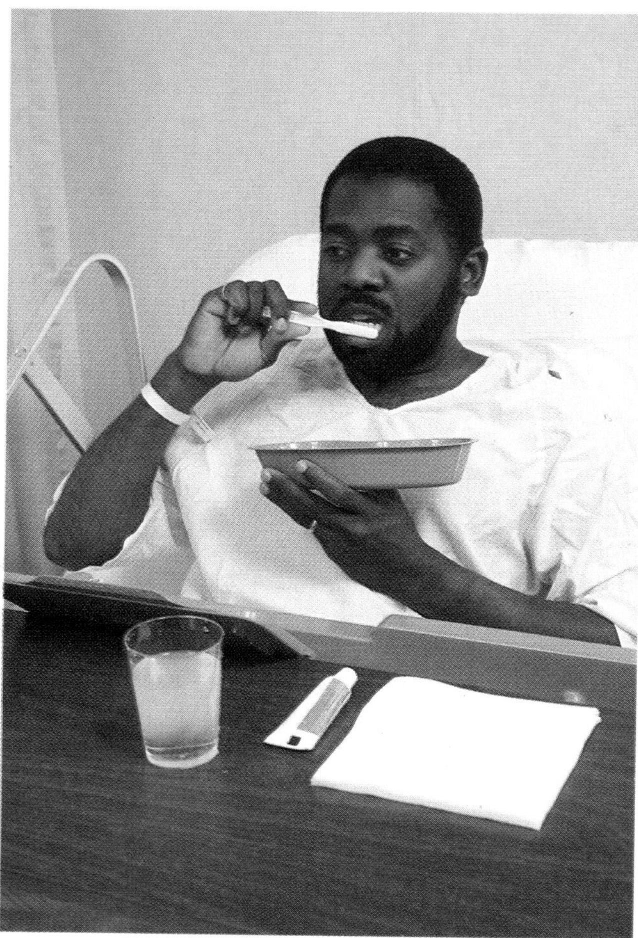

FIGURE 12-3 Oral hygiene is an essential part of daily patient care.

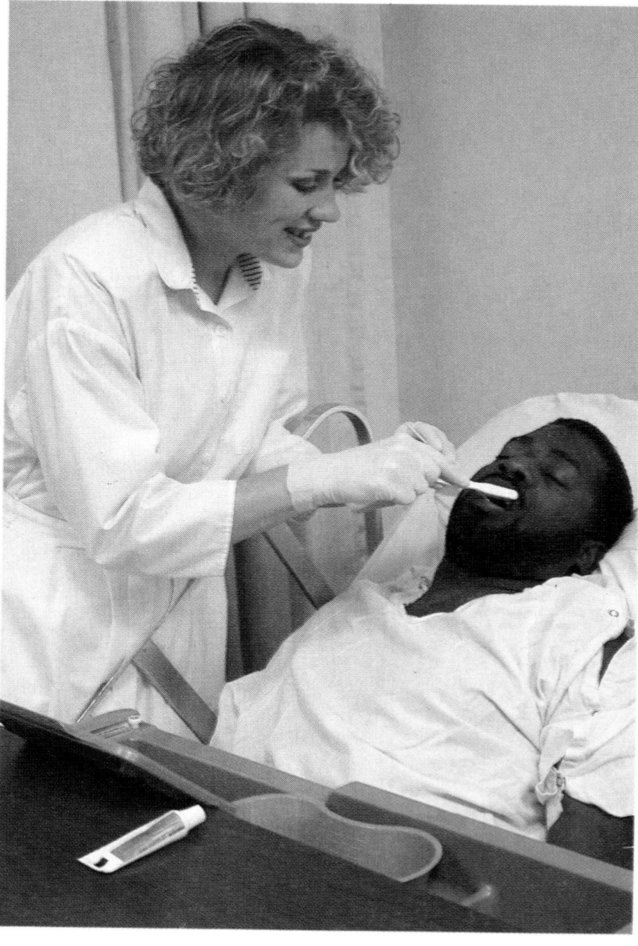

Procedure Oral Hygiene

1. Assemble your equipment on the bedside table:
   a) Mouthwash
   b) Fresh water
   c) Disposable cup
   d) Straw
   e) Toothbrush
   f) Toothpaste
   g) Emesis basin
   h) Face towel
2. Wash your hands.
3. Identify the patient by checking the identification bracelet.
4. Ask visitors to step out of the room, if this is your hospital's policy.
5. Tell the patient you will help her clean her teeth and mouth.
6. Pull the curtain around the bed for privacy.
7. Spread the towel across the patient's chest to protect the gown and top sheets.
8. Mix one-half cup of water with one-half cup of mouthwash in the disposable cup.
9. Let the patient take a mouthful of the mixture if allowed and rinse her mouth.
10. Hold the emesis basin under the patient's chin so she can spit out the mouthwash solution.
11. Put toothpaste on the wet toothbrush.
12. If the patient can do it, let her brush her teeth. If she cannot, brush her teeth for her.
13. Help the patient rinse the toothpaste out of her mouth, using the mouthwash solution or fresh water.
14. Clean and put your equipment in its proper place. Discard disposable equipment.
15. Make the patient comfortable.
16. Lower the bed to a position of safety for the patient.
17. Pull the curtains back to the open position.
18. Raise the side rails where ordered, indicated, and appropriate for patient safety.
19. Place the call light within easy reach of the patient.
20. Wash your hands.
21. Report to your immediate supervisor:
    - That you have assisted the patient with oral hygiene
    - How the patient tolerated the procedure
    - Your observations of anything unusual

Dentures
Artificial teeth. Dentures may replace some or all of a person's teeth; they are described as being partial or complete and upper or lower.

Procedure Cleaning Dentures (False Teeth)

1. Assemble your equipment on the bedside table (Figure 12-4):
   a) Tissues
   b) Mouthwash
   c) Disposable denture cup
   d) Emesis basin
   e) Toothbrush or denture brush
   f) Towel
   g) Denture toothpaste
2. Wash your hands.
3. Identify the patient by checking the identification bracelet.
4. Ask visitors to step out of the room, if this is your hospital's policy.

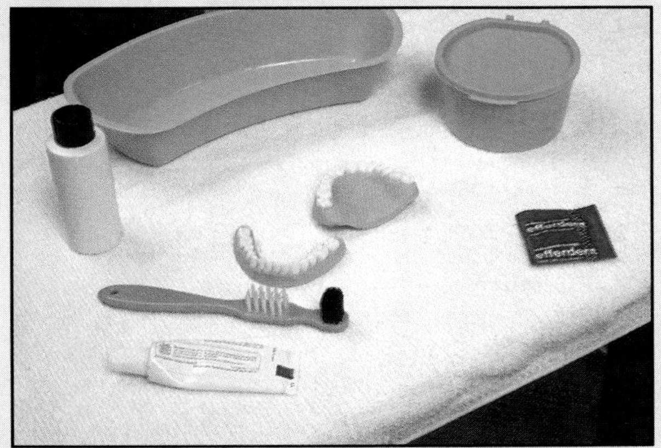

FIGURE 12-4

5. Tell the patient you wish to clean his dentures.

Pull the curtain around the bed for privacy.

7. Spread the towel across the patient's chest to protect the gown and top sheets.
8. Ask the patient to remove his dentures. Have tissue in the emesis basin ready to receive them. Help the patient who is unable to remove his own dentures.
9. Take the dentures to the sink in the lined emesis basin. (Figure 12-5).

FIGURE 12-5

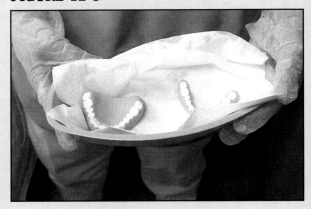

10. Put on gloves.
11. Fill the sink with water to guard against breaking the dentures if you drop them accidentally.
12. Apply toothpaste or denture cleanser. With the dentures in the palm of your hand, brush them until they are clean (Figure 12-6).

FIGURE 12-6

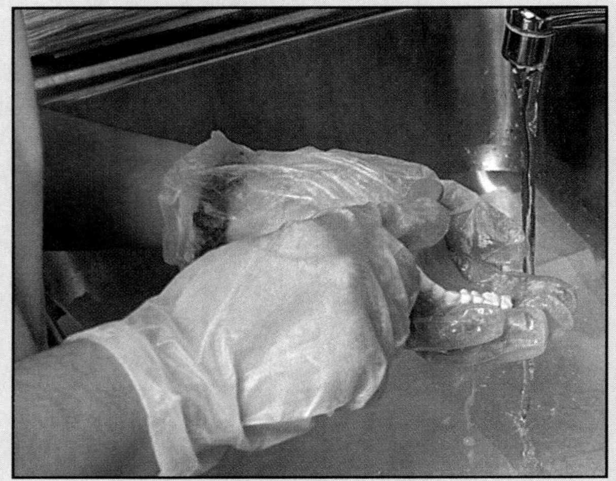

13. Rinse them thoroughly under cool running water (Figure 12-7).

FIGURE 12-7

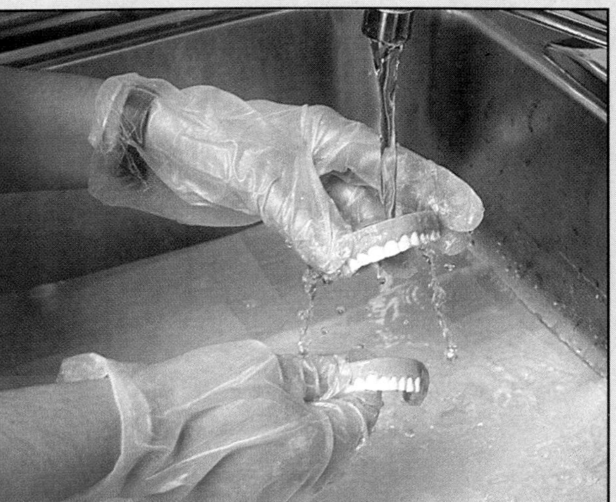

14. Fill the clean denture cup with half cool water and half mouthwash. Or use water and salt, a saline solution. Place the dentures in the cup.
15. Help the patient rinse his mouth with the mouthwash and water solution.
16. Have the patient replace the dentures in his mouth if that is what he wants. Be sure dentures are moist before replacing them.
17. Leave the labeled denture cup with the clean solution on the bedside table where the patient can reach it easily.
18. Clean all your equipment and put it in the proper place. Discard disposable equipment in the proper container.
19. Make the patient comfortable.
20. Lower the bed to a position of safety for the patient.
21. Pull the curtains back to the open position.
22. Raise the side rails where ordered, indicated, and appropriate for patient safety.
23. Place the call light within easy reach of the patient.
24. Wash your hands.
25. Report to your immediate supervisor:
    - That you have cleaned the patient's dentures
    - Your observations of anything unusual

Procedure Oral Hygiene for the Unconscious Patient (Special Mouth Care)

1. Assemble your equipment on the bedside table:
   a) Towel
   b) Emesis basin
   c) Special disposable mouth care kit of commercially prepared swabs. Or if such a kit is not available:
      - Tongue depressor
      - Applicators or gauze sponges
      - Lubricant such as glycerine, petroleum jelly, or a solution of lemon juice and glycerine
2. Wash your hands.
3. Identify the patient by checking the identification bracelet.
4. Ask visitors to step out of the room, if this is your hospital's policy.
5. Tell the patient what you are going to do. Even though a patient seems to be unconscious, he still may be able to hear you.
6. Pull the curtain around the bed for privacy.
7. Stand at the side of the bed. Turn the patient's head to the side facing you.
8. Put a towel on the pillow under the patient's head and partly under the face.
9. Put the emesis basin on the towel under the patient's chin.
10. Ask the patient to open his mouth. If he is in a coma, he will not be able to respond. In this case you will have to hold his mouth open. Press on his cheeks or open the mouth using gentle pressure with hand on chin.
11. Open the commercial package of swabs. Wipe the patient's entire mouth (roof, tongue, and inside the cheeks and lips) with the prepared swab (Figure 12-8).
12. Put used swabs into the emesis basin. Some commercial swabs leave a coating of glycerine solution on the entire inside of the mouth, tongue, and teeth.
13. If a disposable mouth care kit of commercial prepared swabs is not available:
    a) Moisten the applicators with mouthwash solution.
    b) Use your free hand to insert the applicators in the patient's mouth.

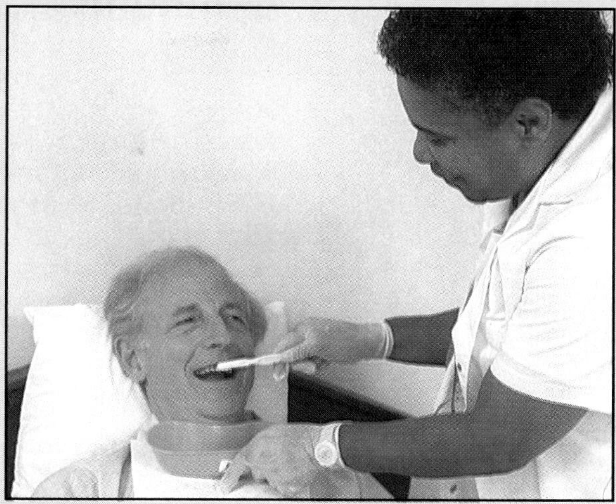

FIGURE 12-8

    c) Thoroughly wipe the roof of the mouth, the teeth, and the tongue.
    d) Change applicators frequently.
    e) Place the used applicators and other supplies in the emesis basin.
    f) Use clear water on more applicators to rinse out the patient's mouth.
14. Dry the patient's face with the towel.
15. Using an applicator, put a small amount of water-soluble lubricant on the patient's lips and tongue and the inside of his mouth (only as necessary).
16. Clean and put your equipment in its proper place. Discard disposable equipment.
17. Make the patient comfortable.
18. Lower the bed to a position of safety for the patient.
19. Pull the curtains back to the open position.
20. Raise the side rails where ordered, indicated, and appropriate for patient safety.
21. Place the call light within easy reach of the patient.
22. Wash your hands.
23. Report to your immediate supervisor:
    - That you have given the patient oral hygiene
    - How the patient tolerated the procedure
    - Your observations of anything unusual

KEY IDEAS

Helping the Patient to Bathe

There are several important reasons for bathing the patient. Bathing gets rid of dirt on the patient's body. It eliminates body odors and cools and refreshes the patient. The bath stimulates circulation and helps to prevent skin breakdown. Bathing requires movements of certain parts of the body; the patient's legs and arms are lifted and the head and torso are turned. This activity exercises muscles that might otherwise remain unused. At this time, the nursing assistant has the opportunity to observe the patient for any unusual body changes, such as skin rashes, pressure ulcers, or reddened areas.

A patient may be bathed in one of four ways, depending on his or her condition. The patient may be given a complete bed bath, a partial bed bath, a tub bath, or a shower.

Types of Baths

- *Complete bed bath:* The patient who is too weak or sick is given a complete bed bath. When you are giving this bath, you will get little or no help from the patient. Sometimes the doctor will write an order placing the patient on complete bed rest. In this case, the patient is not permitted to do anything.
- *Partial bed bath:* A patient may be able to take care of most of his or her own bathing needs. In this case you bathe only the areas that are hard for the patient to reach, such as the back or feet.
- *Tub bath:* The tub bath might be ordered by the doctor for therapeutic reasons.
- *Shower:* Showers may be permitted for patients who are recovering from their illness (convalescent patients). These patients have been judged by their doctor to be strong enough to get out of bed and walk around.

Rules to Follow

BATHING THE PATIENT

- Usually the complete bed bath is given as part of morning care. After the bath, the occupied bed is made, the hair combed, and the gown changed.
- Take everything you will need to the bedside before you start the bath. Clear off the bedside table and put the items you will be using on it.
- Always cover the patient with a bath blanket before giving the complete bed bath.
- Have the patient move or help her or him move close to you so that you can work easily without strain on your back.
- Use good body mechanics. Keep your feet separated, stand firmly, bend your knees, and keep your back straight.
- Raise the patient's bed to a comfortable working position with the side rails up on the far side of the bed.
- Make a mitten for your hand out of the washcloth. This will prevent it from dragging roughly across the patient's skin.
- Change the water during the bed bath as necessary. For example, change the water whenever it becomes soapy, dirty, or cold. Change water before washing the patient's legs, before washing the back, and before washing the perineal area.
- Only one part of the body is washed at a time. Wash, rinse, and dry each part or area very well. Then cover it right away with the bath blanket.

- Soap has a drying effect on the patient's skin. Be sure to rinse off all the soap.
- When you are not using the soap, keep it in the soap dish instead of the basin. In this way, the water will not dissolve the soap and get too soapy.
- Putting the patient's hands and feet into the water makes the patient feel relaxed.
- Observe the condition of the patient's skin when you are giving the bath. Report any redness, rashes, broken skin, or tender places you see on the patient's body.
- Never trim or cut fingernails or toenails without special instructions from the nurse.
- At the beginning of the bath, put the patient's bottle of lotion for the back rub in the basin of water to keep it warm or put lotion on your hands and rub your hands together to warm it up. (All patients have their own bottle of lotion.)
- Deodorant should be used if the patient asks for it. It should be applied after the bath has been completed and before the clean bed has been made.
- Check the patient's gown for personal items or valuables and return them to the patient before putting it in the laundry hamper.

Procedure The Complete Bed Bath

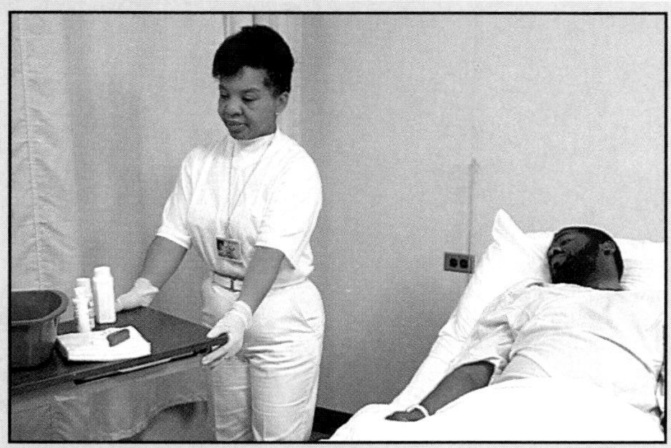

FIGURE 12-9

1. Assemble your equipment on the bedside table (Figure 12-9):
   a) Soap and soap dish
   b) Washcloth
   c) Wash basin
   d) Bath thermometer, if available
   e) Face and bath towels
   f) Talcum powder or corn starch (optional)
   g) Clean gown
   h) Bath blanket
   i) Orange stick for nail care, if used by your health care institution
   j) Lotion
   k) Comb or hair brush
   l) Disposable plastic laundry bags for dirty linen, if used in your institution, or linen laundry bag (a pillow case is sometimes used for dirty linen)
   m) Clean bed linen, stacked on the chair in order of use, if the bed is to be made following the bed bath
   n) Disposable gloves, optional
2. Wash your hands (Figure 12-10).

FIGURE 12-10

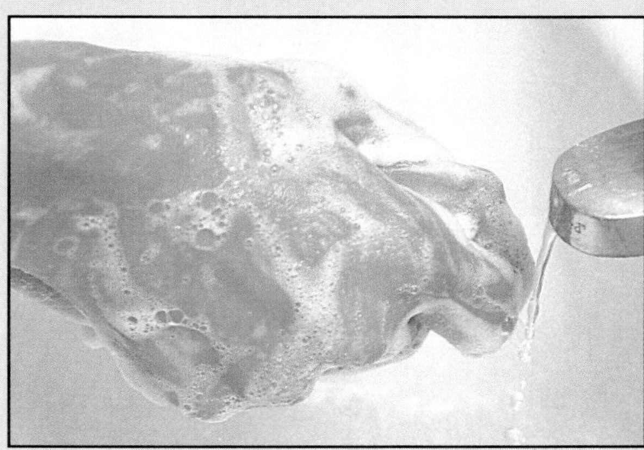

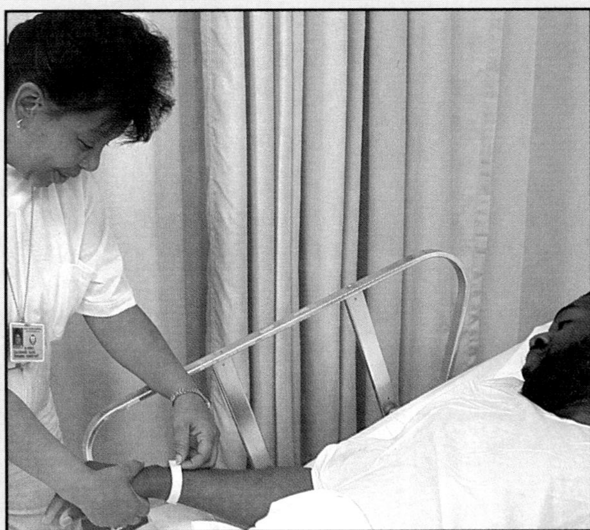

FIGURE 12-11

3. Identify the patient by checking the identification bracelet (Figure 12-11).
4. Ask visitors to step out of the room, if this is your hospital's policy.
5. Tell the patient you are going to give him a bed bath.
6. Pull the curtain around the bed for privacy (Figure 12-12).

FIGURE 12-12

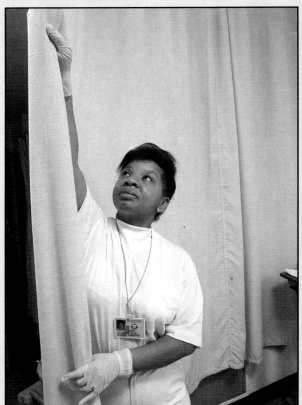

7. Assist the patient with oral hygiene.
8. Offer the bedpan or urinal.
9. Place the laundry bag on a chair near the bed.
10. Pull out all the bedding from under the mattress. Leave it hanging loosely at all four sides of the bed (Figure 12-13).

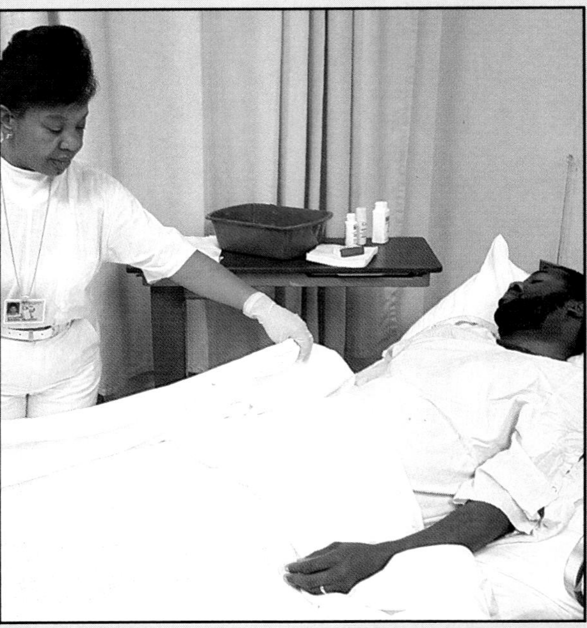

FIGURE 12-13

11. Take the bedspread and regular blanket off the bed. Fold them loosely over the back of the chair, leaving the patient covered with the top sheet.
12. Place the bath blanket over the top sheet. Ask the patient to hold the blanket in place.
13. Remove the top sheet from underneath without uncovering (exposing) the patient. Fold the sheet loosely over the back of the chair if it is to be used again; if not, put it in the laundry bag.
14. Lower the headrest and knee rest of the bed, if permitted. The patient should be in a flat position, as flat as is comfortable for him and as is permitted.
15. Raise the bed to a comfortable working position, and lock it in place (Figure 12-14).
16. Remove the patient's gown and jewelry. Keep the patient covered with the bath blanket. If the gown belongs to the pa-

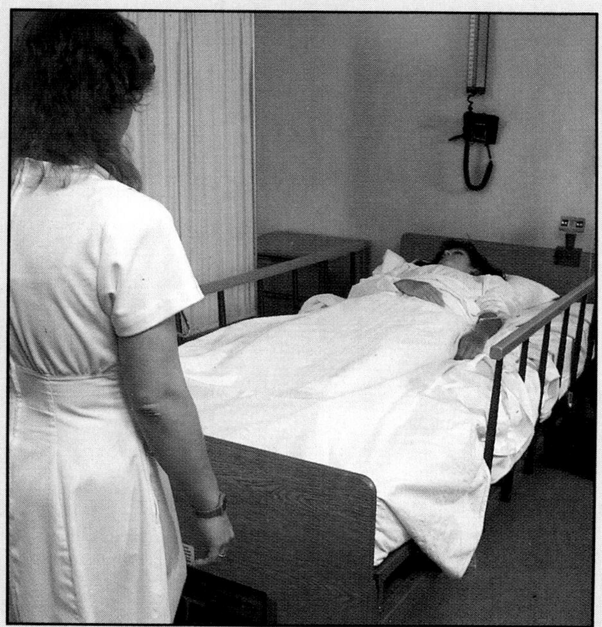

FIGURE 12-14

tient, put it away as requested. Place the hospital gown in the laundry bag. Put the jewelry into the drawer of the bedside table.

17. Fill the wash basin two-thirds full of water at 115°F (46.1°C). Use the bath thermometer to test the temperature of the water.
18. Help the patient to move to the side of the bed closest to you. Use good body mechanics.
19. Put a towel across the patient's chest and make a mitten with the washcloth (Figure 12-15). Wash the patient's eyes from the nose to the outside of the face. Ask the patient if he wants soap used on his face. Wash the face. Be careful not to get soap in his eyes. Rinse and dry

FIGURE 12-15

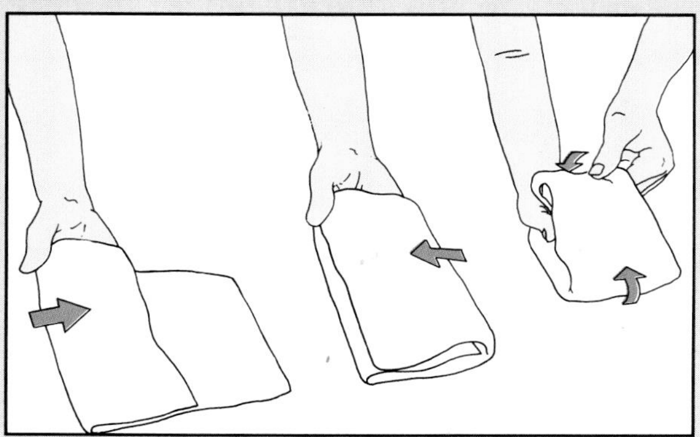

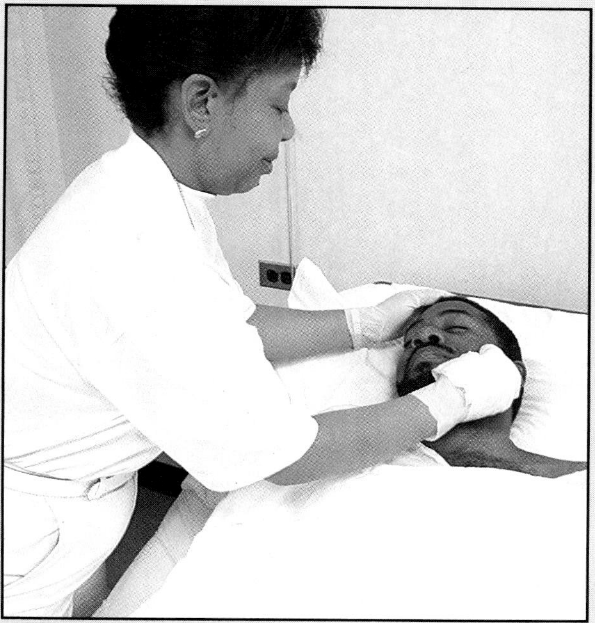

FIGURE 12-16

by patting gently with the bath towel (Figure 12-16).

20. Put a towel lengthwise under the patient's arm farthest from you. This will keep the bed from getting wet. Support the patient's arm with the palm of your hand under his elbow. Then wash his shoulder, armpit (axilla), and arm. Use long, firm, circular strokes. Rinse and dry the area well (Figures 12-17 and 12-18).

FIGURE 12-17

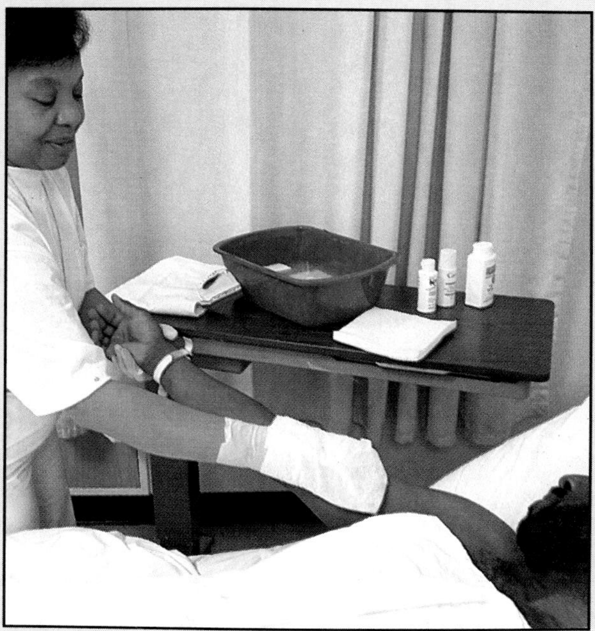

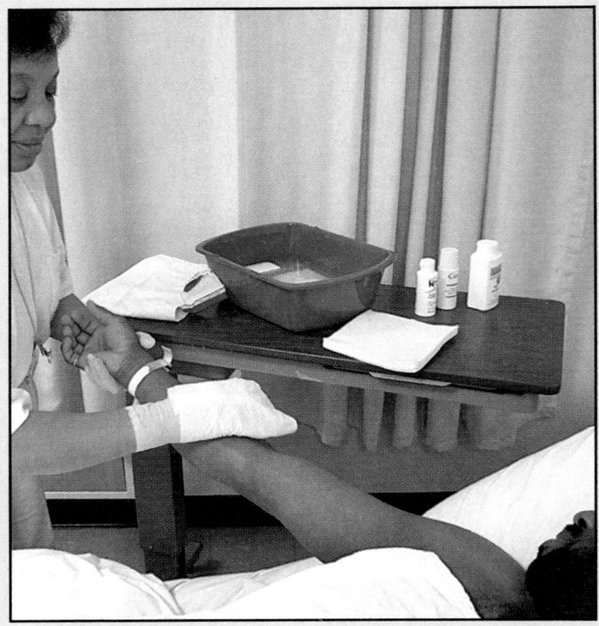

FIGURE 12-18

21. Place the basin of water on the towel. Put the patient's hand into the water. Wash, rinse, and dry the hand well. Place it under the bath blanket.

22. Wash, rinse, and dry the arm, hand, axilla, and shoulder closest to you in the same way.

23. Clean beneath the patient's fingernails with an orange stick, if used by your health care institution.

24. Place a towel across the patient's chest. Fold the bath blanket down to the patient's abdomen. Wash and rinse the patient's ears, neck, and chest. Take note of the condition of the skin under the female patient's breasts. Dry the area thoroughly.

25. Cover the patient's entire chest with a towel. Fold the bath blanket down to the pubic area. Wash the patient's abdomen (Figure 12-19). Be sure to wash the navel (umbilicus) and in any creases of the skin. Dry the patient's abdomen (Figure 12-20). Then pull the bath blanket over the abdomen and chest and remove the towels.

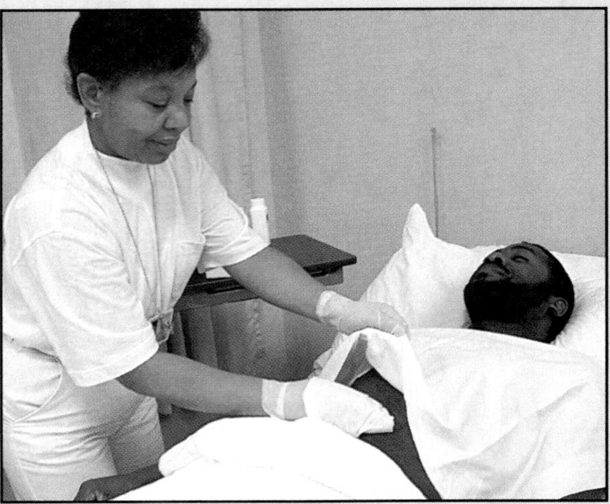

FIGURE 12-19

FIGURE 12-20

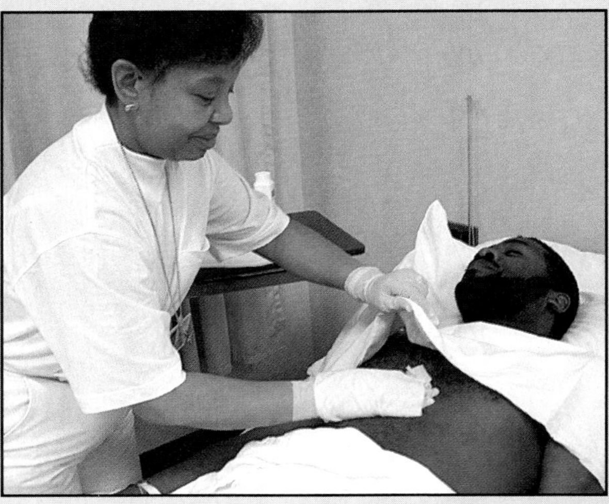

26. Empty the dirty water. Rinse the basin. Fill the basin with clean water at 115°F (46.1°C).

27. Fold the bath blanket back from the patient's leg farthest from you.

28. Put a towel lengthwise under that leg and foot.

29. Bend the knee and wash, rinse, and dry the leg and foot. Take hold of the heel for more support when flexing the knee or place your hand under the knee (Figure 12-21). If the patient can easily bend his knee, put the wash basin on the towel. Then put the patient's foot directly into the basin to wash it.

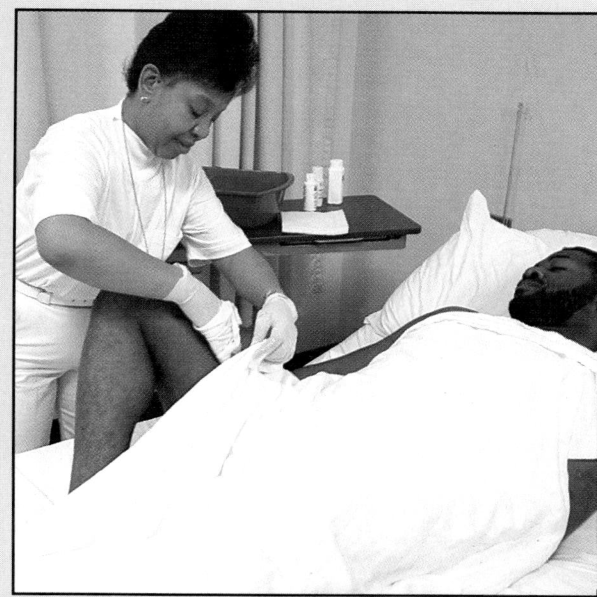

FIGURE 12-21

30. Observe the toenails and the skin between the toes for general appearance and condition. Look especially for redness and cracking of the skin. Take away the basin. Dry the patient's leg and foot and between the toes (Figure 12-22). Cover the leg and foot with the bath blanket and remove the towel.

FIGURE 12-22

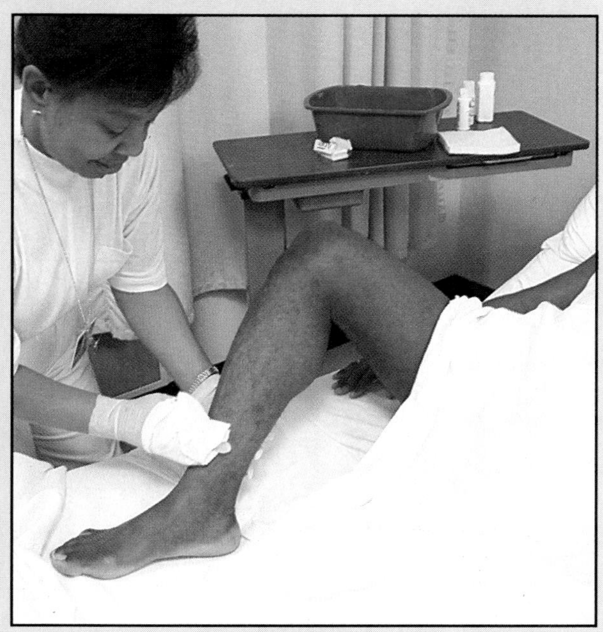

31. Repeat the entire procedure for the leg and foot closest to you. Empty the basin, rinse, and refill it with clean water at 115°F (46.1°C).
32. Ask the patient to turn on his side with his back toward you. If he needs help in turning, assist him. Raise the side rail to the up position so the patient is safe. Return to your working side of the bed (Figure 12-23).

FIGURE 12-23

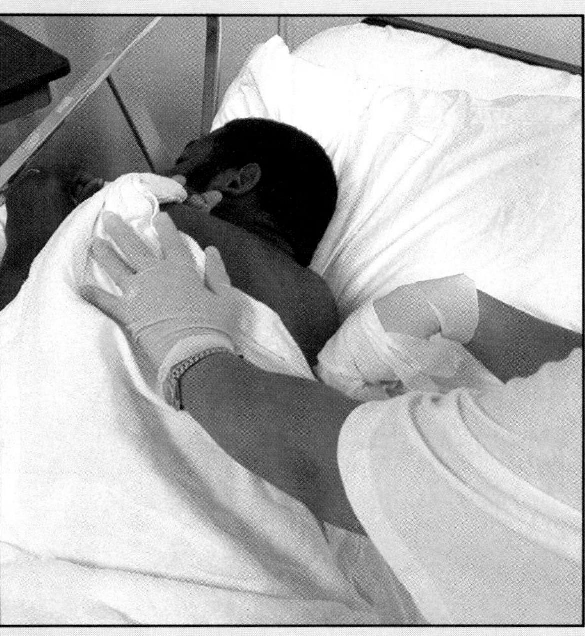

33. Put the towel lengthwise on the bottom sheet near the patient's back. Wash, rinse, and dry his back, buttocks, and back of the neck behind the ears with long, firm, circular strokes. Give the patient a back rub with warm lotion. The patient's back should be rubbed for at least a minute and a half. Give special attention to bony areas (for example, shoulder blades, hips, and elbows). Look for red areas. Dry the patient's back, remove the towel, and turn him on his back.
34. Put on the disposable gloves and wash the patient's genital area with clean soap and water. Dry well. Allow for privacy at all times.

35. Put a clean gown on the patient (Figure 12-24).

FIGURE 12-24

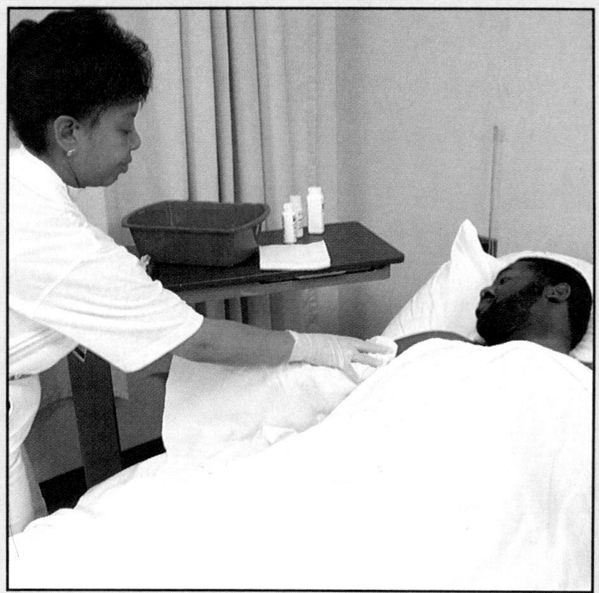

36. Comb the patient's hair if he cannot do this for himself (Figure 12-25).

FIGURE 12-25

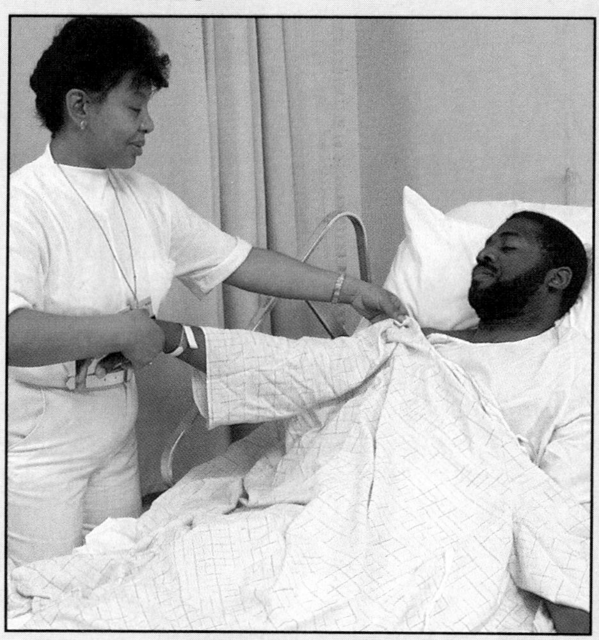

37. Make the patient's bed. Straighten the bedside table. Remove any unneeded articles. Replace the items the patient wants on the table.
38. Raise the backrest and knee rest to suit the patient, if this is allowed (Figure 12-26). Lower the bed to its lowest horizontal position.

FIGURE 12-26

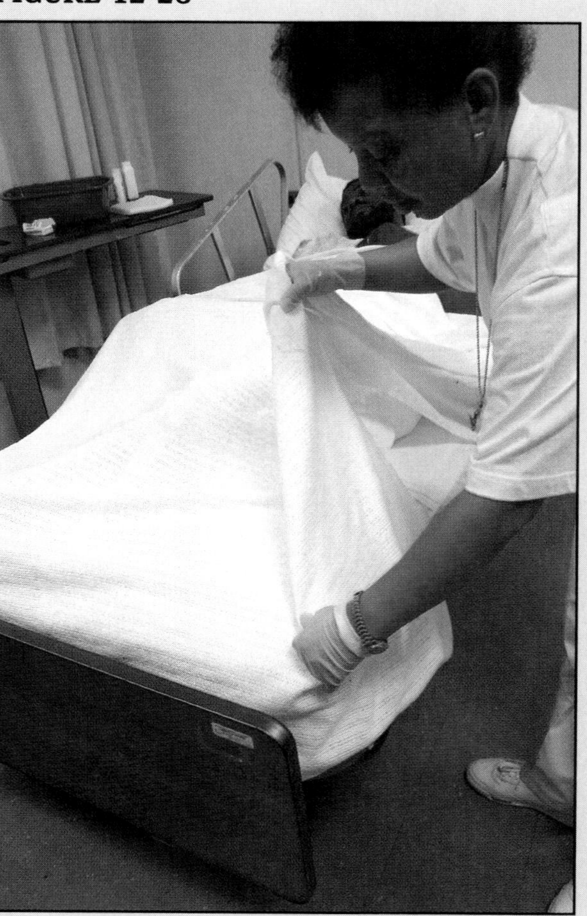

39. Place the signal cord in its proper place where the patient can reach it easily.
40. Clean and put your equipment in its proper place. Discard disposable equipment.
41. Wipe off the bedside table. Discard soiled linen in the dirty linen hamper in the utility room (Figure 12-27).

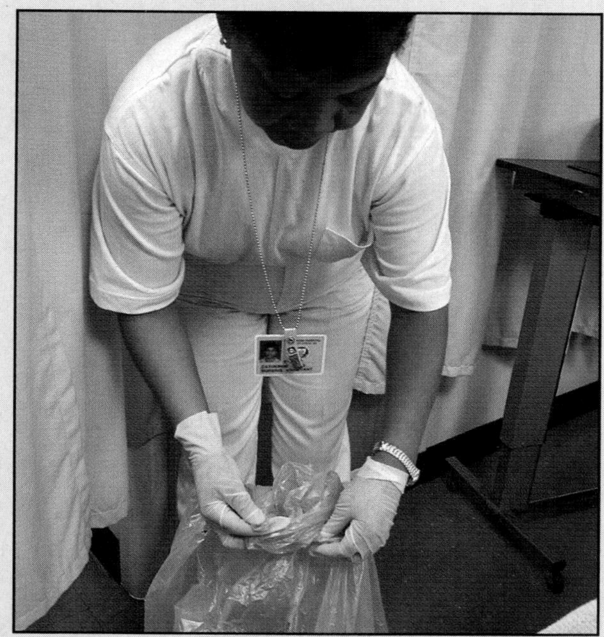

FIGURE 12-27

42. Make the patient comfortable.
43. Lower the bed to a position of safety for the patient.
44. Pull the curtains back to the open position.
45. Raise the side rails where ordered, indicated, and appropriate for patient safety.
46. Place the call light within easy reach of the patient.
47. Wash your hands.
48. Report to your immediate supervisor:
    - That you have given the patient a bed bath
    - How the patient tolerated the procedure
    - Your observations of anything unusual

Procedure The Partial Bed Bath (Partial Self-care)

1. Assemble your equipment on the bedside table:
    a) Soap and soap dish
    b) Washcloth
    c) Wash basin
    d) Bath thermometer
    e) Face and bath towels
    f) Talcum powder or corn starch
    g) Clean gown
    h) Bath blanket
    i) Orange stick for nail care, if used by your health care institution
    j) Lotion for back rub
    k) Comb or hair brush
    l) Disposable plastic laundry bags for dirty linen or a dirty laundry bag
    m) Clean bed linen, stacked on the chair in order of use, if the bed is to be made following the bed bath
2. Wash your hands.
3. Identify the patient by checking the identification bracelet.
4. Ask visitors to step out of the room, if this is your hospital's policy.
5. Tell the patient you are going to help her with a bath.
6. Pull the curtains around the bed for privacy.
7. Assist the patient with oral hygiene.
8. Offer the bedpan or urinal.
9. Place the laundry bag on a chair near the bed.
10. Pull out all the bedding from under the mattress. Leave it hanging loosely at all four sides of the bed.
11. Take the bedspread and regular blanket off the bed. Fold them loosely over the back of the chair, leaving the patient covered with the top sheet.
12. Place the bath blanket over the top sheet. Ask the patient to hold the blanket in place. Remove the top sheet from underneath without uncovering the patient. Fold the sheet loosely over the back of the chair if it is to be used again. Or put it in the laundry bag.

13. Take off the patient's gown and jewelry, keeping her covered with the bath blanket. If the gown belongs to the patient, put it away as requested. Place the jewelry into the drawer of the bedside table. Put the hospital gown into the laundry bag.
14. Fill the wash basin two-thirds full of water at 115°F (46.1°C). Use the bath thermometer to test the temperature.
15. Ask the patient to wash the areas of her body that she can reach easily.
16. Place the signal cord where the patient can easily reach it. Instruct her to signal when she has finished washing herself.
17. Wash your hands and leave the room.
18. When the patient signals that she is finished, go back into the room.
19. Wash your hands.
20. Empty the water, rinse the basin, and fill it with clean water at 115°F (46.1°C).
21. Wash the areas of the body that the patient was unable to reach. Follow the procedure you learned for a complete bed bath. The body parts washed by the patient plus the body parts washed for the patient by the nursing assistant should equal a complete bed bath.
22. Put a clean gown on the patient without exposing her.
23. If the patient is allowed out of bed, assist her to a chair.
24. Make the empty bed.
25. Place the signal cord in its proper place.
26. Clean and put your equipment in its proper place. Discard disposable equipment.
27. Wipe off the bedside table. Discard all soiled linen in the dirty linen hamper in the utility room.
28. Make the patient comfortable.
29. Lower the bed to a position of safety for the patient.
30. Pull the curtains back to the open position.
31. Raise the side rails where ordered, indicated, and appropriate for patient safety.
32. Place the call light within easy reach of the patient.
33. Wash your hands.
34. Report to your immediate supervisor:
    - That you have given the patient a partial bath
    - How the patient tolerated the procedure
    - Your observations of anything unusual

Procedure The Tub Bath

1. Assemble your equipment on a chair near the bathtub.
    a) Bath towels
    b) Washcloths
    c) Soap
    d) Bath thermometer
    e) Wash basin
    f) Chair (place near the bathtub)
    g) Clean gown
    h) Disinfectant solution
2. Wash your hands.
3. Identify the patient by checking the identification bracelet.
4. Ask visitors to step out of the room, if this is your hospital's policy.
5. Tell the patient you are going to give him a tub bath.
6. Pull the curtain around the bed for privacy.
7. Help the patient out of bed. Get him into a bathrobe and slippers and to the room with the bathtub, either by walking or by wheelchair (Figure 12-28).
8. For safety, remove all electrical appliances from near the bathtub.
9. Place the chair next to the bathtub. Assist the patient into the chair.
10. Wash the bathtub with the disinfectant solution (Figure 12-29). You may do this before you get the patient up.

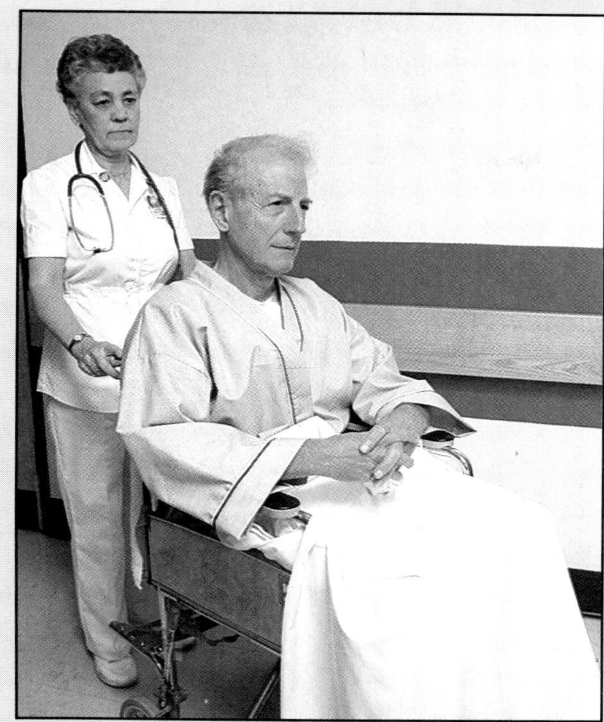

FIGURE 12-28

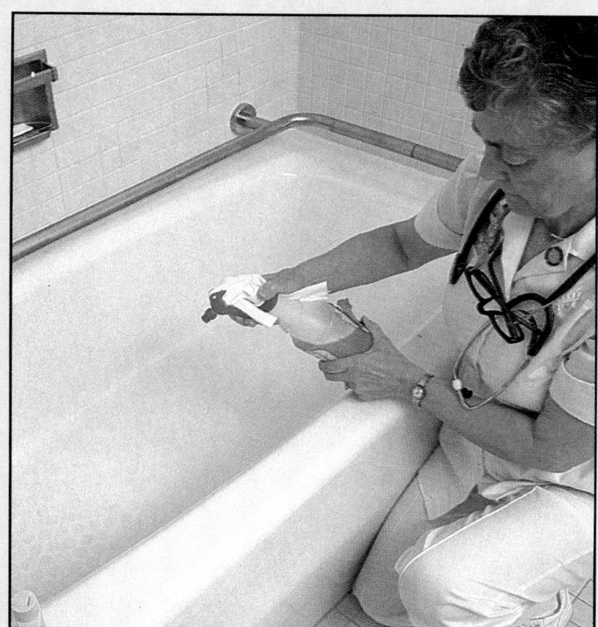

FIGURE 12-29

11. Fill the bathtub half full of water at 105°F (40.5°C). Test the temperature with a bath thermometer.
12. Place one towel in the bathtub for the patient to sit on (Figure 12-30).

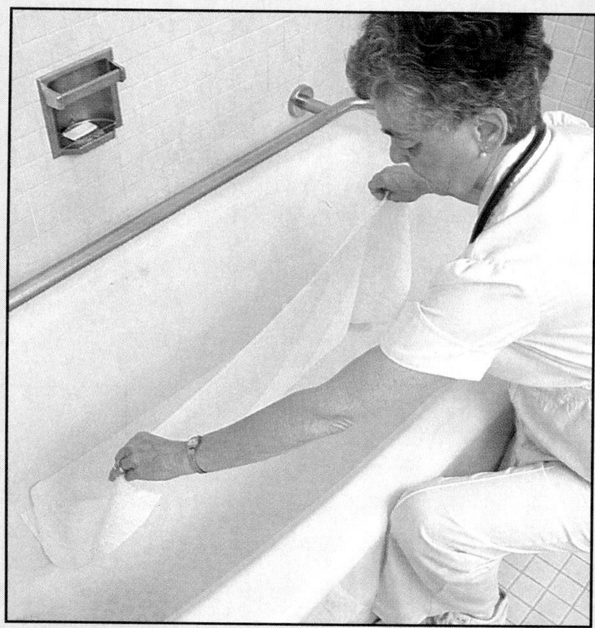

FIGURE 12-30

13. Place one towel or bath mat on the floor where the patient will step out of the tub. This will prevent him from slipping.
14. Assist the patient to get undressed and into the bathtub.
15. Let the patient stay in the bathtub as long as permitted, according to your instructions.
16. Help the patient wash himself, if help is needed (Figure 12-31).

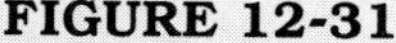

FIGURE 12-31

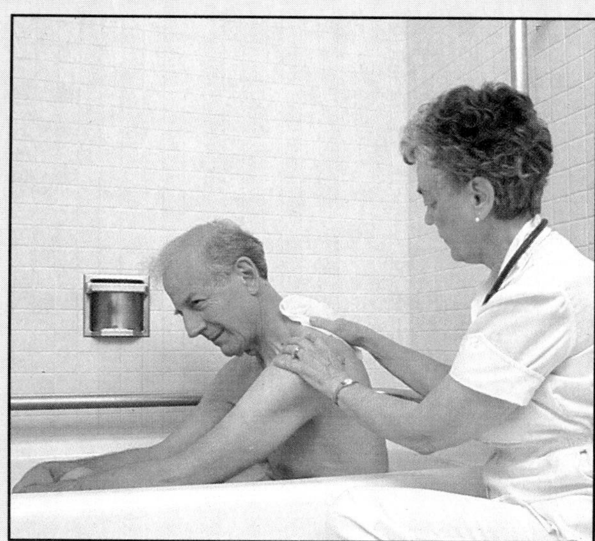

17. Put one towel across the chair.
18. Help the patient out of the bathtub. Seat him on the towel-covered chair, if he needs assistance.
19. Dry the patient well by patting gently with a towel (Figure 12-32). Help him put on pajamas or gown, bathrobe, and slippers.

FIGURE 12-32

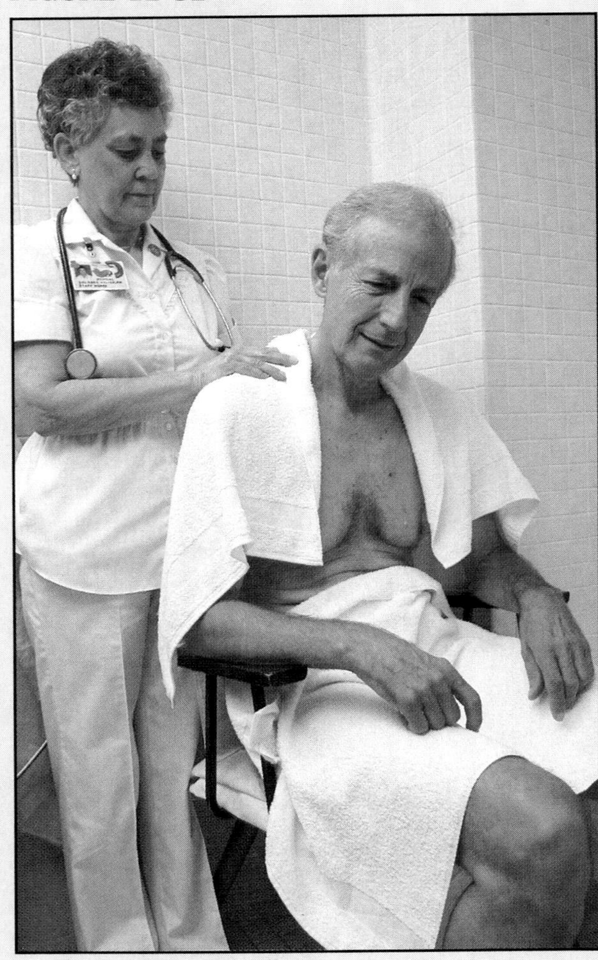

20. Help the patient return to his room and into bed.
21. Make the patient comfortable.
22. Lower the bed to a position of safety for the patient.
23. Pull the curtains back to the open position.
24. Raise the side rails where ordered, indicated, and appropriate for patient safety.
25. Place the call light within easy reach of the patient.
26. Return to the tub room. Clean the bathtub with disinfectant solution (Figure 12-33).

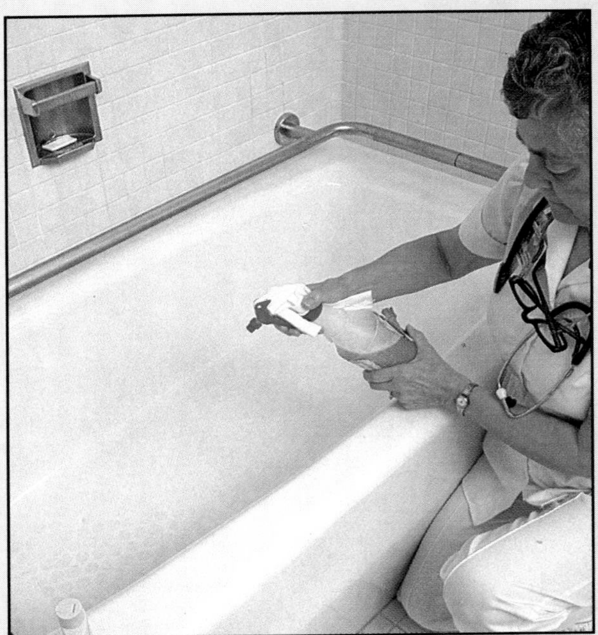

FIGURE 12-33

27. Remove all used linen. Put it in the dirty linen hamper in the utility room.
28. Wash your hands.
29. Report to your immediate supervisor:
    - That you have given the patient a tub bath
    - How the patient tolerated the procedure
    - Your observations of anything unusual

Procedure Helping the Patient Take a Shower

1. Assemble your equipment on a chair near the shower:
   a) Towels
   b) Soap
   c) Showercap
   d) Washcloth
   e) Clean gown
   f) Disinfectant solution
2. Wash your hands.
3. Identify the patient by checking the identification bracelet.
4. Ask visitors to step out of the room, if this is your hospital's policy.
5. Tell the patient that you will assist her with taking a shower.
6. Pull the curtain around the bed for privacy.
7. Help the patient out of bed and into a bathrobe and slippers. Help her to the bathroom with shower, as necessary.
8. For safety, remove all electrical appliances from the shower room.
9. Place one towel on the floor outside the shower.
10. Place one towel on a chair close to the shower. Assist the patient into the chair.
11. Wash the floor of the shower with disinfectant solution (you may do this before you get the patient up).
12. Turn on the shower and adjust the water temperature.
13. Assist the patient into the shower.
14. Give the patient soap and washcloth so that she can wash herself, but wait beside the shower in case the patient needs assistance.
15. Turn off the water and assist the patient out of the shower when she is finished. Seat her on the towel-covered chair.
16. Dry the patient well by patting gently with the towel.
17. Assist her with putting on pajamas or nightgown, bathrobe, and slippers.
18. Help the patient return to her room and into bed, or a chair if permitted.
19. Make the patient comfortable.
20. Lower the bed to a position of safety for the patient.
21. Pull the curtains back to the open position.
22. Raise the side rails where ordered, indicated, and appropriate for patient safety.
23. Place call light within easy reach of the patient.
24. Return to the shower room. Remove all used linen and put it in the dirty linen hamper in the dirty utility room.
25. Wash your hands.
26. Report to your immediate supervisor:
    - That you have helped the patient take a shower
    - How the patient tolerated the procedure
    - Your observations of anything unusual

Self-care

Self-care
Activities or care tasks performed by the patient.

Patients who are ordered to be on **self-care** should be encouraged to do as much as possible for themselves.

KEY IDEAS

The Back Rub

Rubbing a patient's back refreshes him or her, relaxes the muscles, and stimulates circulation. Because of pressure caused by the bedclothes and the lack of movement to stimulate circulation, the skin of a bedridden patient needs special care (Figure 12-34).

Back rubs are usually given during morning care, right after the patient's bath. They also are given (1) as part of evening care, (2) when changing the position of a bedridden patient, (3) for very restless patients who need relaxing, and (4) on a doctor's orders for "special back care."

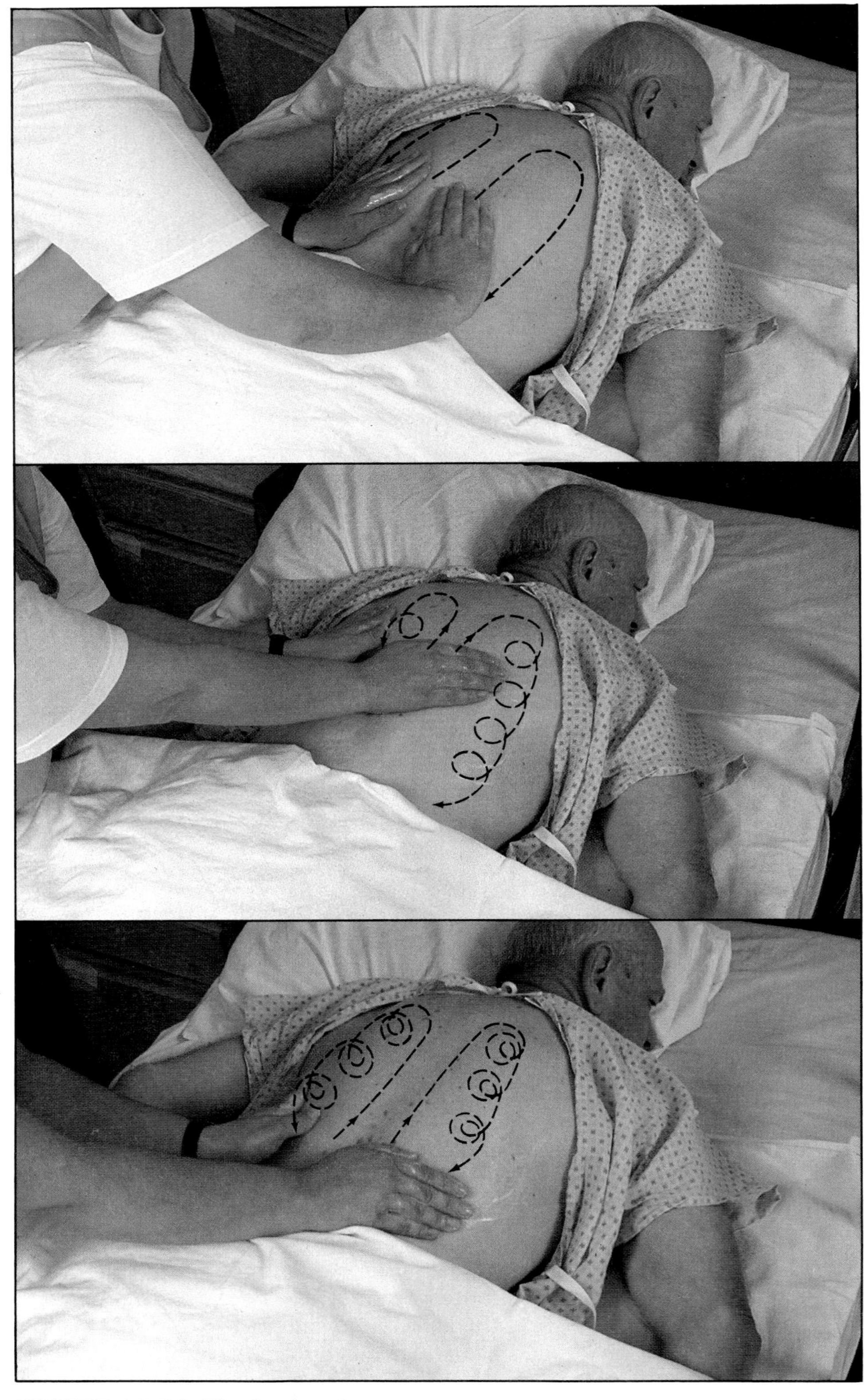

FIGURE 12-34 The back rub.

Procedure Giving the Patient a Back Rub

1. Assemble your equipment on the bedside table:
   a) Towels
   b) Lotion
   c) Basin of warm water at 115°F (46.1°C)
2. Wash your hands.
3. Identify the patient by checking the identification bracelet.
4. Ask visitors to step out of the room, if this is your hospital's policy.
5. Tell the patient you are going to give him a back rub.
6. Pull the curtain around the bed for privacy.
7. Ask the patient to turn on his side so his back is toward you. Or have him turn on his abdomen. Use the position that is most comfortable for the patient and for yourself. Raise bed to a comfortable working position.
8. The side rail should be in the up position on the far side of the bed.
9. Lotion should be warmed by placing the container in a basin of warm water 115°F (46.1°C). Also, warm your hands by running warm water over them (Figure 12-35).
10. Open the ties on the patient's gown.

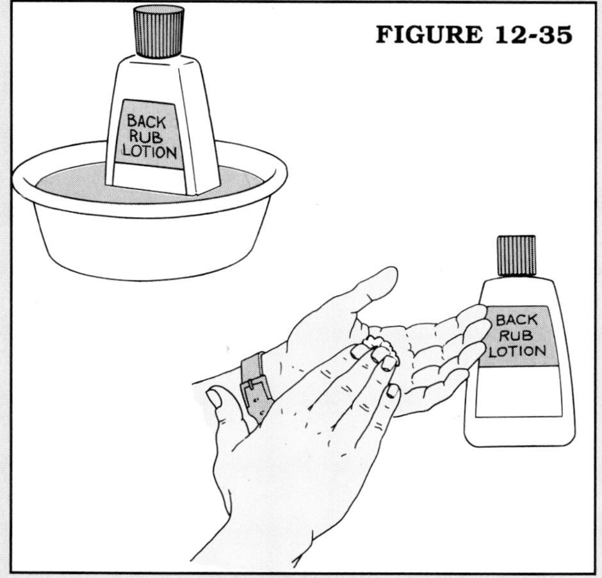

FIGURE 12-35

11. Pour a small amount of lotion into the palm of your hand.
12. Rub your hands together using friction to warm the lotion.
13. Apply lotion to the entire back with the palms of your hands. Use firm, long strokes from the buttocks to the shoulders and back of the neck.
14. Keep your knees slightly bent and your back straight.
15. Exert firm pressure as you stroke upward from the buttocks toward the shoulders. Use gentle pressure as you stroke downward from shoulders to buttocks.
16. Use a circular motion on each bony area.
17. This rhythmic rubbing motion should be continued from one and one-half minutes to three minutes.
18. Dry the patient's back by patting gently with a towel.
19. Close and retie the gown.
20. Assist the patient to turn back to a comfortable position.
21. Arrange the top sheets of the bed neatly.
22. Put your equipment back in its proper place. Discard disposable equipment.
23. Make the patient comfortable.
24. Lower the bed to a position of safety for the patient.
25. Pull the curtains back to the open position.
26. Raise the side rails where ordered, indicated, and appropriate for patient safety.
27. Place the call light within easy reach of the patient.
28. Wash your hands.
29. Report to your immediate supervisor:
    - That you have given the patient a back rub
    - The time it was given
    - How the patient tolerated the procedure
    - Your observations of anything unusual

KEY IDEAS

Changing the Patient's Gown

It is important when you change a patient's gown not to expose his or her body unnecessarily. In this way you avoid chills and prevent embarrassment for the patient.

Procedure Changing the Patient's Gown

1. Assemble your equipment on the bedside table:
   a) A clean gown
2. Wash your hands.
3. Identify the patient by checking the identification bracelet.
4. Ask visitors to step out of the room, if this is your hospital's policy.
5. Tell the patient you are going to change his gown.
6. Pull the curtain around the bed for privacy.
7. Ask the patient to turn on his side with his back toward you so you can untie the tapes.
8. If the patient cannot be turned, you will have to reach under his neck to untie the tapes.
9. Loosen the soiled gown around the patient's body.
10. Get the clean gown ready to put on the patient. Unfold it and lay it across the patient's chest on top of the bath blanket or top sheets.

FIGURE 12-36

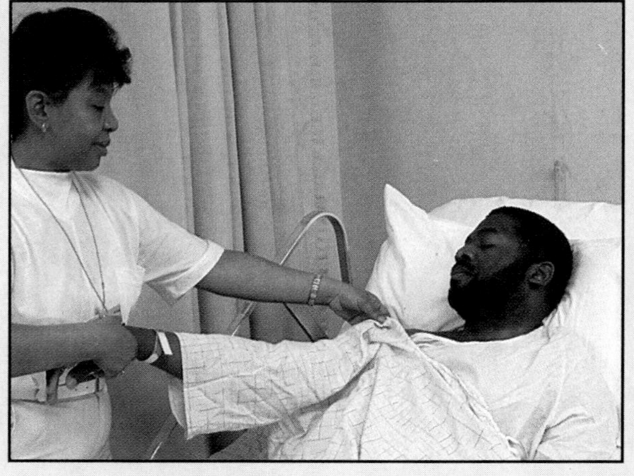

11. Take off one sleeve at a time, leaving the old gown in place on the patient.
12. Slide each arm through one sleeve of the clean gown (Figure 12-36).
13. If the patient cannot hold his arm up, put your hand through the sleeve. Take his hand in yours and slip the sleeve up the patient's wrist and arm. Do this for both arms. Then pull the gown down over the patient's chest. If the patient has a sore arm, remove the sleeve on the unaffected arm first. Then remove the sleeve on the sore (affected) arm. To put the clean gown on, put the sleeve on the sore (affected) arm first. Then slide the unaffected arm through the second sleeve.
14. Remove the soiled gown from under the bath blanket or top sheets.
15. Tie the tapes on the clean gown. Some patients want only the tapes at the neck tied so they will not be lying on knots.
16. Put the soiled gown in the dirty linen hamper in the dirty utility room.
17. Make the patient comfortable.
18. Lower the bed to a position of safety for the patient.
19. Pull the curtains back to the open position.
20. Raise the side rails where ordered, indicated, and appropriate for patient safety.
21. Place the call light within easy reach of the patient.
22. Wash your hands.
23. Report to your immediate supervisor:
    - That you have replaced the patient's soiled gown with a clean one
    - Your observations of anything unusual

KEY IDEAS

Shampooing the Patient's Hair

Patients who will be in the health care institution for a long time may occasionally need to have their hair shampooed. Often the doctor must write the order for a shampoo. The nurse must give you instructions for giving the shampoo. For patients on bed rest, the patient must be in bed when the shampoo is given (Figure 12-37). Other patients may be allowed to shampoo in the tub or shower.

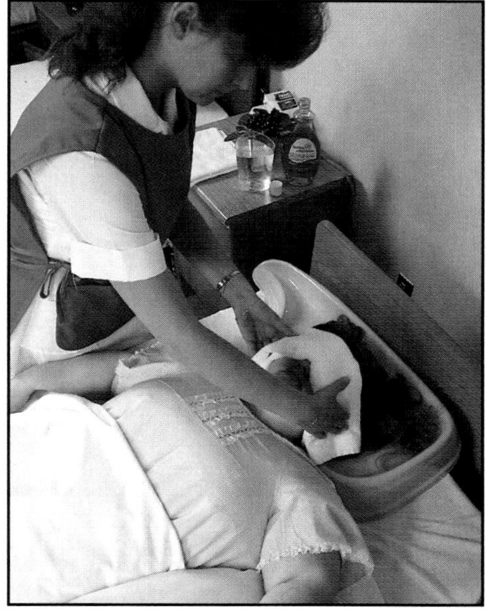

FIGURE 12-37 Giving the patient a shampoo in bed.

Procedure Shampooing the Patient's Hair

1. Assemble your equipment on the bedside table:
   a) Chair
   b) Basin of water at 105°F (40.5°C)
   c) Pitcher of water at 115°F (46.1°C)
   d) Bath thermometer
   e) Large basin
   f) Water trough (shampoo tray) or plastic sheet
   g) Disposable bed protector
   h) Pillow with waterproof case
   i) Bath towels
   j) Washcloth, to cover the patient's eyes
   k) Paper or Styrofoam® cup
   l) Bath blanket
   m) Small towel
   n) Cotton
2. Wash your hands.
3. Identify the patient by checking the identification bracelet.
4. Ask visitors to step out of the room, if this is your hospital's policy.
5. Tell the patient you are going to give her a shampoo.
6. Pull the curtain around the bed for privacy.
7. Raise the bed to its highest horizontal position.
8. Place a chair at the side of the bed near the patient's head. The chair should be lower than the mattress. The back of the chair should be touching the mattress.
9. Place the small towel on the chair. Put the large basin on the chair.
10. Put small amounts of cotton in the patient's ears for protection.
11. Ask the patient to move across the bed so that her head is close to where you are standing.

12. Remove the pillow from under the patient's head. Cover the pillow with the waterproof case. Have the pillow under the small of the patient's back, so that when she lies down, her head is tilted back.
13. Put the bath blanket on the bed. From underneath, fan-fold the top sheets to the foot of the bed without exposing the patient.
14. Place the disposable bed protector on the mattress under the patient's head.
15. Place the shampoo trough under the patient's head. A trough can be made by rolling over the three sides of the plastic sheet three times. This makes a channel for the water to run off. Put the end of the channel under the patient's head. Have the other open end hanging over the side of the bed. This free end of the plastic sheet should be put into the large basin on the chair.
16. Loosen the patient's gown at the neck and turn the neckband under.
17. Ask the patient to hold the washcloth over her eyes.
18. Fill the basin with water at 105°F (40.5°C). Put the basin on the bedside table with the paper or Styrofoam® cup.
19. Fill the pitcher with water at 115°F (46.1°C). Have the pitcher on the bedside table, for extra water, if needed.
20. Brush the patient's hair. Have her turn her head from side to side so the hair can be brushed one exposed side at a time.
21. Fill the paper cup with water from the basin. Pour it over the hair; repeat until completely wet.
22. Apply a small amount of shampoo and, using both hands, wash the hair and massage the patient's scalp with your fingertips. Avoid using fingernails as they could scratch the scalp.
23. Rinse the soap off the hair by pouring water from the cup over the hair. Have the patient turn her head from side to side. Repeat this until the hair is clear of shampoo.
24. Dry the patient's forehead and ears with the face towel.
25. Remove the cotton from the ears.
26. Raise the patient's head and wrap the head with a bath towel.
27. Rub the patient's hair with the towel to dry it as much as possible.
28. Remove your equipment from the bed. Change the patient's gown, if necessary.
29. Comb the patient's hair. Leave a towel wrapped around the head or spread a towel out over the pillow under the head until the hair is completely dry. If a dryer is available, use it to dry the patient's hair.
30. Remove the bath blanket and at the same time bring the top sheets back up to cover the patient.
31. Clean your equipment and put it in its proper place. Discard disposable equipment.
32. Make the patient comfortable.
33. Lower the bed to a position of safety for the patient.
34. Pull the curtains back to the open position.
35. Raise the side rails where ordered, indicated, and appropriate for patient safety.
36. Place the call light within easy reach of the patient.
37. Wash your hands.
38. Report to your immediate supervisor:
    - That you have given the patient a shampoo
    - How the patient tolerated the procedure
    - Your observations of anything unusual

KEY IDEAS

Combing the Patient's Hair

As with other types of personal care, a patient may be too weak or sick to take care of his own hair. It may be difficult for him to raise his arms. Almost always, however, combing and brushing a patient's hair, which makes him look better, will also make him feel better.

Procedure Combing the Patient's Hair

1. Assemble your equipment on the bedside table:
   a) Towel
   b) Comb or brush
   c) Hand mirror, if available
2. Wash your hands.
3. Identify the patient by checking the identification bracelet.
4. Ask visitors to step out of the room, if this is your hospital's policy.
5. Tell the patient you are going to brush or comb his hair.
6. Pull the curtain around the bed for privacy.
7. If possible, comb the patient's hair after the bath and before you make the bed.
8. Lay a towel across the pillow under the patient's head. If the patient can sit up in bed, drape the towel around his shoulders.
9. If the patient wears glasses, ask him to take them off before you begin. Be sure to put the glasses in a safe place.
10. Part the hair down the middle to make it easier to comb.
11. Brush or comb the patient's hair carefully, gently, and thoroughly, combing small amounts of hair at a time.
12. For the patient who cannot sit up, separate the hair into small sections. Comb each section separately, using a downward motion. Ask the patient to turn his head from side to side or turn it for him so you can reach the entire head (Figure 12-38).
13. Comb the patient's hair into the style the patient requests.
14. If the patient has very long hair, suggest braiding it to keep it from getting tangled.
15. Be sure you brush the back of the head.
16. Remove the towel when you are finished.
17. Let the patient use the mirror.

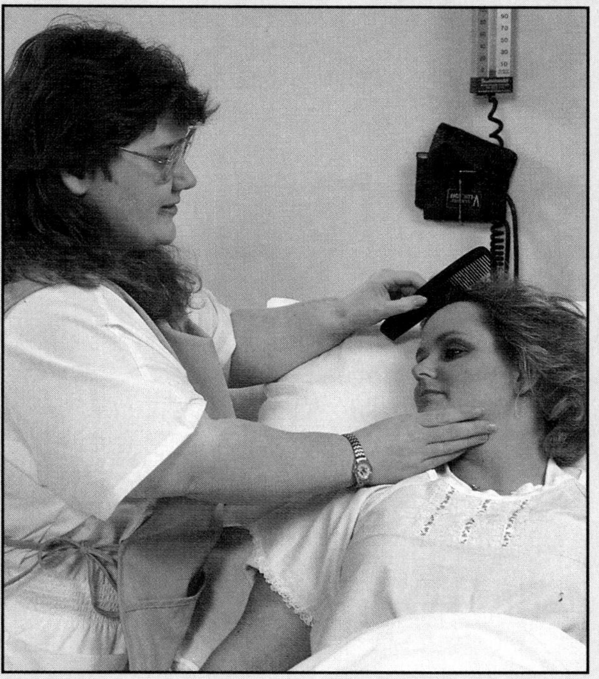

FIGURE 12-38

18. Put your equipment back in its proper place.
19. Make the patient comfortable.
20. Lower the bed to a position of safety for the patient.
21. Pull the curtains back to the open position.
22. Raise the side rails where ordered, indicated, and appropriate for patient safety.
23. Place the call light within easy reach of the patient.
24. Wash your hands.
25. Report to your immediate supervisor:
    - That you have combed the patient's hair
    - How the patient tolerated the procedure
    - Your observations of anything unusual

KEY IDEAS

Shaving the Patient's Beard

A regular morning activity for most men is shaving their beard. A patient is often well enough to shave himself. In this case, you will give him only the help that is necessary, such as being sure he has the equipment he needs. Sometimes patients are too ill or weak to shave themselves. In such cases, you will do it. Before shaving any patient's face, be sure to get permission from your immediate supervisor. Certain patients may not be permitted to shave or be shaved.

Shaving can be done with an electric razor or a safety razor. Often, the patient will have his own electric razor which you will be able to use. Many hospitals have special rules and policies regarding electrical equipment being brought into the hospital. Follow the nurse's instructions regarding electric razors.

Procedure Shaving the Patient's Beard

1. Assemble your equipment on the bedside table:
   a) Basin of water at 115°F (46.1°C)
   b) Shaving brush, shaving cream, and safety razor, or
   c) electric razor
2. Wash your hands.
3. Identify the patient by checking the identification bracelet.
4. Ask visitors to step out of the room, if this is your hospital's policy.
5. Tell the patient you are going to shave his beard.
6. Pull the curtain around the bed for privacy.
7. Adjust a light so that it shines on the patient's face.
8. Raise the head of the bed, if allowed.
9. Spread the face towel under the patient's chin. If the patient has dentures, be sure they are in his mouth.
10. Pat some warm water or use a damp, warm washcloth on the patient's face to soften his beard if using a safety razor.
11. Apply shaving soap generously to the face if using a safety razor.
12. With the fingers of one hand, hold the skin taut (tight) as you shave in the direction that the hairs grow. Start under the sideburns and work downward over the cheeks (Figure 12-39). Continue carefully over the chin. Work upward on the neck under the chin. Use short, firm strokes.
13. Rinse the safety razor often.
14. Areas under the nose and around the lips are sensitive. Take special care in these areas.
15. If you nick the patient's skin, report this to your head nurse or team leader.

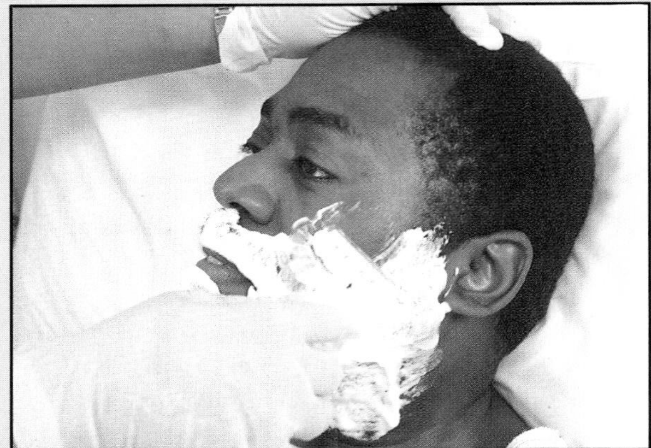

FIGURE 12-39 Some institutions use battery-operated razors. Follow your institution's policies regarding this matter.

16. Wash off the remaining soap when you have finished.
17. Apply aftershave lotion or powder as the patient prefers.
18. Clean your equipment and put it in its proper place. Discard disposable equipment.
19. Make the patient comfortable.
20. Lower the bed to a position of safety for the patient.
21. Pull the curtains back to the open position.
22. Raise the side rails where ordered, indicated, and appropriate for patient safety.
23. Place the call light within easy reach of the patient.
24. Wash your hands.
25. Report to your immediate supervisor:
    - That you have shaved the patient's beard
    - How the patient tolerated the procedure
    - Your observations of anything unusual

KEY QUESTIONS

1. What should be done for the patient during early morning care? morning care? afternoon care? evening care?
2. What should be recorded on the ADL flow sheet?
3. When should the patient receive oral hygiene? Why?
4. Name and describe the four types of baths.
5. Why is a back rub an important part of the daily care of the patient?
6. What is the most important thing to remember when changing the patient's gown? Why?
7. How can you shampoo a patients' hair in bed?
8. How should a patient's beard be shaved?
9. Define: activities of daily living, dentures, flow sheet, oral hygiene, self-care.

CHAPTER

13

Elimination

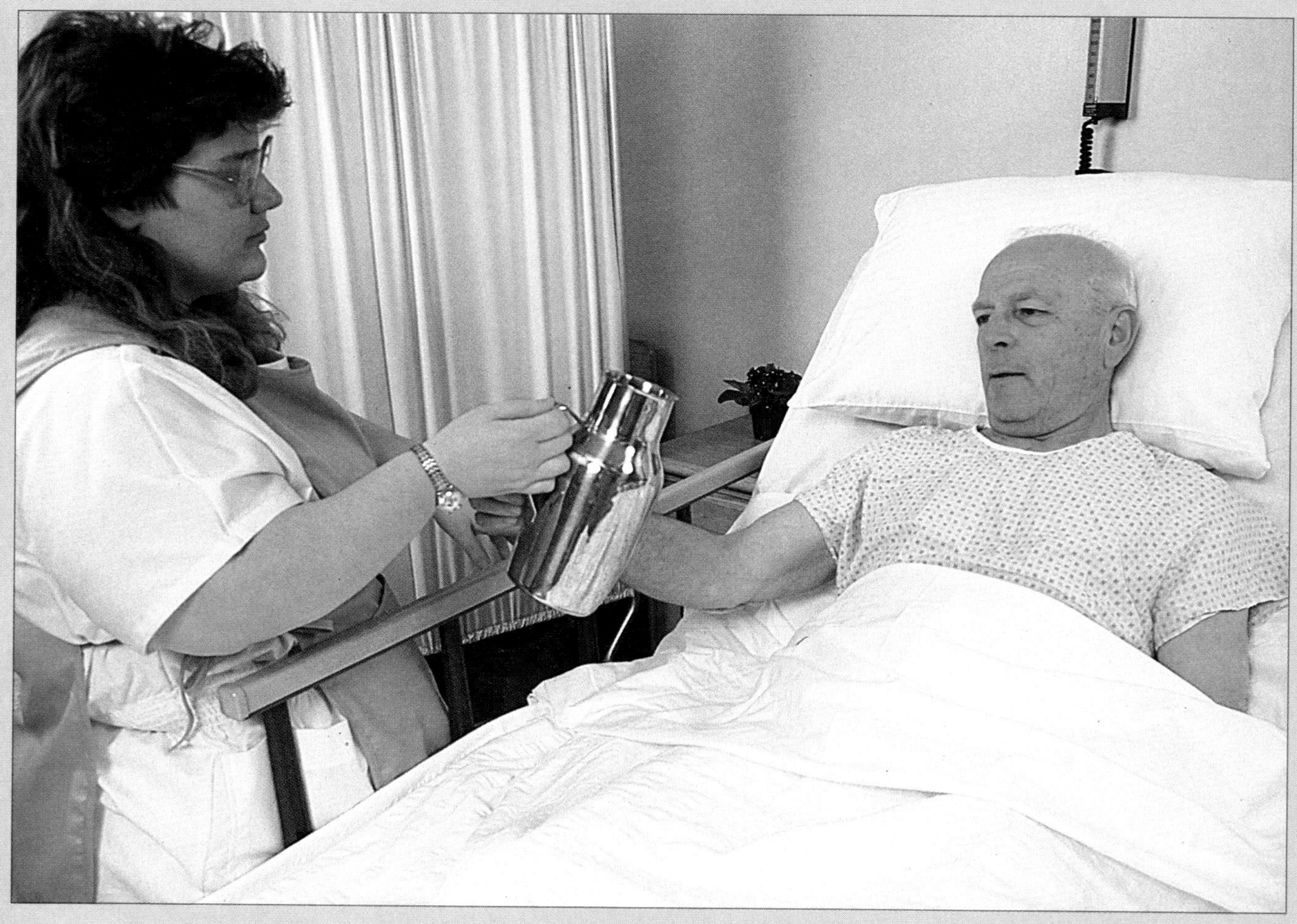

WARNING

For all patient contact, adhere to Universal Precautions (see page 91, 97, or the front cover flap). Wear protective equipment as indicated.

Objectives

What You Will Learn

When you have completed this chapter, you will be able to:

- Help the patient use a bedpan.
- Help the patient use a urinal.
- Help the patient use a bedside commode.
- Define: bedpan, commode, defecate, urinal, urinate.

Urinal
A portable pan given to male patients in bed so that they can urinate without getting out of bed.

Bedpan
A pan used by patients who must defecate or urinate while in bed.

Defecate
To have a bowel movement; to excrete waste matter from the bowels.

Urinate
To discharge urine from the body. Other words for this function are void and micturate.

KEY IDEAS

Offering the Bedpan or Urinal

SOME PATIENTS ARE UNABLE TO GET out of bed to use the bathroom. For these patients a **urinal** and a **bedpan** are required. The urinal is a container into which the male patient **urinates**. The bedpan is a pan into which he **defecates** (moves his bowels). The female patient uses the bedpan for urination and defecation. Wear gloves whenever handling a bedpan or urinal after use. You should always cover the bedpan and remove it from the patient's bedside to the bathroom as quickly as possible after use. At this time you would collect a specimen if required. You would also measure the urine if the patient is on intake and output.

Procedure Offering the Bedpan

1. Assemble your equipment on the bedside table (Figure 13-1).
   a) Bedpan and cover, or fracture bedpan and cover (Figure 13-2)
   b) Toilet tissue
   c) Wash basin with water at 115°F (46.1°C)
   d) Soap
   e) Hand towel
   f) Disposable gloves
2. Wash your hands.

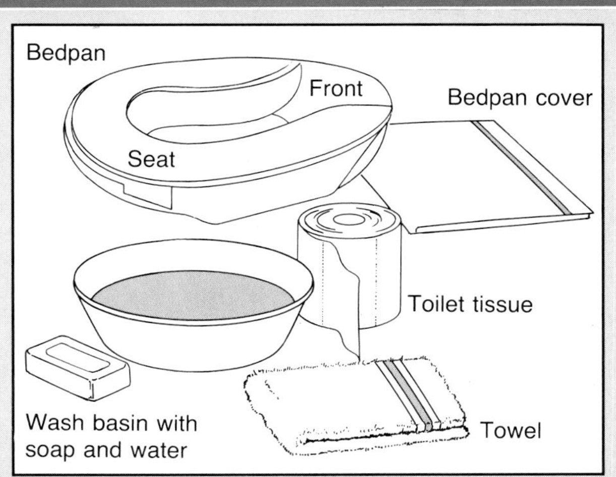

FIGURE 13-1

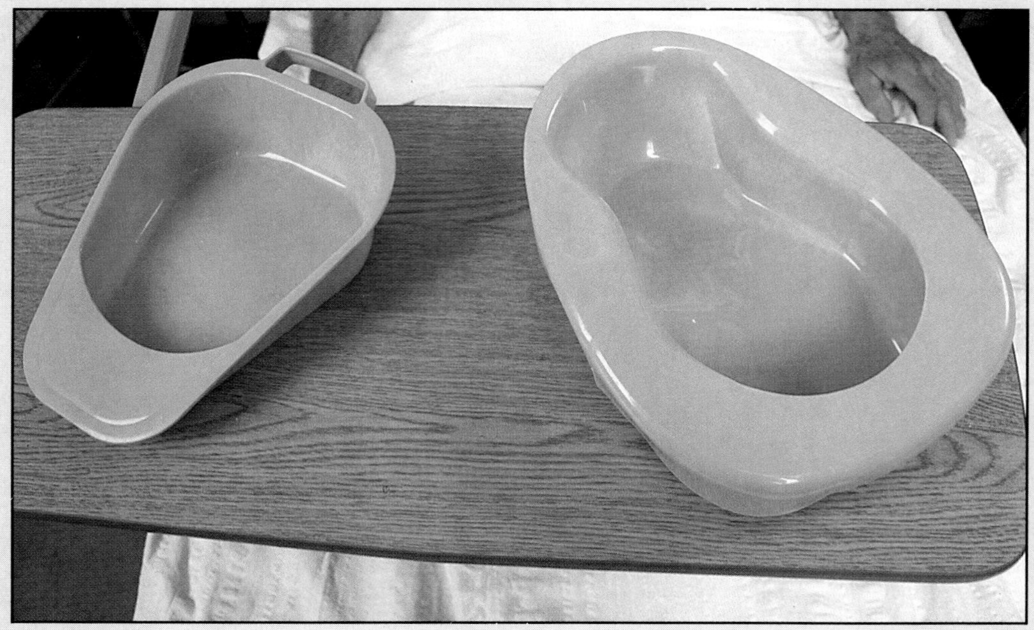

FIGURE 13-2

3. Identify the patient by checking the identification bracelet.
4. Ask visitors to step out of the room, if this is your hospital's policy.
5. Ask the patient if he would like to use the bedpan.
6. Pull the curtain around the bed for privacy.
7. Take the bedpan out of the bedside table. Warm the bedpan if necessary by running warm water inside it and along the rim. Dry the outside of the bedpan with paper towels. Put powder on the bedpan to decrease friction.
8. Fold back the top sheets so that they are out of the way.
9. Raise the patient's gown, but keep the lower part of his body covered.
10. Ask the patient to bend his knees and put his feet flat on the mattress if he is able. Then ask the patient to raise his hips. If necessary, help the patient to raise his buttocks by slipping your hand under the lower part of his back. Place the bedpan in position with the seat of the bedpan under the buttocks (Figure 13-3).

FIGURE 13-3

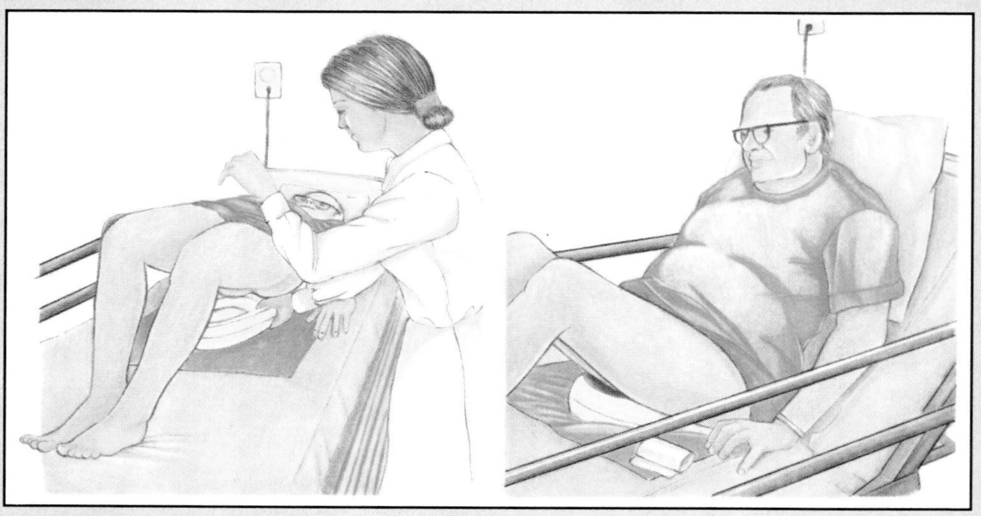

11. Sometimes the patient is unable to lift his buttocks to get on or off the bedpan. In this case, turn the patient on his side with his back to you. Put the bedpan against the buttocks. Then turn the patient onto the bedpan (Figure 13-4).
12. Replace the covers over the patient.
13. Raise the backrest and a knee rest, if allowed, so the patient is in a sitting position.
14. Put toilet tissue and the signal cord where the patient can reach them easily.
15. Ask the patient to signal when he is finished.

FIGURE 13-4

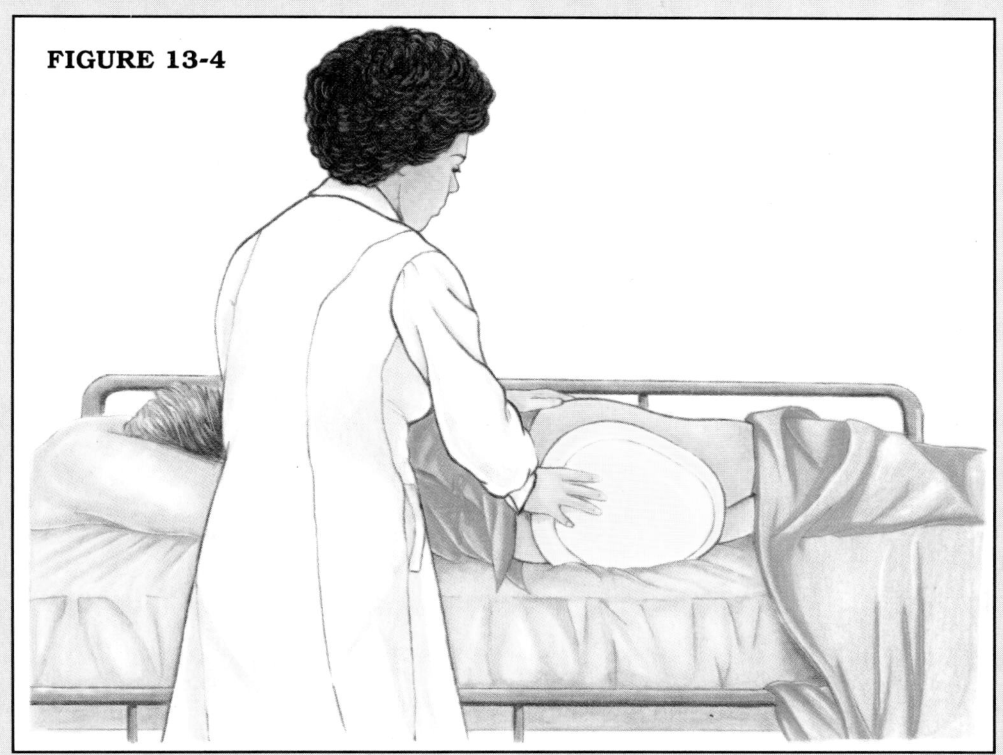

16. Raise the side rails to the up position.
17. Wash your hands. Leave the room to give the patient privacy.
18. When the patient signals, return to the room.
19. Wash your hands and put on gloves.
20. Help the patient to raise his hips so you can remove the bedpan.
21. Cover the bedpan immediately with a disposable pad or a paper towel if no cover is available (Figure 13-5).
22. Help the patient if he is unable to clean himself. Turn the patient on his side. Clean the anal area with toilet tissue.
23. Take the bedpan to the patient's bathroom. Clean your equipment and put it in its proper place. Discard disposable equipment.

FIGURE 13-5

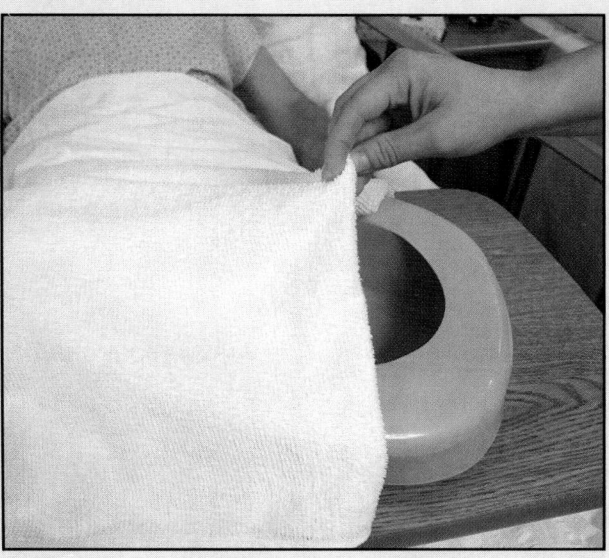

24. If a specimen is required, collect it at this time. Measure the urine if the patient is on intake and output.
25. Check the excreta (feces or urine) for abnormal (unusual) appearance.
26. Empty the bedpan into the patient's toilet.
27. Institutions have different equipment in the bathroom for cleaning the bedpan. Follow your institution's instructions for cleaning the bedpan.
28. Put the clean bedpan and cover back into the bedside table.
29. Help the patient to wash his hands in the basin of water.
30. Make the patient comfortable. Lower the backrest as necessary.
31. Lower the bed to a position of safety for the patient.
32. Pull the curtains back to the open position.
33. Raise the side rails where ordered, indicated, and appropriate for patient safety.
34. Place the call light within easy reach of the patient.
35. Wash your hands.
36. Report to your immediate supervisor:
    - That the patient has urinated or defecated
    - If a specimen was collected
    - How the patient tolerated the procedure
    - Your observations of anything unusual

Procedure Offering the Urinal

1. Assemble your equipment on the bedside table:
    a) Urinal and cover
    b) Basin with water at 115°F (46.1°C)
    c) Soap
    d) Towel
    e) Disposable gloves
2. Wash your hands.
3. Identify the patient by checking the identification bracelet.
4. Ask visitors to step out of the room, if this is your hospital's policy.
5. Ask the patient if he would like to use the urinal.
6. Pull the curtain around the bed for privacy.
7. Give the urinal to the patient (Figure 13-6).
8. Place the signal cord within easy reach.

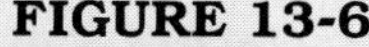

FIGURE 13-6

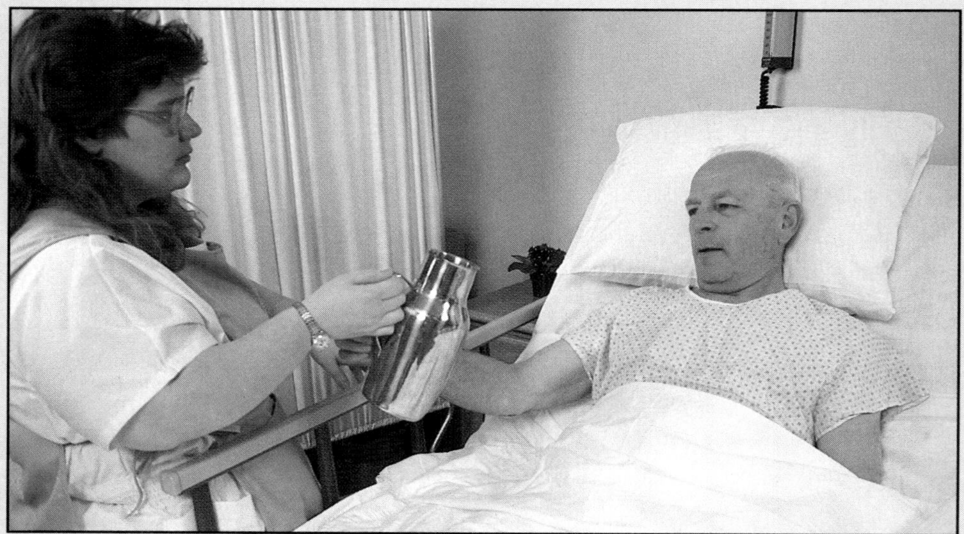

9. Ask the patient to signal when he is finished.
10. Wash your hands. Leave the room to give the patient privacy.
11. When the patient signals, return to the room, wash your hands, and put on gloves.
12. Cover the urinal and take it to the patient's bathroom.
13. Check the urine for abnormal (unusual) appearance.
14. Measure the urine if the patient is on intake and output. Collect a specimen at this time, if required.
15. Empty the urinal into the toilet. Rinse.
16. Put the clean urinal back in the patient's bedside table.
17. Help the patient to wash his hands in the basin of water.
18. Make the patient comfortable.
19. Lower the bed to a position of safety for the patient.
20. Pull the curtains back to the open position.
21. Raise the side rails where ordered, indicated, and appropriate for patient safety.
22. Place the call light within easy reach of the patient.
23. Wash your hands.
24. Report to your immediate supervisor:
    - That the patient has urinated or defecated
    - If a specimen was collected
    - How the patient tolerated the procedure
    - Your observations of anything unusual

Procedure Offering the Portable Bedside Commode

1. Assemble your equipment on the bedside table:
   a) Portable bedside commode next to the bed (Figure 13-7)
   b) Bedpan and cover, or the container used in your institution
   c) Toilet tissue
   d) Basin of water at 115°F (46.1°C)
   e) Soap
   f) Towel
   g) Disposable gloves
2. Wash your hands.
3. Identify the patient by checking the identification bracelet.
4. Ask visitors to step out of the room, if this is your hospital's policy.
5. Tell the patient you will assist him onto the bedside commode.
6. Pull the curtain around the bed for privacy.
7. Put the commode next to the patient's bed. Open the cover and insert a bedpan under the toilet seat if there is not a pan already in place.

Commode
A movable chair enclosing a bedpan or with an opening that can fit over a toilet.

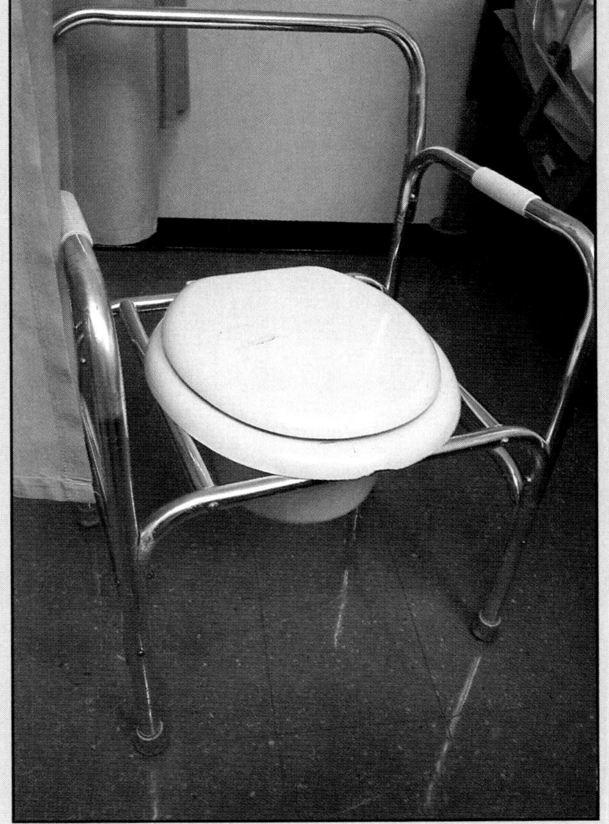

FIGURE 13-7

8. Help the patient put on his slippers and then help him out of bed and onto the commode.
9. Put toilet tissue and the signal cord where the patient can reach them easily.
10. Ask the patient to signal when he is finished.
11. Wash your hands. Leave the room to give the patient privacy.
12. When the patient signals, return to the room. Wash your hands.
13. Put on gloves to help the patient clean himself.
14. Assist the patient back to bed.
15. Close the cover on the commode.
16. Help the patient to wash his hands in the basin of water.
17. Make the patient comfortable.
18. Remove the bedpan from under the commode. Cover it and carry it to the patient's bathroom.
19. Check the excreta (feces or urine) for abnormal (unusual) appearance.
20. Measure output if patient is on intake and output. If a specimen is required, collect it at this time.
21. Empty the bedpan into the toilet.
22. Institutions have different equipment in the bathroom for cleaning the bedpan. Follow your instructions for cleaning the bedpan in your institution.
23. Put the clean bedpan back in the bedside table. Put the commode in its proper place.
24. Make the patient comfortable.
25. Lower the bed to a position of safety for the patient.
26. Pull the curtains back to the open position.
27. Raise the side rails where ordered, indicated, and appropriate for patient safety.
28. Place the call light within easy reach of the patient.
29. Wash your hands.
30. Report to your immediate supervisor:
    - That the patient has voided or defecated
    - If a specimen was collected
    - How the patient tolerated the procedure
    - Your observations of anything unusual

KEY QUESTIONS

1. Which patients should be offered the bedpan?
2. Which patients should be offered the urinal?
3. Which patients should be offered the use of the portable bedside commode?
4. Define: bedpan, commode, defecate, urinal, urinate.

CHAPTER

14

The Human Body

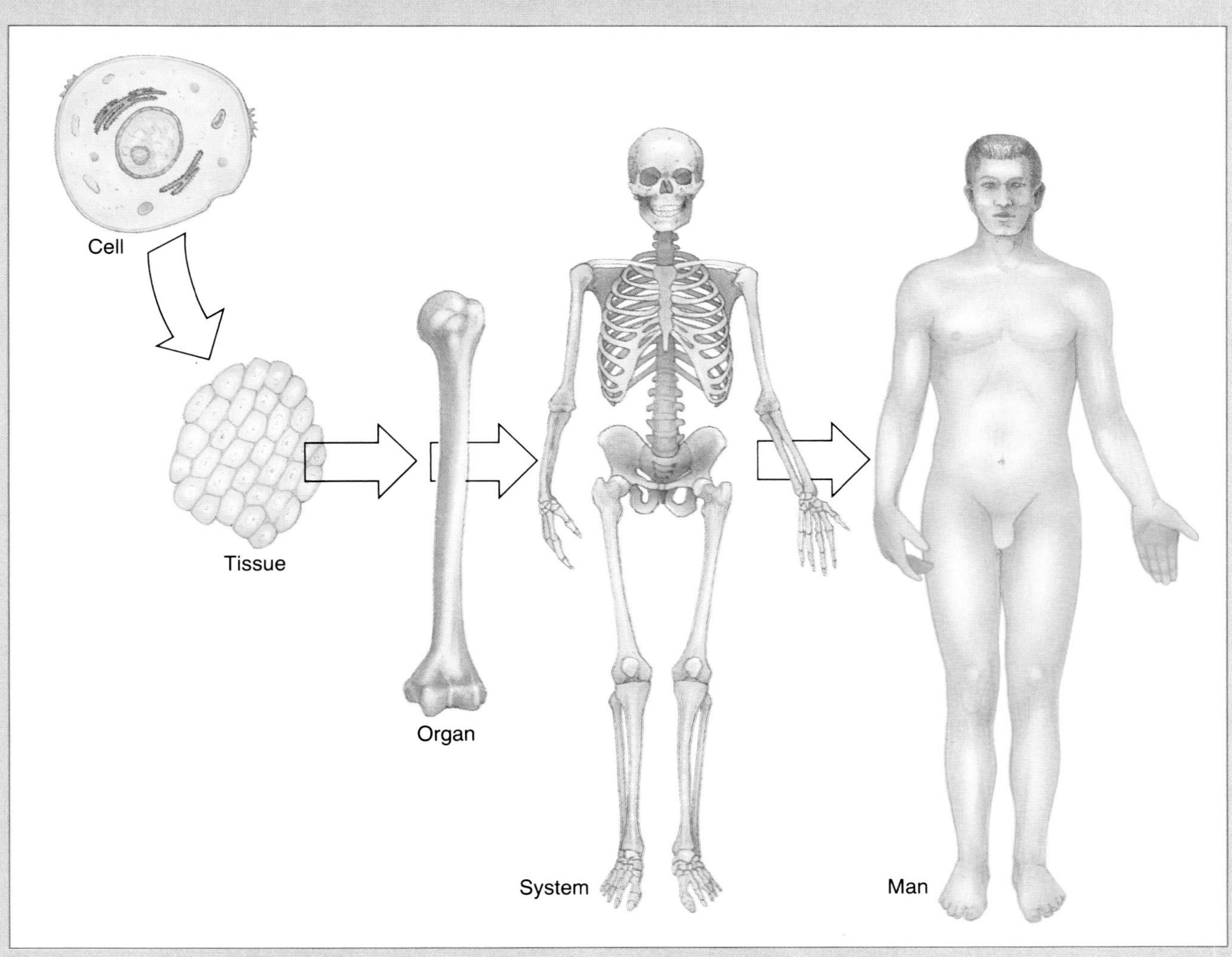

WARNING

For all patient contact, adhere to Universal Precautions (see page 91, 97, or the front cover flap). Wear protective equipment as indicated.

Objectives

What You Will Learn

When you have completed this chapter, you will be able to:

- Name the body areas and cavities.
- List the things all living cells have in common.
- Relate the parts of a cell to their functions.
- Explain the process of cellular reproduction.
- Name the primary kinds of tissues, their duties, and examples of their location in the human body.
- List the basic groupings of cells that build a human being.
- Identify the organs and basic functions of each body system.
- Describe the developmental tasks and typical characteristics of each stage of growth and development.
- Explain the major causes of disease, including an example of each type.
- Contrast benign and malignant tumors.
- List the signs and symptoms of cancer.
- Explain the psychosocial aspects of cancer.
- Define: acute, anatomy, anterior, benign, blood and lymph tissue, cancer, cardiac muscle tissue, cell, chronic, connective tissue, deep, development, dorsal, epithelial tissue, growth, inferior, malignant, metastasis, muscle tissue, neoplasm, nerve tissue, organ, physiology, posterior, superficial, superior, system, tissue, tumor, and ventral.

Anatomy
The study of the structure of an organism.

Physiology
The study of the functions of the body.

KEY IDEAS
Anatomy and Physiology

ANATOMY IS THE STUDY OF THE structure of the body. **Physiology** is the study of the bodily functions. Knowledge of these subjects will help you understand the instructions the nurse gives you. The study of anatomy and physiology is the basis for understanding the clinical procedures you will be doing as a nursing assistant.

KEY IDEAS
Body Areas and Cavities

Anterior
Located in the front; opposite of posterior.

Posterior
Located in the back or toward the rear.

As part of the study of each system, it would be wise to take an overall look at the body and to become familiar with the names given to body areas and cavities. In any demonstration or diagram, the body or body part shown is in the anatomical position (Figure 14-1). The person is standing up straight, facing you, palms out and feet together. When you look at a person in the anatomical position, remember that the left side is always on your right side. This is especially important in studying diagrams. The front of a person is referred to as the **anterior** side. The back, containing the spine (backbone), is called the **posterior** side. The areas of the body closer to the head are called **superior**. Those closer to

Ventral
On the abdominal, anterior, or front side of the body.

Deep
Distant from the surface of the body.

Dorsal
Refers to the back or to the back part of an organ.

Superficial
On or near the surface of the body.

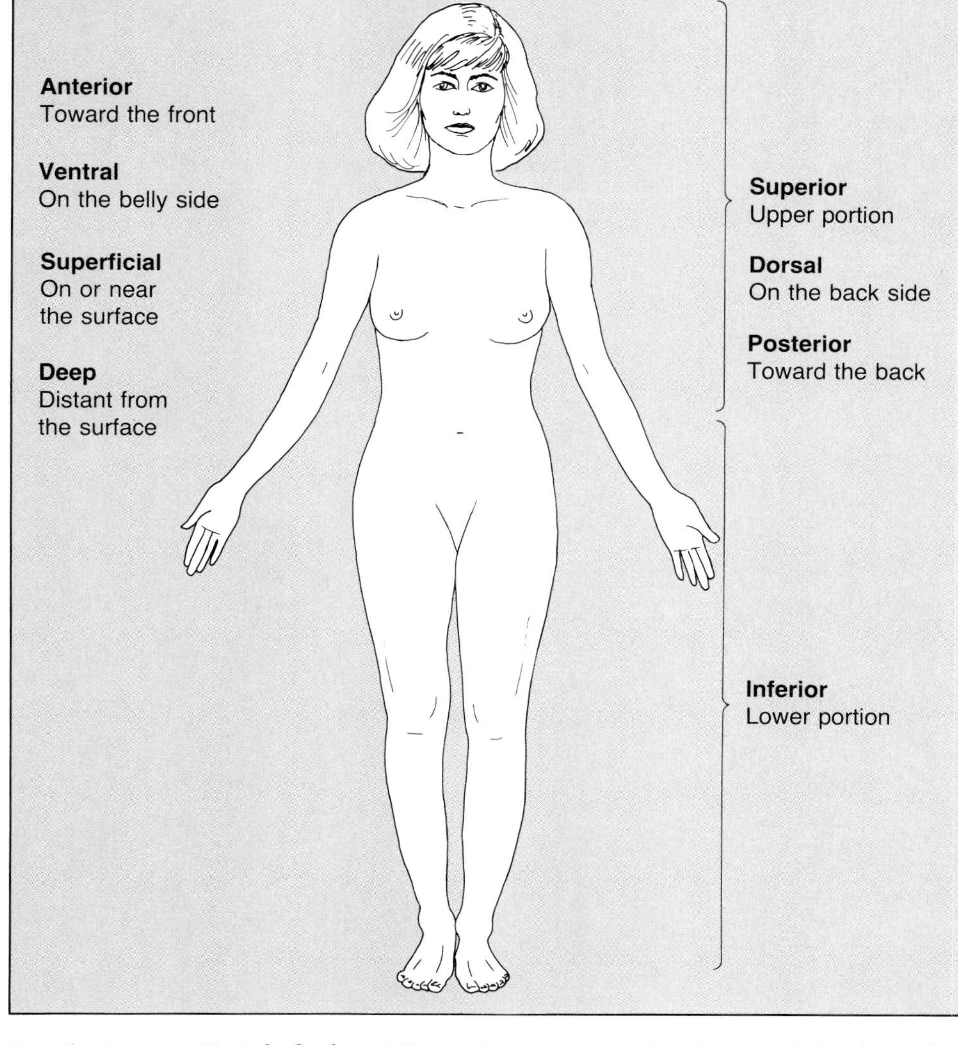

FIGURE 14-1 Where body parts are located.

Superior
The upper portion of the body.

Inferior
Lower portion of the body.

the feet are called **inferior**. These terms may also be used to describe the position of an organ in the body. For example, the liver is inferior to the diaphragm. The shoulder is superior to the elbow.

The body has two major cavities, the dorsal cavity and the ventral cavity (Figure 14-2). The dorsal cavity is divided into the cranial and spinal cavities. The cranial cavity is in the head and contains the brain, its protecting membranes, large blood vessels, and nerves. The spinal cavity contains the spinal cord.

The ventral cavity is divided into the thoracic and abdominal cavities by a large, dome-shaped muscle called the diaphragm. The thoracic cavity is in your chest and contains the lungs, the heart, the major blood vessels, and a portion of the esophagus (the food tube). The esophagus penetrates (passes through) the diaphragm and enters the stomach, which is in the abdominal cavity. Other organs in the abdominal cavity include the liver, spleen, stomach, pancreas, small and large intestines, urinary bladder, and, in the female, the ovaries and uterus. The kidneys are located in the dorsal portion of the abdominal cavity. The kidneys are outside the large membrane (peritoneum) that envelops all the other organs. When this membrane becomes infected, the disease is known as peritonitis. The peritoneum, like all membranes in the body, is made up of both epithelial and connective tissue. It protects organs and prevents friction when they move.

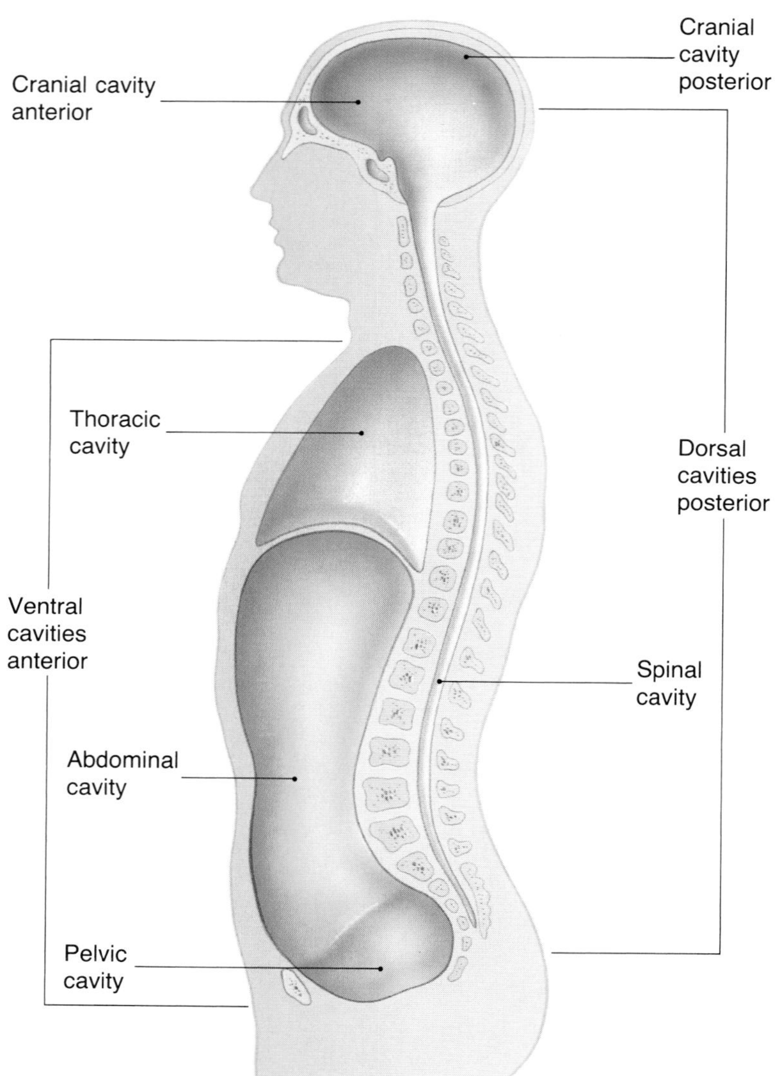

FIGURE 14-2 Body cavities.

Figure 14-3 shows the organs of the body and their approximate locations. The prefixes associated with the organs (cardio, pneumo, gastro, and so on) are combined with roots and suffixes to form the medical terminology discussed in Chapter 5.

KEY IDEAS

The Cell

Cell
The basic unit of living matter.

The microscopic **cell** is the fundamental building block of all living matter. Cells are microscopic in size. They are the living parts of organisms. The human body is made up of millions of cells. There are many kinds of cells and each has a special task within the body. Living cells have many things in common:

- They come from preexisting cells.
- They use food for energy.
- They use oxygen to break down the food.
- They use water to transport various substances.

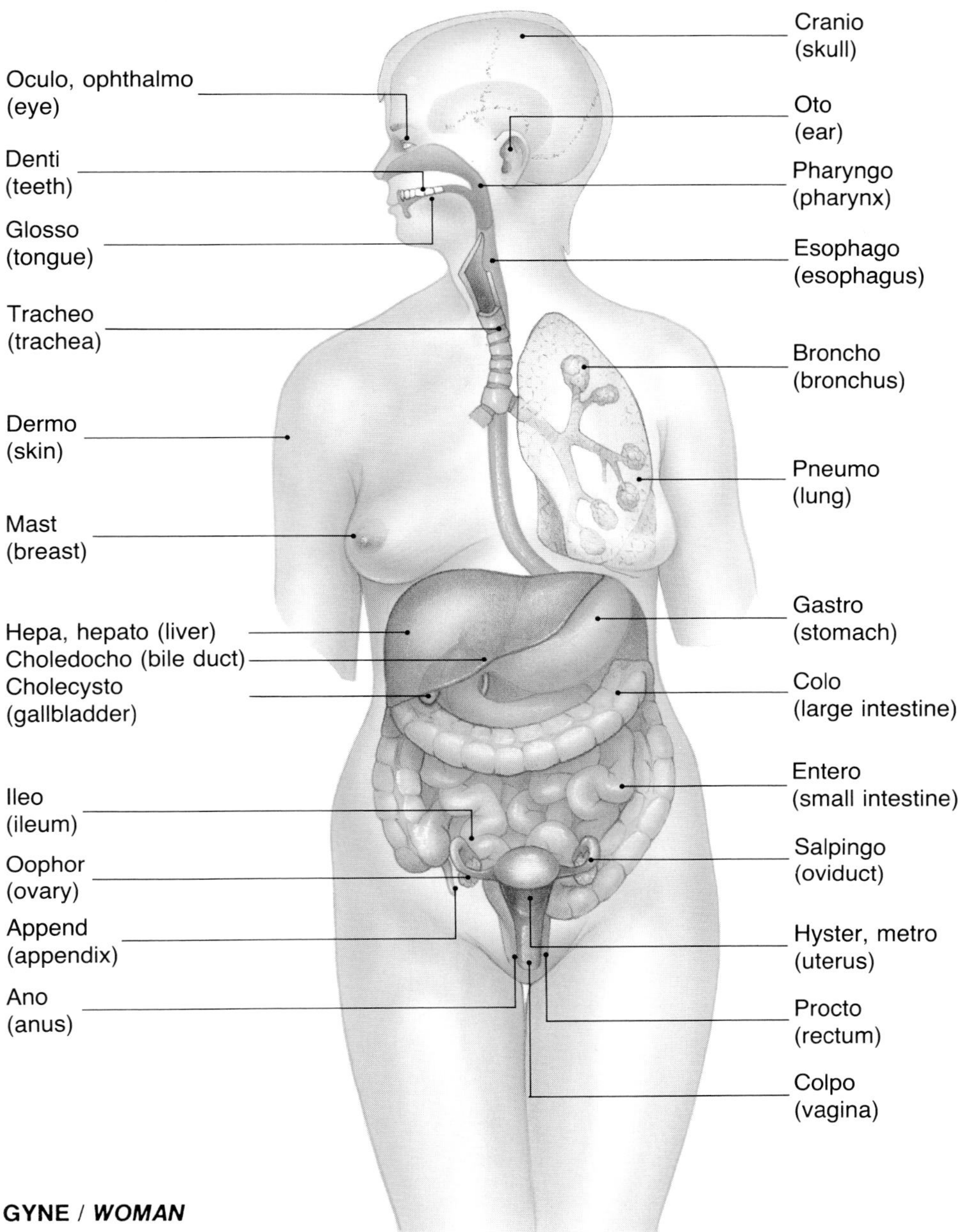

FIGURE 14-3 The organs of the body.

- They grow and repair themselves.
- They reproduce themselves (with the exception of mature neural cells).

Structure of the Cell

Cells consist of three main parts:

- *Nucleus*, which directs cellular activities
- *Cytoplasm*, where the activities of the cell take place
- *Cell membrane*, which keeps the living substance of the cell, called the protoplasm, within bounds and allows certain materials to pass in and out of the cell

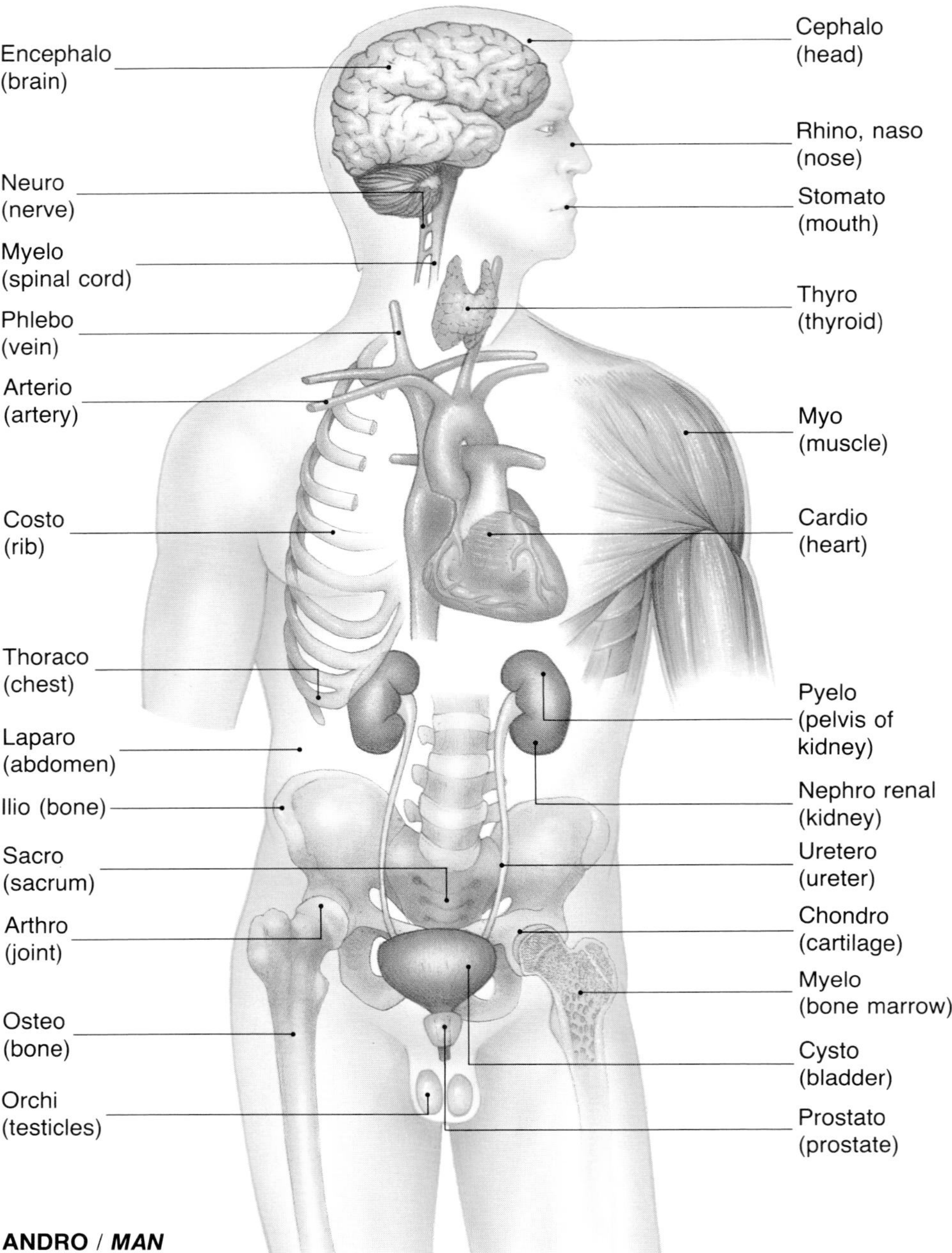

ANDRO / *MAN*

FIGURE 14-3 (Continued)

Cells are made up of two main compartments: a nucleus that contains the chromosomes (the hereditary material) and a surrounding mass of cytoplasm (Figure 14-4). The nucleus is important to the process of heredity, growth, and cell division. The chromosomes are threadlike structures that contain deoxyribonucleic acid (DNA) and control heredity factors.

DNA molecules produce messenger RNA molecules, which are partial copies of the DNA. Each RNA passes into the cytoplasm and directs the formation of the protein molecules necessary to maintain life. Through RNA, the nucleus controls the kinds of chemical reactions carried out by the cell.

Cells reproduce by division. In any cell preparing for division, the nucleus exactly duplicates its chromosomes. As the cell divides, the

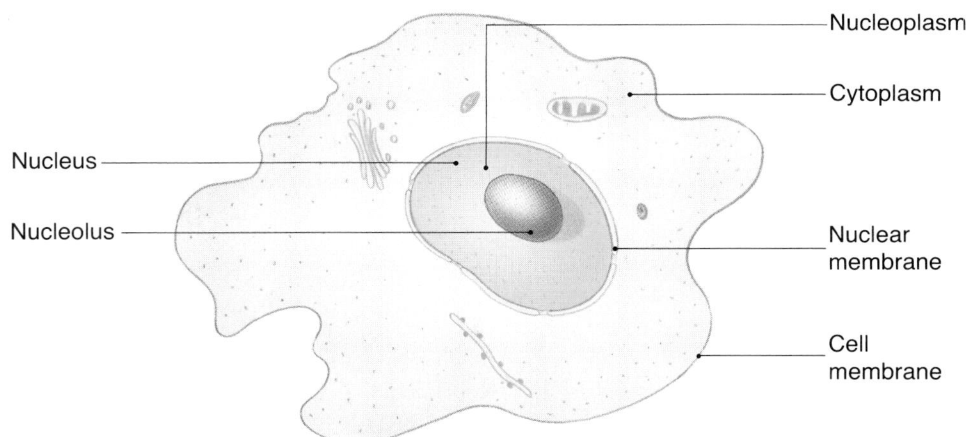

FIGURE 14-4 The cell.

pairs of chromosomes pull apart and move to opposite sides of the nucleus. Then the rest of the cell divides and goes with one or the other set of chromosomes. When division is complete, the new cells are identical.

Current research to discover what is causing diseases involves studying the cell and its immediate environment. We are living in a time when there is an explosion of scientific knowledge about the cell. It is hoped from this kind of study that scientists will someday find out how to cure or prevent many diseases.

Tissues

Tissue
A group of cells of the same type.

Cells usually do not work alone. They are organized together in tissues (Figure 14.5). Groups of cells of the same type that do a particular kind of work are called **tissues**.

Some of the primary kinds of tissues (Table 14-1) in the human body are:

Epithelial Tissue
Tissue that protects, secretes, absorbs, and receives sensations.

Connective Tissue
Tissue that connects, supports, covers, ensheathes, lines, pads, or protects.

Muscle Tissue
Tissue that ensures movement; it is capable of stretching and contracting.

Cardiac Muscle Tissue
Involuntary muscle tissue found only in the heart.

Nerve Tissue
Tissue that carries nervous impulses between the brain, the spinal cord, and all parts of the body.

Blood and Lymph Tissue
Tissue composed of singular cells that move within a fluid to every part of the body, circulating nutrients, oxygen, and antibodies and removing waste products.

- **Epithelial tissue:** Examples are skin, linings of the intestines, linings of the glands. The duty of this tissue is to protect, secrete, absorb, and receive sensations.
- **Connective tissue:** Examples are bone, blood, ligaments, and tendons. The duty of this tissue is to connect, to support, to cover or line, and to pad or protect.
- **Muscle tissue:** The duty of this tissue is movement. Striated tissue is found in voluntary muscles, those you can move consciously. Smooth tissue is found in the involuntary muscles, such as those that push food and water through the gastrointestinal tract. Smooth muscle allows such action as dilation (making opening larger) and contraction (making opening smaller) of the pupil of your eye and of blood vessels.
- **Cardiac muscle tissue:** Involuntary tissue found only in the heart (technically in the family of smooth muscles).
- **Nerve tissue:** The duty of this tissue is to carry nervous impulses from a portion of the brain or spinal cord to all parts of the body and vice versa. The body cannot renew nervous tissue.
- **Blood and lymph tissue:** In this type of tissue the cells are singular and move within a fluid to every part of the body (technically these are in the family of connective tissue).

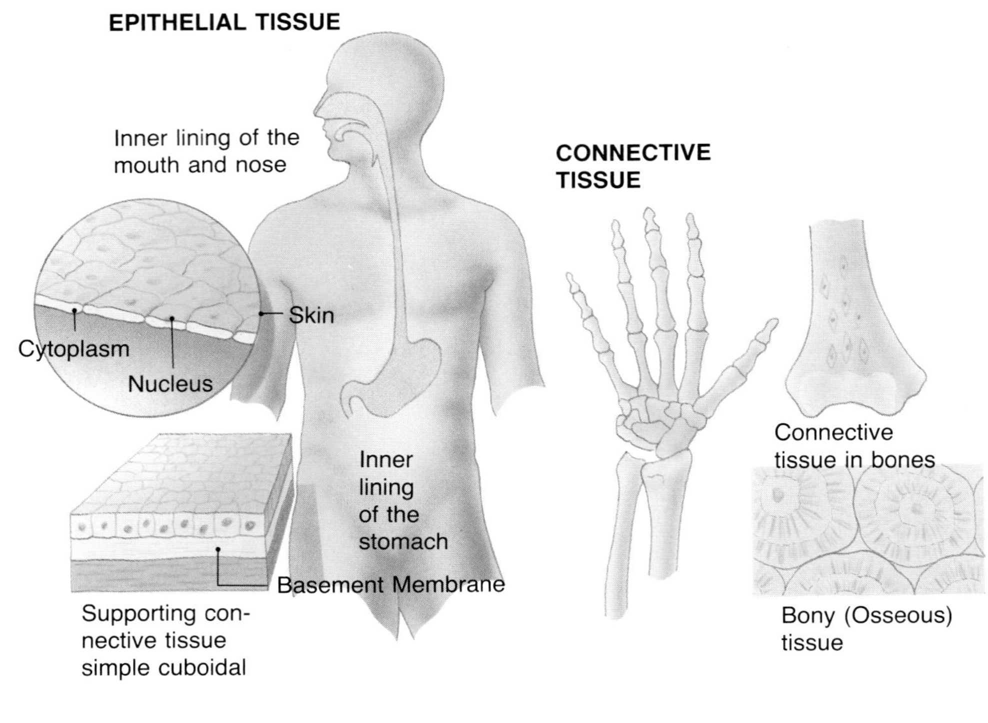
EPITHELIAL TISSUE
Inner lining of the mouth and nose
Skin
Cytoplasm
Nucleus
Inner lining of the stomach
Basement Membrane
Supporting connective tissue simple cuboidal
CONNECTIVE TISSUE
Connective tissue in bones
Bony (Osseous) tissue

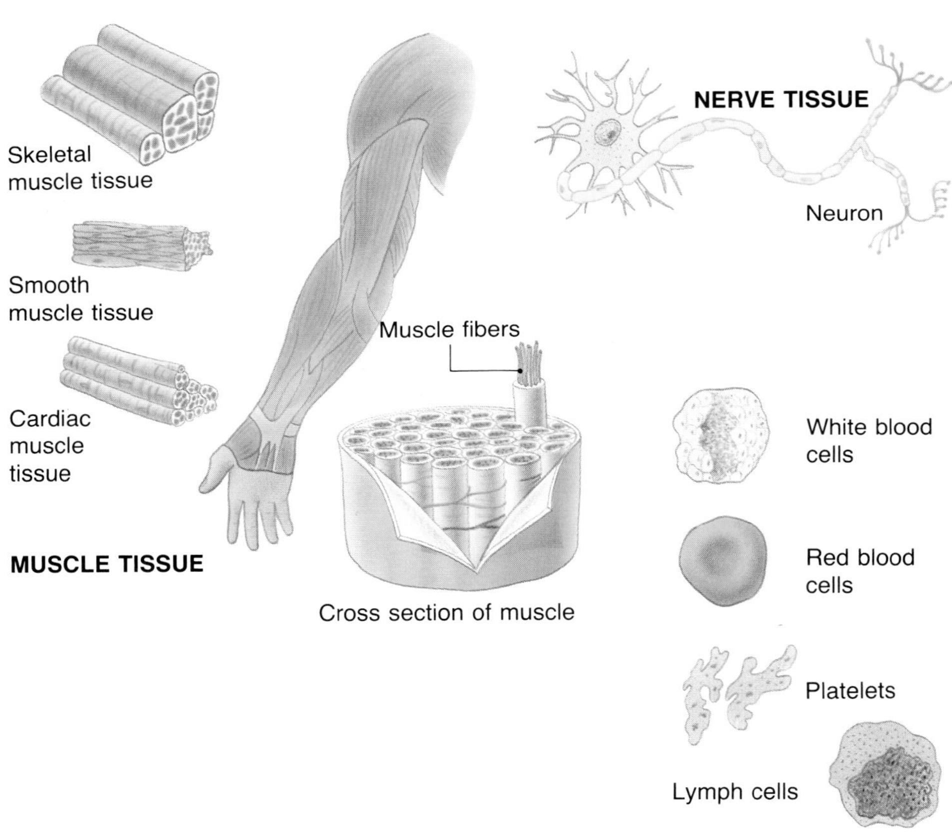
Skeletal muscle tissue
Smooth muscle tissue
Cardiac muscle tissue
MUSCLE TISSUE
Muscle fibers
Cross section of muscle
NERVE TISSUE
Neuron
White blood cells
Red blood cells
Platelets
Lymph cells
BLOOD CELLS

FIGURE 14-5 Types of body tissue.

Table 14-1 Primary Kinds of Tissue

Type of Tissue	Function	Location in the Body
Epithelial	Protect, secrete, absorb, receive sensations	Lining of mouth and nose, skin, lining of stomach
Connective tissue	Connect, support, cover	Tendons, bones, layer of fatty tissue under skin
Muscle tissue (a) striated (b) smooth (c) cardiac	Movement—stretch, contract	Muscle groups in arms, legs, abdomen, back and internal organs
Nerve tissue	Transmit impulses to and from the central nervous system and to and from the body systems	Throughout the body
Blood and lymph tissue	Circulate nutrients, oxygen, and antibodies throughout the body; remove waste products	Circulatory system

Organ
A part of the body made of several types of tissue grouped together to perform a certain function. Examples are the heart, stomach, and lungs.

System
A group of organs acting together to carry out one or more body functions.

Cells to Systems

Tissues are grouped together to form **organs**, such as the heart, lungs, and liver (Figure 14-6). Each organ has specific jobs. Organs that work together to perform similar tasks make up **systems**. It is easier to study anatomy and physiology by systems. Always remember that systems cannot work by themselves but are dependent, one upon the other.

FIGURE 14-6 Cells combine to form tissues, and tissues combine to form organs.

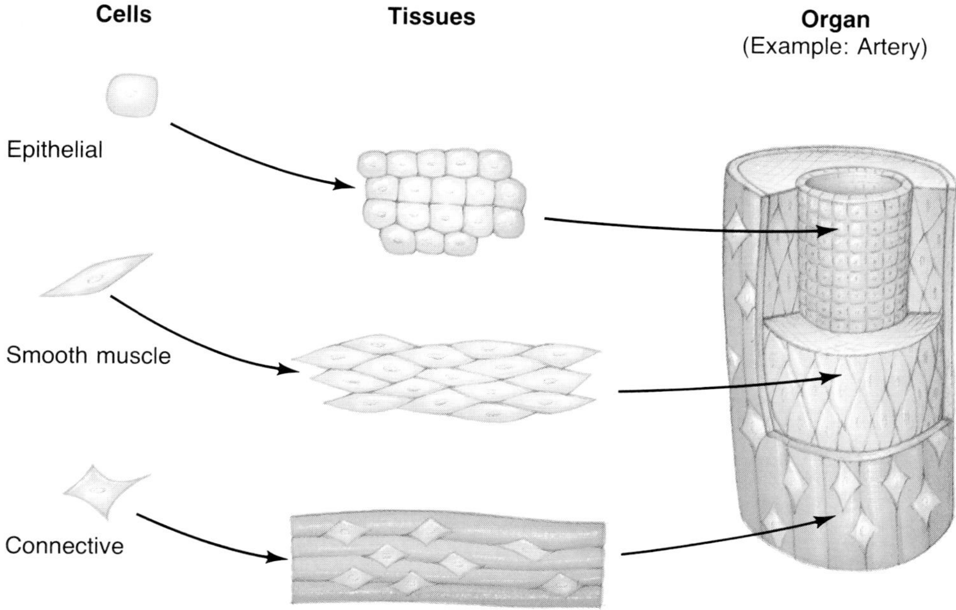

KEY IDEAS

The Body Systems

Body Systems

System	Function	Organs
Skeletal	Supports and protects the body	Bones; joints
Muscular	Gives movement to the body	Muscles; tendons; ligaments
Gastrointestinal (digestive)	Takes in and absorbs nutrients and eliminates wastes	Mouth; teeth; tongue, esophagus; salivary glands; stomach; duodenum; intestines; liver; gallbladder; ascending, transverse, and descending colon; rectum; anus; appendix
Nervous	Controls activities of the body	Brain; spinal cord; nerves
Excretory	Removes wastes from the blood, produces urine, and eliminates urine	Kidneys; ureters; bladder; urethra
Reproductive	To reproduce, allows a new human being to be born; for sexual fulfillment and expression of sexuality	Male: tests, scrotum, penis, prostate glands Female: ovaries, uterus, fallopian tubes, vagina
Respiratory	Gives the body air to supply oxygen to the cells through the blood and eliminates carbon dioxide	Nose; pharynx; larynx; trachea; bronchi; lungs
Circulatory	Carries food, oxygen, and water to the body cells and removes wastes	Heart; blood; arteries; veins; capillaries; spleen; lymph nodes; lymph vessels
Endocrine	Secretes hormones directly into the blood to regulate body function	Thyroid and parathyroid glands; pineal gland; adrenal glands; testes; ovaries; breasts; thymus; pancreas, and pituitary gland
Integumentary	Provides first line of defense against infection, maintains body temperature, provides fluids and eliminates wastes	Skin; hair; nails; sweat and oil glands

KEY IDEAS

Growth and Development

Growth
An increase in physical size.

Development
An increase in the ability to do things.

Growth is an increase in the physical size of the human being. Growth can be measured in centimeters and kilograms (inches and pounds). For example, a 3-year-old child may have grown to a height of 94 centimeters (37 inches) and a weight of 14.5 kilograms (32 pounds). **Development** refers to an increase in the ability to do things. For example, a 2-year-old child develops the ability to walk, which he did not have when he was 6 months old.

Growth and development begin when the baby is conceived and extend through all the stages of life. The child learns to sit up, to walk, and to talk. These are things that require development of his or her body muscles and nervous system, as well as development of the mind. Other kinds of learning require development of the senses: seeing,

KEY IDEAS

Stages of Growth and Development

Stage	Developmental Tasks	Typical Characteristics
Infant: Birth to 1 year	Developing gross and fine motor control (e.g., walking) Developing a sense of self Begins to learn communication skills Forming trusting relationships, especially with the primary care giver(s) Stabilizing eating and sleeping patterns	Needs: food, sucking, warmth, comfort, love, security, sensory stimulation Completely dependent Rapid growth and development Separation anxiety (distressed when parents leave)
Toddler: 1–2½ years	Developing coordination Self-feeding Talking Beginning of independence Forming identity Beginning to control bowel and bladder Beginning to differentiate between right and wrong Beginning to socialize	Curious Possessive Temper tantrums Climbs Plays alongside others Uses "no" frequently Likes to show and tell Explores Objects to discipline Begins to tolerate separation from primary care giver
Preschoolers: 2½–6 years (early childhood)	Developing identity Improving coordination Communicating Distinguishing right and wrong Playing with others Distinguishing between the sexes Developing family relationships Mastering self-care activities such as dressing, feeding, and washing Controls bowel and bladder	Asks many questions Slow to warm up to strangers Needs security, independence, rules, limits, and approval Curious Wants to play with other children Likes drawing, coloring, stories, running, jumping Talks constantly Imitates adults May be modest Can play independently Can dress, eat, and wash alone

(continued)

Stage	Developmental Tasks	Typical Characteristics
School age child: 6–12 years	Getting along with others Working toward a goal Learning to read, write, do math, and study Developing a positive self-concept through achievement Becoming independent Developing friendships Understanding sex roles Developing strength and coordination Developing a conscience	Wants to accomplish things Friends become important Initiates conversation Enjoys group activities Prefers to play with children of the same sex Peer opinions are important Enjoys team sports Physical changes before puberty Need for sex education Rebellion and disagreements are common
Adolescent teen-ager: 12–18 years	Establishing individual identity Preparing for independence Developing satisfying relationships with peers of both sexes Accepting physical changes Clarifying values and attitudes Choosing education and occupation	Peer pressure becomes influence Looks for role models Rebellion Desires independence Uses clothing, hairstyles, or activities to express individuality Desires interaction with peers Mood swings unpredictable
Young adult: 18–40 years	Establishing independence from parents Forming an individual life-style Adjusting to companions Coping with career, social, and economic constraints Selecting a career Choosing a mate Learning to live cooperatively with mate Parenting	Forms appropriate relationships Adjusts to rules Makes decisions independently Works toward goals Desires husband/wife and children Finds employment Adjusts to the world of work and responsibility
Middle-aged adult: 40–65 years	Building socioeconomic status Assists younger and older to cope Fulfilled by work, family, or by giving or caring for others Coping with the physical changes of aging Relating to grown children and the empty nest Dealing with aging parents Coping with the death of parents	Physical changes of aging Stable period Makes decisions independently Increased leisure time Decreased energy and endurance Becoming parents or grandparents Responsible for aging parents Often active in community affairs
Older adult: 65 years and older	Developing mutually supportive relationships with grown children Adjusting to loss of friends and relatives Coping with loss of spouse Adjusting to retirement Adapting to the physical changes of aging Forming new friends Coping with dying Adjusting to a new role in the family	Physical changes of aging Increased leisure time Slower to adapt to new surroundings, foods, routines, and the like Increased risk of illness or injury Reduced income Change in social and family relationships May consult grown children before making decisions

touching, hearing, and recognizing objects or people. People also develop, whether quickly or slowly, the feeling of being cared for, or being loved and having relationships.

Some people develop more quickly than others in certain ways. Some children can speak in sentences several months before other children of the same age begin to talk. Every person is an individual and, in many ways, is different from every other person. Although a child may be called a "typical" teen-ager, this does not mean the child is exactly like all other teen-agers. Both growth and development usually follow patterns and stages, although both may occur at different rates for different individuals. In each developmental stage, there are tasks that must be mastered before the person matures into the next stage. The boundaries between each stage overlap, but there are general characteristics that describe the typical person within that stage.

KEY IDEAS

Classification of Disease

Diseases, conditions, infections, and illnesses can be chronic or acute. These categories often overlap. They are based on the cause of the disease, the body system that has been affected, or the way the disease has been acquired.

Types of Disease or Condition by Cause

Type (cause)	Meaning	Disease or Condition (examples)
Aging	Alterations of all the body systems	Hardening of the arteries Arteriosclerosis
Birth injury	Occurring at birth	Cerebral palsy
Chemical	Foreign substance interfering	Alcoholic cirrhosis of the liver
Congenital/ Hereditary	Occurring during pregnancy or passed on through genes	Cleft palate, sickle-cell anemia
Deficiency	Lacking the right foods or nutrients and/or hormones	Scurvy (lack of vitamin C)
Infectious	Communicable, caused by microorganisms	Measles, chickenpox, mumps
Mechanical blocks	Formation of an obstruction of body wastes, fluids, or natural chemicals	Gallstones, kidney stones, blood clots
Metabolic	Failing to produce or break down substances needed for normal processes	Diabetes (lack of insulin)
Neoplastic	Abnormal growth of tissue; tumors (benign or malignant)	Fibroids (benign); cancer (malignant)
Occupational	Peculiar to a job	Lead poisoning (painter); black lung disease (miner)
Trauma	Injury, usually physical	Fracture, broken bone

Acute
Illness that comes on suddenly.

Chronic
Describing an illness that continues over many years or a lifetime.

- **Acute illness** comes on suddenly and usually runs its course within a short period of time. Examples are appendicitis and pneumonia.
- **Chronic illness** continues over years or a lifetime. Examples are arthritis and diabetes.

Refer students to the neoplastic section of the chart on p. 184.

KEY IDEAS

Cancer and Benign Tumors

Neoplasm
New growth in which the cells grow without any control, organization, or purpose.

Tumor
A growth in or on the body. There are two kinds: (1) benign tumors, and (2) malignant tumors

Benign
A tumor or neoplasm that stays at its site or origin and does not usually regrow once removed.

Cancer
Refers to malignant neoplasms. Cancer cells interfere with normal body function, grow and spread between cells, invade surrounding tissue, and sometimes cause death.

Malignant
Describing a tumor or neoplasm that grows, spreads, invades, and destroys organs.

Metastasis
The spreading of cancer cells through the body systems.

Neoplasm means new growth. Normal cells reproduce because of need; however, when a neoplasm grows, the cells grow without any control, organization, or purpose. Neoplastic growth can be slow or rapid, benign or malignant. The words **tumor** and neoplasm are interchangeable.

A **benign tumor** stays at its site of origin and does not usually regrow once removed. It never invades surrounding tissue and grows slowly. It looks like the tissue it grew from.

Cancer refers to malignant neoplasms. **Malignant** neoplasms grow, spread, invade, and destroy organs. Cancer cells interfere with normal body function. If they are not controlled, they grow and spread between cells, invade surrounding tissues, and sometimes cause death. Malignant neoplasms can recur after surgical removal. **Metastasis** refers to the spreading of cancer cells through the systems of the body.

Changing behavior to decrease risk factors (for example, stop smoking), early detection of cancer can reduce the risk death rate from cancer. Signs and symptoms of malignant tumors include:

- Unaccountable weight loss
- A lesion, ulcer, or rash that does not heal
- Changes in the appearance of a sore
- Hoarseness, coughing, difficulty in breathing
- Unusual bleeding or discharges
- A lump that appears where never felt before
- Change in bowel habits
- Blood in the stool
- Blood in the urine
- Unusual increase in abdominal size
- Pain or pressure
- Nausea
- Weakness, extreme tiring

Psychosocial Aspects

Every patient has a different personality and coping patterns. The patient with cancer goes through the stages of denial, anger, depression, bargaining, and finally acceptance. When the cancer patient must undergo a surgical procedure that results in changes in body function or form, acceptance is not easy to achieve. For example:

- Removal of the rectum due to cancer (including creation of an ostomy in the abdomen) necessitates wearing of an appliance to collect bowel movement.
- Total or partial removal of one or both breasts. Both men and women have difficulty in accepting this body change.
- Amputation of an extremity.
- Removal of the (larynx) voice box. The patient loses the ability to speak.

KEY QUESTIONS

1. What are the names of the body areas and cavities? Where is each located?
2. What are the things all living cells have in common?
3. What are the main parts of the cell? What does each part do?
4. How does a cell reproduce itself?
5. What are the primary kinds of tissues? What does each type of tissue do? Where can each type of tissue be found in the human body?
6. What are the basic ways cells are grouped together, from simple to complex, to form a human being?
7. Name the ten body systems. What is the major job of each system? Which organs are included in each system?
8. List the stages of growth and development. What are the developmental tasks and typical characteristics of each stage?
9. What are the major causes of disease? List them, including an example of each cause.
10. What are the differences between benign and malignant tumors?
11. What are the signs and symptoms of cancer?
12. What are the psychosocial aspects of cancer?
13. Define: acute, anatomy, anterior, benign, blood and lymph tissue, cancer, cardiac muscle tissue, cell, chronic, connective tissue, deep, development, dorsal, epithelial tissue, growth, inferior, malignant, metastasis, muscle tissue, neoplasm, nerve tissue, organ, physiology, posterior, superficial, superior, system, tissue, tumor, ventral.

CHAPTER 15

Anatomy and Physiology of the Musculoskeletal Systems

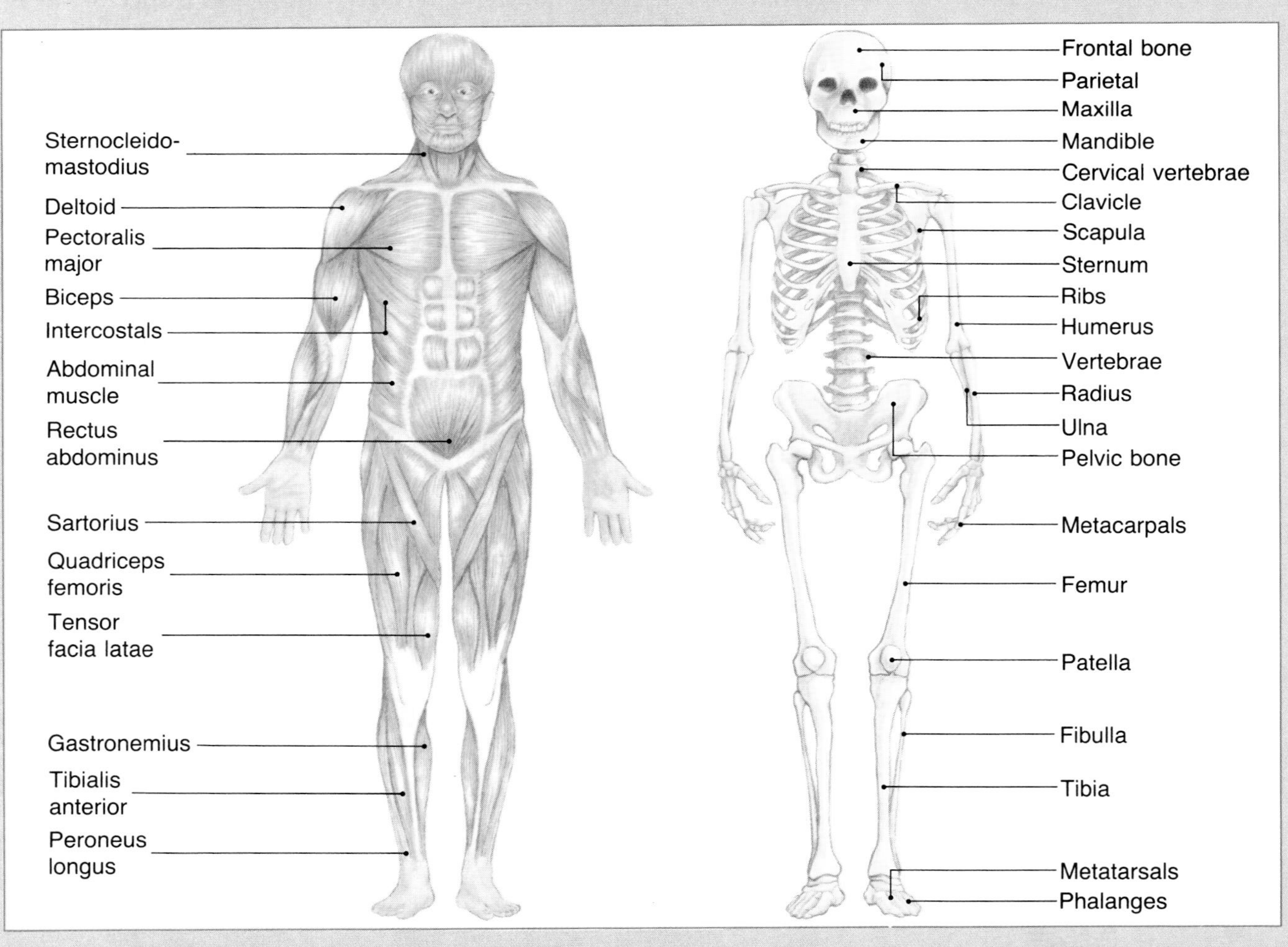

WARNING

For all patient contact, adhere to Universal Precautions (see page 91, 97, or the front cover flap). Wear protective equipment as indicated.

Objectives

What You Will Learn

When you have completed this chapter, you will be able to:

- Identify the function of the muscular system.
- Explain how groups of muscles work together to perform body motion.
- List the functions of the skeletal system.
- Give an example of how several body systems interact.
- List the four general types of bones and give examples of each.
- Name three major types of joints and give examples of each.
- Label a diagram of the skeletal and surface muscles.
- List common diseases and disorders of the musculoskeletal systems.
- Define: abduction, adduction, atrophy, contract, extension, flex, flexion, joint, ligament, relax.

KEY IDEAS

The Muscular System

Flex
To bend.

Relax
In a resting position; the time following contraction of a muscle in which tension decreases, fibers lengthen, and the muscle returns to a resting position.

THE MUSCULAR SYSTEM MAKES ALL MOTION possible, either that of the whole body or that which occurs inside the body. Groups of muscles work together to perform a body motion. Other groups perform the opposite motion. These two groups are called *antagonistic groups.* For example, **flex** your arm, which means bring it toward your shoulder. Your biceps muscle contracts and the triceps muscle **relaxes**. Extend your arm. The biceps relaxes while the triceps contracts. **Flexion** and **extension** are two terms you should know (Figure 15-1). Two others are

Flexion
To bend a joint (elbow, wrist, knee).

FIGURE 15-1 Coordination of muscles.

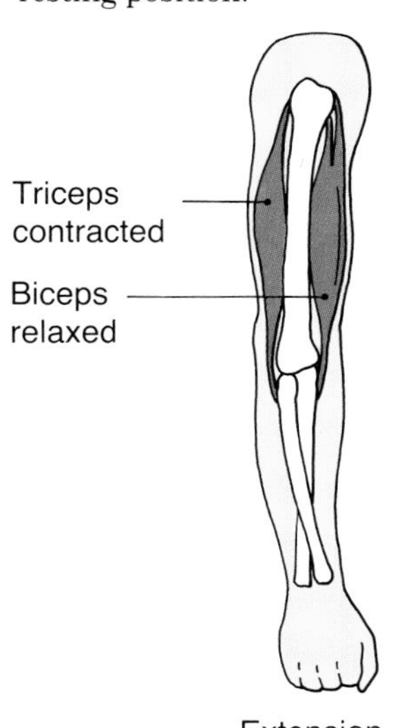

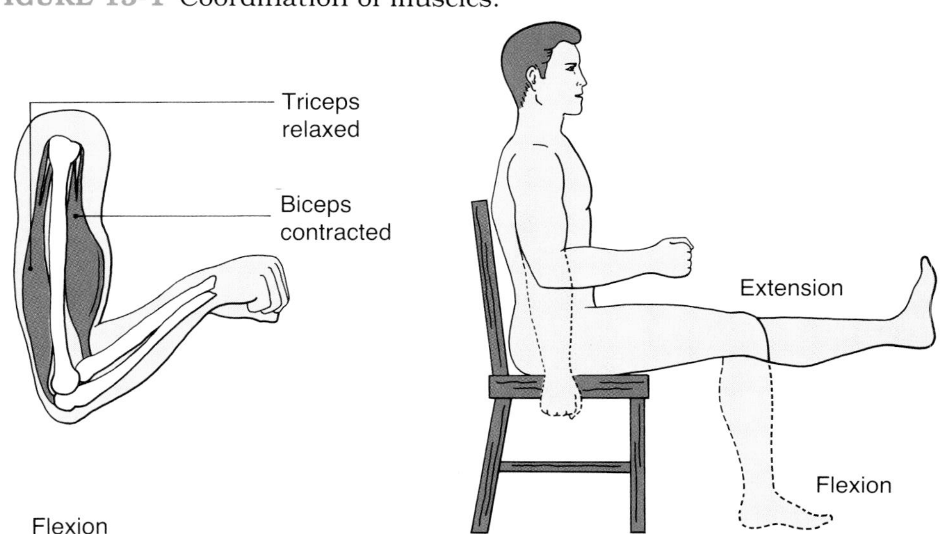

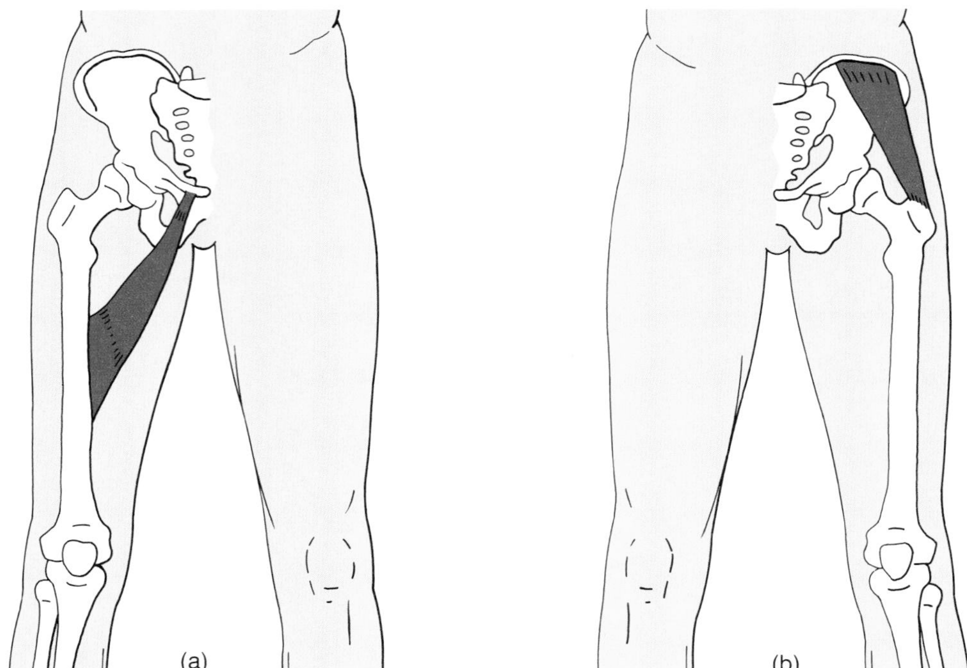

FIGURE 15-2 (a) Adduction and (b) abduction, moving a body part toward and away from the body midline.

Extension
To straighten.

Abduction
To move an arm or leg away from the center of the body.

Adduction
To move an arm or leg toward the center of the body.

Atrophy
Muscles wasting away or decreasing in size.

abduction, which means moving a part away from the body midline, and **adduction**, which means moving it toward the body (Figure 15-2).

Because of a muscle's exceptionally rich blood supply, it is the most infection-free of all the body's basic tissues. Muscles move the body and help to keep the body warm, especially during activity. If a muscle is kept inactive for too long, it tends to shrink and waste away. This is called **atrophy**. Contracture is a permanent muscle shortening, one reason why regular exercise is so important to good health. Range-of-motion exercises are often given to inactive patients to prevent these problems.

When you are helping to lift a patient or when you are making a bed, remember to use the strong muscles of your legs rather than those of your back. This will prevent you from seriously hurting yourself. Use the large thigh muscles, the quadriceps femoris, on the ventral portion of the thigh, and the hamstrings on the dorsal portion. This will also save you from straining your muscles.

KEY IDEAS

The Skeletal System

Contract
Get smaller.

The skeletal system is made up of 206 bones. The bones act as a framework for the body and give it structure and support. They are also the passive organs of motion; they do not move by themselves. They must be moved by muscles, which shorten or contract. A muscle is stimulated to contract by a nerve impulse.

There are four types of bones (Figure 15-3):

- *Long bones*, such as the big bone in your thigh, the femur
- *Short bones*, like the bones in your fingers, the phalanges
- *Irregular bones*, such as the vertebrae that make up the spinal column
- *Flat bones*, like the bones of the rib cage

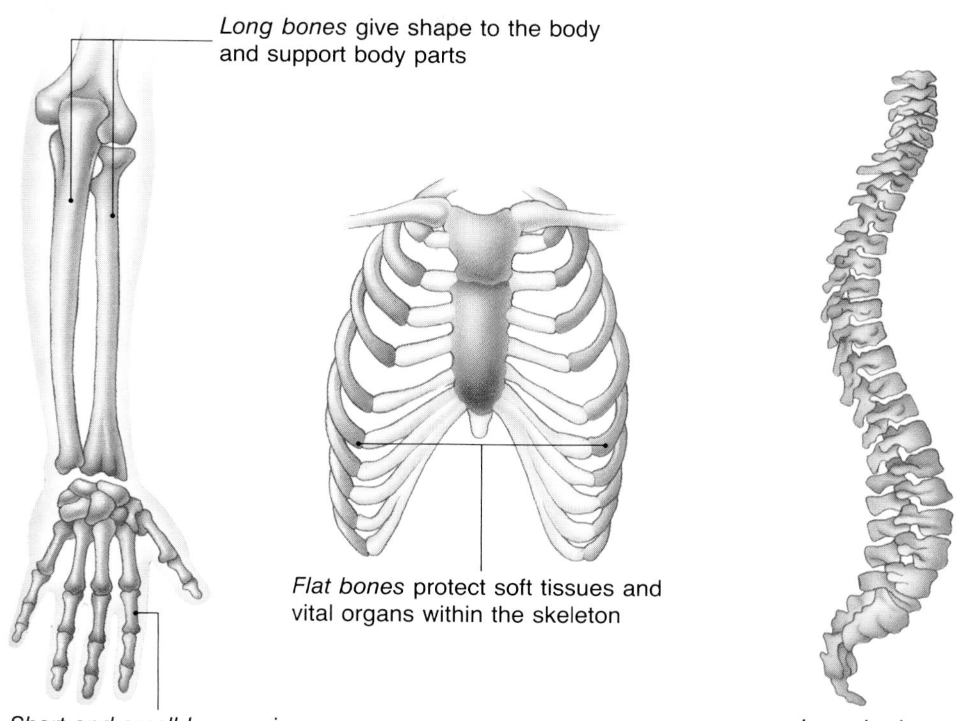

FIGURE 15-3 Types of bones.

Bones store vital minerals that are necessary for many other body activities. The bones of the head are designed to protect the very delicate tissue of the brain (Figure 15-4). They are joined by *sutures*, similar to a zigzag pattern, and totally surround the brain and cranial nerves. Two other bones that protect vital organs include the vertebrae of the spinal column, which protect the spinal nerve cord, and the ribs, which guard the heart and lungs.

FIGURE 15-4 The skull.

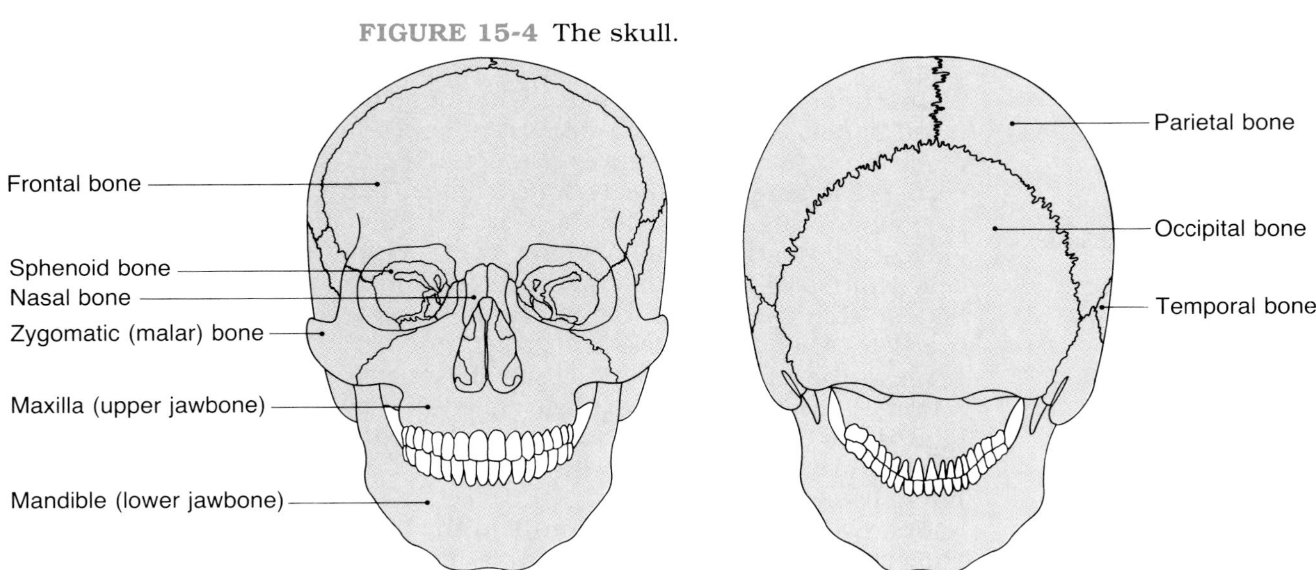

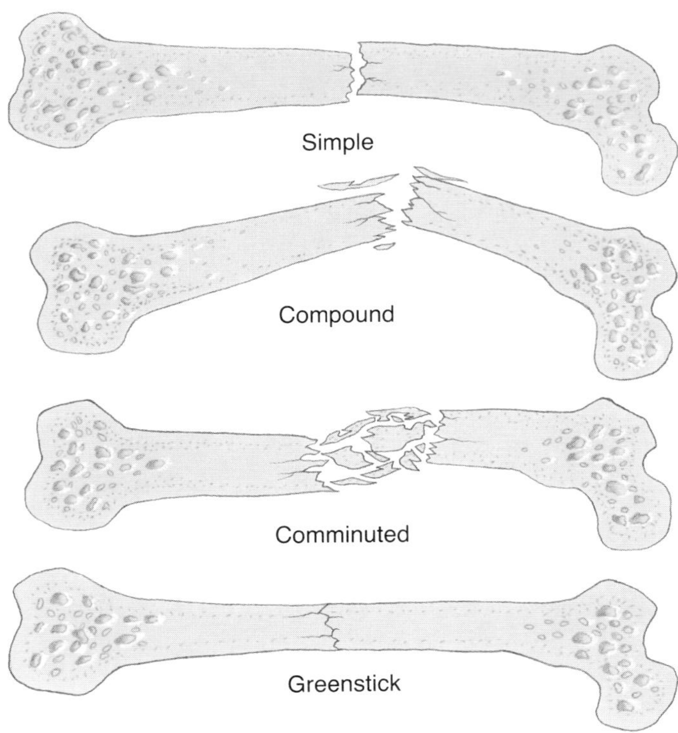

FIGURE 15-5 Types of bone fractures.

Broken bones can mend, but the process is slow and gradual because bone cells grow and reproduce slowly. The hardening of the new bone is a gradual procedure of depositing calcium. Blood supply to bone tissue is poor in comparison to other areas of the body. Therefore, resistance to infection in the bone is relatively low. Figure 15-5 shows four types of bone fractures.

Joints (Motion)

In a healthy human body, all the systems of the body work together. No one system can stand alone. During each body movement, the skeletal system, muscular system, nervous system, and circulatory system are all interacting. This body movement occurs at the joints, a perfect example of how several systems must work together.

Joint
A part of the body where two bones come together.

Ligament
A tough, white fibrous cord that connects bone to bone.

Joints are the meeting place where one bone connects with one or more bones. They are the necessary levers for all motion. Joints are made up of many structures (Figure 15-6). The tough, white fibrous cord, the **ligament**, connects bone to bone. The *tendons* connect muscle to bone. Joints—especially those in the shoulder, hip, and knee—are enclosed in a strong capsule lined by a membrane that secretes a fluid called *synovial fluid.* This fluid acts as a buffer, very much like a water bed, so that the ends of the bones do not get worn out from too much motion. Other structures that protect the bone include the pad of cartilage at the end of the bone, a sac of synovial fluid (which is known as a bursa), and a disk of cartilage called the meniscus. Many such safeguards are built into the body. Injury to joints may cause a ligament or tendon to be strained in what we call a *sprain.* Inflammation of the bursa causes *bursitis.*

There are several kinds of joints in the human body. The hinge joint, such as in the knee, is freely movable. There are also less movable joints,

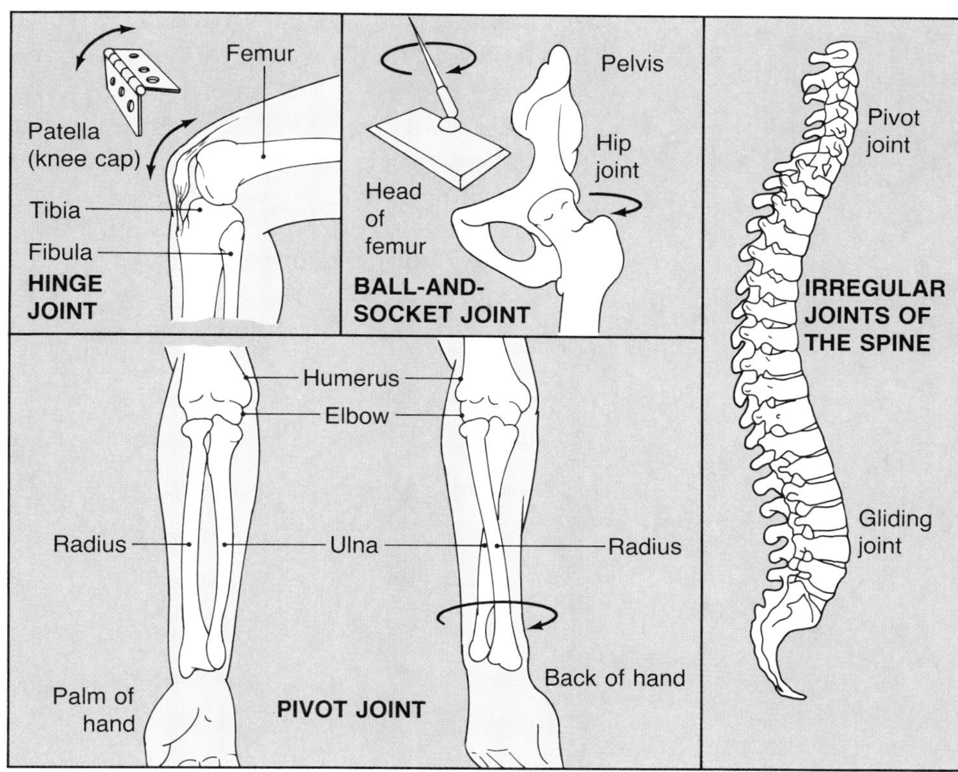

FIGURE 15-6 Synovial (movable) joints.

such as those between the vertebrae. Some joints do not move at all, such as the joints between the bones of the head, which protect the brain.

KEY IDEAS

Common Diseases and Disorders of the Musculoskeletal System

- *Contusion:* injury to soft tissue
- *Sprains:* injury to ligaments surrounding a joint
- *Joint dislocations:* injury in which the bones of the joint are no longer in anatomic position
- *Fractures:* break in the bone
- *Surgical amputation:* removal of a portion of a limb
- *Low back pain:* often with muscle spasms
- *Rheumatoid arthritis:* inflammation of the lining of the joints
- *Osteoarthritis:* degeneration of the cartilage of the joints
- *Osteogenic sarcoma* (cancer): malignant bone tumor
- *Osteoporosis:* reduced amount of normal bone tissue resulting in softening
- *Muscular dystrophy:* a condition characterized by a progressive atrophy of muscular tissue

KEY QUESTIONS

1. What is the main function of the muscular system?
2. How do groups of muscles work together to perform body motion?
3. What are the functions of the skeletal system?

4. How do body systems interact? Give an example.
5. What are the four general types of bones? Give examples of each.
6. What are the three major types of joints?
7. Label a diagram of the skeleton and surface muscles.
8. What are the common diseases and disorders of the musculoskeletal system?
9. Define: abduction, adduction, atrophy, contract, extension, flex, flexion, joint, ligament, relax.

CHAPTER

16

Body Mechanics

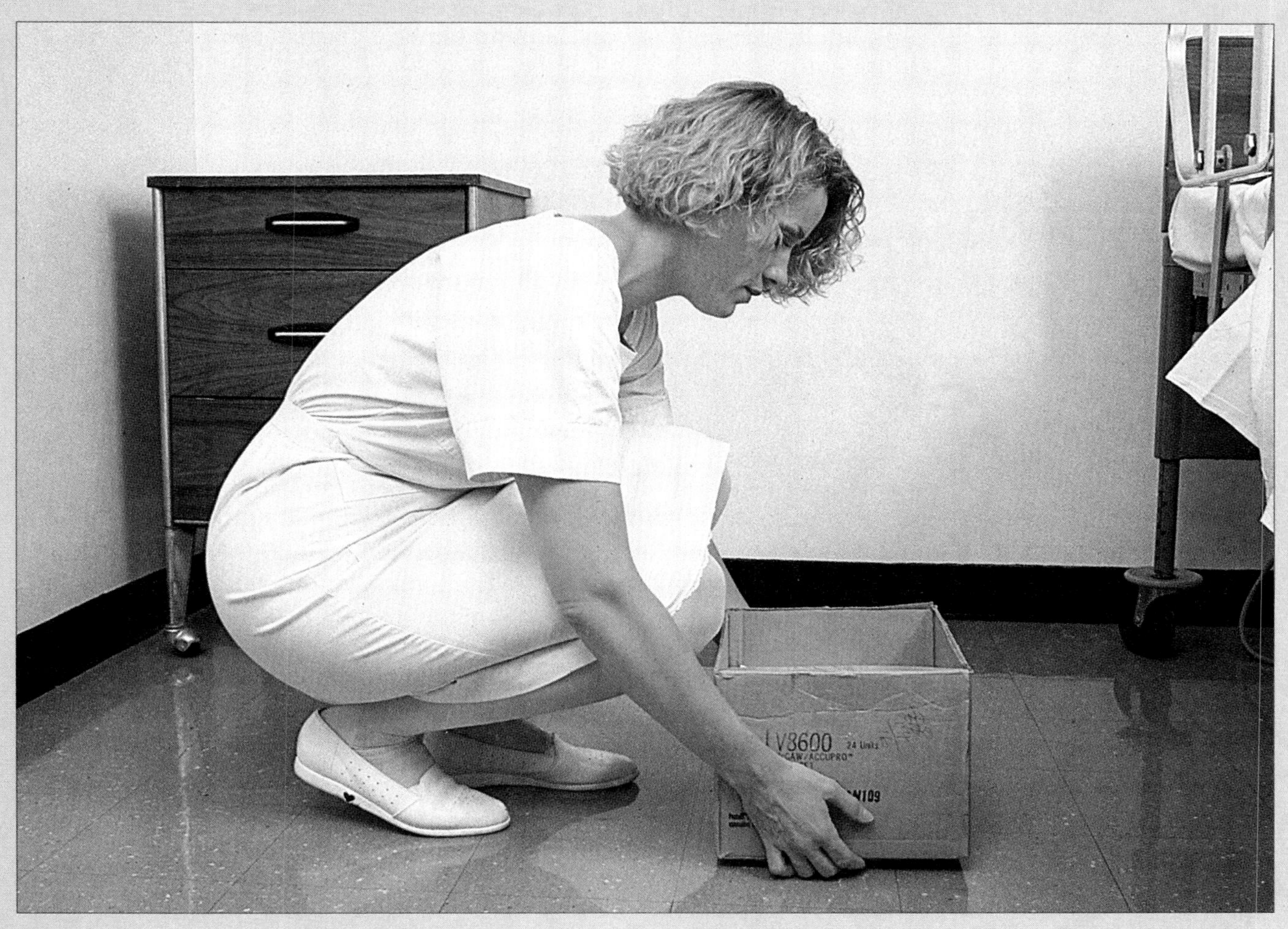

WARNING

For all patient contact, adhere to Universal Precautions (see page 91, 97, or the front cover flap). Wear protective equipment as indicated.

Objectives

What You Will Learn

When you have completed this chapter, you will be able to:

- List the rules to follow for good body mechanics.
- Lift, hold, or move an object or patient using good body mechanics.
- List the rules to follow for lifting and moving patients.
- Lock arms with a patient to raise his or her head and shoulders.
- Move a nonambulatory patient up in bed.
- Move a patient up in bed with his or her help.
- Move the mattress to the head of the bed with the patient's help.
- Move a helpless patient to one side of the bed on his or her back.
- Roll the patient like a log.
- Turn a patient on either side.
- Assist the patient into 11 different positions and drape for privacy.
- Define: bedridden, body alignment, body mechanics, dorsal recumbent position, drape, draping, Fowler's position, knee–chest position, lithotomy (dorsal) position, nonambulatory, prone, side lying, Sims's position, supine, Trendelenburg's position.

KEY IDEAS
Body Mechanics

THE TERM **BODY MECHANICS** REFERS TO special ways of standing and moving one's body to make the best use of strength and avoid fatigue or injury. You should understand the rules of good body mechanics and learn to apply them to your work. You will then find that you will be less tired and will feel better at the end of the day.

Body Mechanics
Special ways of standing and moving one's body to make the best use of strength and avoid fatigue.

Rules to Follow
GOOD BODY MECHANICS

- When an action requires physical effort, try to use larger muscles or groups of muscles whenever possible. For example, use both hands rather than one hand to pick up a heavy piece of equipment.
- Use good posture. Keep your body aligned properly. Keep your back straight. Have your knees bent. Keep your weight evenly balanced on both feet. Always face your work area.
- Check your feet when you are going to lift something. They should be 12 inches apart to give you a broad base of support and good balance.
- Get close to the load that is being lifted.
- When you have to move a heavy object, it is better to push it, pull it, or roll it rather than lift and carry it.
- Use your arms to support the object. The muscles of your legs actually do the job of lifting, not the muscles of your back.

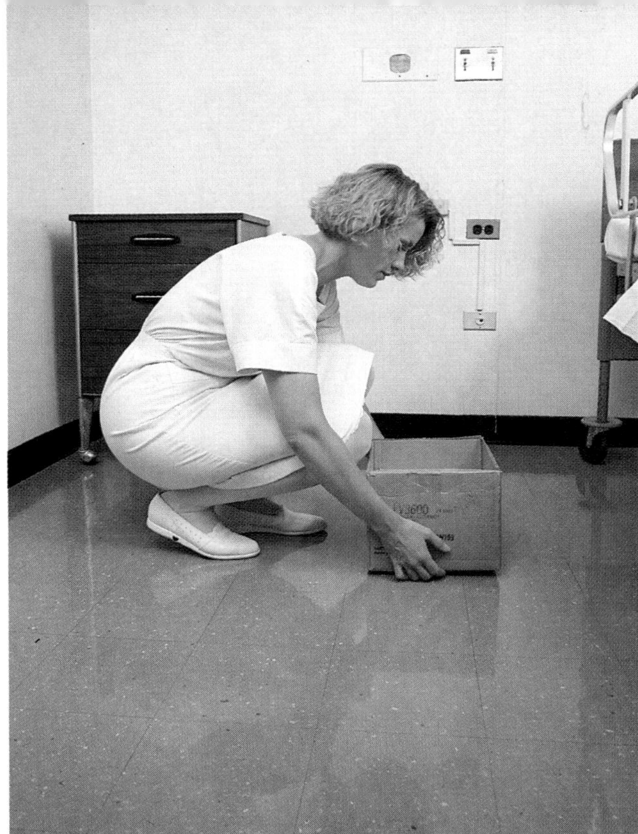
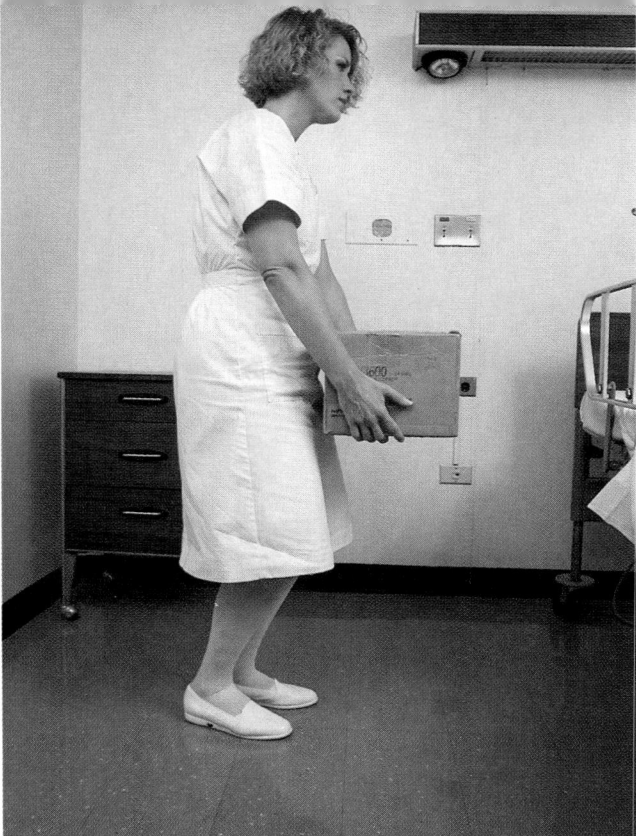

FIGURE 16-1 Good body mechanics: lifting.

- When you are doing work such as giving a back rub, making a corner on a bed, or moving the patient, work with the direction of your efforts, not against it. Avoid twisting your body at the waist. Always turn or pivot completely around.
- When you lift an object (Figure 16-1):
  - Squat close to the load.
  - Keep your back straight.
  - Grip the object firmly.
  - Hold the load close to your body.
  - Lift by pushing up with your strong leg muscles.
- If you think you may not be able to lift the load, if it seems too large or heavy, then get help.
- Lift smoothly to avoid strain. Always count "one, two, three" with the person you are working with. Or say "ready" and "go" so you work in unison. Do this with both the patient and with other health care workers.
- When you want to change the direction of movement:
  - Pivot (turn) with your feet (Figure 16-2).
  - Turn with short steps.
  - Turn your whole body without twisting your back and neck.

KEY IDEAS

Lifting and Moving Patients

Many of your tasks require lifting and moving helpless or nearly helpless patients. A **bedridden** patient must have his or her position changed often. Proper support and alignment of the patient's body are important.

The patient's body should be straight and properly supported; otherwise, his or her safety and comfort might be affected. The correct positioning of the patient's body is referred to as **body alignment**. Body

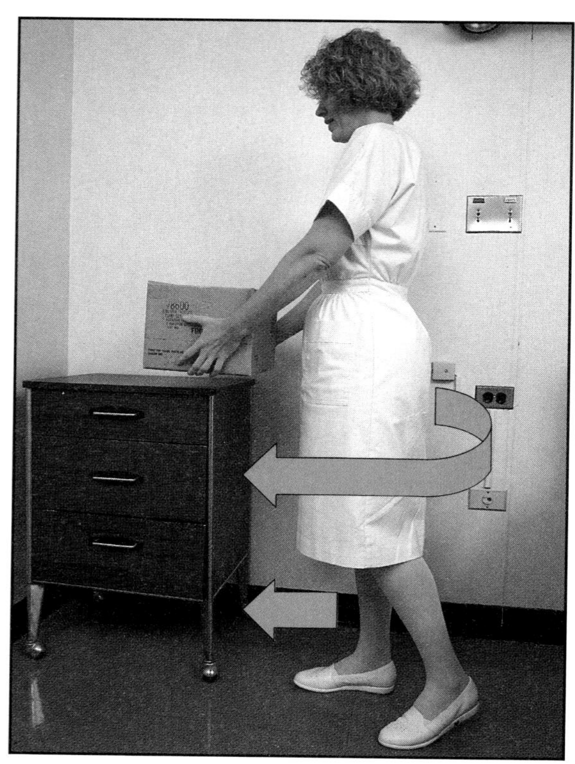

FIGURE 16-2 Good body mechanics: turning.

Bedridden (Bed-bound)
Unable to get out of bed.

Body Alignment
Refers to the arrangement of the body in a straight line; the placing of portions of the body in correct anatomical position.

alignment means the arrangement or adjustment of the patient's body so that all parts of the body are in their proper positions in relation to each other.

Many conditions and injuries, as well as special patient care treatments, make it difficult or even dangerous for a patient to be in a certain position. As a member of the nursing team, you will be responsible for making sure that the patient you are caring for is in the position ordered by the doctor.

A pull or lift sheet can help you move the patient in bed more easily (Figure 16-3). A regular extra sheet folded over many times and placed under the patient can be used as a pull sheet. The cotton draw sheet can also be used as a pull sheet. When moving the patient, roll and pull the sheet up tightly on each side next to the patient's body. Grip the rolled portion to slide the patient into the desired position. By using the pull sheet, friction and irritation to the patient's skin are avoided.

Rules to Follow

LIFTING AND MOVING PATIENTS

- Before you begin each procedure, explain what you are going to do and encourage the patient to participate and help as much as possible.
- Before moving the patient, place tubing from catheters and IVs where they won't be pulled.
- Give the most support to the heaviest parts of the patient's body.
- Hold the patient close to your body for the most support.
- Move the patient with smooth and steady motion. Avoid sudden jerking movements.

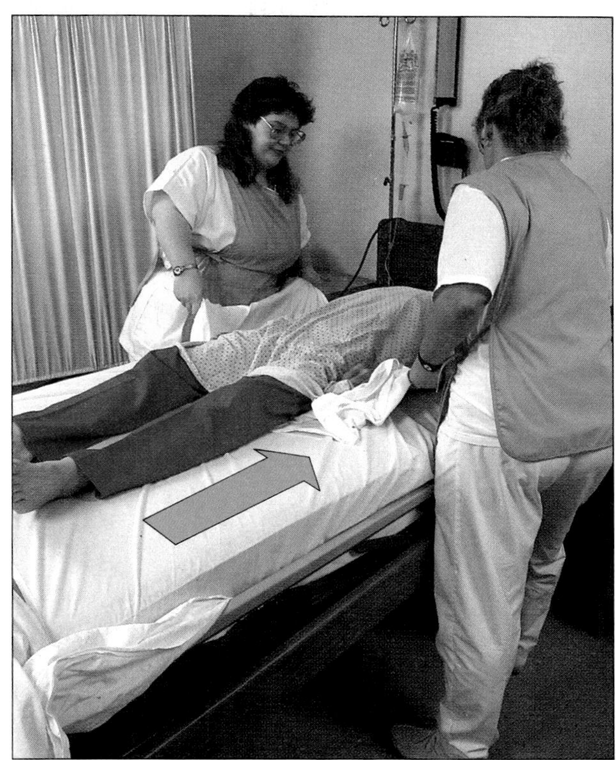

FIGURE 16-3 To move the helpless patient up in bed, use a pull sheet to avoid friction.

Locking Arms with the Patient

To turn the patient's pillow over or to raise his or her head and shoulders, you should lock arms with the patient who is able to help (Figure 16-4). For the **nonambulatory** patient, two nursing assistants should lock arms with the patient to lift him or her.

Nonambulatory
Not able to walk.

FIGURE 16-4 Locking arms with the patient.

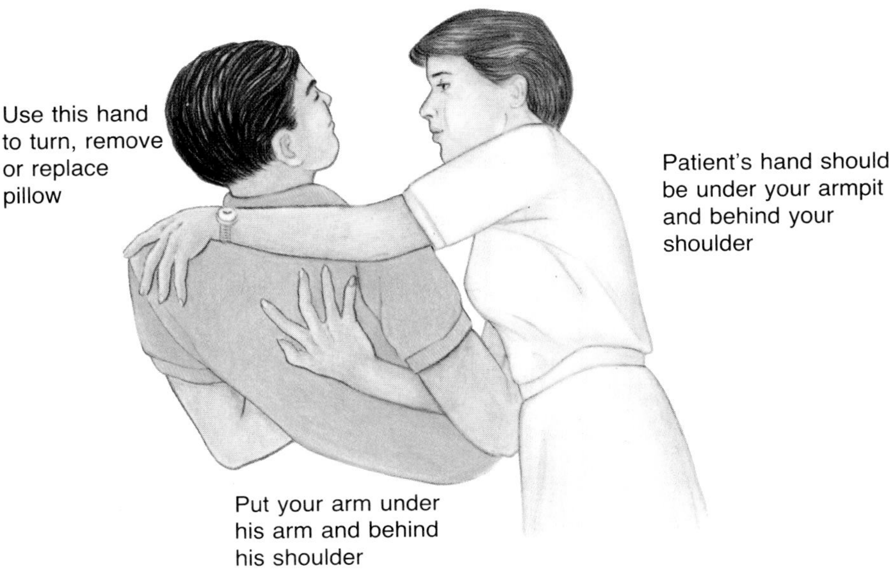
Use this hand to turn, remove or replace pillow
Patient's hand should be under your armpit and behind your shoulder
Put your arm under his arm and behind his shoulder

Procedure Locking Arms with the Patient

1. Wash your hands.
2. Identify the patient by checking the identification bracelet.
3. Ask visitors to step out of the room, if this is your hospital's policy.
4. Tell the patient you are going to help raise him by locking arms.
5. Pull the curtain around the bed for privacy.
6. Lock the wheels on the bed, and adjust the height of the bed to a comfortable working position.
7. Face the head of the bed. Bend your knees. Keep your back straight.
8. Have the patient put his arm under your arm (the arm next to him) and behind your shoulder, with his hand over the top of your shoulder. (If you are standing at his right side, his right hand will be on your right shoulder. If you are on his left, you will be locking your left arm with his left arm.)
9. Put your arm under the patient's arm with your hand on his shoulder.
10. When you say "one, two, three," help the patient pull himself up as you support him. This will raise his head and shoulders.
11. Turn or replace the pillow with your free hand. It is this hand that gives support to the back of the shoulders and head while lifting the patient.
12. To help the patient lie down again, continue supporting him with your locked arm and your free hand. Help the patient gently ease himself down.
13. Make the patient comfortable.
14. Lower the bed to a position of safety for the patient.
15. Pull the curtains back to the open position.
16. Raise the side rails where ordered, indicated, and appropriate for patient safety.
17. Place the call light within easy reach of the patient.
18. Wash your hands.
19. Report to your immediate supervisor:
    - That the patient's position has been changed
    - The time the patient's position was changed
    - How the patient tolerated the procedure
    - Your observations of anything unusual

Procedure Moving the Nonambulatory Patient Up in Bed

1. Ask another nursing assistant to work with you.
2. Wash your hands.
3. Identify the patient by checking the identification bracelet.
4. Ask visitors to step out of the room, if this is your hospital's policy.
5. Tell the patient that you and your partner are going to move him up in the bed, even if he appears to be unconscious.
6. Pull the curtain around the bed for privacy.
7. Remove the pillow from the bed. Put the pillow at the top of the bed against the headboard. This will protect the patient's head.
8. Lock the wheels on the bed.
9. Raise the bed to a comfortable working position.
10. Stand on one side of the bed. The other nursing assistant will stand on the opposite side.
11. Both nursing assistants should stand straight, turned slightly toward the head of the bed with their feet 12 inches apart. The foot closest to the head of the bed should be pointed in that direction. Bend your knees. Keep your back straight (Figure 16-5).
12. Use of a draw, pull, or turning sheet is always preferred for moving a helpless patient up in bed. This is to avoid friction between the patient's skin and bedding and to prevent skin irritation. Roll

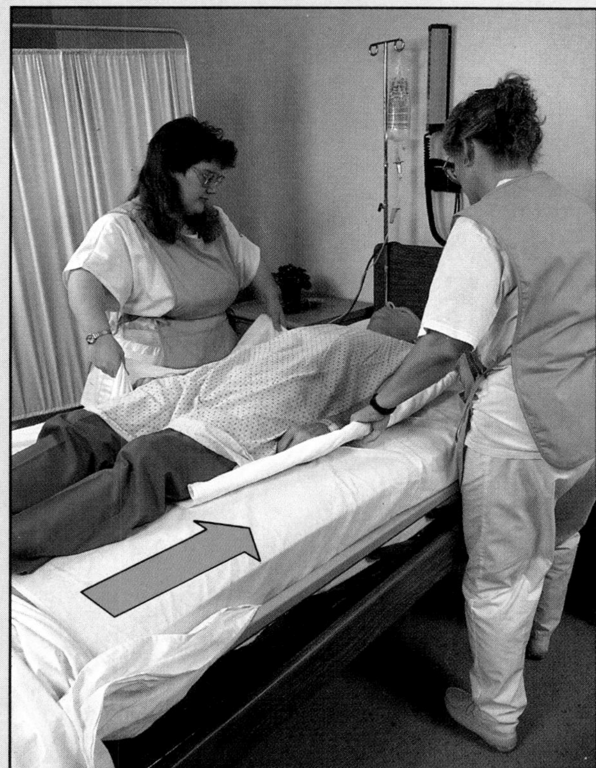

FIGURE 16-5 Moving the helpless patient up in bed with a pull, draw, or turning sheet.

the sides of the sheet to be used as a pull sheet close to the patient. Each nursing assistant then grasps one side of the rolled portion of the sheet firmly so that, when the patient is moved up, the sheet will stay in place under the patient.

13. You will be sliding the patient's body when you move him up in bed. Straighten your knees as you start to slide the patient. Your body is in the correct position for the direction in which you will move. Therefore, you can shift your weight easily from one foot to the other.
14. When you say "one, two, three" in unison, you and your partner will move together to slide the patient gently and move him toward the head of the bed or to the position he should be in.
15. Make the patient comfortable.
16. Replace the pillow, as per the patient's request.
17. Lower the bed to a position of safety for the patient.
18. Pull the curtains back to the open position.
19. Raise the side rails where ordered, indicated, and appropriate for patient safety.
20. Place the call light within easy reach of the patient.
21. Wash your hands.
22. Report to your immediate supervisor:
    - That the patient's position has been changed
    - The time the patient's position was changed
    - How the patient tolerated the procedure
    - Your observations of anything unusual

Procedure Moving a Patient Up in Bed with His Help

1. Wash your hands.
2. Identify the patient by checking the identification bracelet.
3. Ask visitors to step out of the room, if this is your hospital's policy.
4. Tell the patient that you are going to move him up in bed. Before you begin, ask your head nurse or team leader if the patient is a cardiac patient and is allowed to exert himself as much as is necessary for this move.
5. Pull the curtain around the bed for privacy.
6. Lock the wheels on the bed.
7. Raise the bed to a comfortable working position.
8. Lower the backrest, if this is allowed.
9. Lock arms with the patient, and remove the pillow with your free hand. Put the pillow at the top of the bed against the headboard. This will protect the patient's head from hitting the headboard.
10. Put the side rails in the up position on the far side of the bed.

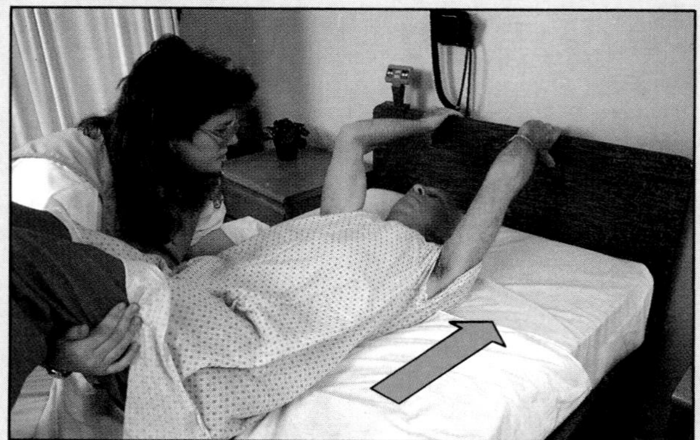

FIGURE 16-6

11. Put one hand under the patient's shoulder. Put your other hand under the patient's buttocks.
12. Ask the patient to bend his knees and brace his feet firmly on the mattress.
13. Ask the patient to grasp the head of the bed (Figure 16-6).
14. Have your feet 12 inches apart. The foot closest to the head of the bed should be pointed in that direction.
15. Bend your knees. Keep your back straight.
16. Bend your body from your hips facing the patient and turned slightly toward the head of the bed.
17. At the signal "one, two, three," have the patient pull with his hands toward the head of the bed and push with his feet against the mattress.
18. At the same time, help him to move toward the head of the bed by sliding him with your hands and arms.
19. Lock arms with the patient and put the pillow back in place, under his head and shoulders.
20. Make the patient comfortable.
21. Lower the bed to a position of safety for the patient.
22. Pull the curtains back to the open position.
23. Raise the side rails where ordered, indicated, and appropriate for patient safety.
24. Place the call light within easy reach of the patient.
25. Wash your hands.
26. Report to your immediate supervisor:
    - That the patient's position has been changed
    - The time the patient's position was changed
    - How the patient tolerated the procedure
    - Your observations of anything unusual

Procedure Moving the Mattress to the Head of the Bed with the Patient's Help

1. Ask another nursing assistant to work with you.
2. Wash your hands.
3. Identify the patient by checking the identification bracelet.
4. Ask visitors to step out of the room, if this is your hospital's policy.
5. Tell the patient that you are going to move his mattress to the head of the bed.
6. Pull the curtain around the bed for privacy.
7. Lock the wheels on the bed.
8. Raise the bed to a comfortable working position.
9. Lower the backrest, if allowed.
10. If you are working alone, put the side rail in the up position on the far side of the bed.
11. Each nursing assistant stands at the side of the bed. The sheets should be loosened.
12. Lock arms with the patient and remove the pillow. Put the pillow on the chair.
13. Ask the patient to grasp the headboard with both hands.
14. Ask the patient to bend his knees and brace his feet firmly on the mattress.
15. Grasp the mattress loops, or grasp the sides of the mattress if there are no loops.

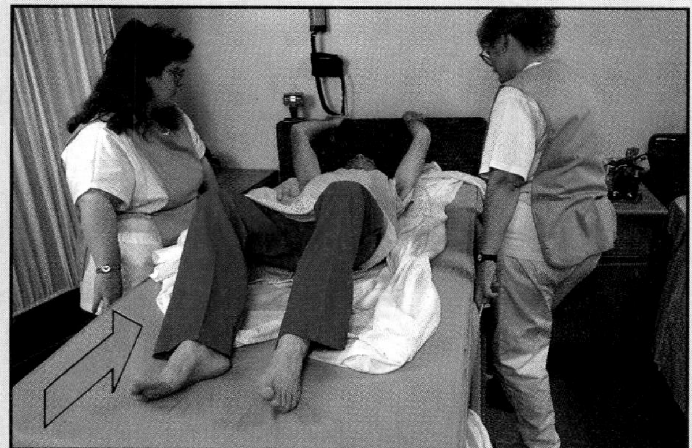

FIGURE 16-7

16. At the signal "one, two, three," have the patient pull with his hands toward the head of the bed and push with his feet against the mattress (Figure 16-7).
17. At the same time, both nursing assistants will slide the mattress toward the head of the bed, keeping their knees bent and their backs straight as they move the mattress.
18. Lock arms with the patient and put the pillow back in place.
19. Make the patient comfortable.
20. Lower the bed to a position of safety for the patient.
21. Pull the curtains back to the open position.
22. Raise the side rails where ordered, indicated, and appropriate for patient safety.
23. Place the call light within easy reach of the patient.
24. Wash your hands.
25. Report to your immediate supervisor:
    - That the mattress was moved to the head of the bed with the patient's help
    - The time the mattress was moved to the head of the bed
    - How the patient tolerated the procedure
    - Your observations of anything unusual

Procedure Moving a Helpless Patient to One Side of the Bed on His Back

1. Wash your hands.
2. Identify the patient by checking the identification bracelet.
3. Ask visitors to step out of the room, if this is your hospital's policy.
4. Tell the patient that you are going to move him to one side of the bed on his back without turning him.
5. Pull the curtain around the bed for privacy.
6. Lock the wheels on the bed.
7. Raise the bed to a comfortable working position.
8. Lower the backrest and footrest, if this is allowed.
9. Put the side rail in the up position on the far side of the bed.
10. Loosen the top sheets, but don't expose the patient.
11. Slide both your arms under the patient's back to his far shoulder; then slide the patient's shoulders toward you on your arms (Figure 16-8).
12. Slide both your arms as far as you can under the patient's buttocks and slide his buttocks toward you. Use a pull (turning) sheet whenever possible.
13. Keep your knees bent and your back straight as you slide the patient.
14. Place both your arms under the patient's lower legs and slide them toward you on your arms (Figure 16-9).
15. Lock arms with the patient and adjust the pillow, if necessary.
16. Remake the top of the bed.
17. Make the patient comfortable.
18. Lower the bed to a position of safety for the patient.
19. Pull the curtains back to the open position.

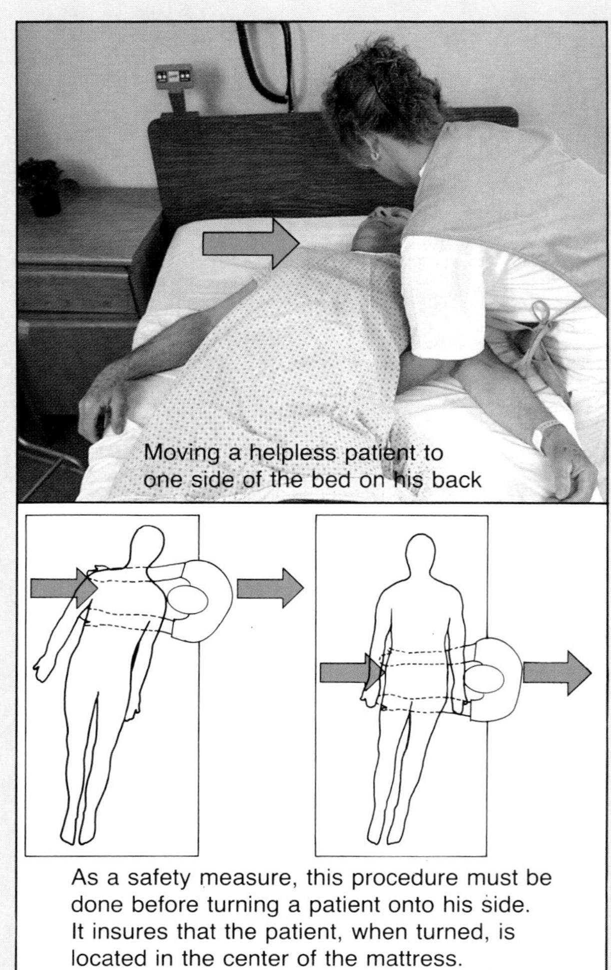
Moving a helpless patient to
one side of the bed on his back

As a safety measure, this procedure must be done before turning a patient onto his side. It insures that the patient, when turned, is located in the center of the mattress.

FIGURE 16-8

FIGURE 16-9

20. Raise the side rails where ordered, indicated, and appropriate for patient safety.
21. Place the call light within easy reach of the patient.
22. Wash your hands.
23. Report to your immediate supervisor:
    - That the patient has been moved to one side of the bed on his back.
    - The time the patient's position was changed
    - How the patient tolerated the procedure
    - Your observations of anything unusual

Procedure Rolling the Patient Like a Log (Log Rolling)

1. Wash your hands.
2. Identify the patient by checking the identification bracelet.
3. Ask visitors to step out of the room, if this is your hospital's policy.
4. Tell the patient that you are going to roll him to his side as if he were a log.
5. Pull the curtain around the bed for privacy.
6. Get help, if necessary.
7. Lock the wheels on the bed.
8. Raise the bed to a comfortable working position.
9. Raise the side rail on the far side of the bed.
10. Remove the pillow from under the patient's head, if allowed. Put the pillow at the foot of the bed or on a chair.
11. Slide both your arms under the patient's back to his far shoulder; then slide the patient's shoulders toward you on your arms.
12. Slide both your arms as far as you can under the patient's buttocks and slide his buttocks toward you. Use a pull (turning) sheet whenever possible.
13. Keep your knees bent and your back straight as you slide the patient.
14. Place both your arms under the patient's lower legs and slide them toward you on your arms.

15. Place a pillow between the patient's knees and cross the patient's legs in the direction of movement.
16. Use the pull (turning) sheets when necessary.
17. Keep your knees apart, your back straight, and your weight balanced evenly on both feet.
18. Roll the patient onto his side like a log, turning his body as a whole unit, without bending his joints. Pull him gently toward you (Figure 16-10).
19. Replace the pillow under the patient's head, if allowed.
20. Use pillows against the patient's back to keep his body in proper alignment (Figure 16-11).
21. Remake the top of the bed.
22. Reverse the procedure to turn the patient on his opposite side.
23. Make the patient comfortable.
24. Lower the bed to a position of safety for the patient.
25. Pull the curtains back to the open position.
26. Raise the side rails where ordered, indicated, and appropriate for patient safety.
27. Place the call light within easy reach of the patient.
28. Wash your hands.
29. Report to your immediate supervisor:
    - That the patient's position has been changed by rolling him or her like a log
    - The time the patient's position was changed
    - How the patient tolerated the procedure
    - Your observations of anything unusual

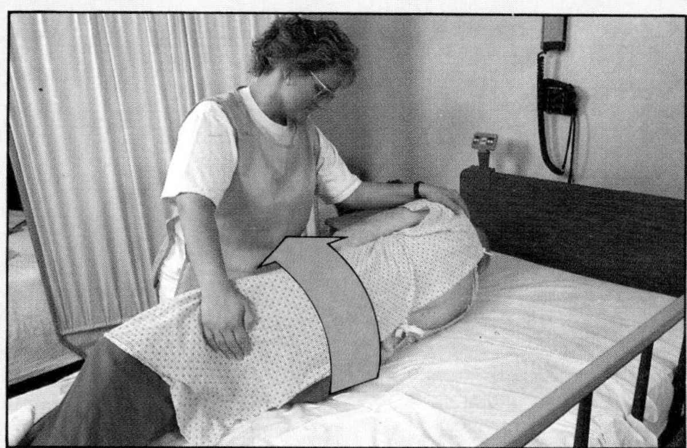

FIGURE 16-10

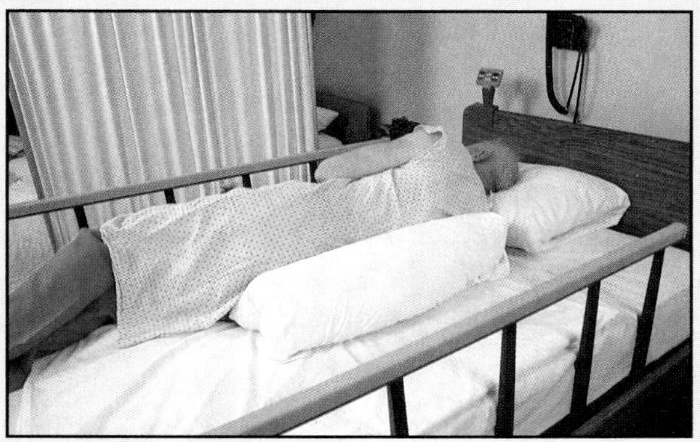

FIGURE 16-11

Procedure Turning a Patient Onto His Side Toward You

1. Wash your hands.
2. Identify the patient by checking the identification bracelet.
3. Ask visitors to step out of the room, if this is your hospital's policy.
4. Tell the patient you are going to turn him on his side.
5. Pull the curtain around the bed for privacy.
6. Lock the wheels on the bed.
7. Raise the bed to a comfortable working position.
8. Lower the backrest and footrest, if this is allowed.
9. Put the side rail in the up position on the far side of the bed.
10. Loosen the top sheets, but don't expose the patient.

11. When you are turning the patient toward you, cross the patient's leg farthest from you over the leg closest to you.
12. Cross the patient's arms over his chest.
13. Reach across the patient and put one hand behind his far shoulder.
14. Place your other hand behind his far hip; gently roll him toward you (Figure 16-12).
15. Fold a pillow lengthwise and place it against the patient's back for support.
16. Support the patient's head with the palm of one hand. With your other hand, slide a pillow under his head and neck.
17. Place the patient's arms and legs in a comfortable position. Be sure the arm nearest the mattress is free from pressure.
18. Remake the top of the bed.
19. Make the patient comfortable.
20. Lower the bed to a position of safety for the patient.
21. Pull the curtains back to the open position.
22. Raise the side rails where ordered, indicated, and appropriate for patient safety.

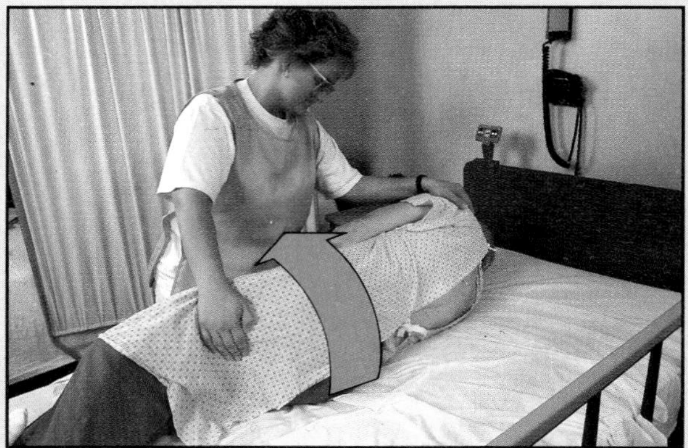

FIGURE 16-12 Turning a patient on his side toward you.

23. Place the call light within easy reach of the patient.
24. Wash your hands.
25. Report to your immediate supervisor:
    - That the patient's position has been changed
    - The time the patient's position was changed
    - How the patient tolerated the procedure
    - Your observations of anything unusual

Procedure Turning a Patient onto His Side away from You

1. Wash your hands.
2. Identify the patient by checking the identification bracelet.
3. Ask visitors to step out of the room, if this is your hospital's policy.
4. Tell the patient you are going to turn him on his other side.
5. Pull the curtain around the bed for privacy.
6. Lock the wheels on the bed.
7. Raise the bed to a comfortable working position.
8. Lower the backrest and footrest.
9. Put the side rail in the up position on the far side of the bed.
10. Loosen the top sheets, but don't expose the patient.
11. Slide both your arms under the patient's back to his far shoulder; then slide the patient's shoulders toward you on your arms.
12. Slide both your arms as far as you can under the patient's buttocks and slide his buttocks toward you. Use a pull (turning) sheet whenever possible.
13. Keep your knees bent and your back straight as you slide the patient.
14. Place both your arms under the patient's lower legs and slide them toward you on your arms.
15. Cross the patient's arms over his chest.
16. When turning a patient away from you, cross the patient's leg closest to you over the leg farthest from you.

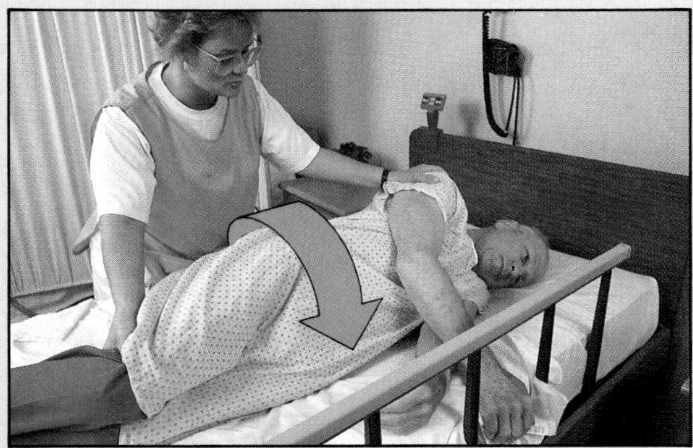

FIGURE 16-13 Turning a patient on his side away from you.

17. Place one hand on the patient's shoulder near you.
18. Put your other hand under his buttocks.
19. Turn him gently on his side, facing away from you (Figure 16-13).
20. Fold a pillow lengthwise. Place it against the patient's back for support.
21. Support the patient's head with the palm of one hand. With your other hand, slide a pillow under his head and neck.
22. Make sure the patient's arms and legs are in a comfortable position. Put a pillow between his knees if this helps to make the patient comfortable. Be sure the arm nearest the mattress is free from pressure.
23. Remake the top of the bed.
24. Lower the bed to its lowest horizontal position.
25. Make the patient comfortable.
26. Lower the bed to a position of safety for the patient.
27. Pull the curtains back to the open position.
28. Raise the side rails where ordered, indicated, and appropriate for patient safety.
29. Place the call light within easy reach of the patient.
30. Wash your hands.
31. Report to your immediate supervisor:
    - That the patient's position has been changed
    - The time the patient's position was changed
    - How the patient tolerated the procedure
    - Your observations of anything unusual

KEY IDEAS

Draping and Positioning the Patient

Draping
Covering a patient or parts of the patient's body with a sheet, blanket, bath blanket, or other material. Draping is usually done during the physical examination of the patient and during surgery.

Drape
A covering used to provide privacy during an examination or an operation.

Supine
Lying on one's back.

Horizontal Recumbent Position (Supine Position)

In this position, the **draping** covers the entire body. The patient lies on the back with the legs together and extended or with the knees bent slightly to relax the muscles of the abdomen. A pillow is placed under the patient's head; the **drape** is spread loosely over the patient's body (Figure 16-14).

FIGURE 16-14 Horizontal recumbent position (supine position).

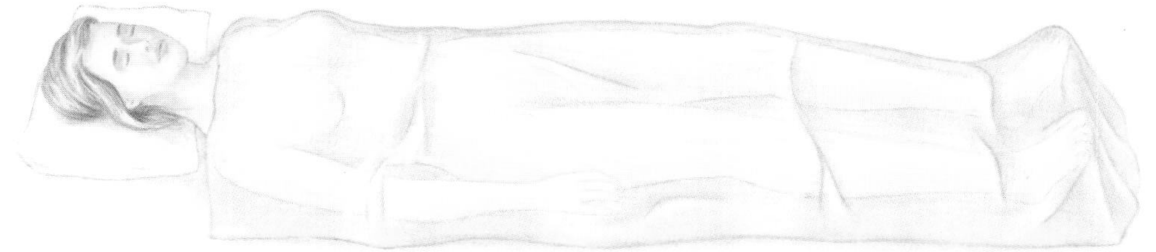

Dorsal Recumbent Position
Refers to the back or to the back part of an organ; the posterior part; lying down or reclining.

Dorsal Recumbent Position

In this position the patient's legs are separated, the knees are bent, and the soles of the feet are flat on the bed. Drape the female patient by putting a sheet, folded once, across her chest. Put a second sheet crosswise over her legs loosely so that the perineal region (the area of the body between the thighs) can be exposed for examination (Figure 16-15).

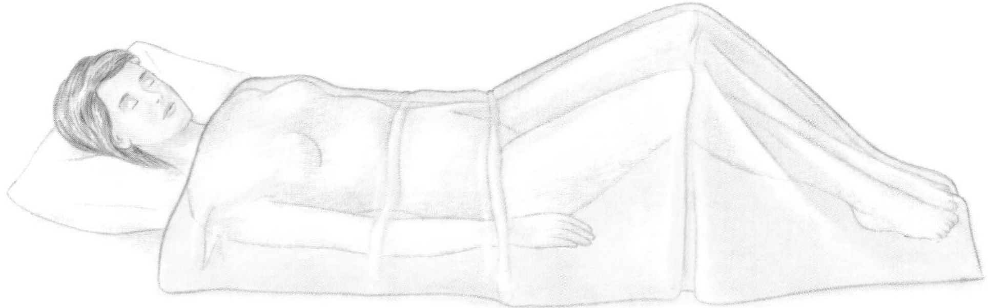

FIGURE 16-15 Dorsal recumbent position.

Fowler's Position
The patient's position when the head of the bed is at a 45-degree angle.

Fowler's Position

This position is also called the *high Fowler's position.* The patient is partly sitting, with the back rest of the bed at a 45-degree angle. The knees are slightly bent. See Figures 16-16 and 16-17.

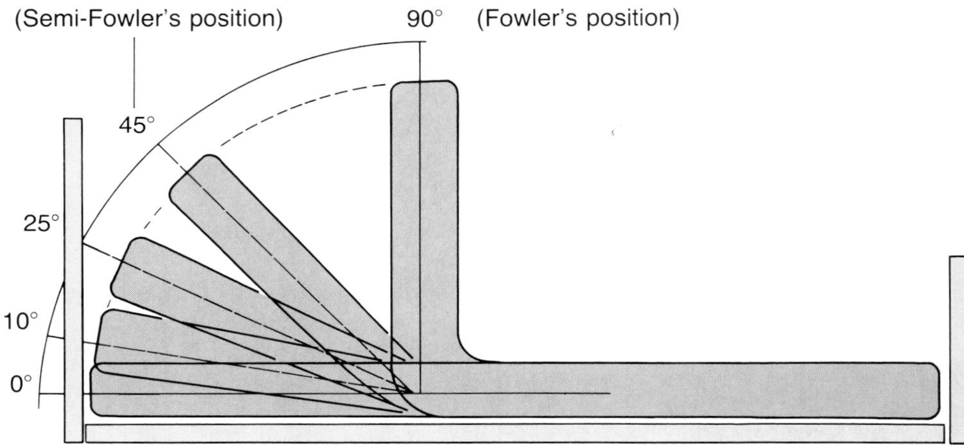

FIGURE 16-16 On electric beds, it is possible to position the patient at any angle ordered by the physician.

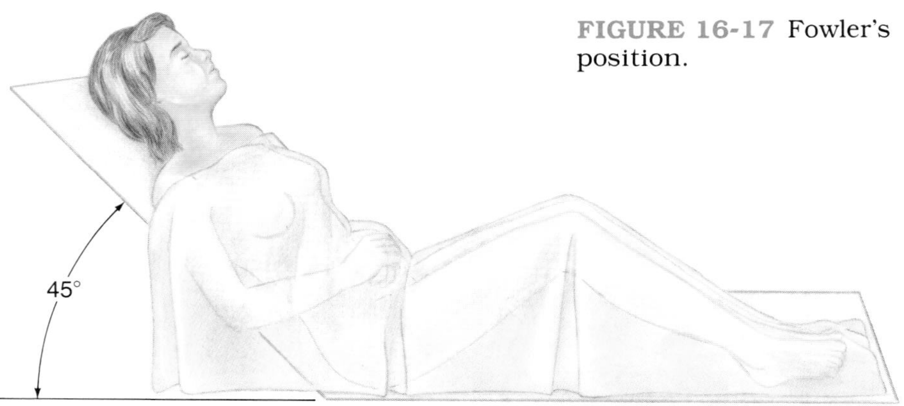

FIGURE 16-17 Fowler's position.

Knee–chest Position
A bent posture with the knees and chest touching the examining table. This position is sometimes used for examining the rectum. It is also used for women who have recently given birth to get the uterus to fall forward into its normal position.

Knee–Chest Position

The patient rests on her knees and chest. The head is turned to one side with the cheek on a pillow. The patient's arms are extended slightly, bent at the elbows. Although the arms help support the patient, the main body weight is supported by the knees and chest. The knees are bent so that they are at right angles to the thighs. Draping is done with two sheets, one for the upper part of the body and one for the lower part (Figure 16-18). This position is used for examining the rectum and vagina.

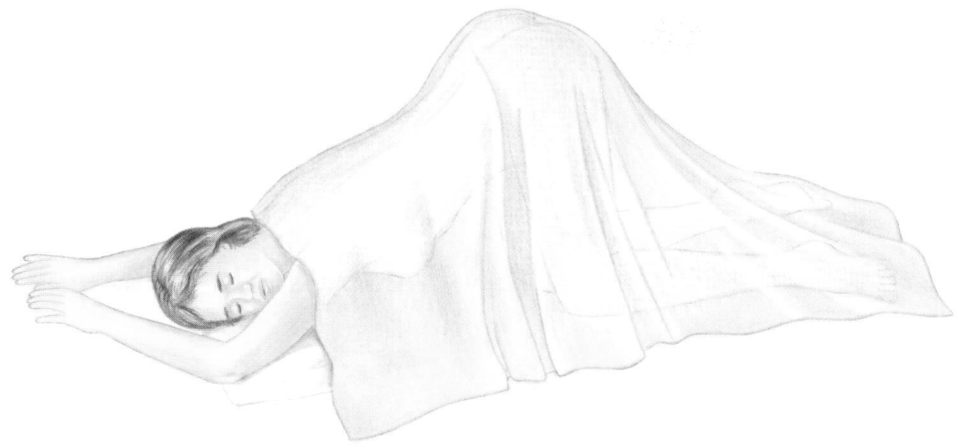

FIGURE 16-18 Knee–chest position.

Side Lying
Lying on one's side.

Side-Lying Positions

Positions of comfort to relieve pressure points are provided by the positions shown in Figure 16-19. Pillows are used to provide support and prevent skin breakdown.

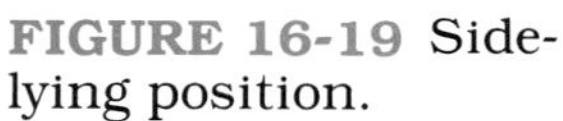

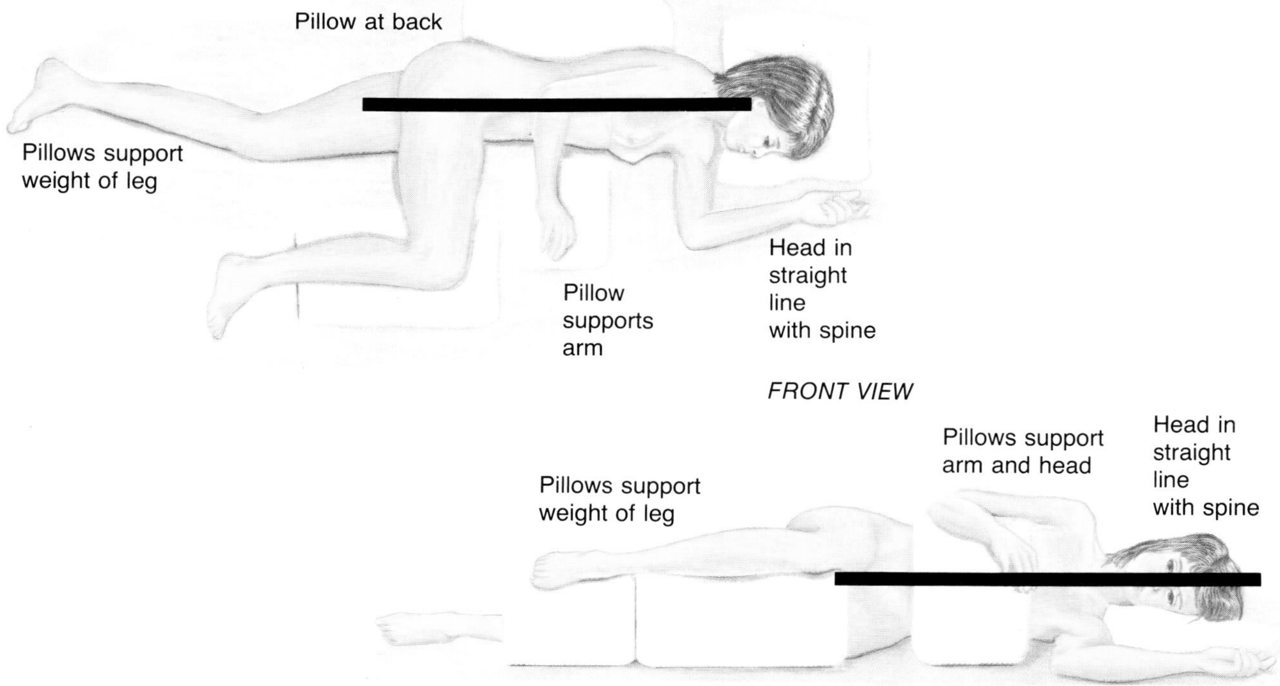

FIGURE 16-19 Side-lying position.

Trendelenburg's Position The bed or operating table is tilted so that the patient's head is about a foot below the level of his or her knees. This position is used to get more blood to the head and prevent shock. Also called the shock position.

Trendelenburg Position

In this position, the draping covers the entire body. The patient's head is low; his or her body is on an incline, carefully supported to prevent the patient from slipping out of position or being injured (Figure 16-20). This position is used for postural drainage, prolapsed cord situations, and so on.

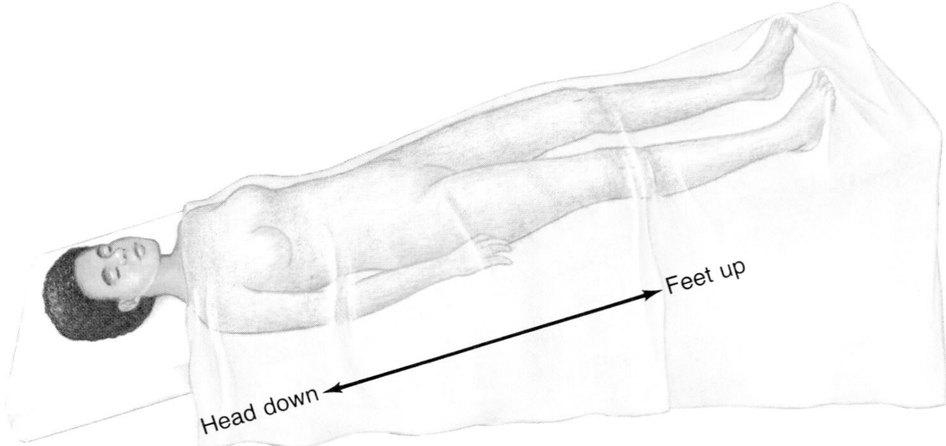

FIGURE 16-20 Trendelenburg position.

Reverse Trendelenburg

In this position, the patient's body is on an incline so that the feet are lower than the head. Again, the body is completely draped (Figure 16-21).

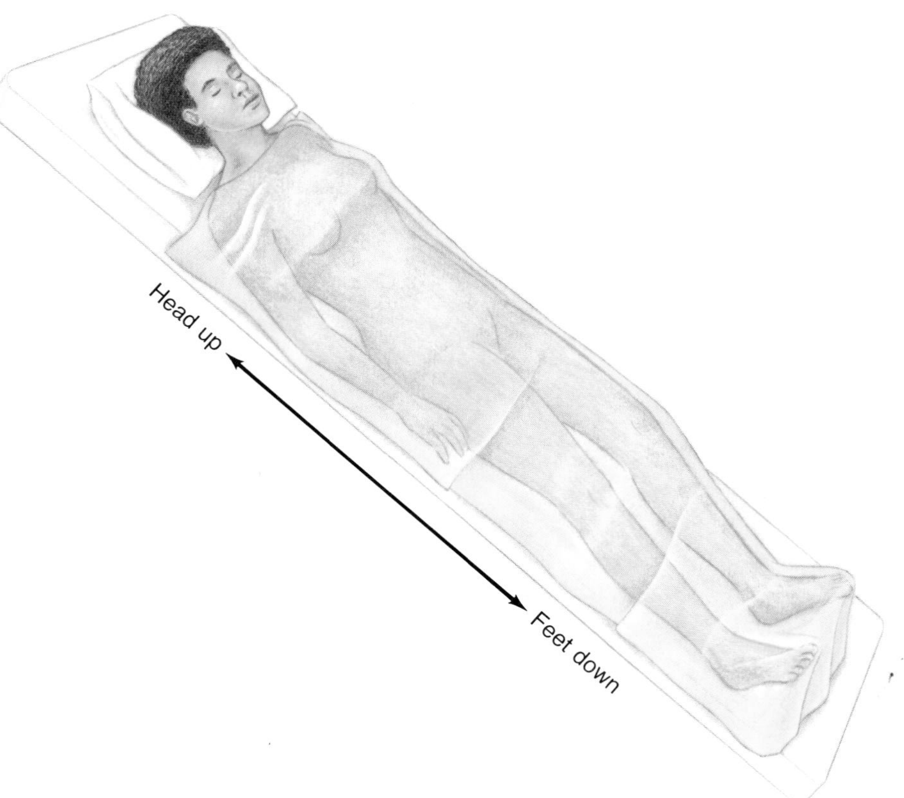

FIGURE 16-21 Reverse Trendelenburg position.

Lithotomy (Dorsal) Position
The patient lies on her back with her legs spread apart and her knees bent. The position is used for performing a pelvic (vaginal) examination.

Dorsal Lithotomy Position

This is the same as the dorsal recumbent position, except that the patient's legs are well separated and the knees are bent more (Figure 16-22). This position is used often for examination of the bladder, vagina, rectum, and perineum. If an examination table is being used, the patient's feet are sometimes placed in stirrups.

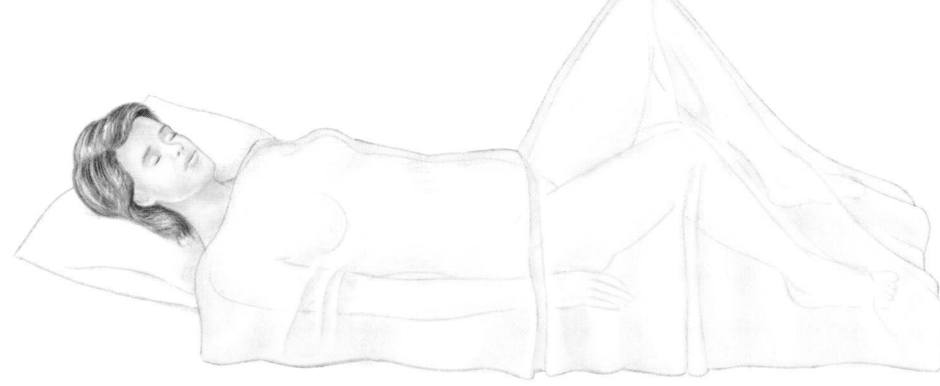

FIGURE 16-22 Dorsal lithotomy position.

Prone
Lying on one's stomach.

Prone Position

The patient lies on the abdomen with the arms at the sides or bent at the elbows. The patient's head is turned to the side (Figure 16-23).

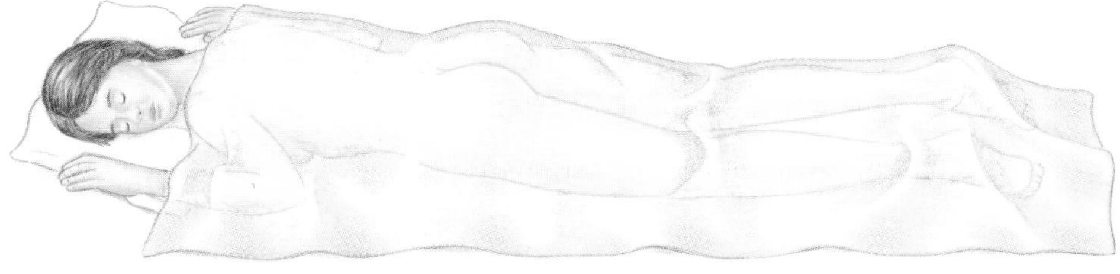

FIGURE 16-23 Prone position.

Sim's Position
The patient lies on the left side with the right knee and thigh drawn up. This position permits a satisfactory rectal examination.

Left Sims's Position

Sims's position is also called the *semiprone* position. The patient lies on the left side. The patient's cheek is resting on a small pillow that is placed under the head. The right knee is bent against the patient's abdomen. The left knee is also bent, but not as much. The left arm is placed behind the body; the right arm rests in a way that is comfortable for the patient (Figure 16-24). This position is used for rectal examinations and enemas. Draping covers the entire body.

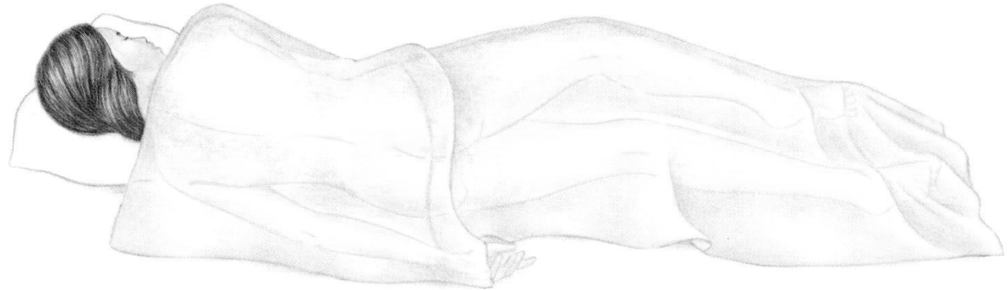

FIGURE 16-24 Left Sims's position.
lateral

Left Lateral Position

The patient lies on the left side. The hips are closer to the edge of the bed than the shoulders. The knees are bent, one more than the other (Figure 16-25).

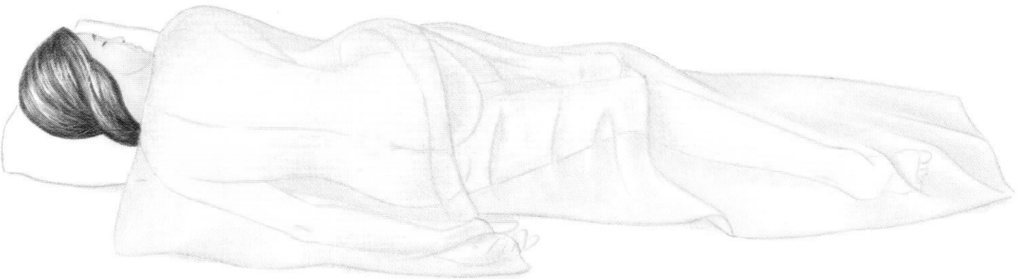

FIGURE 16-25 Left lateral position.

KEY QUESTIONS

1. What are the ten rules for good body mechanics?
2. How should you lift, hold, or move an object or a patient using good body mechanics?
3. What are the rules for lifting and moving patients?
4. How should you lock arms with a patient to raise his head and shoulders?
5. What should you do to move a nonambulatory patient up in bed?
6. How can you move a patient up in bed with his help?
7. Explain how to move the mattress to the head of the bed with the patient's help.
8. How can a helpless patient be moved to one side of the bed on his back?
9. How should you roll a patient like a log?
10. Explain how to turn a patient on either side.
11. How should the patient be draped for privacy in each position in bed? Describe each position.
12. Define: bedridden, body alignment, body mechanics, dorsal recumbent position, drape, draping, Fowler's position, knee–chest position, lithotomy (dorsal) position, nonambulatory, prone, side lying, Sims's position, supine. Trendelenburg's position.

CHAPTER

17

Transporting a Patient

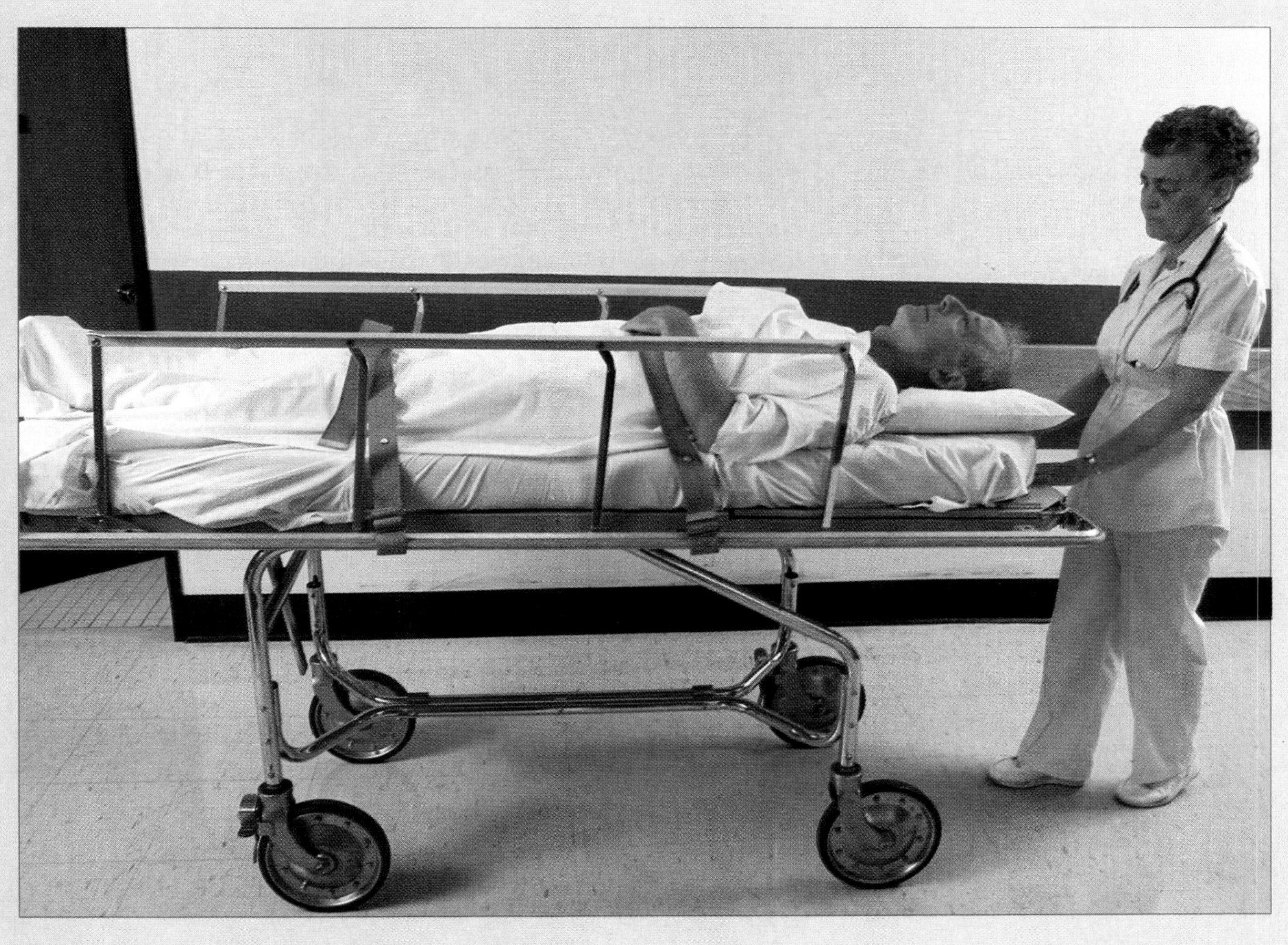

WARNING

For all patient contact, adhere to Universal Precautions (see page 91, 97, or the front cover flap). Wear protective equipment as indicated.

Objectives

What You Will Learn

When you have completed this chapter, you will be able to:

- Transport a patient by wheelchair or stretcher.
- Move a patient from the bed to a wheelchair and back into bed.
- Move the helpless patient using a portable mechanical patient lift.
- Move a patient from the bed to a stretcher and back into bed.
- Define: incontinent and transporting.

KEY IDEAS

Transporting a Patient by Wheelchair

Incontinent
Unable to control the bowels or bladder.

Transporting
Moving from one place to another

THE PATIENT IN A WHEELCHAIR SHOULD be well covered, if she or he is not dressed in a robe and slippers. You may cover the feet as well as the shoulders with a sheet or a blanket, making sure it does not get caught in the wheels. In some institutions the seat of the wheelchair is covered with a piece of linen or with a disposable bed protector if the patient is **incontinent**. The wheelchair must be wiped off with a disinfectant solution after it has been used by each patient.

When you are transporting a patient in a wheelchair, you should push the wheelchair from behind, except when going into or out of elevators (Figure 17-1). When you are entering an elevator, pull the wheelchair into the elevator backward (Figure 17-2). When you are leaving an elevator, ask everyone to step out. Push the button marked "open." Turn the chair around, and pull it out of the elevator backward. This may not be necessary with very wide elevators. Take caution not to make contact with other individuals as you just push the wheelchair out. Don't move the wheelchair while the elevator is in motion.

When you are moving a patient down a steep incline or ramp, you should take the chair down backward (Figure 17-3). To do this, stand behind the chair with your back facing the direction you want to go. Walk backward, holding the chair and moving it carefully down the ramp. Glance back now and then to make sure of your direction and to avoid collisions, as if you were driving a car in reverse.

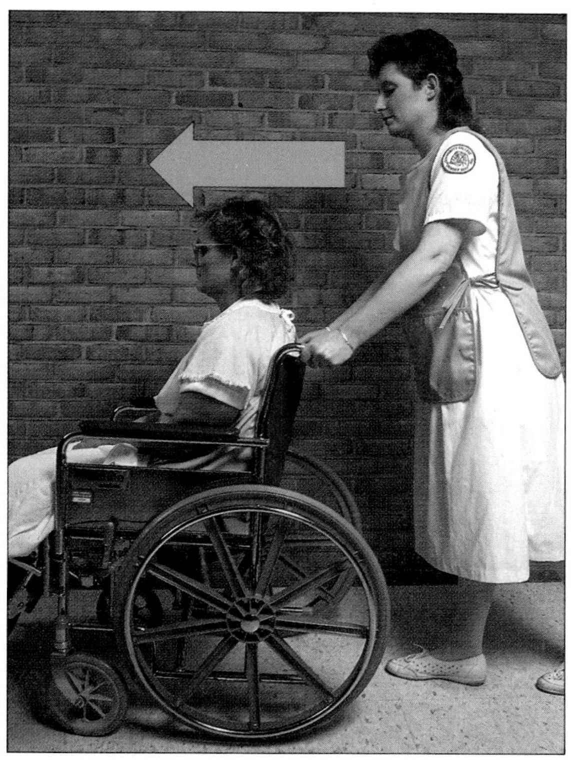

FIGURE 17-1 Transporting the patient by wheelchair.

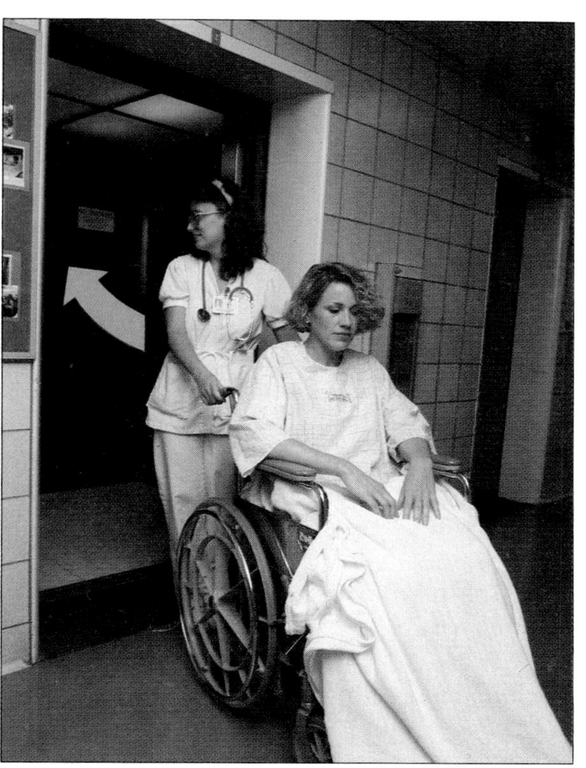

FIGURE 17-2 Entering an elevator with a patient in a wheelchair.

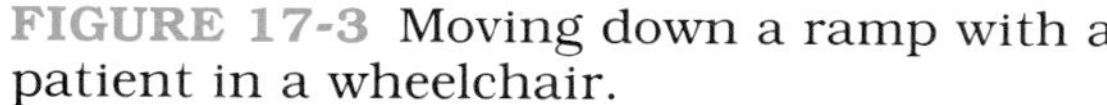

FIGURE 17-3 Moving down a ramp with a patient in a wheelchair.

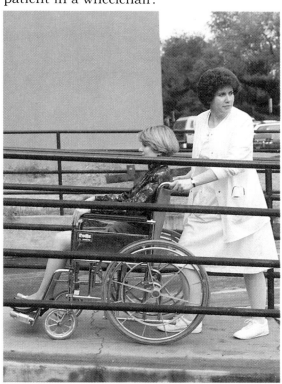

Procedure Helping a Nonambulatory Patient Back into Bed from a Wheelchair or Arm Chair

1. Wash your hands.
2. Identify the patient by checking the identification bracelet.
3. Ask visitors to step out of the room, if this is your hospital's policy.
4. Tell the patient you are getting him back into bed.
5. Ask another nursing assistant to help you.
6. Place a pull sheet on the bottom sheets; fan-fold the top of the bed to the foot.
7. Lock the wheels on the bed.
8. Raise the head of the bed as high as it will go to a sitting position.
9. Lower the bed to its lowest horizontal position.
10. Raise the side rail on the far side of the bed.
11. Bring the wheelchair with the patient to the bedside.
12. Position the wheelchair so that the back of the chair is in line with the footboard of the bed.
13. Lock the brakes on the wheelchair.
14. Raise the footrests of the wheelchair, lifting the patient's feet off them and onto the floor at the same time.
15. Open up the blanket and safety straps that are on the patient in the wheelchair.
16. Both nursing assistants lock arms with the patient, help him to stand, pivot (turn), and sit on the side of the bed.
17. Rest the patient's head and shoulders on the mattress that is in the highest sitting position.
18. One nursing assistant stands next to the patient's head while the other gently lifts both his feet up onto the mattress.
19. Raise that side rail.
20. Lower the head of the bed.
21. Raise the bed to its highest horizontal position.
22. One nursing assistant goes to the far side of the bed.
23. Lower that side rail.
24. Slide both your arms under the patient's back to his far shoulder; then slide the patient's shoulders toward you on your arms.
25. Slide both your arms as far as you can under the patient's buttocks and slide his buttocks toward you. Use a pull (turning) sheet whenever possible.
26. Keep your knees bent and your back straight as you slide the patient.
27. Place both your arms under the patient's lower legs and slide them toward you on your arms.
28. Both nursing assistants then roll the pull sheet toward the patient and slide the patient up in bed using the pull sheet.
29. Put a pillow under the patient's head.
30. Remake the top of the bed.
31. Make the patient comfortable.
32. Lower the bed to a position of safety for the patient.
33. Pull the curtains back to the open position.
34. Raise the side rails where ordered, indicated, and appropriate for patient safety.
35. Place the call light within easy reach of the patient.
36. Wipe the wheelchair with disinfectant solution and return the chair to its proper place.
37. Wash your hands.
38. Report to your immediate supervisor:
    - That the patient has been put back into bed
    - The time the patient was put back into bed
    - How the patient tolerated the procedure
    - Your observations of anything unusual

Procedure Moving the Nonambulatory Patient into a Wheelchair or Arm Chair from the Bed

1. Assemble your equipment:
   a) Wheelchair or arm chair
   b) Blanket or sheet
2. Wash your hands.
3. Identify the patient by checking the identification bracelet.
4. Ask visitors to step out of the room, if this is your hospital's policy.
5. Tell the patient you are going to help him into a wheelchair.
6. Pull the curtain around the bed for privacy.
7. Lock the wheels on the bed.
8. Place the wheelchair at the bedside with the back of the chair in line with the footboard of the bed (Figure 17-4). Lock the wheels on the chair.
9. Fold up the footrests of the wheelchair so they are out of the way. If the wheelchair has leg rests, adjust them to hang straight down.
10. Lock the brakes on the wheelchair.
11. Spread a blanket or sheet on the chair. Have the corner of the blanket between the handles over the back so the opposite corner will be at the patient's feet.

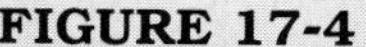

FIGURE 17-4

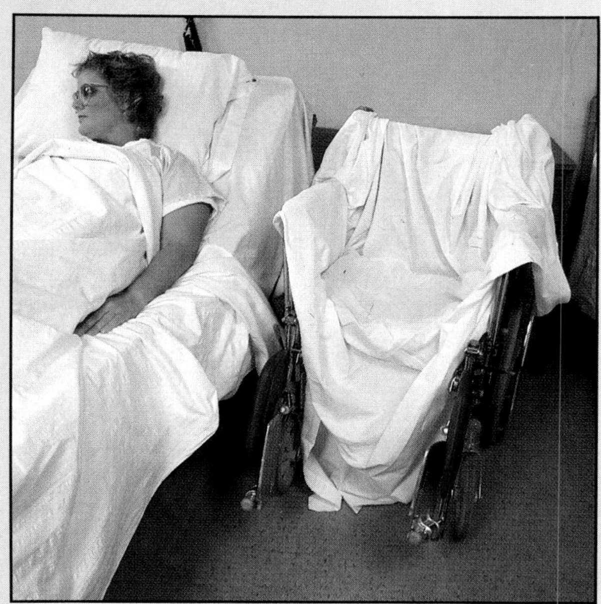

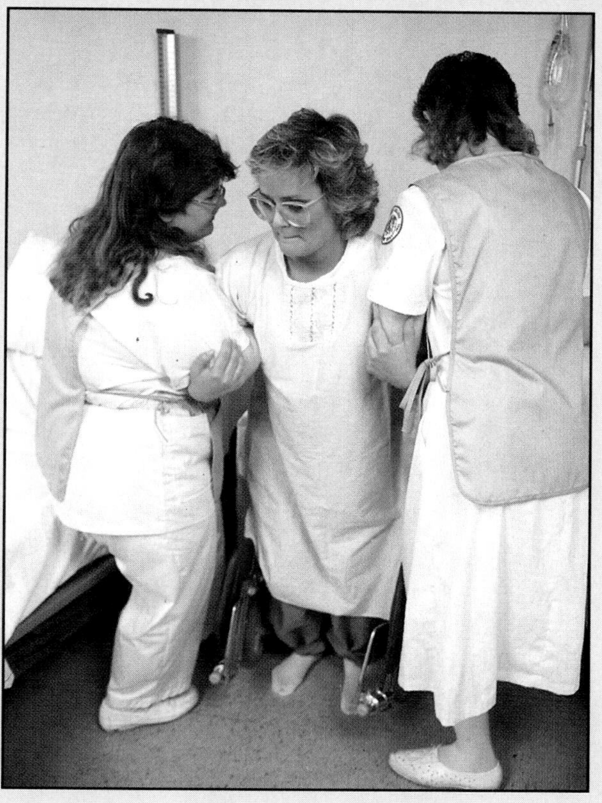

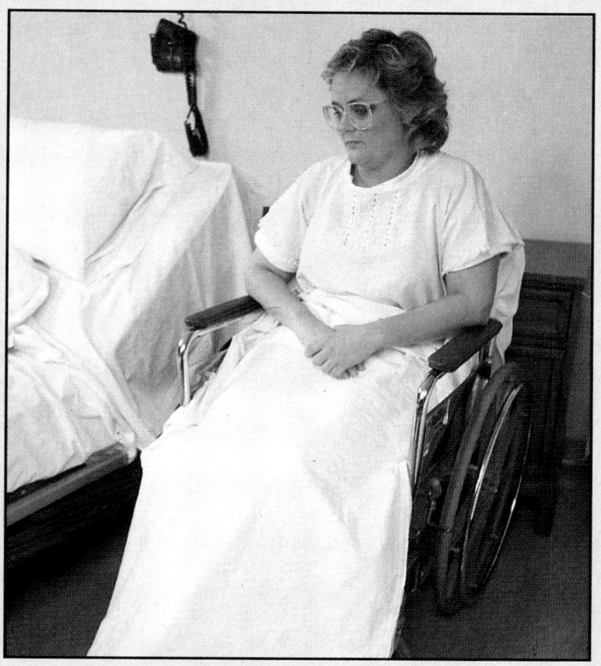

12. Ask another nursing assistant to help you.
13. Put the patient's robe and slippers on while he is in bed.
14. a) Move the patient to the edge of the bed by sliding both your arms under the patient's back to his far shoulder; then slide the patient's shoulders toward you on your arms.
    b) Slide both your arms as far as you can under the patient's buttocks and slide his buttocks toward you. Use a pull (turning) sheet whenever possible.
    c) Place both your arms under the patient's lower legs and slide them toward you on your arms.
15. Raise the side rail.
16. Lower the bed to its lowest horizontal position so that when you dangle the patient his feet will touch the floor when he sits up.
17. Raise the back rest so the patient is in a sitting position in bed.
18. Lower the side rail on the side where you and the other nursing assistant will be working.
19. Place both hands under the patient's legs and turn them to the dangling position. His feet should be firmly on the floor. One nursing assistant supports the patient's back and head and raises them at the same time. The other nursing assistant supports the patient's back while he is in the dangling position with her arm around the patient's shoulders. Give the patient a minute to adjust. Observe the patient's color.
20. Each nursing assistant locks arms with the patient. At the count of three they both lift the patient gently to a standing position, pivot (turn) the patient, and sit him in the wheelchair.
21. Fasten the safety straps around the patient to keep him from falling out of the chair.
22. Arrange the blanket snugly but firmly around the patient. Make sure that no part of the blanket can possibly get caught in the wheels.
23. Adjust the footrests so that the patient's feet are resting on them.
24. Use the signal cord to call your immediate supervisor and take the patient's pulse and blood pressure if you observe any of the following:
    a) The patient becomes very pale.
    b) The patient seems to be perspiring a lot.
    c) The patient says something like "I feel weak," "I feel dizzy," or "I feel faint."
25. Adjust the chair to a comfortable angle.
26. Put a pillow behind the patient's back or shoulders, if needed.

    Wash your hands.

28. Report to your immediate supervisor:
    - That the patient has been moved out of bed into a chair or wheelchair
    - The time the patient's position was changed
    - How the patient tolerated the procedure
    - Your observations of anything unusual

Procedure Helping a Patient Who Can Stand and Is Ambulatory Back into Bed from a Chair or a Wheelchair

1. Wash your hands.
2. Identify the patient by checking the identification bracelet.
3. Ask visitors to step out of the room, if this is your hospital's policy.
4. Tell the patient you are getting him back into bed.
5. Pull the curtain around the bed for privacy.
6. Lock the wheels on the bed.
7. Bring the wheelchair very close to the bed.
8. Lock the brakes on the wheelchair.
9. Raise the head of the bed to a sitting position.
10. Lower the bed to its lowest horizontal position.

11. Raise the footrests of the wheelchair, placing the patient's feet on the floor.
12. Open up the safety straps on the wheelchair.
13. Help the patient out of the wheelchair to stand, pivot (turn), and sit on the side of the bed. His feet should be resting firmly on the floor.
14. Lean the patient against the backrest.
15. Put one arm around the patient's shoulders for support. Put the other arm under his knees (Figure 17-5).

FIGURE 17-5 Helping a patient out of or into the bed.

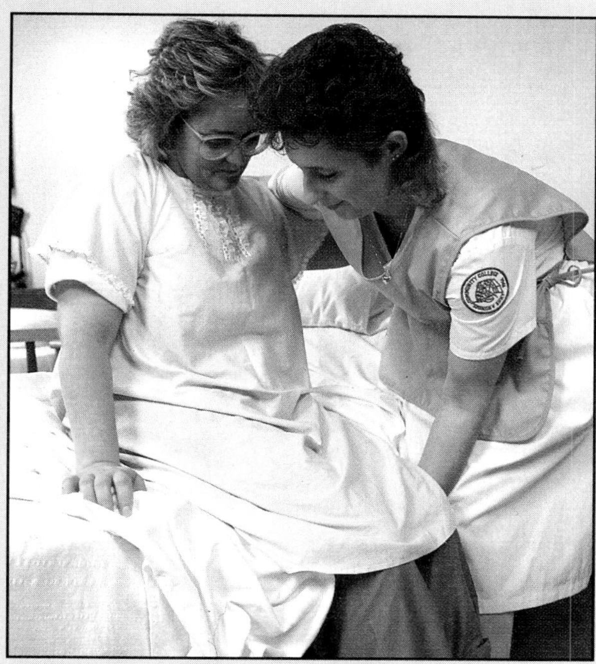

16. Swing his body slowly around, helping him to lift his legs onto the bed.
17. Raise the side rail.
18. Lower the head of the bed.
19. Help the patient move to the center of the bed.
20. Place a pillow under the patient's head.
21. Take off the patient's robe and slippers.
22. Remake the top of the bed.
23. Make the patient comfortable.
24. Lower the bed to a position of safety for the patient.
25. Pull the curtains back to the open position.
26. Raise the side rails where ordered, indicated, and appropriate for patient safety.
27. Place the call light within easy reach of the patient.
28. Fold the blanket from the wheelchair and put it in its proper place.
29. Wash the wheelchair with an antiseptic or disinfectant solution and return it to its proper place.
30. Wash your hands.
31. Report to your immediate supervisor:
    - That you have helped the patient back into bed
    - The time you helped the patient back into bed
    - How the patient tolerated the procedure
    - Your observations of anything unusual

Procedure Using a Portable Mechanical Patient Lift to Move the Helpless Patient

1. Assemble your equipment (Figure 17-6):
   a) Mechanical patient lift
   b) Sling
2. Wash your hands.
3. Identify the patient by checking the identification bracelet.
4. Ask visitors to step out of the room, if this is your hospital's policy.
5. Tell the patient you are going to get him out of bed by using the portable mechanical patient lift. (You may need the help of a second nursing assistant as a partner.)
6. Pull the curtain around the bed for privacy.
7. Position the chair next to the bed with the back of the chair in line with the headboard of the bed. Lock the wheels of the bed and the mechanical lift.
8. Cover the chair with a blanket or sheet.

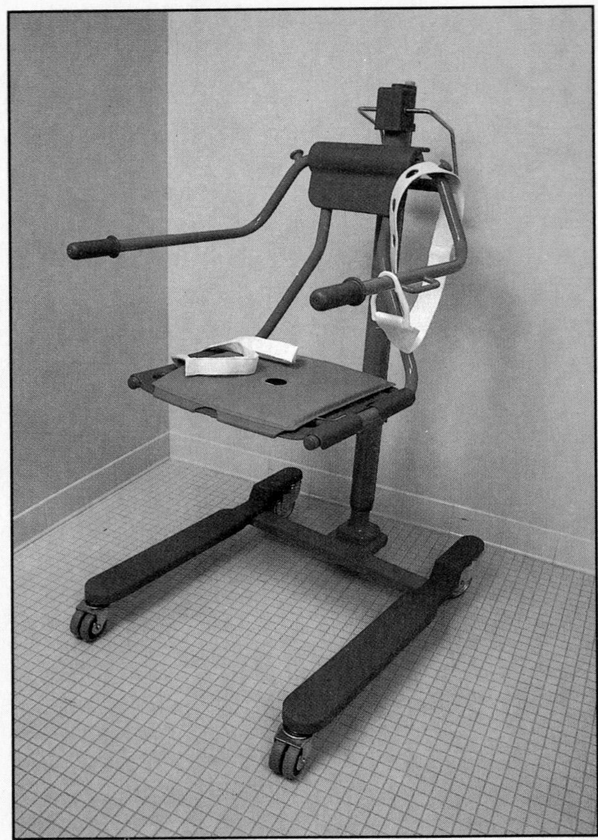

FIGURE 17-6 Portable mechanical patient lift.

9. By turning the patient from side to side on the bed, slide the sling under the patient.
10. Attach the sling to the mechanical lift with the hooks in place through the metal frame. Be sure to apply hooks with open, sharp ends away from the patient.
11. Have the patient fold both arms across his chest, if possible.
12. Using the crank, lift the patient from the bed.
13. Have your partner, a second nursing assistant, guide the patient's legs.
14. Lower the patient into the chair.
15. Remove the hooks from the frame of the portable mechanical patient lift.
16. Wrap the patient with the blanket.
17. Secure the patient to the chair with safety straps, if necessary.
18. Leave the patient safe and comfortable in the chair for the proper amount of time, according to your instructions.
19. To get the patient back to bed, put the hooks through the metal frame of the sling, which is still under the patient.
20. Raise the patient by using the crank on the mechanical patient lift. Lift him from the chair into the bed. Have your partner guide the patient's legs.
21. Lower the patient into the center of the bed.
22. Remove the hooks from the frame.
23. Remove the sling from under the patient by having him turn from side to side on the bed.
24. Put a pillow under the patient's head.
25. Remake the top of the bed.
26. Make the patient comfortable.
27. Lower the bed to a position of safety for the patient.
28. Pull the curtains back to the open position.
29. Raise the side rails where ordered, indicated, and appropriate for patient safety.
30. Place the call light within easy reach of the patient.
31. Wash the mechanical patient lift with an antiseptic or disinfectant solution and return it to its proper place.
32. Wash your hands.
33. Report to your immediate supervisor:
    - That the patient was taken out of bed by means of the portable mechanical patient lift
    - The time the patient was taken out of bed
    - The prescribed length of time that the patient sat in a chair
    - That the patient was put back into bed by means of the portable mechanical patient lift
    - The time the patient was put back into bed
    - How the patient tolerated the procedure
    - Your observations of anything unusual

KEY IDEAS

Using a Stretcher

A hospital stretcher is a wheeled cart on which patients are moved from one place to another. When moving a helpless patient from her or his bed to a stretcher, you will need a second nursing assistant working as your partner. Whenever you are moving the stretcher, you should stand at the end where the patient's head is and push the stretcher so the patient's feet are moving first. Be careful to protect the patient's head at all times. When entering an elevator, push the stop button so the doors of the elevator will not close until you are ready. Pull the stretcher into the elevator with the head end first (Figure 17-7). Stand at the patient's head while the elevator is in motion. When you leave the elevator, press the stop button and push the stretcher out foot-end first.

Use siderails or restraining straps whenever you move a patient on a stretcher. Check the straps before you move the stretcher. Guide the stretcher from the foot end when going down a ramp (Figure 17-8).

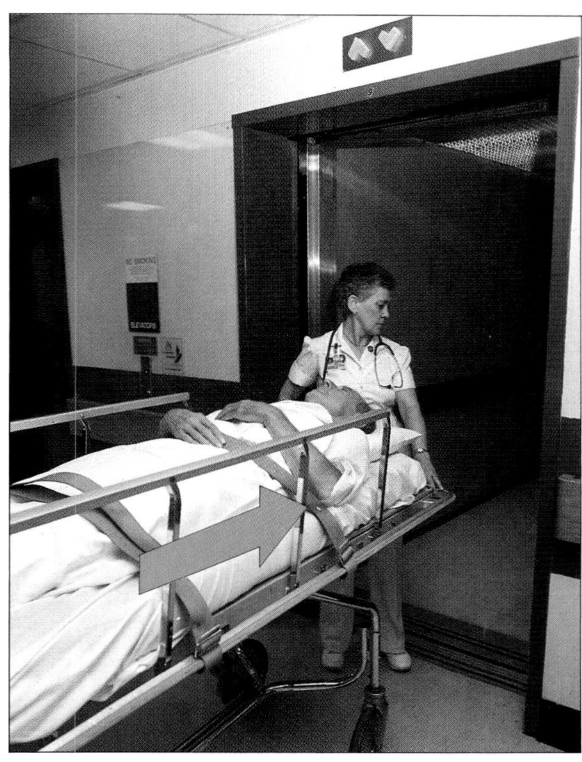

FIGURE 17-7 Entering an elevator with a stretcher.

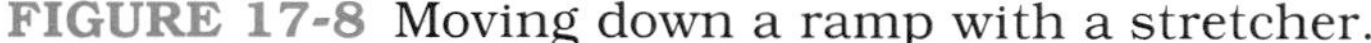

FIGURE 17-8 Moving down a ramp with a stretcher.

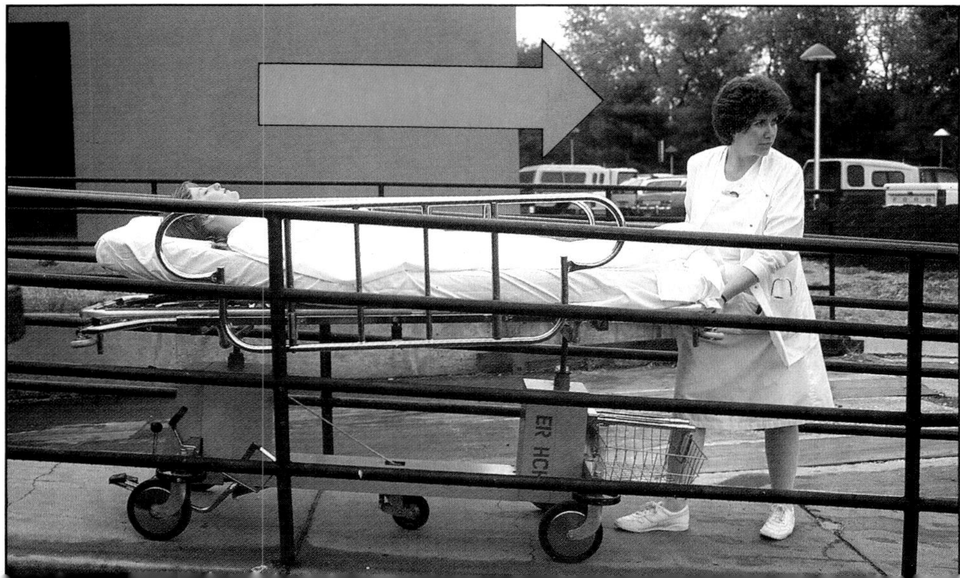

Procedure Moving a Patient from the Bed to a Stretcher

1. Assemble your equipment:
   a) Stretcher
   b) Sheet or blanket
2. Ask another nursing assistant to help you. The two of you should work in unison to move the patient from the bed to a stretcher.
3. Wash your hands.
4. Identify the patient by checking the identification bracelet.
5. Tell the patient you are going to move him from the bed to a stretcher.
6. Ask visitors to step out of the room, if this is your hospital's policy.
7. Pull the curtain around the bed for privacy.
8. Loosen the top sheets.
9. Cover the patient with a blanket or sheet. Remove the top sheets without exposing the patient.
10. Bring the stretcher next to the bed.
11. Raise the bed so that it is the same height as the stretcher. Lock the wheels on the bed.
12. Lock the wheels on the stretcher.
13. You will stand on the far side of the bed using your body to hold the bed in place.
14. Your partner will stand on the far side of the stretcher using his or her body to hold the stretcher in place.
15. You should both have your knees bent, your backs straight, and your weight balanced on both feet.
16. At the signal "one, two, three," push, pull, and slide the patient from the bed to the stretcher. Use a pull (turning) sheet whenever possible (Figure 17-9).
17. Support the patient's head and feet and keep his body covered with a loose blanket or sheet.
18. Fasten the stretcher straps around the patient at his hips and shoulders.
19. Put the side rails of the stretcher in the up position for the patient's safety.
20. Wash your hands.
21. Report to your immediate supervisor:
   - That you have moved the patient from the bed to a stretcher
   - The time you moved the patient to the stretcher
   - How the patient tolerated the procedure
   - Your observations of anything unusual

FIGURE 17-9

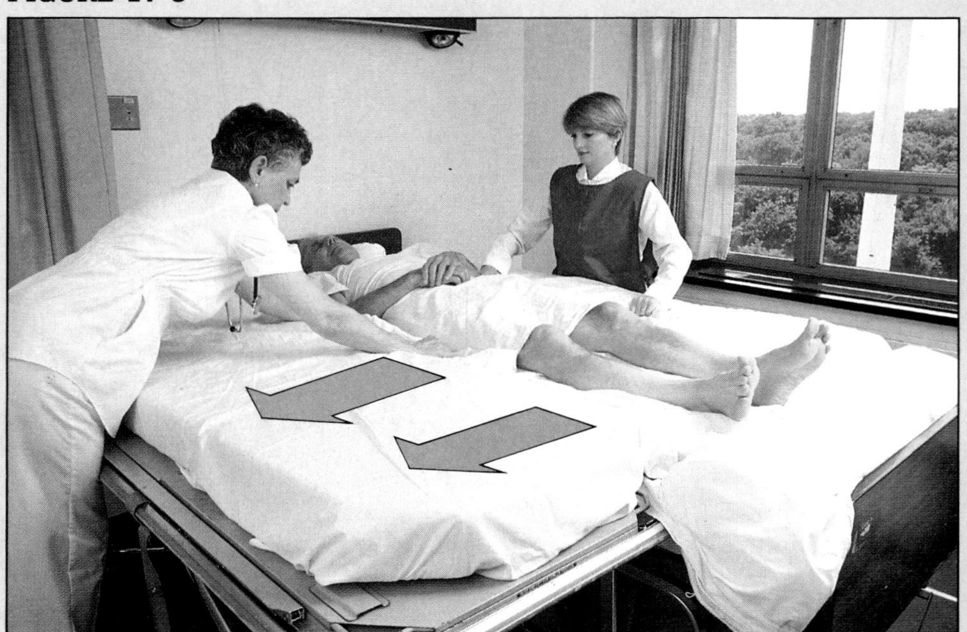

Procedure Moving a Patient from a Stretcher to the Bed

1. Assemble your equipment:
   a) Stretcher
   b) Sheet or blanket
2. Ask another nursing assistant to help. You should work in unison to move the patient from the bed to a stretcher.
3. Wash your hands.
4. Identify the patient by checking the identification bracelet.
5. Tell the patient you are going to move him from the stretcher to the bed.
6. Ask visitors to step out of the room, if this is your hospital's policy.
7. Pull the curtain around the bed for privacy.
8. Lock the wheels on the bed.
9. Fan-fold the top sheet to the bottom of the bed.
10. Bring the stretcher next to the bed.
11. Raise the bed so that it is even with the stretcher.
12. Lock the wheels on the stretcher.
13. One nursing assistant stands on the far side of the bed using his or her body to hold the bed in place.
14. The other nursing assistant stands on the far side of the stretcher using his or her body to hold the stretcher in place.
15. Open the stretcher straps.
16. Both of you should have your knees bent, your backs straight, and your weight balanced on both feet.
17. At the signal, "one, two, three," slide the patient from the stretcher to the bed. Use a pull (turning) sheet whenever possible.
18. Keep the patient covered with a loose blanket or sheet and support his head and feet.
19. Make the patient as comfortable as possible.
20. Make sure the signal cord is within the patient's easy reach.
21. Replace the top sheets, removing the blanket without exposing the patient.
22. Lower the bed to a position of safety for the patient.
23. Pull the curtains back to the open position.
24. Raise the side rails where ordered, indicated, and appropriate for patient safety.
25. Place the call light within easy reach of the patient.
26. Wash your hands.
27. Report to your immediate supervisor:
    - That you have moved the patient from the stretcher to the bed
    - The time you moved the patient from the stretcher to the bed
    - How the patient tolerated the procedure
    - Your observations of anything unusual

KEY QUESTIONS

1. What should you do to transport a patient by wheelchair or stretcher?
2. How should a patient be moved from the bed to a wheelchair and back into bed?
3. How can you move the helpless patient using a portable mechanical patient lift?
4. What should be done to move a patient from the bed to a stretcher and back into bed?
5. Define: incontinent and transporting.

CHAPTER

18

Care of the Orthopedic Patient

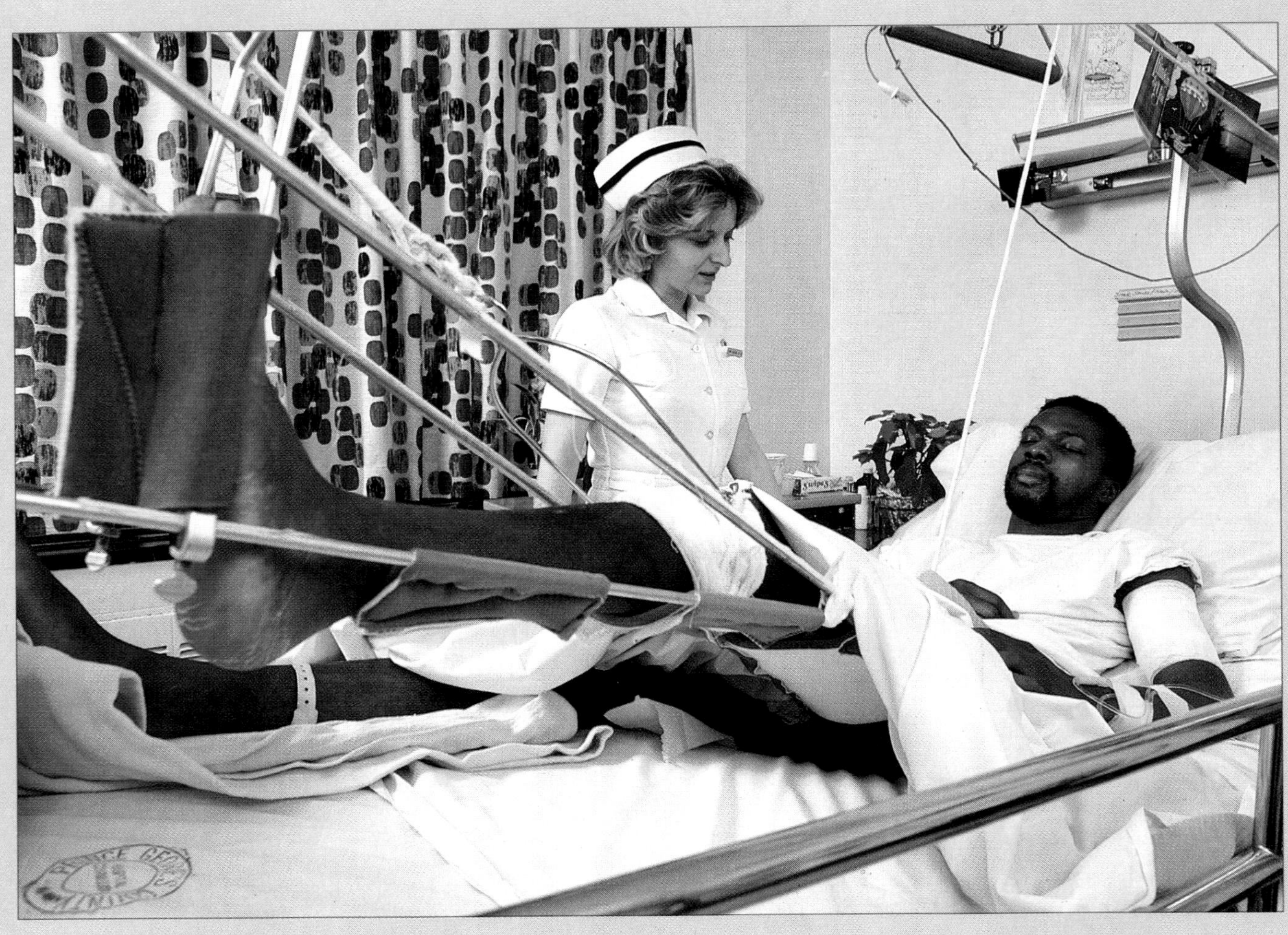

WARNING

For all patient contact, adhere to Universal Precautions (see page 91, 97, or the front cover flap). Wear protective equipment as indicated.

Objectives

What You Will Learn

When you have completed this chapter, you will be able to:

- Describe the scope of orthopedic nursing care and the purposes of orthopedic equipment.
- List the common diseases and disorders of the orthopedic patient.
- Explain the reasons for and describe special skin care for the orthopedic patient.
- List important points to observe while performing any nursing task involving patients in traction.
- List important points to observe while performing any nursing task involving patients in plaster casts.
- Define: fracture, immobile, orthopedics, traction device, trapeze.

KEY IDEAS

Scope of Orthopedics

Orthopedics (orthopaedics)
The medical specialty that covers the treatment of broken bones, deformities, or diseases that attack the bones, joints, and muscles.

ORTHOPEDICS (ALSO SPELLED ORTHOPAEDICS) IS THE science of the prevention and correction of deformities and the treatment of diseases of the bones, muscles, joints, and fasciae (supporting membranes) either by manipulation, special apparatus, or surgery. Orthopedic nursing requires special knowledge and skills, in addition to routine patient care. To care for the orthopedic patient, the nursing assistant will need knowledge of body mechanics and specialized procedures peculiar to the treatment of this type of patient. Nursing assistants will need to be familiar with special equipment, such as splints, casts, and traction devices.

Common Diseases and Disorders of the Orthopedic Patient

Fracture
A break in the bone.

1. **Fractures:**
   (a) *Simple:* The bone is broken but there is no external wound.
   (b) *Compound:* The bone is broken and there is an external wound or fragment of bone protruding through the skin.
2. Dislocations: Pulling out (displacement) of a bone end that forms part of a joint
3. Sprains: An injury in which ligaments are partially torn
4. Bone diseases:
   (a) Osteomyelitis
   (b) Tuberculosis

5. Joint diseases:
   (a) Arthritis
   (b) Inflammation
6. Central nervous system injury, which may be neurological in nature:
   (a) Poliomyelitis (not seen often)
   (b) Trauma or accidental injury damaging the spinal cord and resulting in paralysis of some area of the body
   (c) Guillain–Barre syndrome: a disease of the nervous system.

Orthopedic Nursing Care

Orthopedic care offers a double challenge to the nursing assistant:

- Routine nursing care is difficult to give when a patient is in a cast or traction. It will be necessary to carry out some procedures with the least possible disturbance to these orthopedic devices.
- The patient presents a challenge. (Because of long hospitalization and the fear of deformity, the patient may become unduly depressed or discouraged.) Encourage the patient to do as much for himself or herself as possible. Offer the patient help only when he or she asks for it and needs it, as the patient should try to be self-reliant. No patient should feel isolated or useless.

Orthopedic Equipment

Modern science is constantly developing new ways and means to help the orthopedic patient. Some of these methods involve the use of special equipment. All devices of orthopedic equipment have a twofold aim:

1. To provide support for the injured part until it heals
2. To prevent deformity and weakness in the injured muscles and joints

Support for the injured part may be provided by bandages, adhesive strapping, splints, or plaster casts applied externally. Support may also be applied directly to a bone by using pins, metal plates, or prosthetic devices (for example, the replacement of a joint). These specialized *prostheses* (artificial aids) are applied in the operating room using specialized surgical procedures. To prevent stiffness or deformity, the patient will be asked to use the affected part within limits ordered by the doctor. Frequently, the patient needs the support of a brace, crutches, or a walker.

KEY IDEAS

Special Skin Care for the Orthopedic Patient

Immobile
Unable to move.

Besides routine nursing care, the orthopedic patient needs special skin care. Since the patient is often confined to his or her bed or **immobile** because of a cast or traction, the patient is particularly susceptible to pressure sores. You should change the patient's position every 2 hours following the doctor's instructions, give special back care, and change the area of pressure as often as is possible to prevent pressure ulcers. Providing a smooth, clean, dry bed and keeping the cast clean can aid patient comfort and prevent pressure sores.

Trapeze
A metal bar suspended over the bed. It is used by a patient to help him or her raise or move the body more easily.

Patients in casts often suffer feelings of restriction and fatigue. A **trapeze**, suspended from an over-the-bed frame, allows the patient to move or lift himself, to aid in back care, and to use the bedpan.

KEY IDEAS

Care of the Patient in Traction

Traction Device
Equipment for pulling and stretching parts of the patient's body by using pulleys and weights. Traction is used to keep broken bones in proper alignment while healing.

Traction means the exertion of pull by means of weights and pulleys. Countertraction (exertion of pull in the opposite direction) must be present to maintain body alignment. Traction is used to promote and maintain the alignment of broken (fractured) bones and for other orthopedic conditions and treatment. It may be applied to the skin externally or to the bone internally through surgery. It is maintained by the use of a special frame on the bed (Figure 18-1).

If the patient is uncomfortable, tell your immediate supervisor. Sand bags (cloth bags filled with sand to make them heavy) are often used with traction. Ask for permission before moving the bags. If your immediate supervisor tells you they may be moved, follow her or his instructions. When you have finished, be sure to put the bags back in the same position they were in before, very slowly. Never change the patient's body position without permission from your immediate supervisor.

A nursing assistant will never set or adjust any of the equipment in use on a patient in traction. This is strictly a function of the physician, licensed nurse, or orthopedic technician. The nursing assistant, however, is expected to check continually on the traction apparatus and to report any defect to the immediate supervisor. The following questions concern points that nursing assistants should observe as they perform any nursing task involving patients in traction.

- Is the rope dragging on the floor?
- Is the bag of weights resting on the floor or against the bed?
- Is a rope off its pulley?
- Has the patient slid down in the bed?
- If there is a cast, is it causing pain?
- Is the skin on the body part where the cast ends blue in color? Is the part cold to the touch?
- Does the patient complain of pain?

IF THE ANSWER TO ANY OF THESE QUESTIONS IS YES, REPORT THE SITUATION TO YOUR IMMEDIATE SUPERVISOR AT ONCE, AS THESE ARE ALL CONDITIONS THAT SHOULD NOT EXIST AND SHOULD RECEIVE PROMPT ATTENTION.

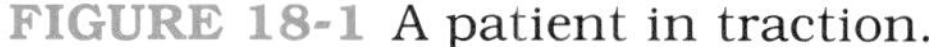

FIGURE 18-1 A patient in traction.

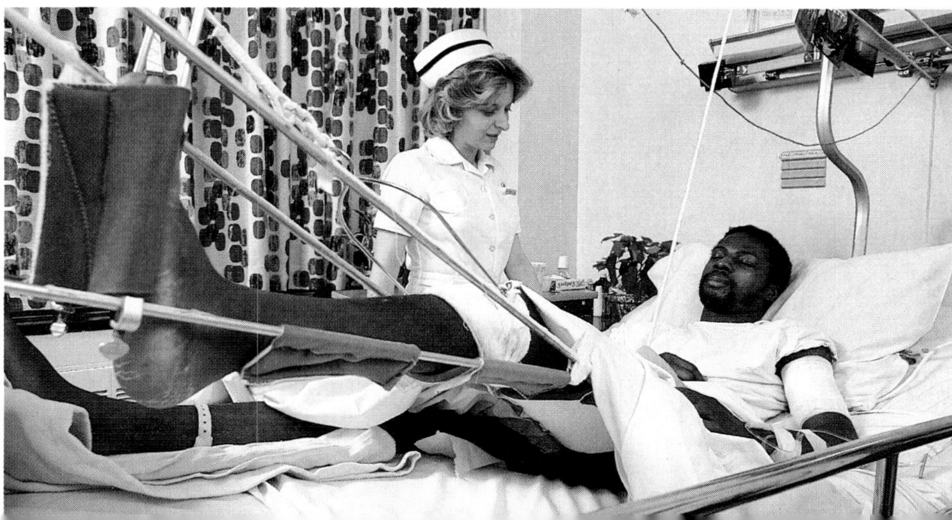

KEY IDEAS

Purpose and Types of Casts

Casts are, in reality, a form of bandage. They are used as a support to hold injured bones in alignment while they are healing. Casts are wet when applied and then allowed to dry. They harden as they dry, and the whole cast becomes rigid. Plastic or fiber-glass casts perform the same task but are lighter, cleaner, and easier to use and remove.

While a cast is drying, the patient's position must be maintained and the cast left uncovered. Pillows are placed to support the cast so it will not bend or move while still soft. Often ice packs are applied to the cast at the area of incision to reduce swelling.

Observing Patients in Casts

Casts are confining and can be very uncomfortable. The skin area near the edges of the cast can become irritated and develop pressure bedsores from chafing.

Casts should not restrict circulation. The nursing assistant should observe patients in casts for signs of pain, pallor, bluish color, and coldness to the touch. You should ask the patient for signs of tingling or numbness, which are signs of poor circulation. The extremities should be compared for size, color, and warmth. The nursing assistant should feel the exposed part of the limb to note whether or not it is cold. Any symptom of circulatory impairment should be reported immediately to your immediate supervisor.

Patients may complain of itching. These effects should be noted and reported to your immediate supervisor.

Nursing assistants should be sure that casts are not soiled while bedpans and urinals are being used. Keeping the cast clean helps greatly to avoid discomfort and other skin irritations.

Unusual odors coming from the cast or stains on the cast should be reported to the head nurse or team leader at once. This could be a sign that a pressure ulcer or infection is forming under the cast.

KEY QUESTIONS

1. What is the purpose of orthopedic equipment?
2. What are the common diseases and disorders of the orthopedic patient?
3. Why does the orthopedic patient need special skin care?
4. Which observations are especially important when giving nursing care to a patient in traction?
5. Which observations are especially important when giving nursing care to a patient in a cast?
6. Define: fracture, immobile, orthopedics, traction device, trapeze.

CHAPTER 19

Anatomy and Physiology of the Integumentary System

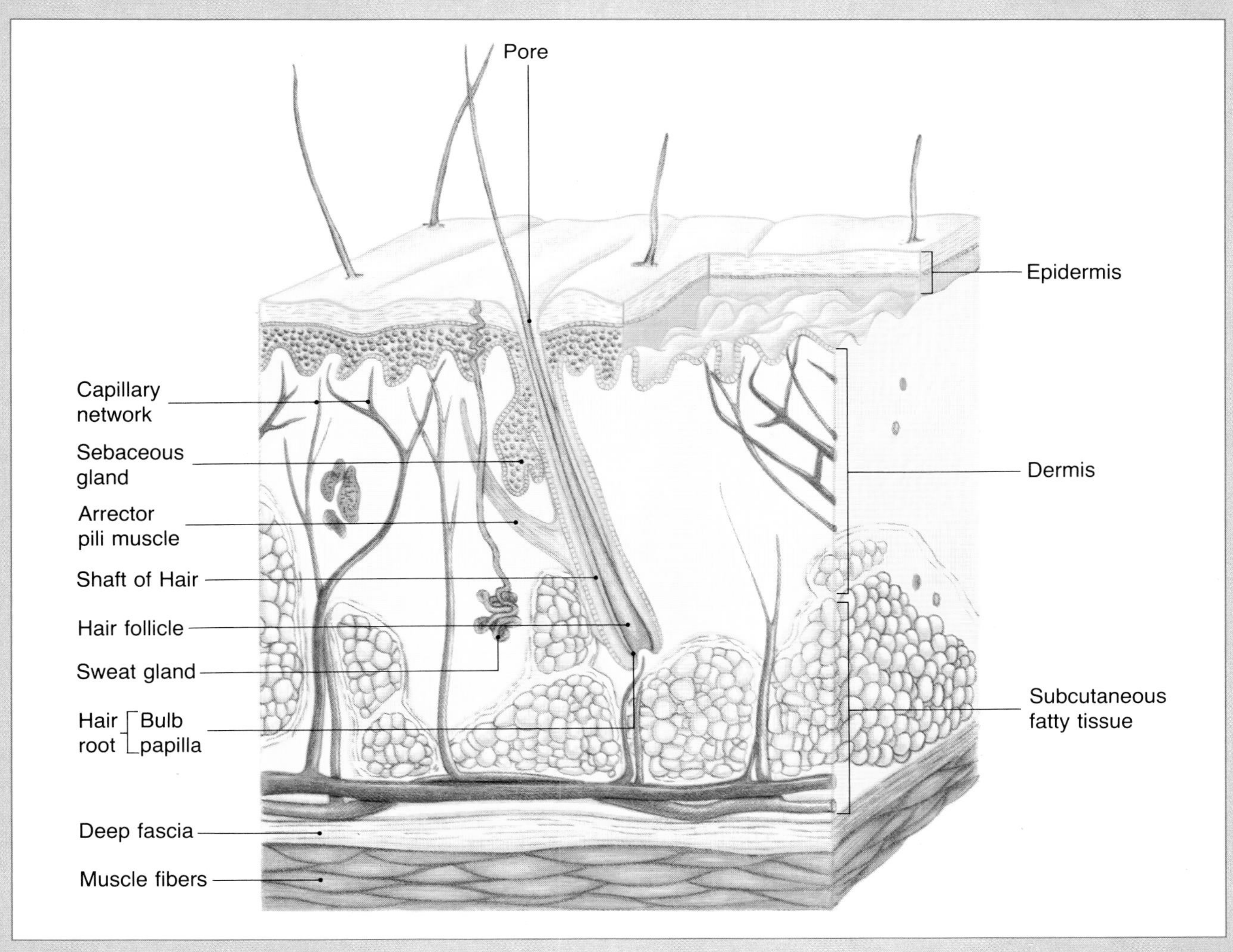

WARNING

For all patient contact, adhere to Universal Precautions (see page 91, 97, or the front cover flap). Wear protective equipment as indicated.

Objectives

What You Will Learn

When you have completed this chapter, you will be able to:

- Label a diagram of a cross section of the skin.
- List the five primary functions of the skin.
- Explain the role of the skin in regulating body temperature.
- Observe the skin for signs of cyanosis.
- List common diseases and disorders of the integumentary system.
- Define: cyanosis, dermis, epidermis, integumentary system, ulcer.

KEY IDEAS

The Integumentary System (the Skin)

Integumentary System
The group of body organs, including the skin, hair, nails, and sweat and oil glands, that provides the first line of defense against infection, maintains body temperature, provides fluids, and eliminates wastes.

THE SKIN COVERS AND PROTECTS UNDERLYING structures from injury or bacterial invasion. Skin also contains nerve endings from the nervous system. A cross section of the skin is shown in Figure 19-1.

The skin helps regulate the body temperature by controlling the loss of heat from the body. To increase heat loss, the blood vessels near the skin dilate, and the increased blood flow brings more heat to the skin's surface. Then the skin temperature rises and more heat is lost from the hot skin to the cooler environment. Even more important in heat loss is the evaporation of sweat (perspiration) that carries heat away from the skin. When the body is conserving heat, sweating stops and blood vessels contract. This prevents the blood from carrying heat to the skin. The skin temperature falls, decreasing heat loss. In this way, the body temperature is kept almost constant.

Perspiration is released from the body through *sweat glands*, which are distributed over the entire skin surface. The glands open by ducts or pores. The body rids itself of certain waste products through perspiration. Skin also secretes a thick, oily substance through the ducts that lead to *oil glands*. In this way, the skin is lubricated and kept soft and pliable. The oil also provides a protective film for the skin, which limits the absorption and evaporation of water from the surface. During the aging process, these oil glands sometimes fail to function properly and the skin becomes quite dry, scaly, and delicate.

Appendages of the Skin

Appendages of the skin, in addition to the sweat and oil glands, include the hair and the nails. Each hair has a root embedded in the skin into which the oil glands of the skin open. Fingernails and toenails grow from the nail bed at the base underneath. If the nail bed is destroyed, the nail stops growing.

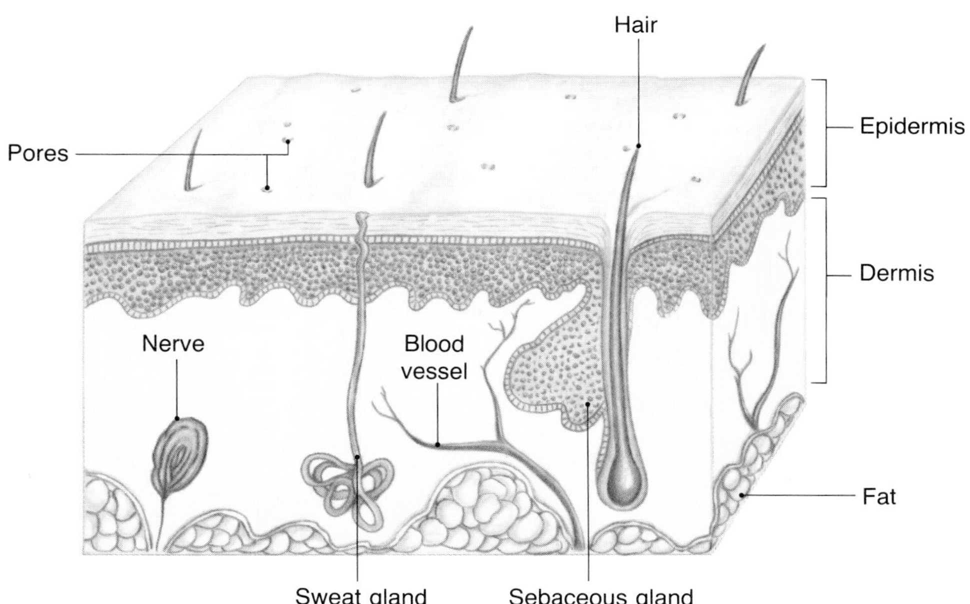

FIGURE 19-1
Magnified cross section of the skin.

Epidermis
The outer layer or surface of the skin.

Dermis
The inner layer of skin.

The skin covers the entire body. The outer layer of the skin (the layer you can see) is called the **epidermis**. Cells are constantly flaking off or being rubbed off this outer layer of skin. Beneath the epidermis is the **dermis**. In this layer of skin are the new cells that will replace the cells that are lost from the epidermis. *Pigment* is found in the epidermis and is responsible for the color of the skin. In sunlight, through a chemical reaction, the amount of pigment increases and a sun tan results.

Moisture on the skin can pick up dust and dirt from the air. Moisture can also mix with the skin particles being flaked off the epidermis. This process causes a condition that promotes the growth and spread of bacteria, which is the main reason for keeping the skin clean. The skin is where the battle for asepsis (being free of disease-causing organisms) begins.

Cyanosis
When the skin looks blue or gray, especially on the lips, nailbeds, and under the fingernails. In a black patient, it may appear as a darkening of color. This occurs when there is not enough oxygen in the blood.

Cyanosis

Watch for changes in the color of the patient's skin, especially a blueness or darkening (cyanosis) of the lips, fingernails, or eyelids. **Cyanosis** is a sign of impaired circulation and one of the effects of shock.

Primary Functions of the Skin

The primary functions of the skin are:

- To cover and protect underlying body structures from injury and microorganism invasion
- To help regulate body temperature by controlling loss of heat from the body
- To provide a first line of defense against infection
- To store energy in the form of fat and vitamins
- To eliminate wastes by perspiration
- To allow sensory perception, that is, the sense of touch (the skin can sense heat, cold, pain, and pressure)

KEY IDEAS

Common Diseases and Disorders of the Integumentary System

Ulcer
A local destruction of the epidermis and dermis.

- Initial lesions (a lesion is an abnormality, either benign or cancerous, of the tissues of the body, such as a wound, sore, rash, or boil)
  - Macule: discoloration that is flat
  - Papule: elevated area
  - Vesicle: elevated area filled with fluid
  - Pustule: elevated area filled with pus
- Secondary lesions
  - Scales: layers of dead skin
  - Excoriations: scratched, broken areas
  - **Ulcer:** local destruction of the epidermis and dermis
- Dermatoses: abnormal skin conditions
- Acne vulgaris: chronic condition of the oil glands
- Furuncle: acute inflammation that starts in a hair follicle
- Impetigo: superficial infection caused by streptococci, staphylococci, or bacteria
- Fungus: caused by plantlike organisms, which include:
  - Athlete's foot
  - Ringworm
- Parasitic diseases
  - *Pediculosis capitus* (head lice)
  - *Pediculosis corporis* (body lice)
- Herpes zoster: inflammatory condition caused by virus that produces painful eruptions
- Dermatitis: reaction to irritating or allergenic materials
- Psoriasis: chronic condition of circular patches for which the cause is unknown
- Cancer of the skin: cutaneous neoplasm, the most curable malignancy
- Malignant melanoma: tumor of the skin that produces a high rate of mortality (death rate)
- Lupus erythematosus: inflammatory disease of unknown origin
- Burns: excessive exposure to heat or fire

KEY QUESTIONS

1. Label a diagram of a cross section of the skin.
2. What are the five primary functions of the skin?
3. How does the skin help to regulate body temperature?
4. What are the signs of cyanosis?
5. What are the common diseases and disorders of the integumentary system?
6. Define: cyanosis, dermis, epidermis, integumentary system, ulcer.

CHAPTER 20

Care of the Patient with Potential Skin Problems

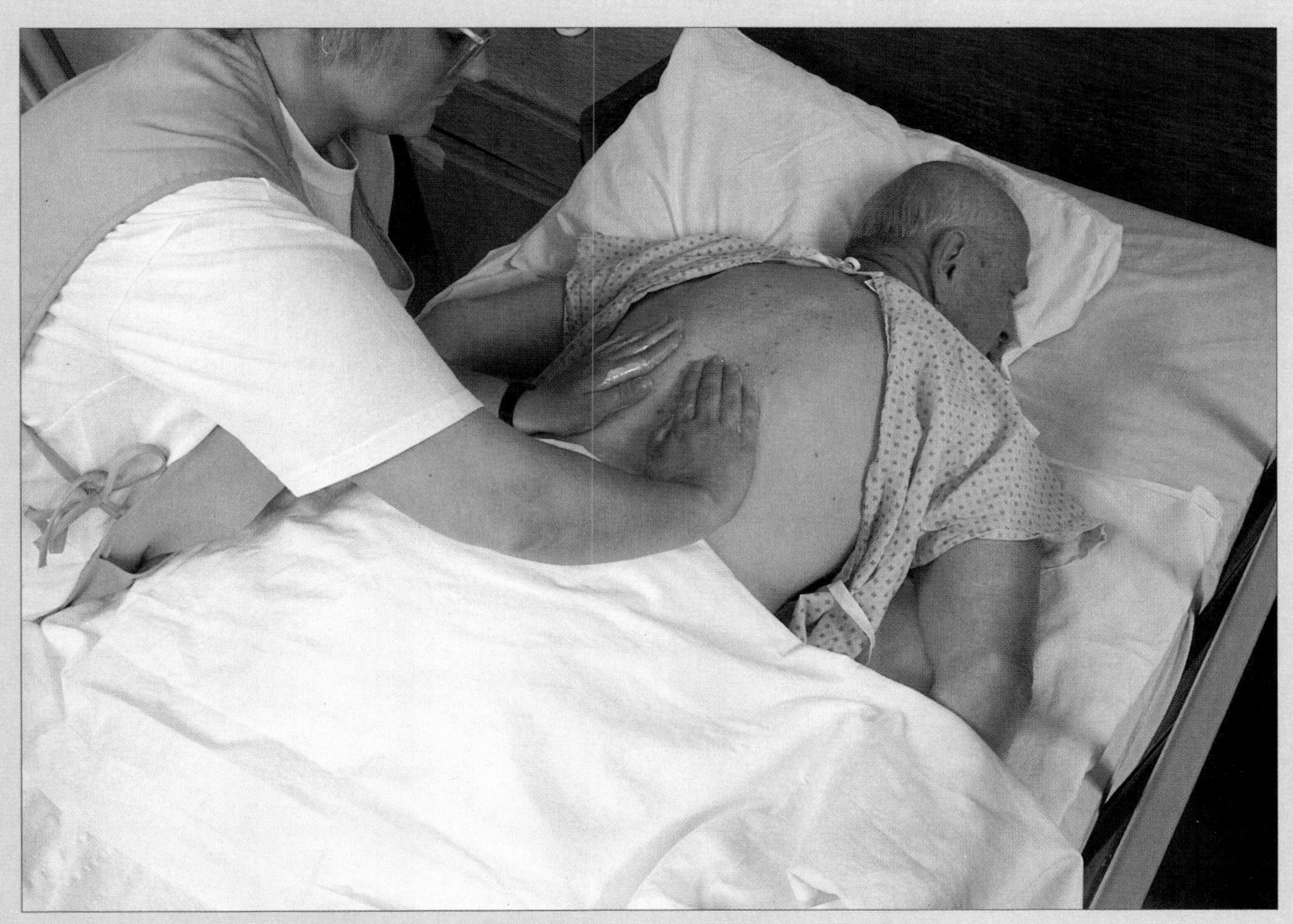

WARNING

For all patient contact, adhere to Universal Precautions (see page 91, 97, or the front cover flap). Wear protective equipment as indicated.

Objectives

What You Will Learn

When you have completed this chapter, you will be able to:

- Explain the cause of bedsores.
- Recognize the signs of a bedsore (pressure ulcer).
- Care for the patient's skin to help prevent bedsores.
- Care for the incontinent patient to prevent decubitus ulcers.
- Provide special back care to prevent pressure ulcers.
- Define: pressure ulcers, incontinent, obese, prevent, prominences.

KEY IDEAS

Decubitus Ulcers

Pressure Ulcers
Also called bedsores; areas of the skin that become broken and painful; caused by continuous pressure on a body part and usually occur when a patient is kept in bed for a long period of time.

Prominences:
Places where bones are close to the surface of the body.

DECUBITUS ULCERS, CALLED *BEDSORES*, ***PRESSURE ULCERS***, or pressure sores, are areas where the skin has broken down because of prolonged underlying pressure (Figure 20-1). Injury to the skin comes from pressure on a part of the body where there is loss of circulation (blood flow), which destroys tissues. If decubitus ulcers are not treated, they quickly get larger, and become very painful. This circulatory interference is usually caused by pressure over the bony **prominences**. These are places where bones are close to the surface of the body. The pressure can come from the weight of the body lying in one position for too long or from splints, casts, or bandages. Even wrinkles in the bed linen can be a cause of bedsores.

FIGURE 20-1 Decubitus ulcers or bedsores are broken areas of the skin caused by the loss of circulation to that area and are the result of continual pressure when the patient remains in the same position too long.

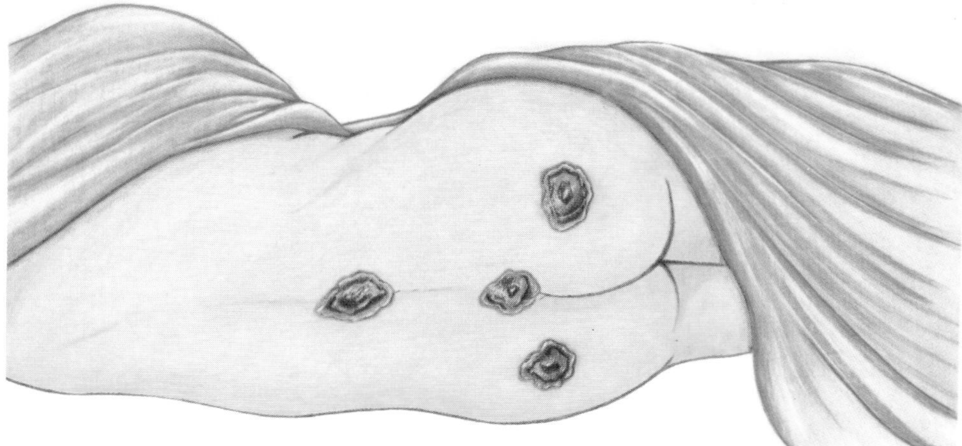

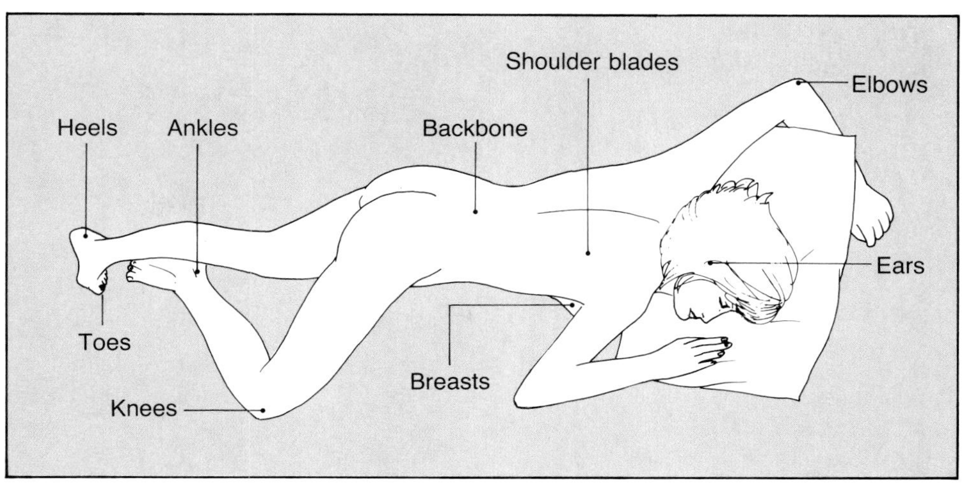

FIGURE 20-2 Places to check for signs of bedsores.

Bedsores are often made worse by continued pressure, heat, moisture, and lack of cleanliness. Irritating substances on the skin such as perspiration, urine, feces, material from wound discharges, or soap that has been left on the skin after a bath all tend to make bedsores worse.

Signs of a Decubitus Ulcer or Bedsore

The signs of a decubitus ulcer on the skin are heat, redness, tenderness, discomfort, and a feeling of burning. When the skin is broken, a bedsore has formed. Specific treatment for a bedsore is prescribed by a doctor. The wound, however, must be kept clean and the rules of asepsis must be followed. As you have learned, the skin is where the battle for asepsis begins.

Places to check on the body for signs of bedsores are the bony areas (Figure 20-2). These are, for example, the shoulder blades, elbows, knees, heels, sides of ankles, back of the head over the ears, and the lower tip of the spine. Usually these areas are covered only by a thin layer of skin. Since these areas receive a smaller supply of blood than other areas of the body, they are the areas where bedsores are most likely to occur when patients lie or sit on them continually.

Preventing Decubitus Ulcers or Bedsores

Preventing bedsores is the responsibility of the entire nursing team. These sores are usually the result of a lack of knowledge and skill in caring for the patient. Once even a mild bedsore has formed, it is very hard to cure. Therefore, as a nursing assistant, you have to know how to prevent bedsores and how to recognize them when they do occur. Report the first sign of a bedsore to your immediate supervisor so that steps can be taken to **prevent** further damage.

Prevent
To keep from happening.

Special Devices and Equipment and the Use of Pillows

The doctor may order special equipment to reduce the pressure on the skin. One way is to use an air cushion or a sponge rubber cushion under

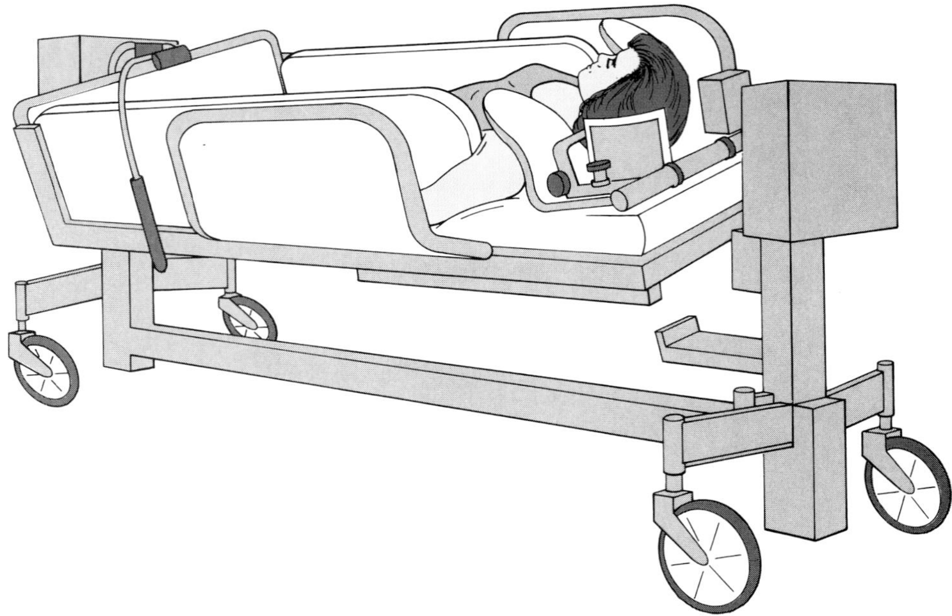

FIGURE 20-3 Specialty bed.

the base of the spine, sacrum, or lower back. If you do use an air cushion, do not fill it more than half full.

There are special devices that can be used to reduce the pressure on the heels, the elbows, and the back of the head, such as sheepskin booties and sheepskin elbow pads. Also used are pillows, pads, air mattresses, alternating pressure mattresses, flotation beds or pads, and commode flotation pads. The specialty bed (Figure 20-3), which constantly turns the patient, is an excellent device to minimize pressure points.

Obese
Very fat.

Obese patients tend to develop bedsores where body parts rub against each other, causing friction. Places to check on **obese** patients are the folds of the body where skin touches skin, such as under the breasts, between the folds of the buttocks, and between the thighs. Pillows are used to provide support and prevent skin breakdown.

Pressure Sore Prevention Devices

Device	Purpose	Precautions for Use
Eggcrate-type mattress Eggcrate-type wheelchair cushion 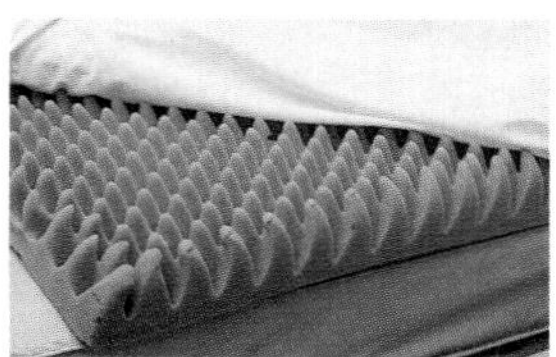	Provides cushioning and a slight redistribution of pressure, as well as some circulation of air beneath patient.	Not as effective for incontinent patients unless a very thin plastic sleeve covering is used to protect the mattress. The mattress will retain a urine odor unless protected. It is most effective when used with only one loosely applied sheet between the patient and the mattress.

(continued)

Device	Purpose	Precautions for Use
Water mattress	Redistributes the body weight during any movement. Conforms to body shape and weight.	Do not puncture. Must not be over- or underfilled.
Air mattress 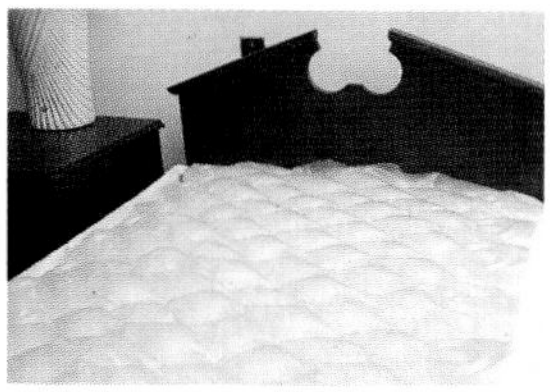	Redistributes pressure on a timed automatic basis.	Must be careful not to puncture. Be sure motor and mattress are working correctly. Use only one loosely applied sheet between the patient and the mattress.
Foam ring or "donut"	Eliminates or reduces pressure on area in center of ring only.	Tends to raise pressure on edge of ring and around opening.
Inflatable rubber or plastic ring 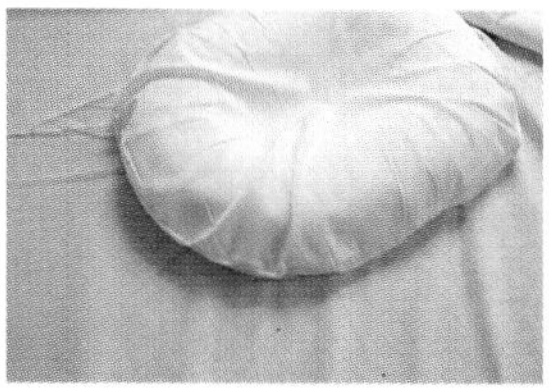	DO NOT USE. These devices increase pressure in the center of the ring and may actually cause pressure sores.	
Sheepskin pad 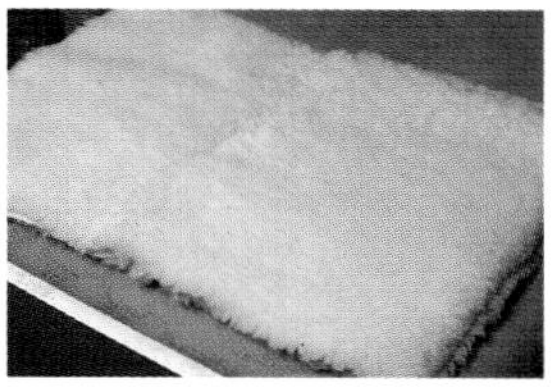	Reduces friction or rubbing against sheets.	Does not eliminate pressure.
Heel protector or elbow protector 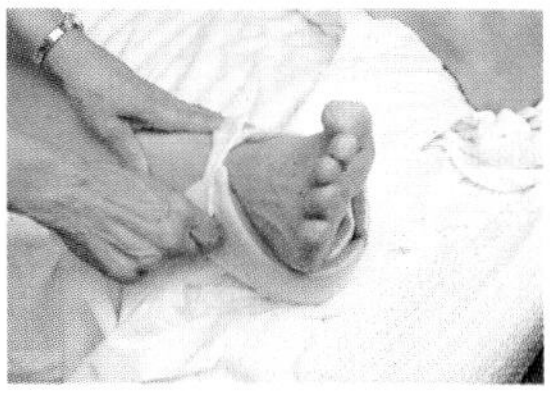	Cushions against trauma. Decreases friction on rubbing against bedlinens.	Must be removed for daily washing of feet and elbows and for inspection of the skin. Creates warm, moist environment favoring growth of bacteria.
Foot elevator 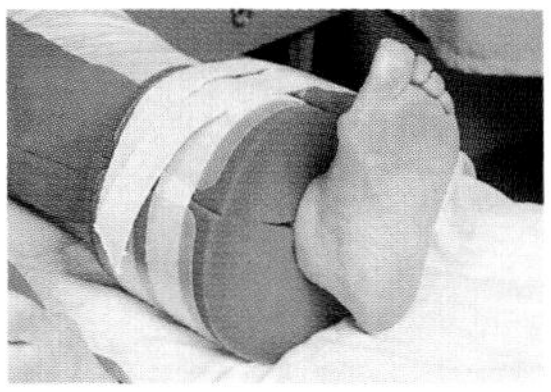	Reduces pressure on heels.	Must be properly applied. Check skin for rubbing.
Wheelchair cushion (solid)	Conforms to body when sitting. Provides comfort.	Place properly in chair. Cover with cloth.
Foot cradle	To keep bed coverings off legs and feet.	Be sure bed covering is off legs. Patient may feel cold, requiring extra blankets to provide additional warmth.

Rules to Follow
PREVENTING BEDSORES (DECUBITUS ULCERS)

You, the nursing assistant, can help to prevent bedsores by doing the following:

- Turn the patient often. You should change the patient's position every 2 hours.
- Be careful when using bedpans. Pressure from sitting on the rim and friction when putting the patient on and off the pan can create or worsen bedsores. Never leave the patient on the bedpan longer than necessary. Use care when removing the bedpan to avoid spilling urine on the skin. Urine could irritate and cause further damage to the reddened or tender area. Covering the bedpan with pads can reduce some pressure, and powdering the rim will minimize friction.
- Keep the patient's body as clean and dry as possible. Change the patient's gown if it is damp. Wash the patient's skin with mild soap to remove urine or feces. Use lotion on the skin to prevent contact with discharged materials from wounds, which can cause irritation.
- If a part of the patient's body shows signs of developing a decubitus, gently rub the area with skin lotion. This should be done every 2 hours. Rub with a circular motion, away from the affected part of the body, but not directly on the affected area as too much rubbing may break the skin. Rubbing, that is, friction, stimulates the circulation of blood in the affected area.
- Use powder or corn starch sparingly where skin surfaces come together and form creases. Examples are under the breasts of women patients, between the buttocks, and in the folds of skin on the abdomen. Corn starch helps keep these areas dry. When bathing the patient, be sure to wash the corn starch off completely. This is especially important in caring for obese patients.
- Keep linen wrinkle-free and dry at all times.
- Remove crumbs, hair pins, and any other hard objects from the bed promptly.
- If the patient is **incontinent** (unable to control urine or defecation), use a disposable bed protector. This allows the area that is soiled to be cleaned easily and often, and it protects the linen the patient has to lie on. Be sure that plastic never touches the patient's skin, and change the bed protector immediately when it becomes wet.

Incontinent:
Unable to control the bowels or bladder.

FIGURE 20-4 Use of the whirlpool bath is a special measure to prevent decubitus ulcers.

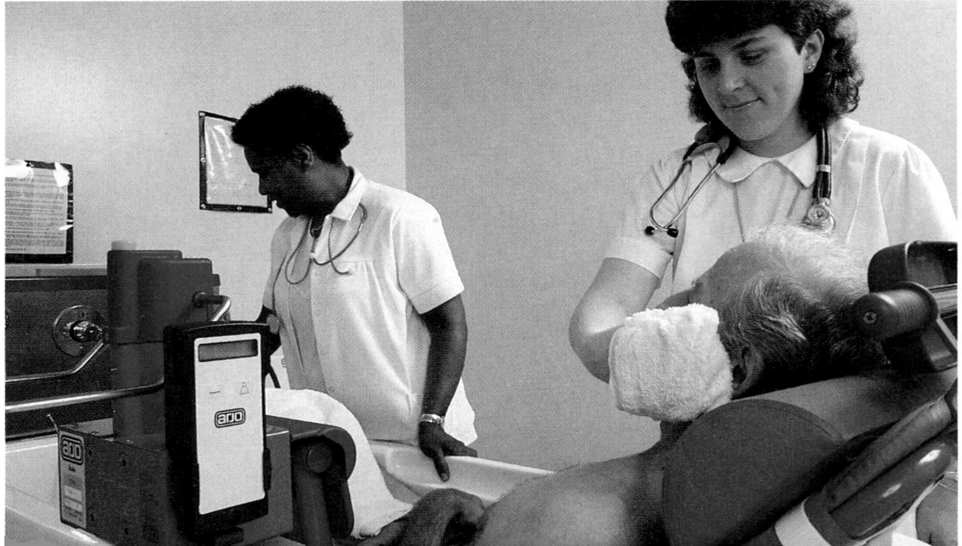

- In some institutions, a large disposable diaper is used for the incontinent patient. However, the skin underneath must be watched carefully for a reaction to the diaper material and to irritations caused by urine and feces touching the skin. The diaper prevents the urine and bowel movement from spreading to the entire body of the patient. However, it needs to be changed immediately when soiled or wet.
- If a pressure ulcer occurs, a protective dressing may be applied.
- In some institutions, a whirlpool bath may be used to prevent and/or treat pressure ulcers (Figure 20-4).
- In some institutions ointments are used to protect the skin of incontinent patients. Follow the instructions of your immediate supervisor.

Procedure Preventing Decubitus Ulcers (Bedsores) in the Incontinent Patient

1. Assemble your equipment:
   a) Basin of water at 115°F (46.1°C)
   b) Soap
   c) Corn starch or powder
   d) Towels
   e) Disposable gloves
   f) Lotion
   g) Washcloths
   h) Bedpan
2. Wash your hands.
3. Identify the patient by checking the identification bracelet.
4. Ask visitors to step out of the room, if this is your hospital's policy.
5. Tell the patient that you are going to wash him.
6. Pull the curtain for privacy.
7. Raise the bed to a comfortable working position.
8. Raise the side rail on the far side of the bed.
9. Put on the disposable gloves.
10. Using the toilet tissue, wipe away as much feces as possible; then wash the area that has urine or feces on it very well, removing all waste material from the skin. Place soiled tissue into the bedpan.
11. Rinse with water, changing the water frequently.
12. Dry with a circular motion to stimulate blood circulation.
13. Apply lotion to the buttocks and back, massaging to stimulate blood circulation.
14. Wipe off any excess lotion.
15. Apply corn starch or powder only where skin surfaces touch other skin surfaces (creases). Dust lightly, not allowing any to cake together.
16. Leave the top sheets loose so air can get to every part of the patient's body.
17. Turn the patient to a different position every 2 hours.
18. Keep the patient dry at all times by checking the patient every 2 hours. Remake the bed as necessary.
19. Make the patient comfortable.
20. Lower the bed to a position of safety for the patient.
21. Pull the curtains back to the open position.
22. Raise the side rails where ordered, indicated, and appropriate for patient safety.
23. Place the call light within easy reach of the patient.
24. Discard disposable equipment.
25. Place dirty soiled linen in the laundry bag, and then place the bag into the dirty linen hamper in the utility room.
26. Remove and discard gloves.
27. Wash your hands.
28. Report to your immediate supervisor:
    - That the patient is incontinent of urine and/or feces
    - That the patient was washed and his or her skin is now clean and dry
    - That the patient's position was

changed every 2 hours and the time of each position change

- Any signs of decubitus ulcers
- The color, amount, and consistency of the feces and urine you cleaned
- How the patient tolerated the procedure
- Your observations of anything unusual

Procedure Special Back Care (Back Rub) to Prevent Decubitus Ulcers

1. Assemble your equipment (Figure 20-5):
   a) Towels
   b) Lotion, standing in a basin of warm water 115°F (46.1°C)

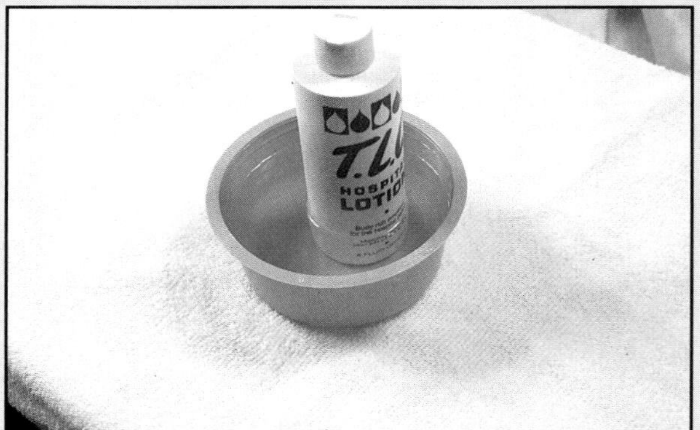

FIGURE 20-5

2. Wash your hands.
3. Identify the patient by checking the identification bracelet.
4. Ask visitors to step out of the room, if this is your hospital's policy.
5. Tell the patient that you are going to give him a back rub (Figure 20-6).

FIGURE 20-6

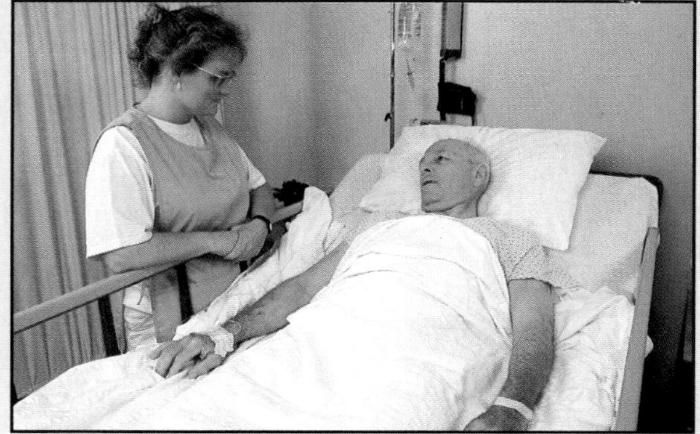

6. Pull the curtain for privacy.
7. Raise the bed to a comfortable working position.
8. Ask the patient to turn on his side so that his back is toward you or have him turn on his abdomen. If he is unable to turn, turn him into whichever of these two positions is most comfortable for the patient and yourself.
9. The side rail should be in the up position on the far side of the bed.
10. Lotion should be warmed by placing the container in a basin of warm water 115°F (46.1°C).
11. Open the ties on the gown. Put a towel lengthwise on the mattress close to the patient's back.
12. Pour a small amount of lotion into the palm of your hand (Figure 20-7).

FIGURE 20-7

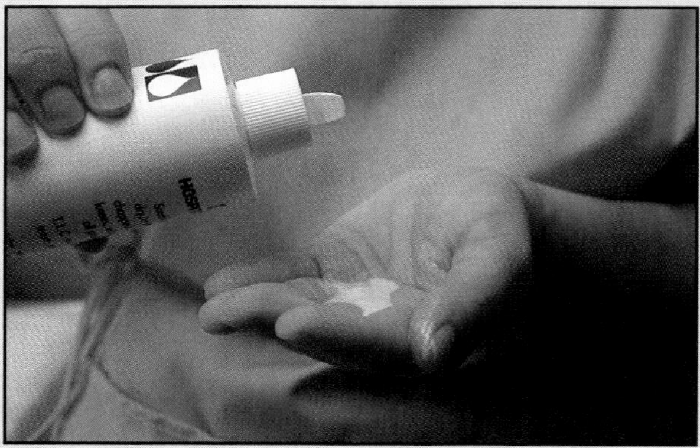

13. Rub your hands together to warm the lotion using friction (Figure 20-8).
14. Apply lotion to the entire back with the palms of your hands. Use long, firm strokes from the buttocks to the shoulders and back of the neck (Figure 20-9).

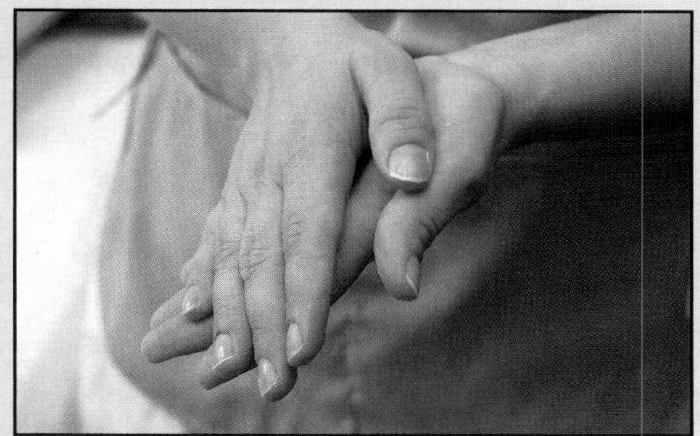

FIGURE 20-8

FIGURE 20-9

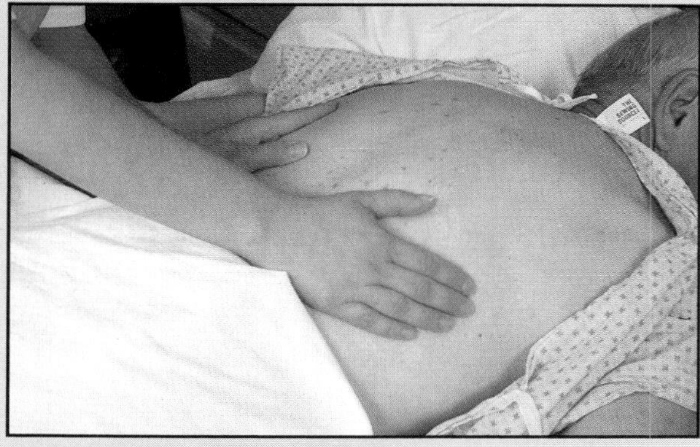

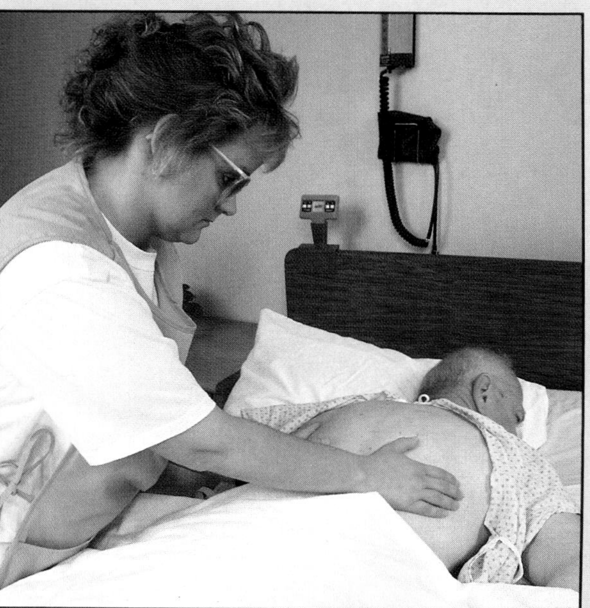

FIGURE 20-10

15. Keep your knees slightly bent and your back straight.
16. Exert firm pressure as you stroke upward from the buttocks to the shoulders. Use gentle pressure as you stroke downward from shoulders to buttocks.
17. Use a circular motion on each bony area (Figure 20-10).
18. This rhythmic rubbing motion should be continued for 1½ to 3 minutes.
19. Dry the patient's back by patting gently with a towel.
20. Close and retie the gown.
21. Remove the towels.
22. Assist the patient to turn back to a comfortable position.
23. Arrange the top sheets of the bed neatly.
24. Lower the bed to a position of safety for the patient.
25. Pull the curtains back to the open position.
26. Raise the side rails where ordered, indicated, and appropriate for patient safety.
27. Place the call light within easy reach of the patient.
28. Put your equipment back in its proper place.
29. Wash your hands.
30. Report to your immediate supervisor:
    - That you have given the patient back care
    - The time the care was given
    - The number of times this care was given on your shift (this is done if the special back care is ordered every 2 hours)
    - Your observations of anything unusual

KEY QUESTIONS

1. What are the causes of bedsores?
2. What are the signs of bedsores?

3. What should you do when caring for the patient's skin to help prevent bedsores?
4. What are the most important things to do for the incontinent patient so that his skin will not develop bedsores?
5. How should special backcare be provided?
6. Define: decubitus ulcers, incontinent, obese, prevent, prominences.

CHAPTER 21

Anatomy and Physiology of the Circulatory and Respiratory Systems

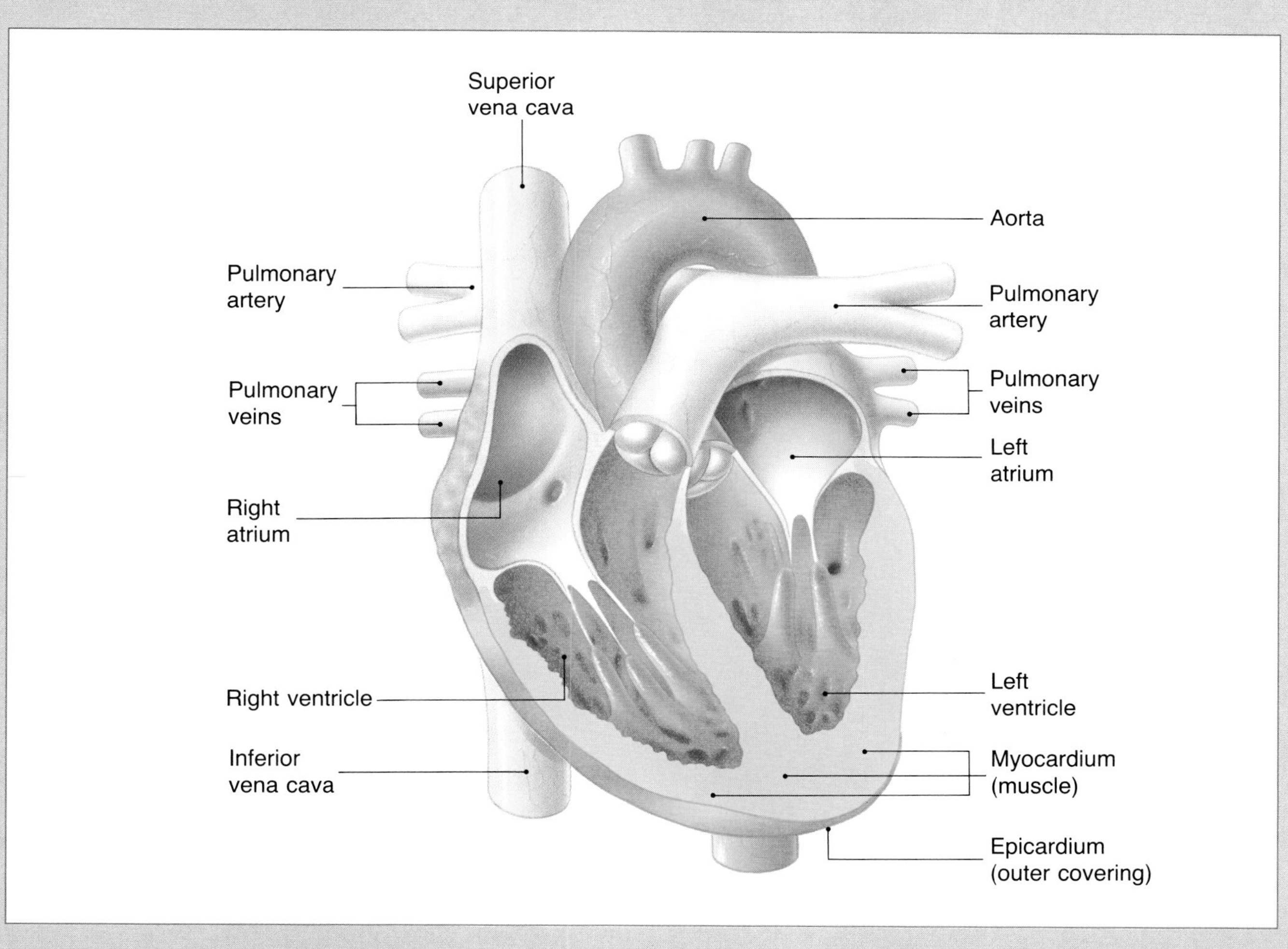

WARNING

For all patient contact, adhere to Universal Precautions (see page 91, 97, or the front cover flap). Wear protective equipment as indicated.

Objectives

What You Will Learn

When you have completed this chapter, you will be able to:

- Describe the functions of blood.
- Compare and contrast pulmonary circulation, systemic circulation, and coronary circulation.
- Label a diagram with the organs of the circulatory and respiratory systems.
- Describe the functions of the respiratory system.
- List common diseases and disorders of the respiratory and circulatory systems.
- Explain vital signs.
- State the average adult normal rates for temperature, pulse, and respiration.
- Define: artery, blood pressure, cardiac, circulation, circulatory system, heart, pulmonary, pulse, respiration, respiratory system, temperature, vein, vital signs.

KEY IDEAS

The Circulatory System

Circulatory System
The heart, blood vessel, blood, and all the organs that pump and carry blood and other fluids throughout the body.

Heart
A four-chambered, hollow, muscular organ that lies in the chest cavity, pointing slightly to the left. It is the pump that circulates the blood through the lungs and into all parts of the body.

THE CIRCULATORY SYSTEM IS MADE UP of the blood, the heart, and the blood vessels (arteries, veins, and capillaries). The heart actually acts as a pump for the blood, which carries the nutrients, oxygen, and other elements needed by the cells. Important facts to know about the blood include:

- The blood carries oxygen from the lungs to the cells.
- Carbon dioxide is carried by the blood from the cells to the lungs.
- Nutrients (food) are picked up (absorbed) by the blood from the duodenum (small intestine) and brought to the cells.
- Waste products from the cells are carried by the blood to the kidneys to be eliminated in urine.
- The hormones from the endocrine glands are transported by the blood.
- Dilation (enlargement) and contraction (narrowing) of the blood vessels help regulate body temperatures.
- The blood helps maintain the fluid balance of the body.
- The white cells of the blood defend the body against disease.

The **heart** (Figure 21-1) is made up of four chambers: two atria and two ventricles. The atria are the two smaller chambers. The right ven-

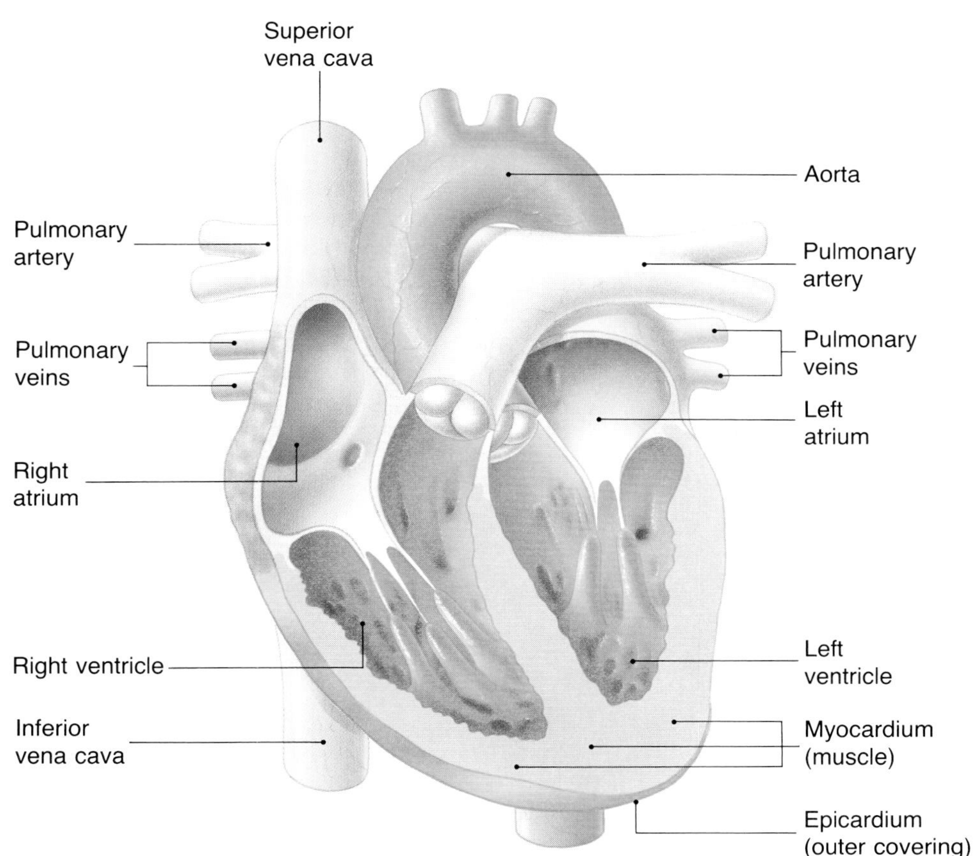

FIGURE 21-1 The heart.

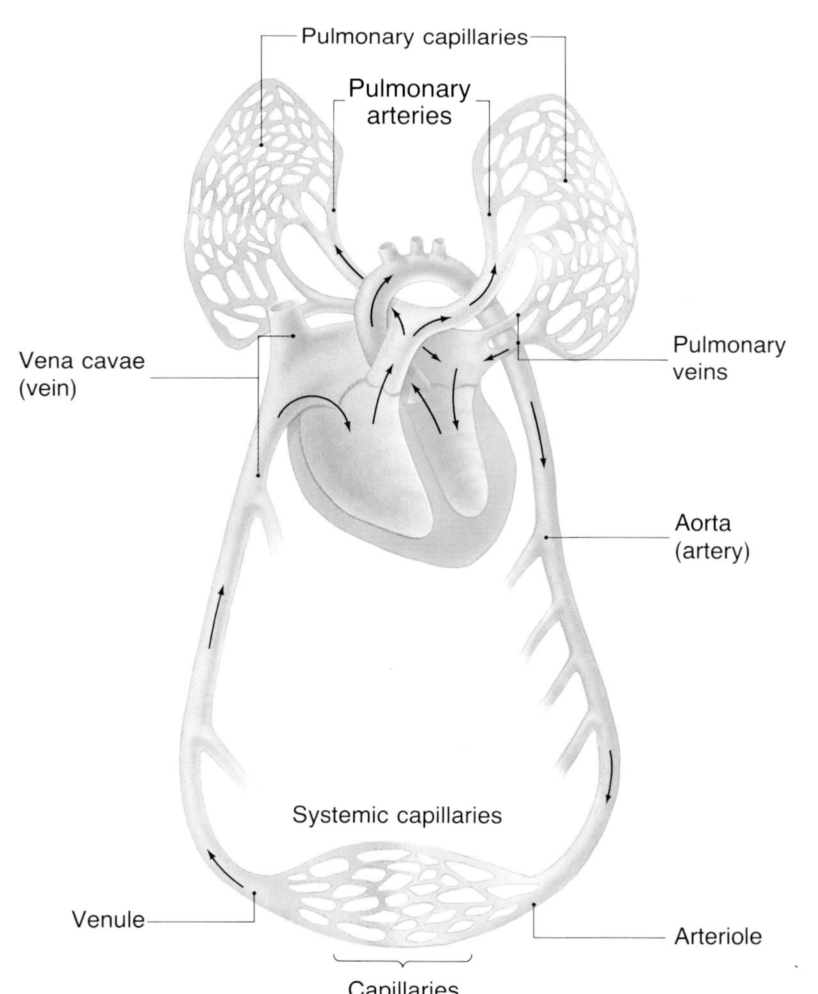

FIGURE 21-2 The circulatory system.

Pulmonary
Refers to the lungs.

Circulation
The continuous movement of blood through the heart and blood vessels to all parts of the body.

Artery
A blood vessel that carries blood away from the heart.

tricle sends the blood only as far as the lungs. Here, in the **pulmonary** circulation (circulation that begins in the heart), the blood picks up oxygen and gets rid of carbon dioxide. This blood then returns to the heart, carrying its load of oxygen, which is pushed into systemic **circulation** by the left ventricle.

The ventricles have thick walls of muscle. When they contract, the left ventricle pushes the blood through the largest blood vessel, the aorta, to all parts of the body. The blood vessels that carry oxygenated (having a lot of oxygen) blood are called **arteries**. The only exception is the pulmonary artery, which carries the blood to the lungs. Arteries branch into a vast network throughout the body (Figure 21-2). As they branch, the blood vessels become smaller and smaller until finally they are so

FIGURE 21-3 The system of arteries.

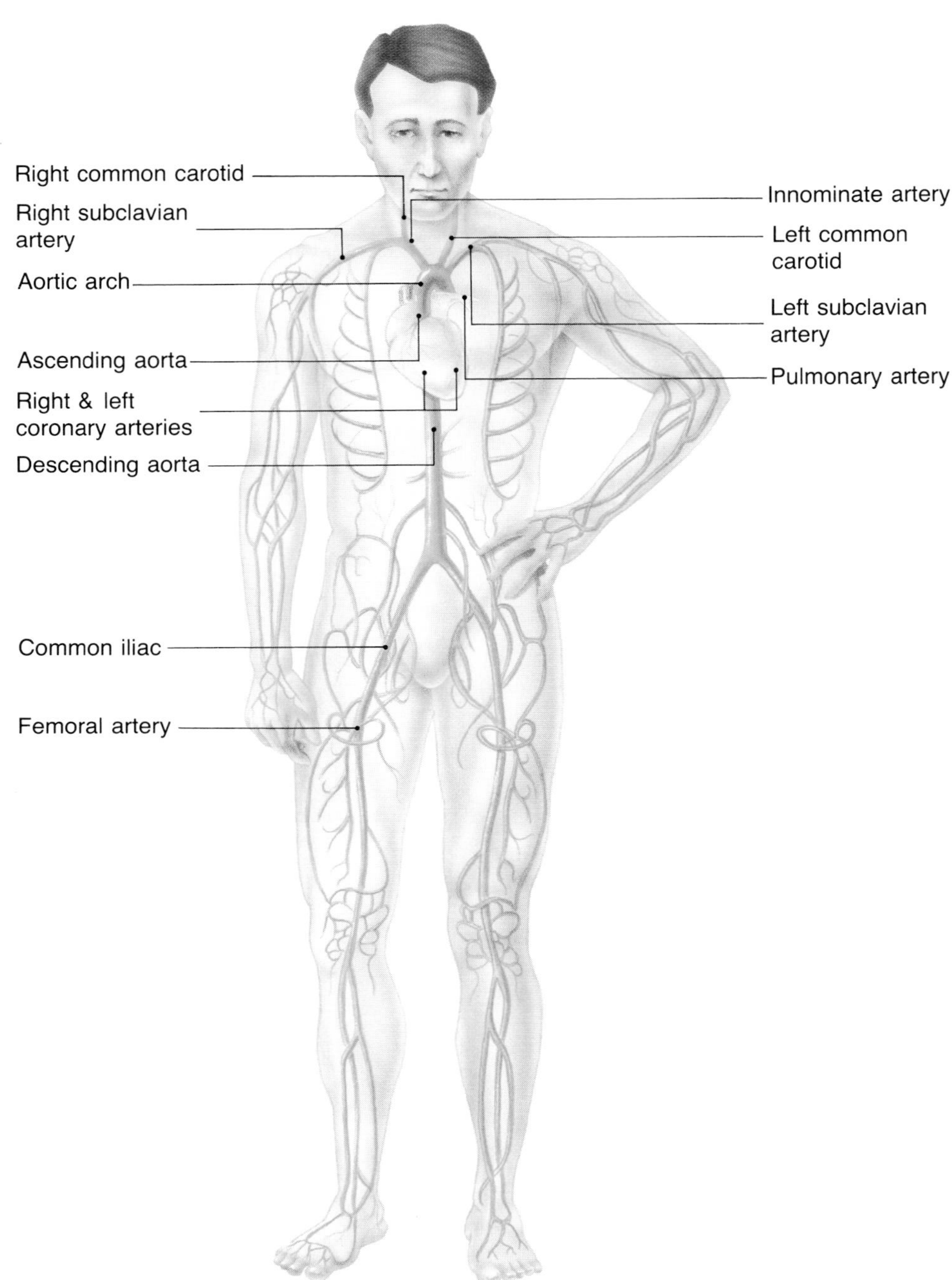

thin they become capillaries. The walls of the capillaries are only one cell-layer thick. Through these walls, gases, nutrients, waste products, and other substances are exchanged among the blood in the capillaries, the tissue fluid, and the individual cell. After the blood has given up its oxygen, which is carried on the surface of the red blood cells, it is returned to the heart through the **veins**. Other important points are:

Vein
A blood vessel that carries blood from parts of the body back to the heart.

- All arteries carry blood away from the heart (Figure 21-3).
- All veins carry blood back to the heart (Figure 21-4).
- All arteries carry oxygenated blood except the pulmonary artery.
- All veins carry deoxygenated blood except the four pulmonary veins.

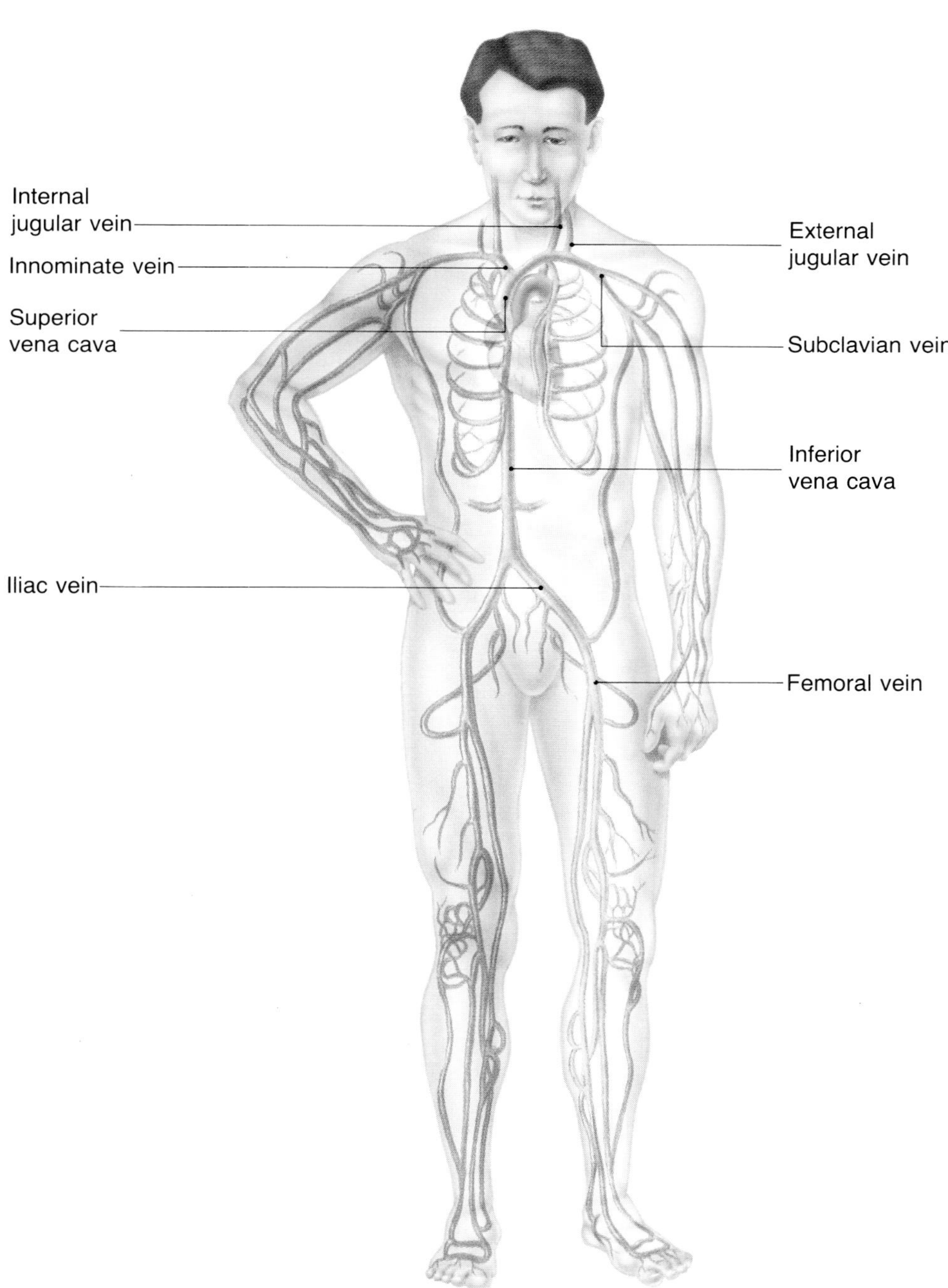

FIGURE 21-4 The system of veins.

It is necessary that the heart muscle be supplied with blood-carrying oxygen. The first branches of the aorta, the coronary arteries, come from the heart's left ventricle. These arteries surround the heart and carry needed oxygen to **cardiac** (heart muscle) tissue. If one of these coronary branches is blocked by a blood clot *(embolism)*, the patient has a heart attack, which can result in the death of some heart tissue. The event is called a *myocardial infarction* (MI).

Cardiac
Pertaining to the heart.

The liquid portion of the blood is called *plasma*. The cells are red blood cells, which carry oxygen, and white blood cells, which fight infection. If a patient has an inflammation in some area of the body, a physician often prescribes warm, moist compresses. These are applied to dilate (widen) the blood vessels in the area and to bring more of the important white blood cells to the place of infection to help fight it. People who have too few red blood cells have some type of *anemia*. People who have too few white blood cells have a lowered resistance to disease. An increase in white blood cells in the blood can mean that an infection is present somewhere in the body.

A patient's blood circulation tends to slow down when she or he is inactive. Sometimes this can cause clotting of the blood. A blood clot is dangerous and can cause a life-threatening situation.

If you have orders to help a patient out of bed for the first time after an illness or after surgery, remember that his or her circulation is slower. Therefore, be sure the patient moves carefully and slowly. Allow the patient to sit at the edge of the bed and dangle his or her legs until the circulation stabilizes (that is, comes back to normal). Then assist the patient carefully to a standing position. Sometimes this procedure will cause the blood to leave the brain suddenly, and the patient may be dizzy or feel faint.

The circulatory system is responsible for getting all the necessary ingredients to a cell for its metabolism and for carrying away its products and waste material. The circulatory system works in close harmony with the respiratory system.

Common Diseases and Disorders of the Circulatory System

- *Arteriosclerosis:* Hardening of the arteries.
- *Angina pectoris:* Pain resulting from insufficient blood flow to the heart muscle.
- *Myocardial infarction (MI):* Obstruction of a blood vessel in the heart muscle, which results in heart tissue death due to lack of oxygen.
- *Endocarditis:* Inflammation of the inner lining of the heart.
- *Rheumatic heart disease:* Damage due to rheumatic fever.
- *Congestive heart failure:* The heart is unable to pump enough blood.
- *Hypertension:* Elevation of the arterial blood pressure.
- *Leukemia:* Cancer of the blood.
- *Anemia:* Decrease in the quantity and quality of red blood cells.
- *Cerebral vascular accident (CVA):* A stroke caused by blockage or rupturing of arteries in the brain.

KEY IDEAS

The Respiratory System

The **respiratory system** (Figure 21-5) provides a route or pathway for oxygen to get from the air into the lungs, where it can be picked up by the blood. The organs that make up this system include the nose and mouth, pharynx (throat), trachea (windpipe), larynx (voicebox), bronchi, and lungs. Because we must have oxygen to live, it is necessary to

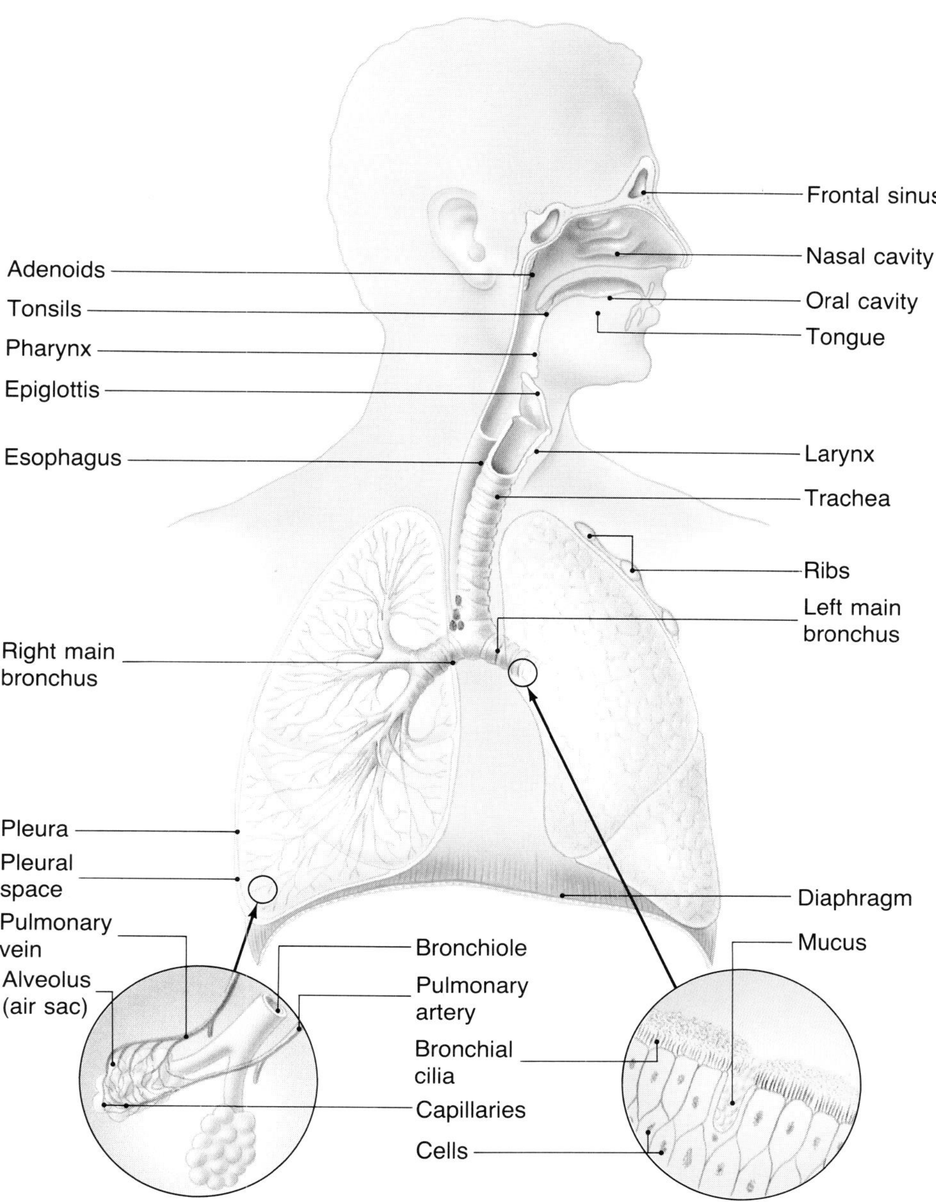

FIGURE 21-5 The respiratory system.

Respiratory System
The group of body organs that carries on the body function of respiration. The system brings oxygen into the body and eliminates carbon dioxide.

keep this pathway open. The structures themselves help to do this. The trachea and bronchi are kept open by incomplete cartilage rings.

On the top of the trachea, opening from the pharynx (the throat), is a structure known as the larynx. In addition to being the opening to the trachea, it also contains the vocal cords, which make it possible for us to talk. An important piece of cartilage, the epiglottis, covers the opening to the trachea when food is swallowed, preventing the food from going into the lungs. A very weak patient or one who is having trouble breathing must be watched carefully during feeding so that food does not get into the trachea. This is known as *aspiration* of food. An unconscious patient who vomits may also be in danger of aspirating that material. Turn the patient's head to one side at once. You must watch the patient with great care, because if the pathway for oxygen is blocked, the patient will not live without immediate treatment.

As in our other systems, the important work of the respiratory system is done at the level of the cell. The exchange of oxygen and carbon dioxide occurs in an area of the lungs that is so small you must use a microscope to see it. The last branch of the bronchus is called the alveolar duct. At its end is a small sac, the alveolus. Many oxygen molecules fill this sac after you breathe in air. The blood has less oxygen and therefore is able to pick up a large amount of oxygen from the alveolar sac. The blood is then returned to the heart to be sent around the body, beginning in the largest artery, the aorta.

The respiratory system, then, is responsible for getting oxygen to the blood. Internal respiration occurs when those cells that need the oxygen receive it in exchange for carbon dioxide, which is the cells' gas waste product. Both functions are equally important.

Breathing is regulated by a center in the medulla, a part of the brain. Often, especially after surgery, a patient must be encouraged to breathe deeply in order to keep all the air sacs open and inflated. Sometimes you will be asked to help the patient cough, especially if there is inflammation of the lung tissue. Placing one of your hands gently under the diaphragm and the other on the patient's back will assist the muscles of respiration. In many of the larger health care institutions the Pulmonary Medicine Department (Respiratory Therapy) will, by a doctor's order, institute a treatment that will force the patient to breathe deeply and cough. An incentive spirometer is used in most hospitals postoperatively.

Common Diseases and Disorders of the Respiratory System

- *Infection of the upper respiratory tract:* The common cold.
- *Sinusitis:* Inflammation of the sinuses.
- *Pharyngitis:* Inflammation of the throat.
- *Cancer of the larynx* (voice box).
- *Pneumonia:* Infection of the lung.
- *Lung cancer.*
- *Chest injuries:* Trauma.
- *Tuberculosis:* Caused by a microorganism that is easily transmitted from one person to another.
- *Chronic obstructive pulmonary disease* (COPD):
  - *Bronchitis:* Inflammation of the bronchi.
  - *Emphysema:* Obstruction of airflow in the lungs.
  - *Asthma:* Allergy with wheezing and dyspnea (difficulty breathing).

KEY IDEAS

Vital Signs

Vital Signs
Temperature, pulse, respiration, and blood pressure.

Temperature
A measurement of the amount of heat in the body at a given time. The normal body temperature is 98.6°F (37°C).

WHEN THE BODY IS NOT FUNCTIONING normally, changes happen in the measurable rates of the **vital signs**. Everyone who is measuring and recording information about patients' vital signs must be accurate. When you record the readings, write carefully. Make sure your handwriting is legible, clear, and easy to read. If you are not sure of your reading or if the readings seem unusual, tell your immediate supervisor. Common abbreviations for the vital signs are:

- Temperature = T
- Pulse = P
- Respiration = R
- Blood pressure = BP
- Vital signs (VSs) = TPR and BP

Pulse
The rhythmic expansion and contraction of the arteries caused by the beating of the heart. The expansion and contraction show how fast, how regular, and with what force the heart is beating.

Respiration
The body process of breathing; inhaling and exhaling air.

Blood Pressure
How much effort the heart is exerting to circulate the blood.

When your immediate supervisor says:

- "Take temps," she or he means measure the patient's temperature, pulse, and respiration.
- "Take vital signs," she or he means measure the patient's temperature, pulse, respiration, and blood pressure.
- "Take blood pressure," she or he means measure the patient's blood pressure, pulse, and respiration.

Write down the numbers for the patient's temperature, pulse, respiration, and blood pressure right away on the form indicated for that purpose, often called the "vital sign sheet." The columns have certain hours of the day written at the top, for example, 8 A.M. or 12 noon. Check the patient's name. Be sure you are writing the vital signs at the right time. Report to your immediate supervisor any time the patient's temperature, pulse, respiration, or blood pressure are not within normal limits, as listed below.

Average Normal Adult Rates

- Temperature: 98.6°F or 37°C
- Pulse: 72 to 80 beats per minute
- Respiration: 16 to 20 per minute

KEY QUESTIONS

1. What are the functions of the blood?
2. What are the differences between pulmonary circulation, systemic circulation, and coronary circulation?
3. Which organs make up the circulatory system? The respiratory system?
4. What are the functions of the respiratory system?
5. What are the common diseases and disorders of the respiratory and circulatory systems?
6. What are the four vital signs? Explain what each means.
7. What are the average adult normal rates for temperature, pulse, and respiration?
8. Define: artery, blood pressure, cardiac, circulation, circulatory system, heart, pulmonary, pulse, respiration, respiratory system, temperature, vein, vital signs.

CHAPTER

22

Measuring the Temperature

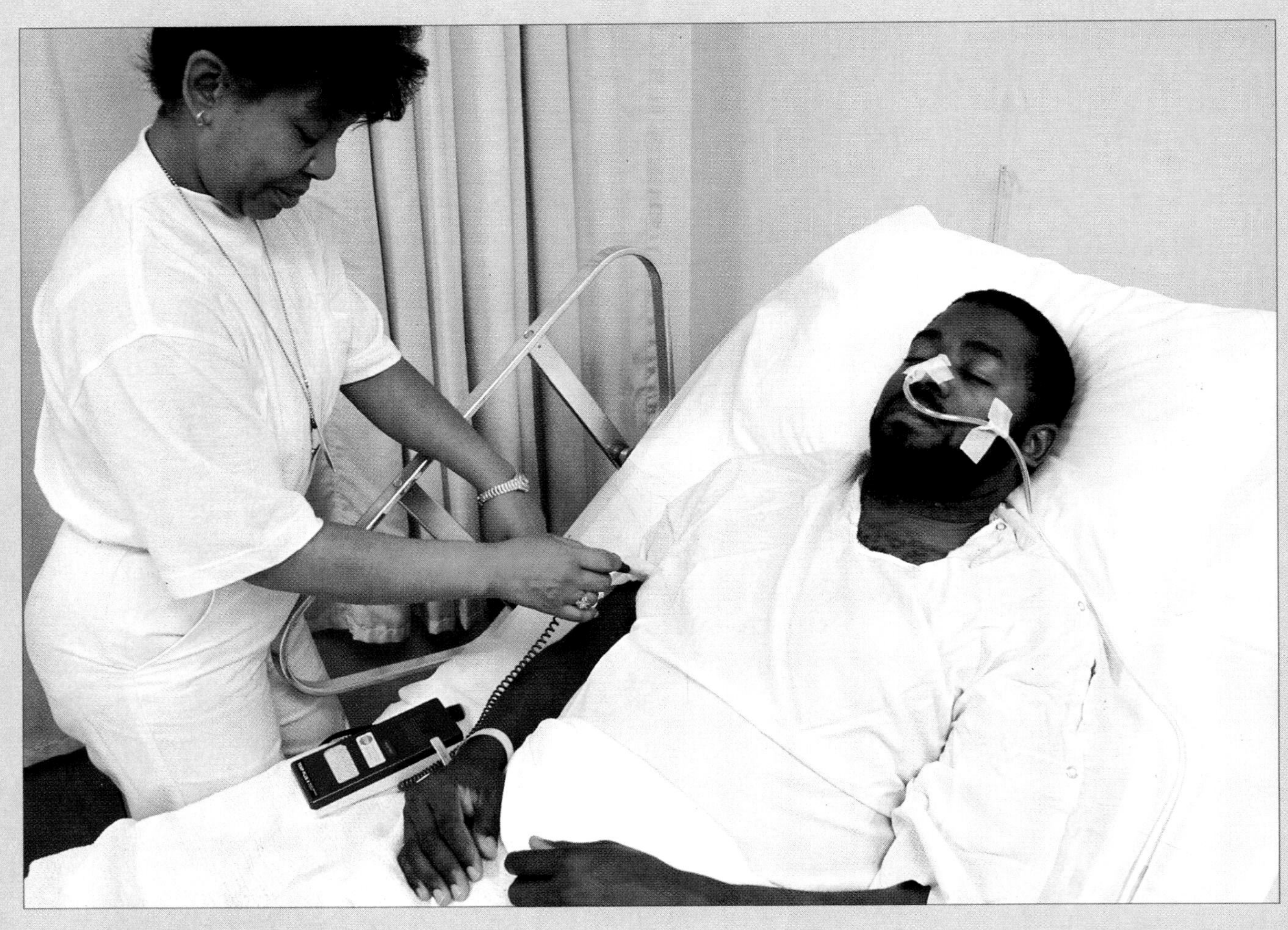

WARNING

For all patient contact, adhere to Universal Precautions (see page 91, 97, or the front cover flap). Wear protective equipment as indicated.

Objectives

What You Will Learn

When you have completed this chapter, you will be able to:

- List and describe the different types of thermometers.
- Read a Fahrenheit and centigrade (Celsius) thermometer accurately.
- Demonstrate the procedure for measuring oral temperatures.
- Demonstrate the procedure for measuring rectal temperatures.
- Demonstrate the procedure for measuring axillary temperatures.
- Demonstrate the proper use of a battery-operated electronic thermometer.
- Define: axillary, centigrade, Fahrenheit, oral, rectal, thermometer.

KEY IDEAS

Body Temperature

Body temperature is a measurement of the amount of heat in the body. The body creates heat in the process of changing food to energy. The body can also lose heat through perspiration, respiration (breathing), and excretion. The balance between the heat produced and the heat lost is the body temperature. The normal adult body temperature is 98.6° **Fahrenheit** or 37° **centigrade** (Celsius). There is a normal range in which a person's body temperature may vary and still be considered normal.

Centigrade
A system for measurement of temperature using a scale divided into 100 units or degrees. In this system, the freezing temperature of water is 0°C and water boils at 100°C. Often referred to as Celsius.

Fahrenheit
A system for measuring temperature. In the Fahrenheit system, the temperature of water at boiling is 212°. At freezing, it is 32°. These temperatures are usually written 212°F and 32°F.

Thermometer
An instrument used for measuring temperature.

Oral
Anything to do with the mouth; examples are eating and speaking.

Rectal
Pertaining to the rectum.

Axillary
The area under the arms; the armpits.

Types of Thermometers

The body temperature is measured with an instrument called a **thermometer**. There are several different types of thermometers.

- *Glass thermometer:* This is a delicate, hollow glass tube with a liquid metal called mercury sealed inside it, an element that is very sensitive to temperature. Mercury expands (gets larger) when the temperature goes up and contracts (gets smaller) when the temperature goes down. Even if the temperature rises only slightly, the mercury will expand and travel up the tube, reflecting the change. The outside of the glass thermometer is marked with lines, or calibrations, and numbers. These markings help us measure exactly the temperature readings displayed by the level of the mercury. There are three types of glass thermometers (Figure 22-1):
  - *Oral:* used to measure the patient's temperature by mouth and also the *axillary* (armpit) temperature.
  - *Rectal:* used to measure temperature by inserting the thermometer into the patient's rectum.
  - *Security:* used for taking an infant's rectal temperature. Many institutions use the security or stubby type with a red knob at the

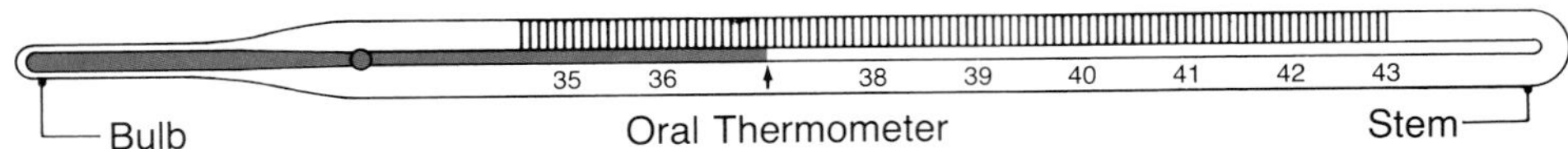

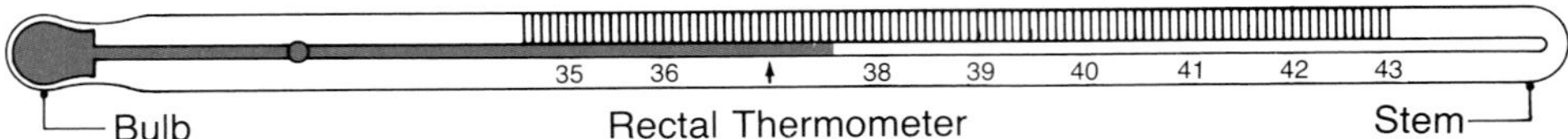

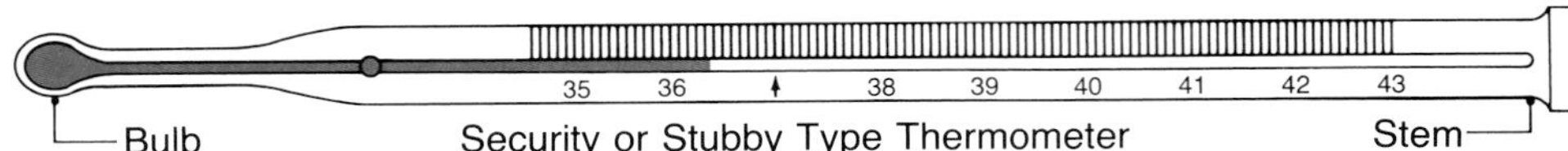

FIGURE 22-1 Types of glass thermometers.

stem for rectal temperatures and with a green or blue knob at the stem for oral temperatures. Follow your institution's policy.

- *Battery-operated electronic thermometers* (Figure 22-2): This type of thermometer eliminates human error and variation that occur in reading a glass thermometer. Electronic thermometers have both a blue (oral) and red (rectal) attachment called a *probe.* A disposable plastic cover (sheath) is used over the probe for each patient.
- *Chemically treated paper or plastic thermometers:* Some health care institutions use plastic or chemically treated single-use paper thermometers that change color to indicate the patient's temperature.
- *The latest electronic thermometers* instantly calculate the body temperature when a sheath-covered probe is inserted into the opening of the outer ear canal. This type of thermometer is available for industrial and home use.

FIGURE 22-2 Battery-operated electronic thermometer.

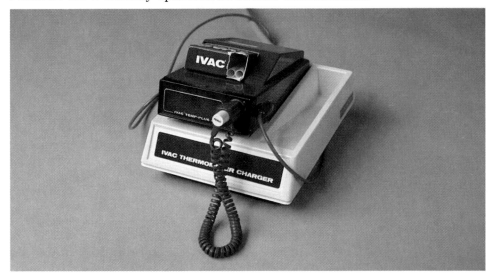

Rules to Follow

CARE OF GLASS THERMOMETERS

- Because glass thermometers break and shatter easily, we must handle them with care. Be especially careful to avoid breaking a thermometer while it is in a patient's mouth or rectum.
- The liquid metal, mercury, inside the thermometer is a poison; that is, it may be harmful if it is ingested (taken into the body by mouth) or if it has contact with the skin for a prolonged period of time.
- Check the containers in which the thermometers are kept. Follow your instructions for cleaning these containers.
- Never clean a glass thermometer with hot water as it will cause the mercury to expand so much that the thermometer will break.

Procedure Shaking Down the Glass Thermometer

1. Assemble your equipment on the bedside table:
   a) Thermometer in container
2. Wash your hands.
3. Before using the thermometer, check to make sure that it is not cracked or that the bulb is not chipped.
4. Hold the thermometer firmly between your fingers and your thumb at the stem and farthest from the bulb. The bulb is the end that is inserted into the patient's body. Never touch the bulb end of the thermometer.
5. Stand clear of any hard surfaces such as counters and tables to avoid striking and breaking the thermometer while you are shaking it. For practice, you might stand with your arm over a pillow or mattress in case you accidentally drop the thermometer.
6. When you are sure that you have a good hold on the thermometer, shake your hand loosely from the wrist. Do it as if you were shaking water from your fingers (Figure 22-3).
7. Snap your wrist again and again. This will shake down the mercury to the lowest possible point. This should be below the numbers and lines (calibrations).
8. Always do this before and after using a thermometer.

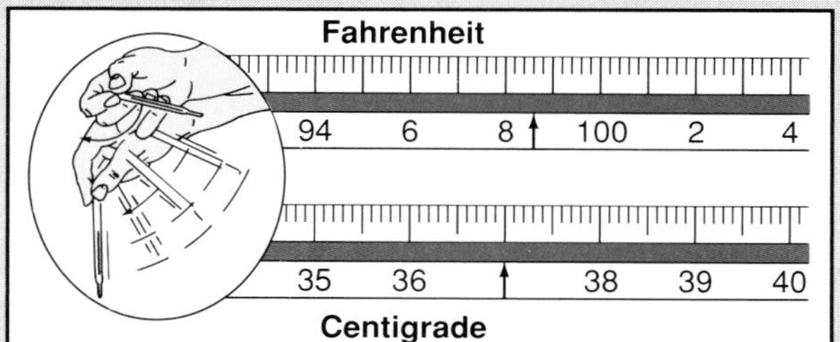

FIGURE 22-3 Method for shaking down the mercury in a thermometer. Shake the mercury down to the lowest point below the numbers and lines.

Procedure Reading a Fahrenheit Thermometer

1. With your thumb and first two fingers, hold the thermometer at the stem. Never touch the bulb end.
2. Hold the thermometer at eye level. Turn the thermometer back and forth between your fingers until you can clearly see the column of mercury.
3. Notice the scale or calibrations. Each long line stands for 1 degree.
4. There are 4 short lines between each of the long lines. Each short line stands for two-tenths (or 0.2) of a degree.
5. Between the long lines that represent 98° and 99°, look for a longer line with an ar-

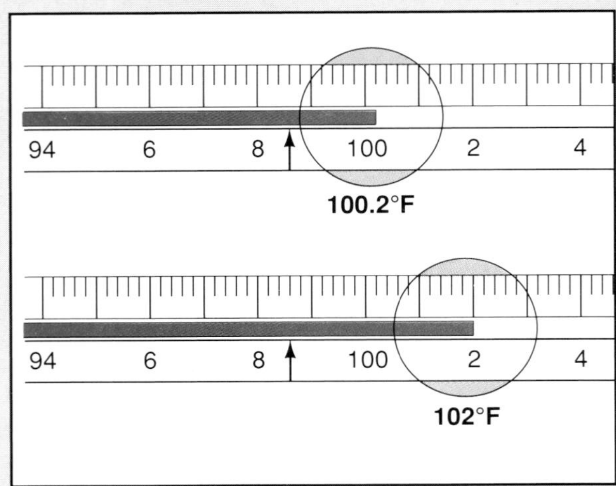

FIGURE 22-4 A Fahrenheit thermometer. Accuracy is extremely important. Look at the mercury carefully when reading a thermometer.

row directly beneath it. This special line points out normal body temperature.

6. Look at the end of the mercury. Notice the first line or number where the mercury ends (Figure 22-4). If it is one of the short lines, notice the previous longer line toward the silver tip that goes into the patient's mouth. The temperature reading is the degree marked by that long line plus 2, 4, 6, or 8 tenths of a degree. For example, if the mercury ends after the 99 line, but on the second short line, the temperature is 99.4°F. If the mercury ends between the two lines, take the line it is closer to:
7. Write down the patient's temperature right away. If you are using a TPR book, check to find the right column next to the patient's name and the right time of day. Write the patient's temperature using the figure you read on the thermometer. Some institutions will write 99.4°F. Others will write $99^{\underline{4}}$. Follow the method used in your institution.

Procedure Reading a Centigrade (Celsius) Thermometer

1. With your thumb and first two fingers, hold the thermometer at the stem.
2. Hold the thermometer at eye level. Turn the thermometer back and forth between your fingers until you can clearly see the column of mercury.
3. Notice the scale or calibrations. Each long line shows one degree.
4. There are 9 short lines between each number. These short lines are 1, 2, 3, 4, 5, 6, 7, 8, and 9 tenths of a degree. If the mercury ended after the 36 and on the third short line, the temperature would read 36.3°C (Figure 22-5). If the mercury ended after the long line 37 and on the eighth short line, the temperature would read 37.8°C. If the mercury ends after line 37 on the fifth short line, the temperature would be referred to as 37.5°C.
5. Write down the patient's temperature right away. If you are using a TPR book, check to find the right column next to the patient's name and the right time of day.

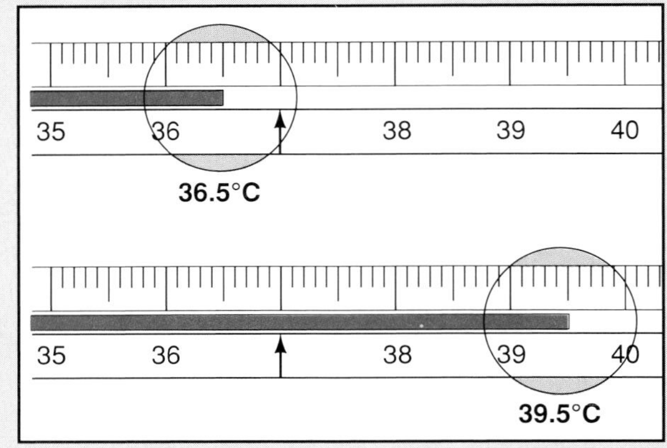

FIGURE 22-5 A centigrade (Celsius) thermometer. Accuracy is extremely important. Look at the mercury carefully when reading a thermometer.

Write the patient's temperature using the figure you read on the thermometer. Some hospitals write 37°C. Others will write 37. Follow the method used in your hospital.

KEY IDEAS

Recording the Patient's Temperature

For recording the patient's temperature, three symbols are used:

° = degrees
F = Fahrenheit
C = centigrade or Celsius

You will record the patient's temperatures according to the method used in your institution (Figures 22-6 and 22-7).

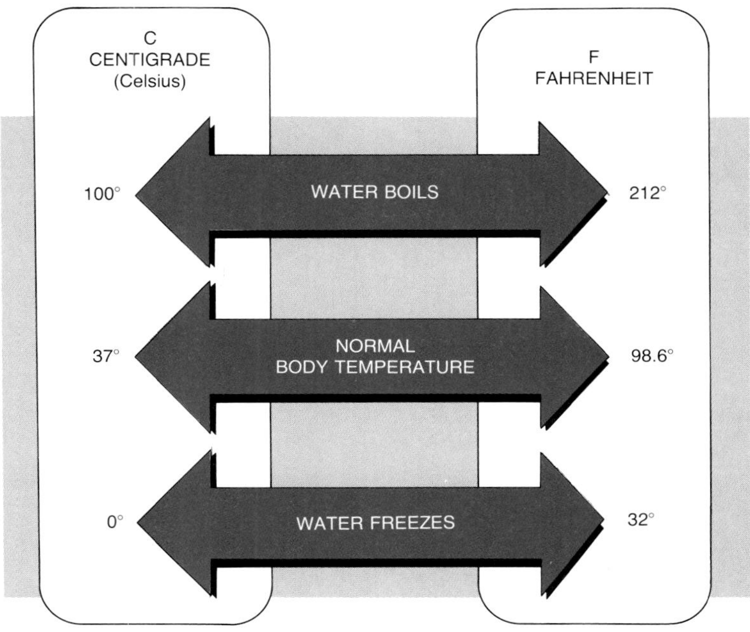

FIGURE 22-6 The two major scales used in the United States for measuring temperature.

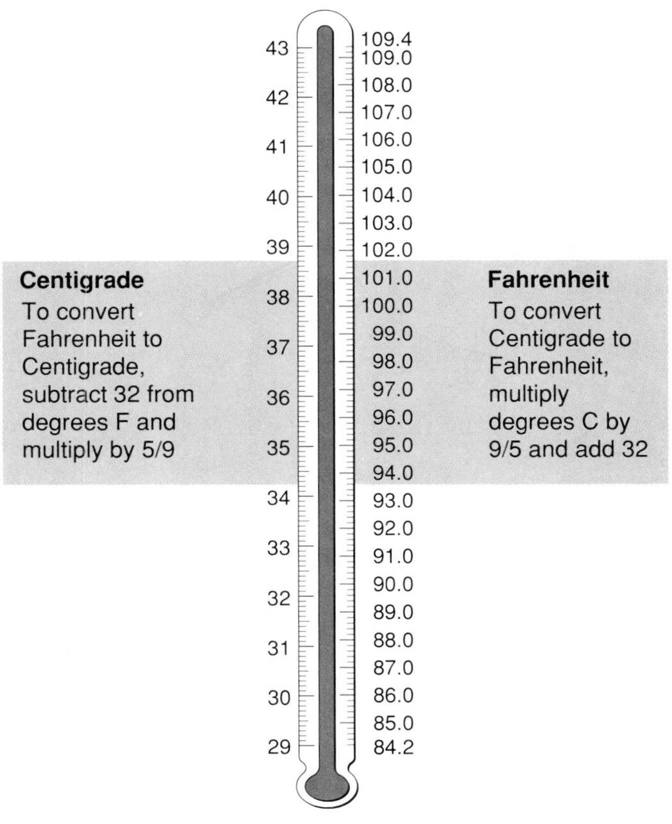

FIGURE 22-7 Temperature conversion.

Fahrenheit temperature can be written in two ways:

98.6°F or $98\frac{6}{}$°F

If you are using a centigrade (Celsius) thermometer, the temperature would be written

37°C or 37.3°C or $37\frac{3}{}$°C

Write an R in front of the temperature reading if a rectal temperature was taken. Write an A if an axillary temperature was taken. Write an O if an oral temperature was taken:

Normal Readings

Methods of Measuring Temperature	Normals °C	Normals °F
Oral	37.0°	98.6°
Axillary	36.4°	97.6°
Rectal	37.5°	99.6°

Procedure Measuring an Oral Temperature

1. Assemble your equipment.
   a) Oral thermometer (Figure 22-8)
   b) Tissue or paper towel
   c) Temperature board, TPR book, or the form used in your institution
   d) Pen or pencil

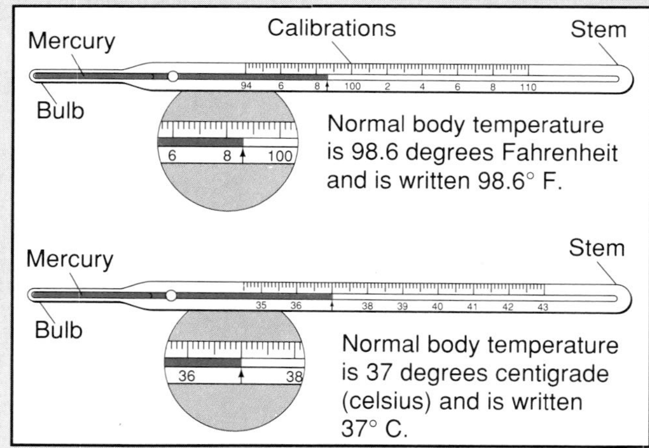

Mercury
Calibrations
Stem
Bulb
Normal body temperature is 98.6 degrees Fahrenheit and is written 98.6° F.
Mercury
Stem
Bulb
Normal body temperature is 37 degrees centigrade (celsius) and is written 37° C.

FIGURE 22-8 Using an oral thermometer.

2. Wash your hands.
3. Identify the patient by checking the identification bracelet.
4. Tell the patient you are going to take his temperature.
5. Ask the patient if he has recently had hot or cold fluids or if he has been smoking. If the answer is yes, wait 10 minutes before taking an oral temperature.
6. Ask visitors to step out of the room, if this is your hospital's policy.
7. Pull the curtain around the bed for privacy.
8. The patient should be in bed or sitting in a chair.
9. Take the thermometer out of its container. Dry with a paper towel.
10. Shake the mercury down.
11. Gently put the bulb end in the patient's mouth under the tongue (Figure 22-9). Ask him to keep his mouth and lips closed.
12. Leave the thermometer in the patient's mouth for 8 minutes. (*Note:* The latest research states that oral temperature is more accurate when the oral thermometer remains in the mouth for 8 minutes. However, if in your institution the policy is for 3 to 5 minutes, follow the procedure of your institution.)

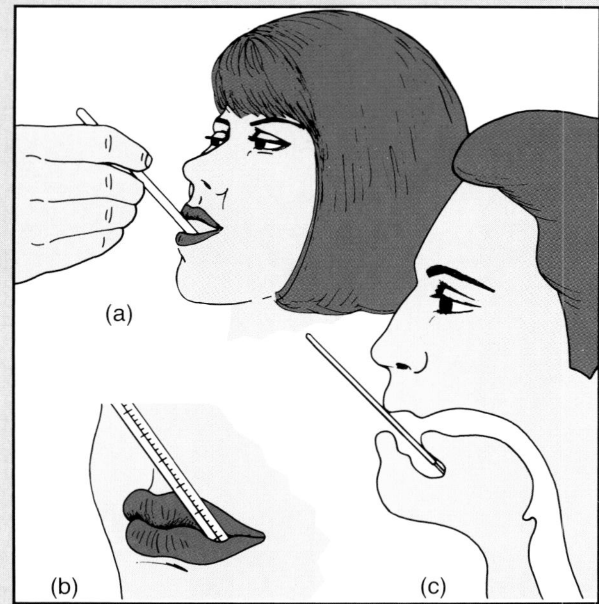

FIGURE 22-9 Inserting the oral thermometer. (a) Insert the thermometer gently into the patient's mouth under the tongue. (b) Position the thermometer to the side of the mouth. (c) Instruct the patient to keep the thermometer under the tongue by gently closing the lips around the thermometer.

13. Take the thermometer out of the patient's mouth. Hold the stem end and wipe the thermometer with a tissue. Wipe the stem of the thermometer toward the bulb end.
14. Read the thermometer.
15. Record the temperature in the TPR book, temperature board, or the form used in your institution.
16. Shake the mercury down. Rinse in cold water. Wipe with alcohol and replace the thermometer in its container.
17. Make the patient comfortable.
18. Lower the bed to a position of safety for the patient.
19. Pull the curtains back to the open position.
20. Raise the side rails where ordered, indicated, and appropriate for patient safety.
21. Place the call light within easy reach of the patient.
22. Wash your hands.
23. Report to your immediate supervisor:
    - If the oral temperature was above 100°F or 37.8°C.
    - Your observations of anything unusual

Procedure Using a Battery-Operated Electronic Oral Thermometer

1. Assemble your equipment:
   a) Disposable plastic probe cover
   b) Battery-operated electronic thermometer
   c) Oral (blue) attachment
   d) Temperature board, TPR book, or the form used in your institution
   e) Pen or pencil
2. Wash your hands.
3. Identify the patient by checking the identification bracelet.
4. Ask visitors to step out of the room, if this is your hospital's policy.
5. Tell the patient you are going to take her temperature.
6. Pull the curtain around the bed for privacy.
7. Check to be sure that the oral (blue top) probe connector is properly placed in its receptacle on the base of the unit.
8. Remove the probe from its stored position. Insert it into a sheath or probe cover.
9. Insert the covered probe into the patient's mouth slowly until the metal tip is at the base under the tongue to the back of the patient's mouth (Figure 22-10).
10. Hold the probe in the patient's mouth. It is much heavier than a glass thermometer and some patients are unable to hold it.
11. Wait about 15 seconds for the buzzer to ring for a computed temperature read-

ing. Then remove the probe from the patient's mouth.

12. Record the temperature on the temperature board, the TPR book, or the form used in your institution. This is very important because when you return the probe to its stored position the reading automatically returns to zero.
13. Discard the used probe cover (sheath) immediately without touching it.
14. Return the probe to its stored position in the face of the thermometer.
15. Store the thermometer in its charging stand whenever it is not in use.
16. Make the patient comfortable.
17. Lower the bed to a position of safety for the patient.
18. Pull the curtains back to the open position.
19. Raise the side rails where ordered, indicated, and appropriate for patient safety.
20. Place the call light within easy reach of the patient.
21. Wash your hands.
22. Report to your immediate supervisor:
    - If the oral temperature was over 100°F (37.8°C)
    - Your observations of anything unusual

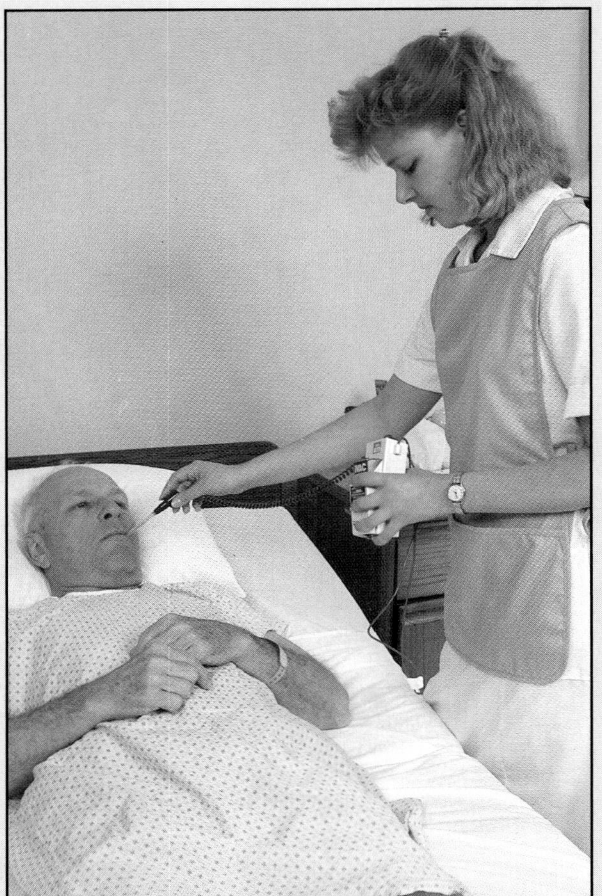

FIGURE 22-10

KEY IDEAS

Measuring Rectal Temperature

Remember that you will always use a rectal thermometer for taking rectal temperatures. Notice that the rectal thermometer has a small round bulb on one end. This bulb prevents the thermometer from injuring the sensitive lining of the patient's rectum. Under the following conditions you might take a rectal temperature. Ask your supervisor for verification.

- When the patient is an infant or child. Follow the policies of your employing health care institution for pediatric patients.
- When the patient is having warm or cold applications on the face or neck.
- When the patient cannot keep his or her mouth closed on the thermometer.
- When the patient finds it hard to breathe through the nose.
- When the patient has sneezing or coughing spells.
- When the patient's mouth is dry or inflamed (red).
- When the patient is restless, delirious, unconscious, or confused.

- When the patient is getting oxygen by cannula, catheter, face mask, or oxygen tent.
- When the patient has a nasogastric tube (Levine's tube, NG tube) in place.
- When the patient has had major surgery in the area of the face or neck.
- When the patient's face is partially paralyzed, as from a stroke.

Procedure Measuring Rectal Temperature

1. Assemble your equipment:
   a) Rectal thermometer
   b) Tissue or paper towel
   c) Lubricating jelly
   d) Temperature board, TPR book, or the form used in your institution
   e) Disposable gloves
2. Wash your hands.
3. Identify the patient by checking the identification bracelet.
4. Ask visitors to step out of the room, if this is your hospital's policy.
5. Tell the patient that you are going to take his temperature by rectum.
6. Pull the curtain around the bed for privacy. Lower the backrest on the bed, if allowed. Put on gloves.
7. Take the thermometer out of its container. Hold the thermometer only by the stem.
8. Inspect the bulb of the thermometer carefully for cracks or chipped places. A broken thermometer could seriously injure the patient's rectum. Do not use a chipped, cracked, or broken thermometer.
9. Hold the thermometer at the stem end. Shake it down until the mercury is below the numbers and lines.
10. Put a small amount of lubricating jelly on a piece of tissue. Then lubricate the bulb of the thermometer with the lubricated tissue. This makes insertion easier and also makes it more comfortable for the patient.
11. Ask the patient to turn on his side. Assist or turn patient, if necessary. Turn back the top covers just enough so that you can see the patient's buttocks. Avoid overexposing him.

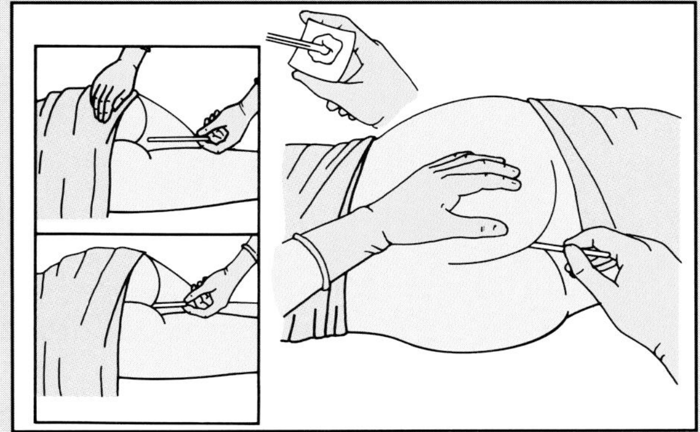

FIGURE 22-11

12. With one hand, raise the upper buttock until you can see the anus, the opening to the rectum. With the other hand gently insert the bulb 1 inch through the anus into the rectum (Figure 22-11). Never use force.
13. If the patient is an infant, remove the diaper. Lay the baby on his abdomen. Insert the thermometer with the other hand one-half inch into the rectum. Always hold the thermometer while it is in the child's rectum.
14. Hold the thermometer in place for 3 minutes. Do not leave any patient with a rectal thermometer in the rectum, no matter what his condition.
15. Remove the thermometer from the patient's rectum. Holding the stem end of the thermometer, wipe it with a tissue from stem to bulb to remove particles of feces (Figure 22-12).
16. Read the thermometer.
17. Record the temperature right away in the TPR book, temperature board, or form used in your institution. Note that this is a rectal temperature by writing an

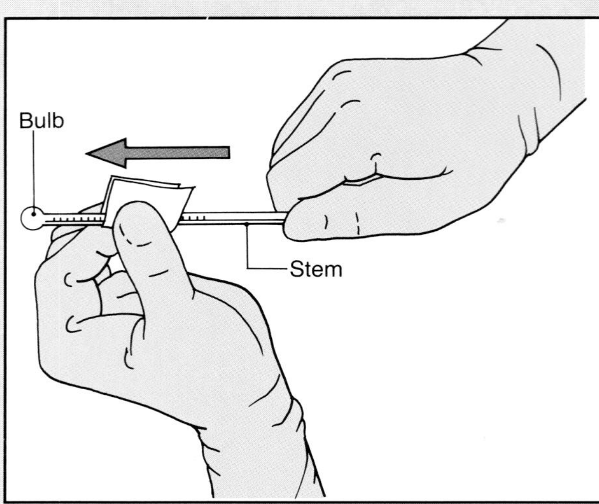

FIGURE 22-12

R in front of the figure. This is necessary because an average rectal temperature is slightly higher than an oral one.

18. Shake the mercury down until it is below the numbers and lines.
19. Clean with alcohol and replace the thermometer in its container. Remove gloves.
20. Make the patient comfortable.
21. Lower the bed to a position of safety for the patient.
22. Pull the curtains back to the open position.
23. Raise the side rails where ordered, indicated, and appropriate for patient safety.
24. Place the call light within easy reach of the patient.
25. Wash your hands.
26. Report to your immediate supervisor:
    - If the rectal temperature is higher than 101°F or 38.3°C. (Many institutions report the rectal temperature 101°F or 38.3°C by circling the figure in red on the temperature board, TPR book, or on the form used in the institution.)
    - Your observations of anything unusual.

Procedure Using a Battery-operated Electronic Rectal Thermometer

1. Assemble your equipment:
   a) Plastic disposable probe cover (sheath)
   b) Battery-operated electronic thermometer
   c) Rectal (red) attachment
   d) Temperature board, TPR book, or the form used in your institution
   e) Pen or pencil
2. Wash your hands.
3. Identify the patient by checking the identification bracelet.
4. Ask visitors to step out of the room, if this is your hospital's policy.
5. Tell the patient you are going to take his temperature.
6. Pull the curtain around the bed for privacy.
7. Check to be sure that the rectal (red top) probe connector is seated properly in its receptacle on the base of the thermometer. Put on gloves.
8. Remove the probe from its stored position and insert it into a probe cover (sheath). Lubricate tip of sheath.
9. Insert the covered probe slowly through the patient's anus into the rectum one-half inch.
10. Hold the probe in the patient's rectum.
11. Wait for the buzzer to ring for a computed temperature reading. Then remove the probe from the rectum. Remove gloves.
12. Record the temperature on the temperature board, TPR book, or form used in your institution. This is very important, because when you return the probe to its stored position the reading automatically returns to zero.
13. Discard the used probe cover immediately without touching it.
14. Return the probe to its stored position in the face of the thermometer.
15. Store the thermometer in its charging stand whenever it is not in use.

16. Make the patient comfortable.
17. Lower the bed to a position of safety for the patient.
18. Pull the curtains back to the open position.
19. Raise the side rails where ordered, indicated, and appropriate for patient safety.
20. Place the call light within easy reach of the patient.
21. Wash your hands.
22. Report to your immediate supervisor:
    - If the rectal temperature was over 101°F (38.3°C)
    - Your observations of anything unusual

Procedure Measuring Axillary Temperature

1. Assemble your equipment:
   a) Oral thermometer in container with proper disinfectant solution
   b) Tissue or paper towel
   c) Temperature board, TPR book, or the form used in your institution
   d) Pen or pencil
2. Wash your hands.
3. Identify the patient by checking the identification bracelet.
4. Ask visitors to step out of the room, if this is your hospital's policy.
5. Tell the patient that you have to take his temperature.
6. Pull the curtain around the bed for privacy.
7. Holding the stem end, remove the oral thermometer from its container.
8. Rinse the thermometer with cool tap water and dry it with tissue.
9. Inspect the bulb of the thermometer carefully for cracks or chipped places. A broken thermometer could seriously injure the patient. Do not use a chipped, cracked, or broken thermometer.
10. Remove the patient's arm from the sleeve of his gown. If the axillary region is moist with perspiration, pat it dry with a towel.
11. Place the bulb of the oral thermometer in the center of the armpit (axilla). The thermometer then should be held upright by the arm and the chest, in contact with the skin (Figure 22-13).
12. Put the patient's arm across his chest or abdomen.
13. If the patient is unconscious or is too weak to help, you will have to hold the thermometer in place.

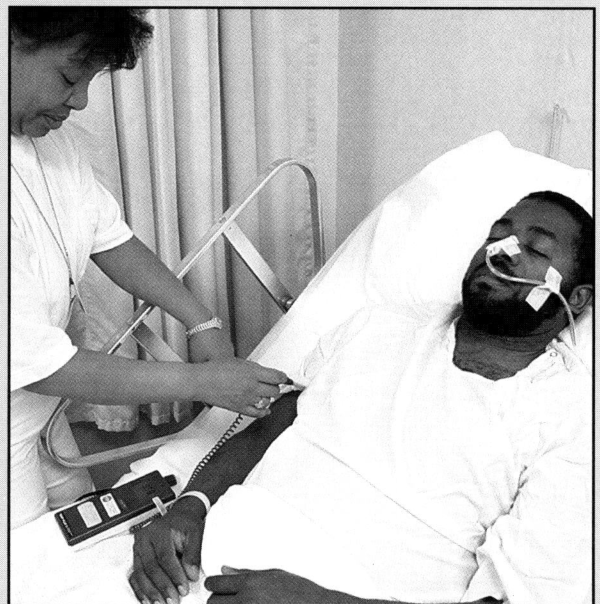

FIGURE 22-13

14. Leave the thermometer in place for 10 minutes. Stay with the patient.
15. Remove the thermometer. Wipe it off with tissue from the stem to the bulb.
16. Read the thermometer.
17. Shake the mercury down until it is below the numbers and lines.
18. Clean with alcohol and replace the thermometer in its container.
19. Record the temperature right away on the temperature board, TPR book, or the form used in your institution. Note that this is an axillary temperature by writing an A in front of the figure.
20. Put the patient's arm back in the sleeve of his gown.
21. Make the patient comfortable.

22. Lower the bed to a position of safety for the patient.
23. Pull the curtains back to the open position.
24. Raise the side rails where ordered, indicated, and appropriate for patient safety.
25. Place the call light within easy reach of the patient.
26. Wash your hands.
27. Report to your immediate supervisor:
    - If the axillary temperature was over 99°F (37.2°C). Many institutions report an axillary temperature over 99°F (37.2°C) by circling the figure in red on the temperature board, TPR book, or form used in your institution.
    - Your observations of anything unusual

Procedure Using a Battery-operated Electronic Oral Thermometer to Measure Axillary Temperature

1. Assemble your equipment:
   a) Plastic disposable probe cover (sheath)
   b) Battery-operated electronic thermometer
   c) Oral (blue) attachment
   d) Temperature board, TPR book, or the form used in your institution
   e) Pen or pencil
2. Wash your hands.
3. Identify the patient by checking the identification bracelet.
4. Ask visitors to step out of the room, if this is your hospital's policy.
5. Tell the patient you are going to take his temperature.
6. Pull the curtain around the bed for privacy.
7. Check to be sure that the oral (blue) probe connector is properly seated in its receptacle on the base of the unit.
8. Remove the probe from its stored position. Insert it into a probe cover (sheath).
9. Put the covered probe in the center of the patient's armpit (axilla).
10. Put the patient's arm across his chest. Hold the probe in place.
11. Wait about 15 seconds for the buzzer to ring for a computed temperature reading. Then remove the probe from the patient's axilla.
12. Record the temperature on the temperature board, TPR book, or form used in your institution. This is very important, because when you return the probe to its stored position the reading automatically returns to zero.
13. Discard the used probe cover immediately without touching it.
14. Return the probe to its stored position in the face of the thermometer.
15. Store the thermometer in its charging stand whenever it is not in use.
16. Make the patient comfortable.
17. Lower the bed to a position of safety for the patient.
18. Pull the curtains back to the open position.
19. Raise the side rails where ordered, indicated, and appropriate for patient safety.
20. Place the call light within easy reach of the patient.
21. Wash your hands.
22. Report to your immediate supervisor:
    - If the axillary temperature was over 99°F (37.2°C)
    - Your observations of anything unusual

KEY QUESTIONS

1. What are the different types of thermometers? Describe them.
2. What is the difference between reading a Fahrenheit and a centigrade (Celsius) thermometer?
3. How should oral temperatures be measured?
4. How should a patient's temperature be measured rectally?
5. What should you do to measure an axillary temperature?
6. How should a battery-operated electronic thermometer be used?
7. Define: axillary, centigrade, Fahrenheit, oral, rectal, thermometer.

CHAPTER

23

Measuring the Pulse

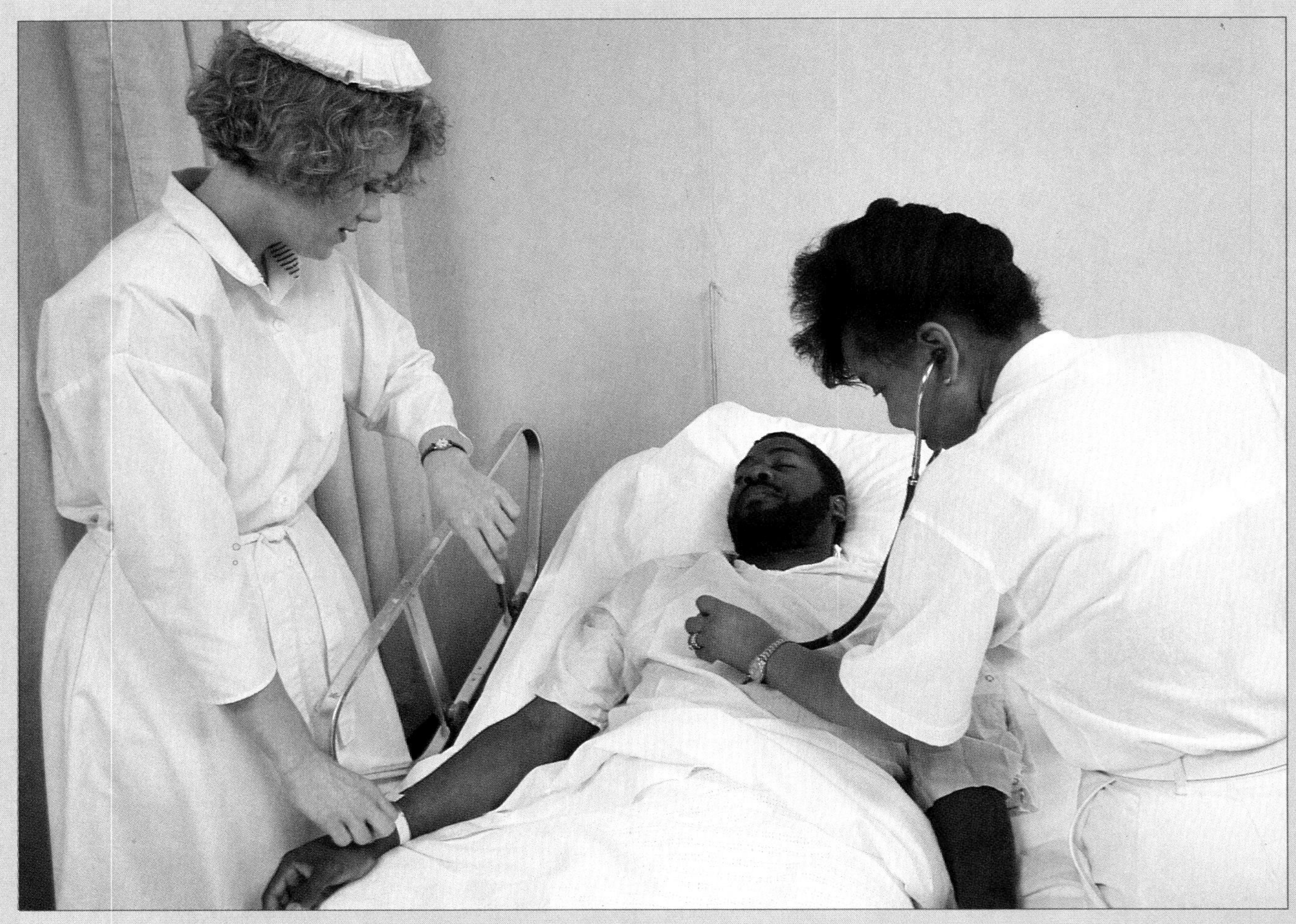

WARNING

For all patient contact, adhere to Universal Precautions (see page 91, 97, or the front cover flap). Wear protective equipment as indicated.

Objectives

What You Will Learn

When you have completed this chapter, you will be able to:

- Count the radial and apical pulse.
- Report the rate and rhythm of the pulse accurately.
- Define: apical pulse, force, pulse, pulse deficit, radial pulse, rate, rhythm.

KEY IDEAS

The Pulse

Pulse
The rhythmic expansion and contraction of the arteries caused by the beating of the heart. The expansion and contraction show how fast, how regular, and with what force the heart is beating.

EACH TIME THE HEART BEATS, IT pumps a certain amount of blood into the arteries. This causes the arteries to expand (get bigger). Between heartbeats, the arteries contract and return to their normal size. The heart pumps the blood in a steady rhythm. The rhythmic expansion and contraction of the arteries, which can be measured to show how fast the heart is beating, is called the **pulse**. Measuring the pulse is a simple method of observing how the circulatory system is functioning. The pulse can be measured at a number of places on the body (Figure 23-1).

Radial Pulse

Radial Pulse
This is the pulse felt at a person's wrist at the radial artery.

The pulse measures how fast the heart is beating. At certain places on the body, the pulse can be felt easily under a person's fingers. One of the easiest and most common places to feel the pulse is at the wrist. This is called a **radial pulse** because you are feeling the radial artery (Figure 23-2). When taking the pulse, you must be able to report accurately the following:

Rate
Used to describe the number of pulse beats per minute.

Rhythm
Used to describe the regularity of the pulse beats.

Force
Strength or power; used to describe the beat of the pulse.

- **Rate:** the number of pulse beats per minute.
- **Rhythm:** the regularity of the pulse beats, that is, whether or not the length of time between the beats is steady and regular.
- **Force** of the beat (weak or bounding).

The average normal rate of pulse for adults is from 72 to 80 beats per minute (Figure 23-3). Always report an adult pulse rate of under 60 and over 100 beats per minute to your supervisor.

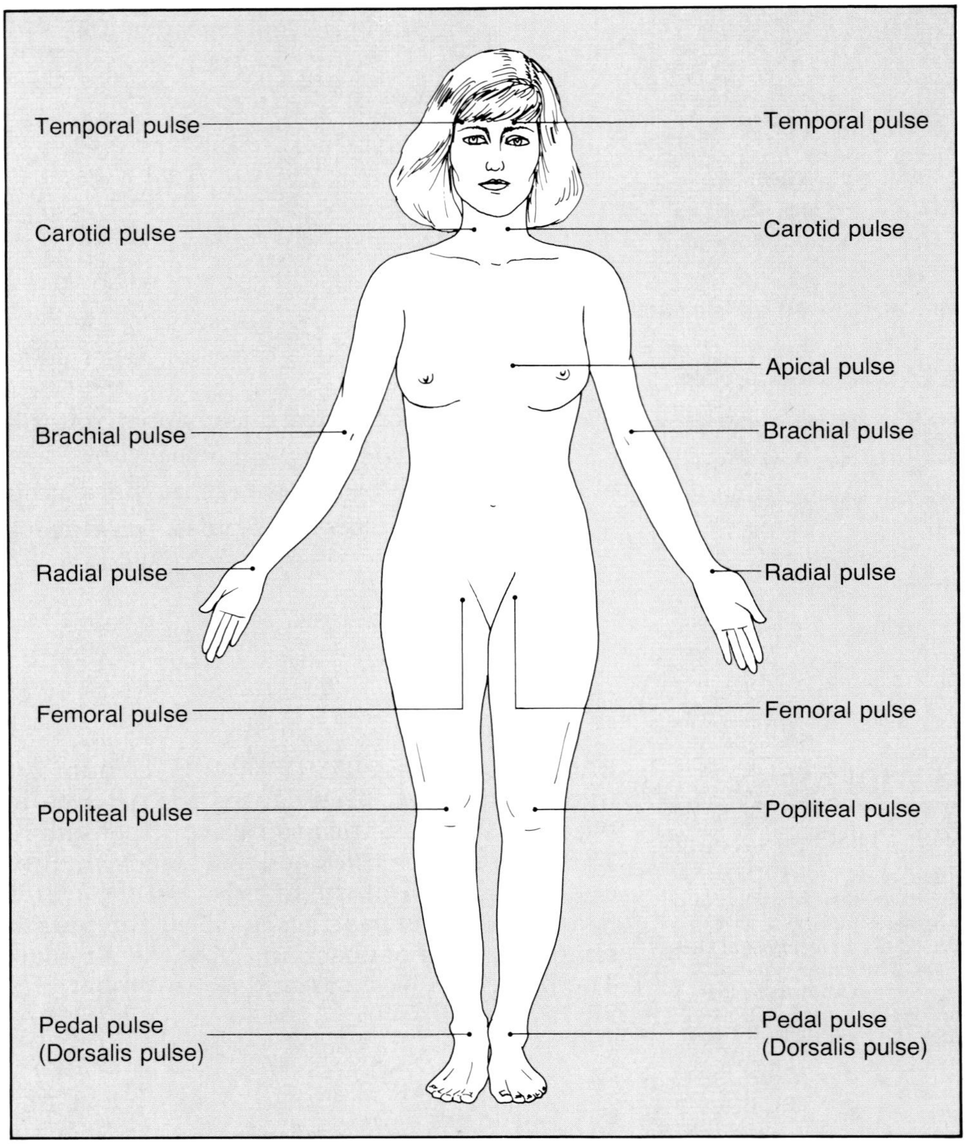

FIGURE 23-1 Points on the human body where pulse may be taken.

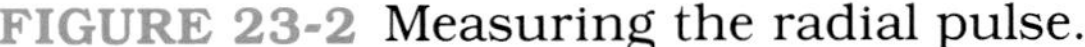

FIGURE 23-2 Measuring the radial pulse.

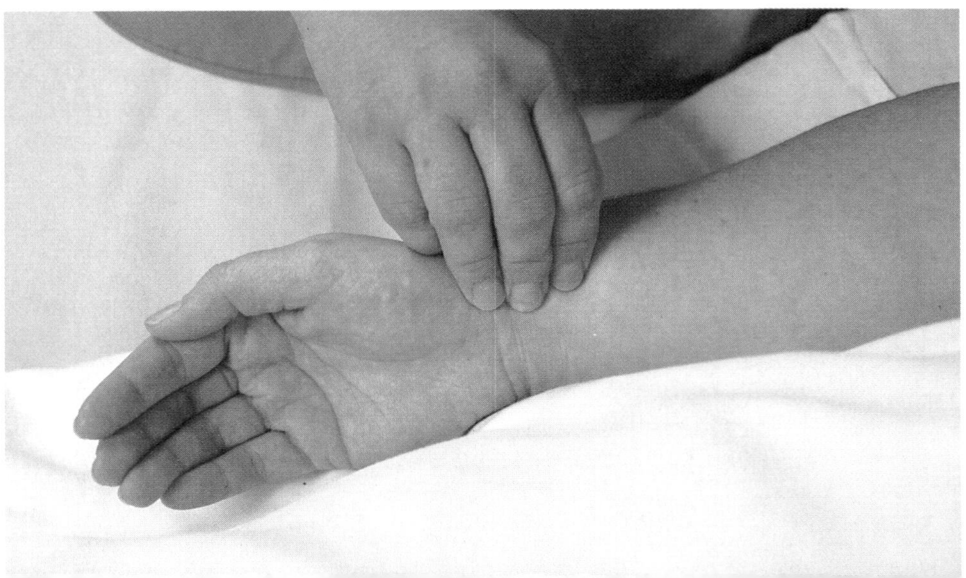

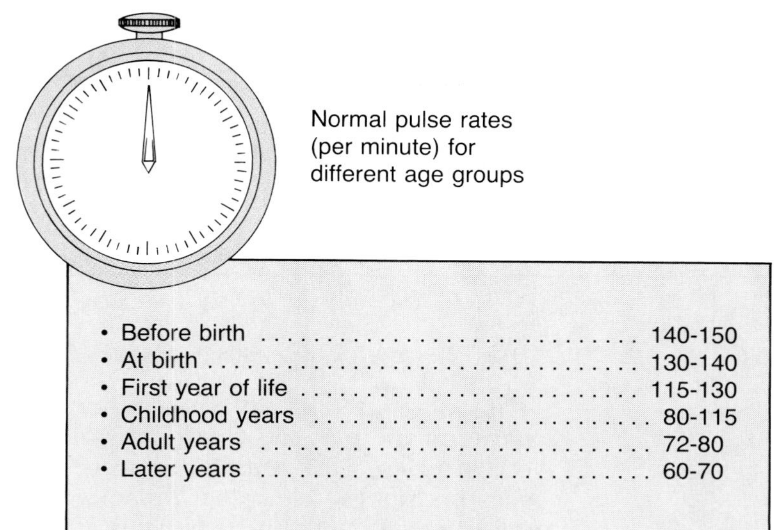

• Before birth	140-150
• At birth	130-140
• First year of life	115-130
• Childhood years	80-115
• Adult years	72-80
• Later years	60-70

FIGURE 23-3 Normal pulse rates per minute for different age groups.

Procedure Measuring the Radial Pulse

1. Assemble your equipment:
   a) Watch with a second hand
   b) Vital-signs form used in your institution
   c) Pen or pencil
2. Wash your hands.
3. Identify the patient by checking the identification bracelet.
4. Ask visitors to step out of the room, if this is your hospital's policy.
5. Tell the patient you are going to take his pulse.
6. If the patient is standing, ask him to sit down. Or have him lying in a comfortable position in bed.
7. The patient's hand and arm should be well supported and resting comfortably.
8. Find the pulse by placing the tips of your first three fingers on the palm side of the patient's wrist in a line with his thumb directly next to the bone. Press lightly until you feel the beat. If you press too hard, you may stop the flow of blood and not feel the pulse. Never use your thumb. Your thumb has its own pulse and you would be counting your own pulse instead of the patient's. When you have found the pulse, notice the rhythm. Notice if the beat is steady or irregular. Notice the force of the beat.
9. Look at the position of the second hand on your watch. Then start counting the pulse beats (what you feel) until the second hand comes back to the same number on the clock.
   - *Method A:* Count the pulse beats for one full minute and report the full minute count. This is always done if the patient has an irregular beat.
   - *Method B:* Count for 30 seconds, until the second hand on the watch is opposite its position when you started. Then multiply the number of beats by 2. This is the number you record. For example, if you count 35 beats for 30 seconds, the count for one full minute is 70.
10. Record the pulse count on the vital-signs form used in your institution. Be sure you write in the correct column next to the patient's name.
11. Make the patient comfortable.
12. Lower the bed to a position of safety for the patient.
13. Pull the curtains back to the open position.
14. Raise the side rails where ordered, indicated, and appropriate for patient safety.

15. Place the call light within easy reach of the patient.
16. Wash your hands.
17. Report to your immediate supervisor:
    - If the pulse rate was under 60 or over 100 for an adult.
    - If the pulse was irregular by circling in red the number on the vital-signs form used by your institution. Sometimes "irr." is written near the number.
    - Your observations of anything unusual.

The Apical Pulse and Pulse Deficit

Apical Pulse
A measurement of the heartbeats at the apex of the heart, located just under the left breast.

Pulse Deficit
A difference between the apical heartbeat and the radial pulse rate.

The pulse rate should be the same as the heart rate. However, in some patients the heartbeats are not strong enough to be transmitted along the arteries. This may be because of some forms of heart disease. For these patients, an apical pulse would be taken. An **apical pulse** is a measurement of the heartbeats at the apex of the heart, located just under the left breast.

Sometimes the patient has a **pulse deficit**, a difference between the apical heartbeat and the radial pulse rate. To determine this, the apical pulse (heart rate) is counted with a stethoscope over the apex of the heart. At the same time, the pulse rate is counted at the radial pulse. The two figures are compared. The difference between the apical heartbeat and the radial pulse beat is the pulse deficit. This is called the *apical pulse deficit.* For maximum accuracy, both pulses should be taken at the same time by two nursing assistants. A different method calls for one nursing assistant, who first takes the apical pulse and then takes the radial pulse. This second method is not considered as accurate as the first method.

Procedure Measuring the Apical Pulse

1. Assemble your equipment:
   a) Stethoscope and antiseptic swabs
   b) Watch with a second hand
   c) Vital-signs form used in your institution (*Note:* In many institutions, this reading is reported directly to your immediate supervisor rather than writing it on the form used.)
   d) Pen or pencil and note paper
2. Wash your hands.
3. Identify the patient by checking the identification bracelet.
4. Ask visitors to step out of the room, if this is your hospital's policy.
5. Explain to the patient that you are going to take her apical pulse.
6. Pull the curtain around the bed for privacy.
7. Clean the earplugs on the stethoscope with antiseptic solution. Put the earplugs in your ears. Warm the bell or diaphragm of the stethoscope by holding it tightly for a few seconds.
8. Uncover the left side of the patient's chest. Avoid overexposing the patient.
9. Locate the apex of the patient's heart by placing the bell or diaphragm of the stethoscope under the patient's left breast. Listen for the heart sounds.
10. Count the heart sounds for a full minute.
11. Write the full minute count on the note paper.
12. Cover and make the patient comfortable.
13. Lower the bed to a position of safety for the patient.

14. Pull the curtains back to the open position.
15. Raise the side rails where ordered, indicated, and appropriate for patient safety.
16. Place the call light within easy reach of the patient.
17. Clean the earplugs of the stethoscope. Return the equipment to its proper place.
18. Wash your hands.
19. Report to your immediate supervisor:
    - That you have taken the patient's apical pulse
    - What the apical pulse rate was
    - Your observations of anything unusual

Procedure Measuring the Apical Pulse Deficit

1. Assemble your equipment:
    a) Stethoscope and antiseptic swabs
    b) Watch with a second hand
    c) Vital-signs form used in your institution (*Note:* In many situations, this reading is reported directly to your immediate supervisor rather than writing it on the form used.)
    d) Note paper, pen, or pencil
2. Wash your hands.
3. Identify the patient by checking the identification bracelet.
4. Ask visitors to step out of the room, if this is your hospital's policy.
5. Explain to the patient that you are going to take his pulse.
6. Pull the curtain around the bed for privacy.
7. There are two methods of taking the apical pulse deficit.
    - *Method A:* Two nursing assistants do this procedure together at the same time (Figure 23-4). One counts the radial pulse. The other counts the apical pulse for one full minute. The difference between the two pulses is known as the apical pulse deficit. This method is used for maximum accuracy.
    - *Method B:* The nursing assistant first takes the apical pulse and then the radial pulse. The difference between the two pulses is known as the apical pulse deficit. However, since the readings are not taken at the same time, it is not considered as accurate as the first method.

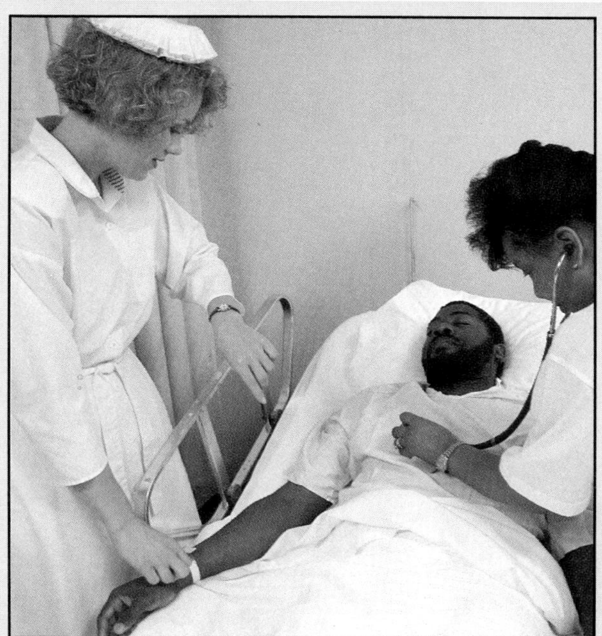

FIGURE 23-4

8. Count the apical pulse and the radial pulse for one full minute and record both figures.
9. Record the figure for the pulse deficit.
10. Make the patient comfortable.
11. Lower the bed to a position of safety for the patient.
12. Pull the curtains back to the open position.
13. Raise the side rails where ordered, indicated, and appropriate for patient safety.
14. Place the call light within easy reach of the patient.

15. Clean the equipment and return it to its proper place.
16. Wash your hands.
17. Report to your immediate supervisor:
    - That you have taken the patient's apical pulse deficit
    - The apical pulse rate
    - The radial pulse rate
    - The pulse deficit
    - Your observations of anything unusual

KEY QUESTIONS

1. How should the radial and apical pulse be counted?
2. What information should be reported about the pulse?
3. Define: apical pulse, force, pulse, pulse deficit, radial pulse, rate, rhythm.

CHAPTER

24

Measuring Respirations

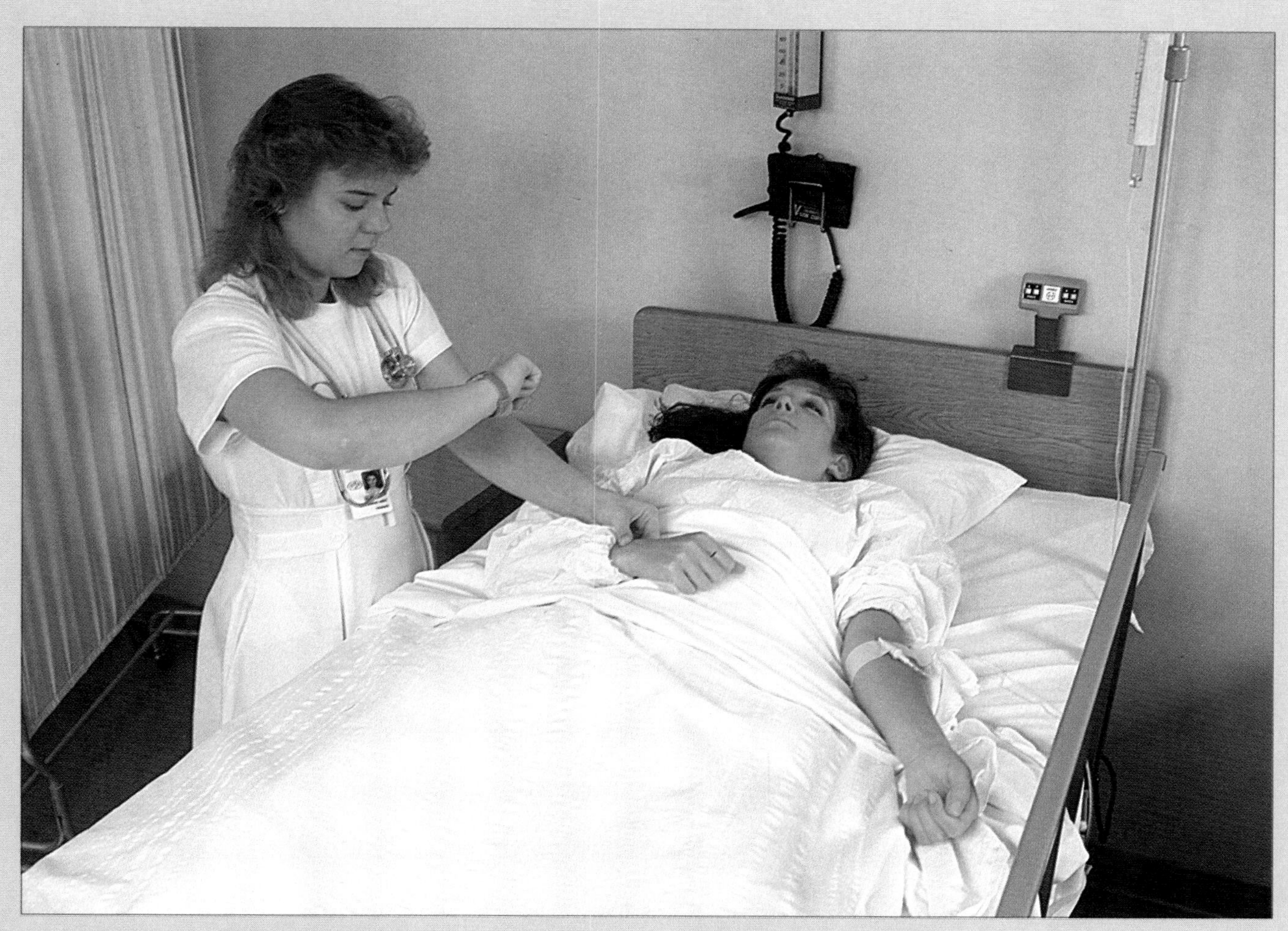

WARNING

For all patient contact, adhere to Universal Precautions (see page 91, 97, or the front cover flap). Wear protective equipment as indicated.

Objectives

What You Will Learn

When you have completed this chapter, you will be able to:

- Count a patient's respirations accurately.
- Determine if the patient's breathing is labored or abnormal.
- Define: abdominal respiration, Cheyne–Stokes respiration, exhaling, inhaling, irregular respiration, labored respiration, shallow respiration, stertorous respiration.

KEY IDEAS

Measuring Respirations

Inhaling
The process of breathing in air in respiration.

Exhaling
The process of breathing out air in respiration.

Labored Respiration
Working hard to breathe.

THE HUMAN BODY MUST HAVE A steady supply of air. The body needs oxygen from the air in order to change food into heat and energy. When you breathe in, air is drawn into the lungs. In the lungs, oxygen is taken out of the air and absorbed into the blood. The blood then carries the oxygen to the body cells. In the body cells, the oxygen is used to produce energy for the body (oxidation).

Respiration is the process of **inhaling** (breathing in) and **exhaling** (breathing out). One respiration includes breathing in once and breathing out once. When a person breathes in, the chest gets larger (expands). When a person breathes out, the chest gets smaller (contracts). When you count respirations, the patient should be lying on his or her back. You watch the chest rise and fall as the patient breathes. Or you feel the chest rise and fall with your hand. Either way, you should count respirations without the patient knowing it (Figure 24-1). If the patient thinks that breathing is being counted, he or she will not breathe naturally. What you want to count is natural breathing. Besides counting respirations, you will be noticing whether the patient seems to breathe easily or seems to be working hard to get his or her breath. When a person is working hard to get breath, it is called **labored respiration**. You must also notice whether the breathing is noisy.

Normally, adults breathe at a rate of from 16 to 20 times a minute. Children breathe more rapidly. The elderly breathe more slowly. Exercise, digestion, emotional stress, disease conditions, some drugs, stimulants, heat, and cold can all affect the number of times per minute that a person breathes.

Abnormal Respiration

While you are counting the patient's respirations, it is important to observe and make note of anything about his or her breathing that

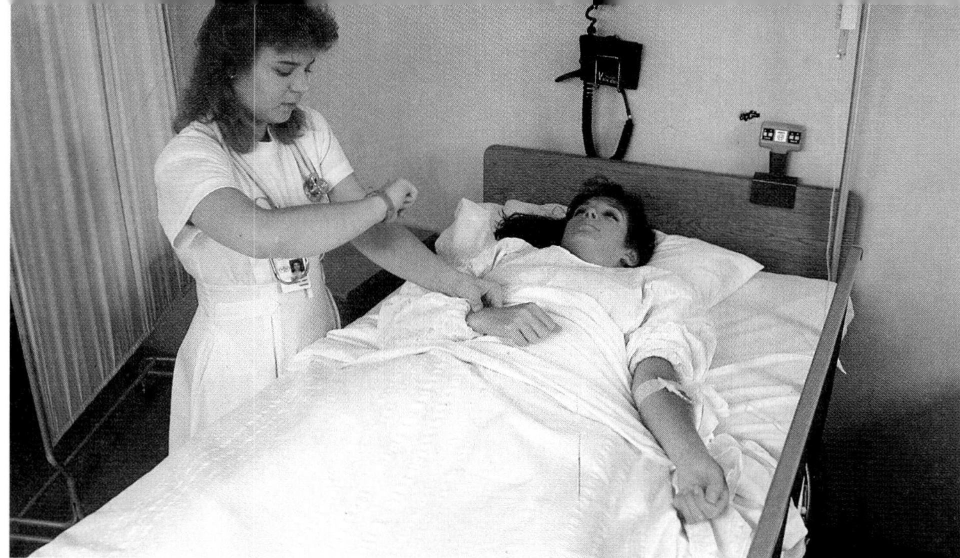

FIGURE 24-1 The patient must be unaware that you are counting his respirations.

Stertorous Respiration
The patient makes abnormal noises like snoring sounds when breathing.

Abdominal Respiration
Breathing in which the patient is using mostly her or his abdominal muscles.

Shallow Respiration
Breathing with only the upper part of the lungs.

Irregular Respiration
The depth of breathing changes and the rate of the rise and fall of the chest is not steady.

Cheyne–Stokes Respiration
One kind of irregular breathing. At first the breathing is slow and shallow; then the respiration becomes faster and deeper until it reaches a peak. The respiration then slows down and becomes shallow again. The breathing may then stop completely for 10 seconds and then begin the pattern again. This type of respiration may be caused by certain cerebral (brain), cardiac (heart), or pulmonary (lung) diseases or conditions.

appears to be abnormal. Different types of abnormal respiration that you should be familiar with are:

1. **Stertorous respiration:** The patient makes abnormal noises like snoring sounds when breathing.
2. **Abdominal respiration:** Breathing in which the patient is using mostly the abdominal muscles.
3. **Shallow respiration:** Breathing with only the upper part of the lungs.
4. **Irregular respiration:** The depth of breathing changes and the rate of the rise and fall of the chest is not steady.
5. **Cheyne–Stokes respiration:** One kind of irregular breathing. At first the breathing is slow and shallow; then the respiration becomes faster and deeper until it reaches a peak. The respiration then slows down and becomes shallow again. The breathing may then stop completely for 10 seconds and then begin the pattern again. This type of respiration may be caused by certain cerebral (brain), cardiac (heart), or pulmonary (chest) diseases or condition.
6. Dyspnea: Insufficient oxygenation of the blood resulting in labored or difficult breathing.

Procedure Measuring Respiration

1. Assemble your equipment:
   a) Watch with a second hand
   b) TPR book, temperature board, or the form used in your institution
   c) Pen or pencil
2. Wash your hands.
3. Identify the patient by checking the identification bracelet.
4. Ask visitors to step out of the room, if this is your hospital's policy.
5. Hold the patient's wri… were taking his pulse…

not know you are watching his breathing. Count the patient's respirations, without him knowing it, immediately after counting his pulse rate.

6. If the patient is a child who has been crying or is restless, wait until he is quiet before counting respirations. If a child is asleep, count his respirations before he wakes up. Always count a child's pulse and respirations before you measure his temperature. (Most children get upset when you measure their temperature.)
7. One rise and one fall of the patient's chest counts as one respiration.
8. If you cannot clearly see the chest rise and fall, fold the patient's arms across his chest. Then you can feel his breathing as you hold his wrist.
9. Check the position of the second hand on the watch. Count "one" when you see the patient's chest rising as he breathes in. The next time his chest rises, count "two." Keep doing this for a full minute. Report the number of respirations you count.
10. You may be permitted to count for 30 seconds. Count the respirations for one-half minute and then multiply the number you counted by 2. For example, if you count 8 respirations in 30 seconds (a half-minute), your number for a full minute is 16.
11. If the patient's breathing rhythm is irregular, always count for a full minute. Observe the depth of the breathing while counting the respirations.
12. Write down the number you counted immediately on the temperature board, TPR book, or form used by your institution. Be sure you are in the proper column, opposite the correct patient's name.
13. Note whether the respirations were noisy or labored.
14. Make the patient comfortable.
15. Lower the bed to a position of safety for the patient.
16. Pull the curtains back to the open position.
17. Raise the side rails where ordered, indicated, and appropriate for patient safety.
18. Place the call light within easy reach of the patient.
19. Wash your hands.
20. Report to your immediate supervisor:
    - Whether the respirations were noisy or labored
    - Whether the respirations were irregular
    - The time they were measured
    - If the respirations were less than 14 or more than 28 a minute
    - Your observations of anything unusual

KEY QUESTIONS

1. How should respirations be counted?
2. Name and describe the abnormal types of respiration.
3. Define: abdominal respiration, Cheyne–Stokes respiration, exhaling, inhaling, irregular respiration, labored respiration, shallow respiration, stertorous respiration.

CHAPTER 25

Measuring Blood Pressure

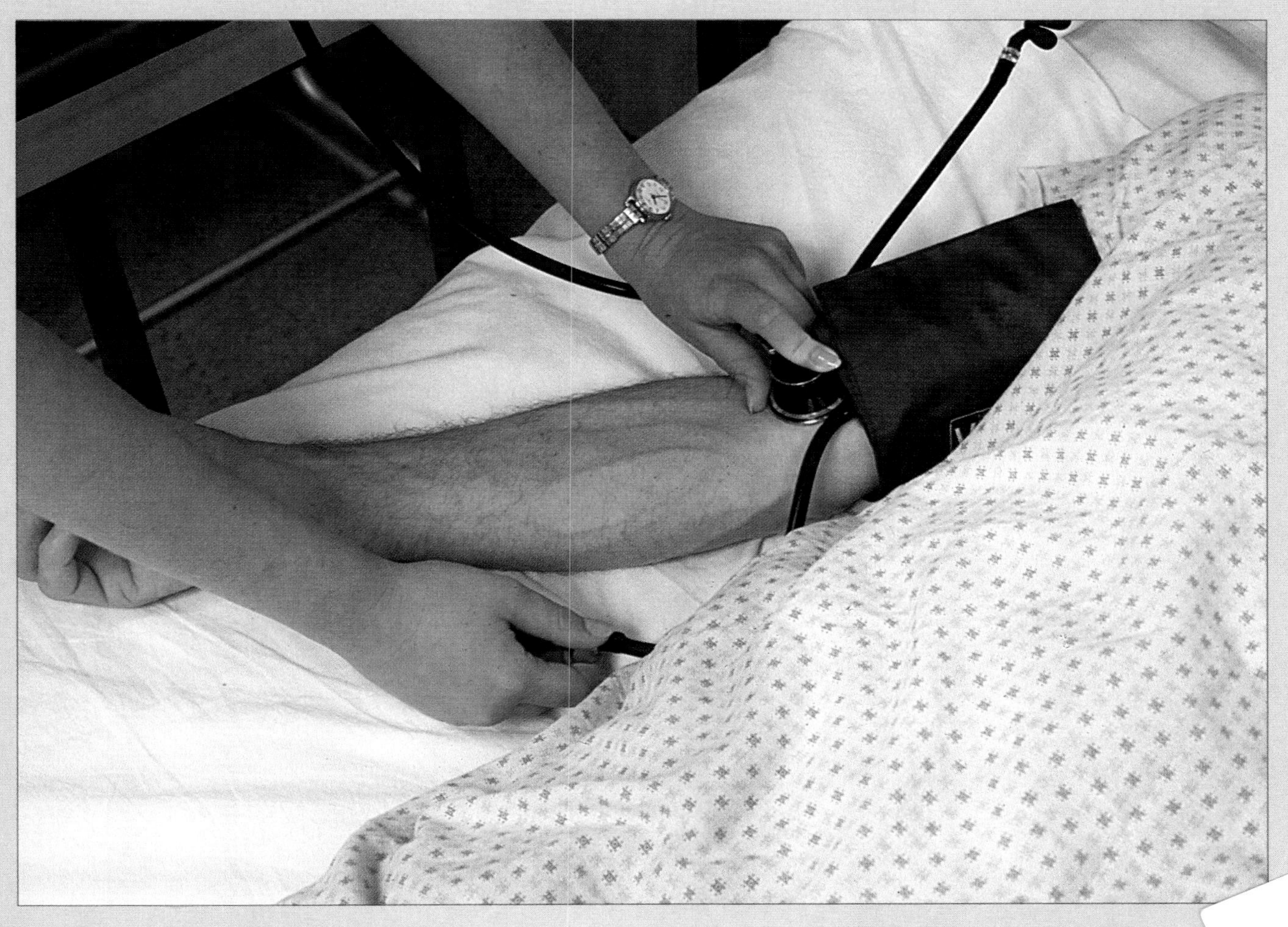

WARNING

For all patient contact, adhere to Universal Precautions (see page 91, 97, or the front cover flap). Wear protective equipment as indicated.

Objectives

What You Will Learn

When you have completed this chapter, you will be able to:

- Explain systolic pressure.
- Explain diastolic pressure.
- Demonstrate the use of aneroid, mercury, and electronic types of blood pressure equipment accurately and efficiently.
- Measure a patient's blood pressure accurately.
- Define: aneroid sphygmomanometer, blood pressure, diastolic blood pressure, mercury sphygmomanometer, stethoscope, sphygmomanometer, systolic blood pressure.

KEY IDEAS

Blood Pressure

Blood Pressure
The force of the blood exerted on the inner walls of the arteries, veins, and chambers of the heart as it flows or circulates through them.

Systolic Blood Pressure
The force with which blood is pumped when the heart muscle is contracting. When taking a patient's blood pressure, the systolic blood pressure is recorded as the top number.

Diastolic Blood Pressure
In taking a patient's blood pressure, one records the bottom number as the reading for the diastolic pressure. This is the relaxing phase of the heartbeat.

BLOOD PRESSURE IS THE FORCE OF the blood pushing against the walls of the blood vessels. When you take a patient's blood pressure, you are measuring this force of the blood flowing through the arteries.

There is always a certain amount of pressure in the arteries. This is because the heart, by pumping blood, is constantly forcing it to circulate. The blood goes first into the arteries. It then circulates through the whole body. The amount of pressure in the arteries depends on two things.

1. The rate of heartbeat
2. How easily the blood flows through the blood vessels

The heart contracts as it pumps the blood into the arteries. When the heart is contracting, the pressure is highest. This pressure is called the **systolic pressure**. As the heart relaxes between each contraction, the pressure goes down. When the heart is most relaxed, the pressure is lowest. This pressure is called the **diastolic pressure**. When you take a patient's blood pressure, you are measuring these two rates, the systolic pressure and the diastolic pressure.

In young, healthy adults, the normal blood pressure range is between 100 and 140 millimeters (mm) mercury (Hg) systolic pressure. It is between 60 and 90 millimeters (mm) mercury (Hg) diastolic pressure. The way these figures are written is:

$$120/80 \quad \text{or} \quad \frac{120}{80} \begin{array}{l} = \text{Systolic} \\ = \text{Diastolic} \end{array}$$

When a patient's blood pressure is higher than the normal range for his or her age and condition, it is referred to as high blood pressure or *hypertension*. When a patient's blood pressure is lower than the normal range for his or her age or condition, it is referred to as low blood pressure or *hypotension.*

Instruments for Measuring Blood Pressure

Sphygmomanometer
An apparatus for measuring blood pressure.

When you take a patient's blood pressure, you will be using an instrument called a **sphygmomanometer**, which is a combination of three Greek words:

- sphygmo, meaning pulse
- mano, meaning pressure
- meter, meaning measure

This instrument, however, is usually referred to as the blood pressure cuff. The four main parts of this instrument are the manometer, valve, cuff, and bulb.

Two kinds of instruments are used for taking blood pressure. One is the mercury type. The other is the aneroid (dial) type. Both kinds have an inflatable, cloth-covered rubber bag or cuff that is wrapped around the patient's arm. Both kinds also have a rubber bulb for pumping air into the cuff. The procedure for measuring blood pressure is the same, except for measuring the reading. When you use the mercury type, you will be watching the level of a column of mercury on a measuring scale (Figure 25-1). When you use the dial (aneroid) type, you will be watching a pointer on a dial (Figure 25-2).

Mercury Sphygmomanometer
Blood pressure equipment containing a column of mercury.

Aneroid Sphygmomanometer
Dial-type blood pressure equipment.

Stethoscope
An instrument that allows one to listen to various sounds in the patient's body, such as the heartbeat or breathing sounds.

When you measure a patient's blood pressure, you will be doing two things at the same time. You will listen to the brachial pulse as it sounds in the brachial artery in the patient's arm. You also will watch an indicator (either a column of mercury or a dial) in order to take a reading.

You will use a stethoscope (Figure 25-3) to listen to the brachial pulse. The stethoscope is an instrument that makes it possible to listen to various sounds in the patient's body, such as the heartbeat or breathing sounds in the chest. The stethoscope is a tube with one end that picks

FIGURE 25-1 Mercury sphygmomanometer.

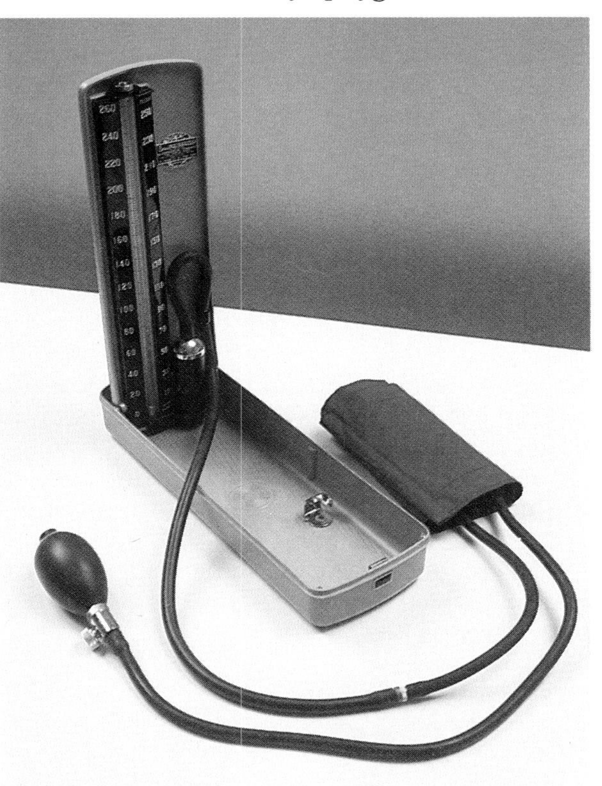

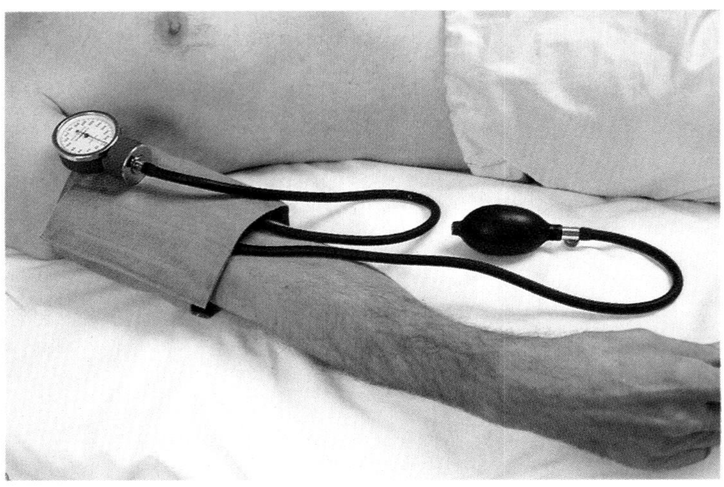

FIGURE 25-2 Aneroid sphygmomanometer.

FIGURE 25-3 Stethoscope.

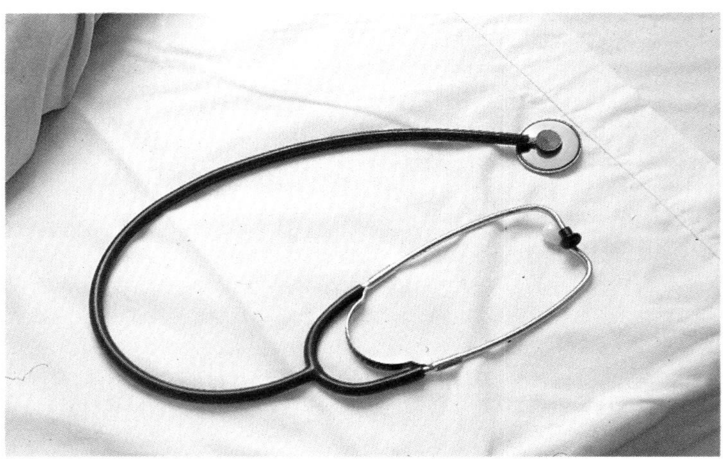

up sound when it is placed against a part of the body. This end is either bell shaped, and is called a bell, or it is round and flat, and is called a diaphragm. The other end of the tube splits into two parts. These parts have tips on the ends and fit into the listener's ears.

In many institutions, the blood pressure equipment hangs on the wall over the bed. A smaller-sized cuff must be used for children or a larger-sized for obese (overweight) patients. Do not take blood pressure on an arm that has an IV (intravenous) setup in it, or surgical site on it, or from a patient with an A.V. shunt.

KEY IDEAS

Electronic Blood Pressure Monitoring Apparatus

The latest development in the electronic blood pressure apparatus is an infrared photoelectric system in which a miniature cuff is placed around the left index finger, inflating to the correct pressure necessary to obtain a proper reading and then deflating once the measurement has been determined. Use of this type of equipment eliminates the use of a stethoscope and human error.

With an automatic digital blood pressure monitor a cuff is placed around the wrist. The arm must be at the level of the heart, and no stethoscope is needed.

Procedure Measuring Blood Pressure

1. Assemble your equipment:
    a) Sphygmomanometer (blood pressure cuff)
    b) Stethoscope
    c) Antiseptic pad
    d) BP board, blood pressure book, or the form used in your institution
    e) Pen or pencil

    Wash your hands.

    Identify the patient by checking the identification bracelet.

    Ask visitors to step out of the room, if this is your hospital's policy.
5. Tell the patient that you are going to measure his blood pressure.
6. Wipe the earplugs of the stethoscope with antiseptic pads.
7. Have the patient resting quietly. He should be either lying down or sitting in a chair.
8. If you are using the mercury apparatus, the measuring scale should be level with your eyes.
9. The patient's arm should be bare up to the shoulder, or the patient's sleeve should be well above the elbow without limiting or constricting circulation.
10. The patient's arm from the elbow down should be resting fully extended on the bed. Or it might be resting on the arm of the chair or your hip, well supported, with the palm upward.
11. Unroll the cuff and loosen the valve on the bulb. Then squeeze the compression bag to deflate it completely.
12. Wrap the cuff around the patient's arm above the elbow snugly and smoothly. But do not wrap it so tightly that the patient is uncomfortable from the pressure. You may need to use a different-size cuff for a patient with very thin arms (a child, for example) or very large arms.
13. Leave the area clear where you will place the bell or diaphragm of the stethoscope.
14. Be sure the manometer is in position so you can read the numbers easily.
15. Put the earplugs of the stethoscope into your ears.
16. With your fingertips, find the patient's brachial pulse at the inner aspect of the arm above the elbow (brachial artery).

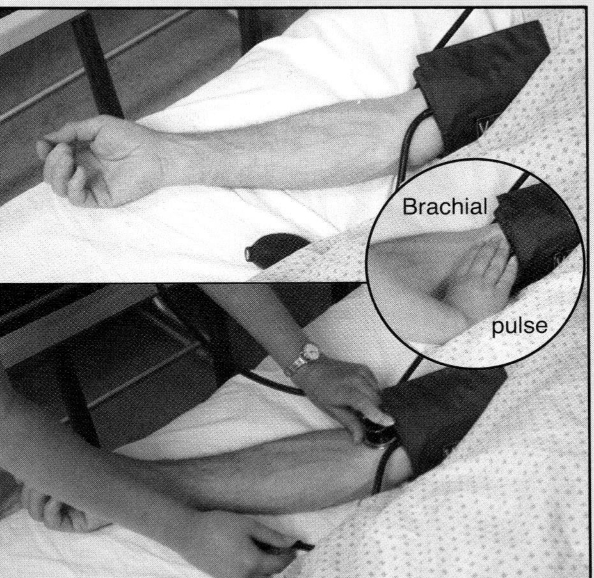

FIGURE 25-4

This is where you will place the diaphragm or bell of the stethoscope (Figure 25-4). The diaphragm should be held firmly against the patient's skin, but it should not touch the cuff of the apparatus.

17. Tighten the thumbscrew of the valve to close it. Turn it clockwise. Be careful not to turn it too tightly. If you do, you will have trouble opening it.
18. Hold the stethoscope in place. Inflate the cuff until the dial points to 170.
19. Open the valve counterclockwise. This allows the air to escape. Let it out slowly until the sound of the pulse comes back. A few seconds must go by without sounds. If you do hear pulse sounds immediately, you must stop the procedure and completely deflate the cuff. Wait a few seconds. Then inflate the cuff to a much higher calibration, above 200. Again, loosen the thumbscrew to let the air out. Listen for a repeated pulse sound. At the same time, watch the indicator.
20. Note the calibration (number) that the pointer passes as you hear the first sound (Figure 25-5). This point indicates the systolic pressure (or the top number).
21. Continue releasing the air from the cuff. When the sounds change to a softer or

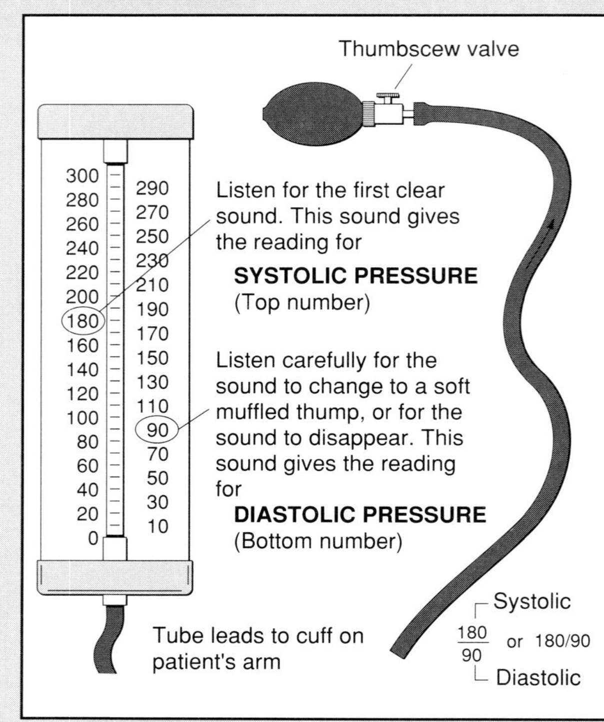

FIGURE 25-5

muffled and faster thud or disappear, note the calibration. This is the diastolic pressure (or bottom number).

22. Deflate the cuff completely. Remove it from the patient's arm.
23. Record your reading on the BP board, BP book, or form used in your institution.
24. After using the blood pressure cuff, roll it up over the manometer and replace it in the case.
25. Wipe the earplugs of the stethoscope again with an antiseptic swab. Put the stethoscope back in its proper place.
26. Make the patient comfortable.
27. Lower the bed to a position of safety for the patient.
28. Pull the curtains back to the open position.
29. Raise the side rails where ordered, indicated, and appropriate for patient safety.
30. Place the call light within easy reach of the patient.
31. Wash your hands.
32. Report to your immediate supervisor:
    - That you have measured the patient's blood pressure
    - The time that you measured the blood pressure
    - Your observations of anything unusual

KEY QUESTIONS

1. What is systolic pressure?
2. What is diastolic pressure?
3. How should aneroid and mercury types of blood pressure equipment be used?
4. What should you do when you measure a patient's blood pressure?
5. Define: aneroid sphygmomanometer, blood pressure, diastolic blood pressure, mercury sphygmomanometer, stethoscope, sphygmomanometer, systolic blood pressure.

CHAPTER 26

Anatomy and Physiology of the Gastrointestinal System

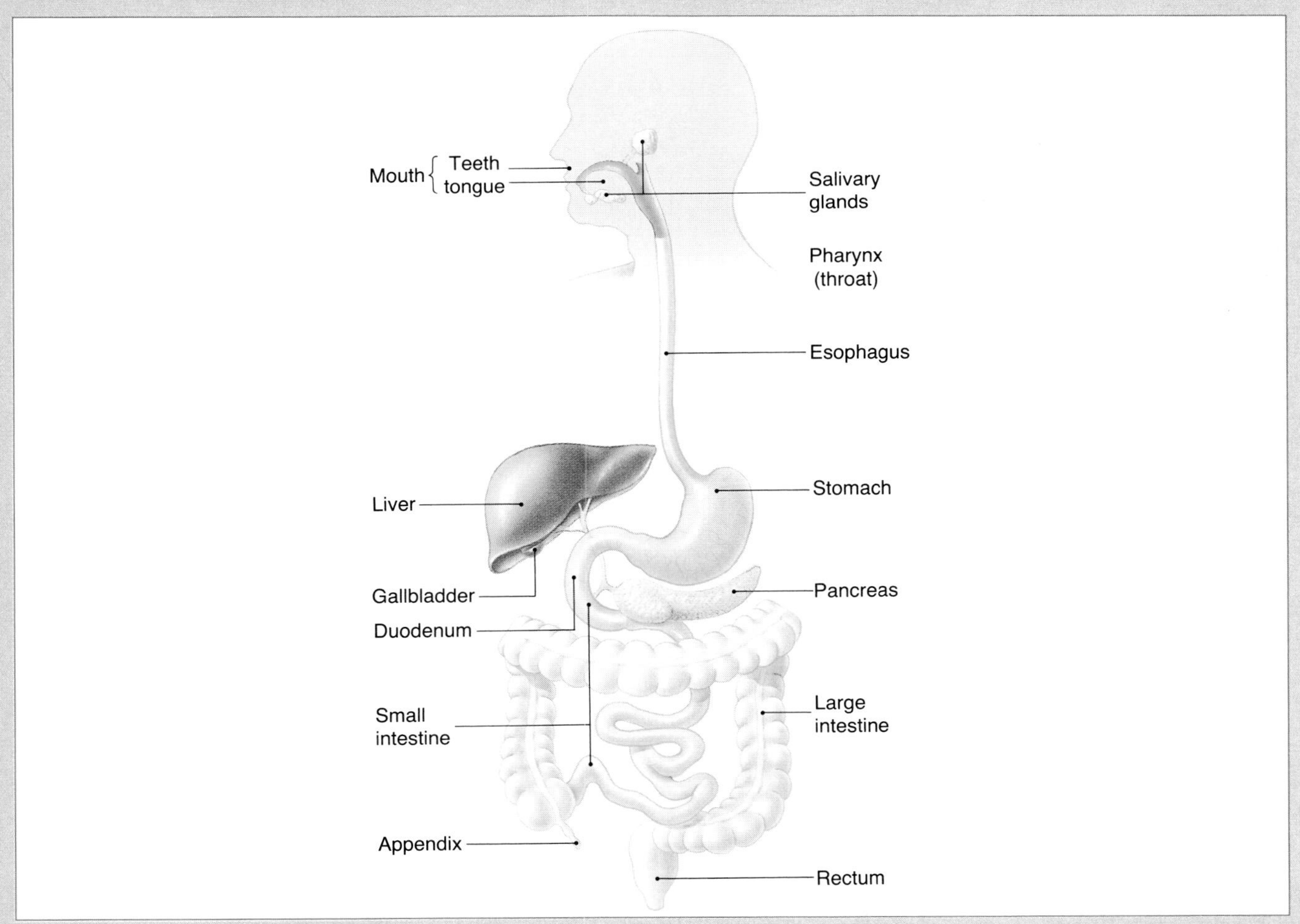

WARNING

For all patient contact, adhere to Universal Precautions (see page 91, 97, or the front cover flap). Wear protective equipment as indicated.

Objectives

What You Will Learn

When you have completed this chapter, you will be able to:

- Label a diagram showing the organs of the digestive system.
- Explain how each organ helps in the process of digestion.
- List the end products of digestion.
- Describe the responsibilities of the liver.
- List common diseases and disorders of the gastrointestinal system.
- Define: digestion, gastrointestinal system, liver, rectum, saliva, villus.

KEY IDEAS

The Digestive System (Gastrointestinal System)

Gastrointestinal System
The group of body organs that carries out digestion; the digestive system. Sometimes called the GI system; an abbreviation for gastro (stomach) and intestinal.

Digestion
The process in the body in which food is broken down mechanically and chemically and is changed into forms that can enter the bloodstream and be used by the body.

Saliva
The secretion of the salivary glands into the mouth. Saliva moistens food and helps in swallowing. It also contains an enzyme (chemical) that helps digest starches.

Absorption
The process of the end products of digestion entering the blood stream.

THE **GASTROINTESTINAL SYSTEM** is responsible for breaking down the food that is eaten into a form that can be used by the body cells. This action is both chemical and mechanical. The digestive tract is about 30 feet long. All of it is important in reducing food to simple compounds.

Digestion begins in the mouth, where food is chewed and mixed with the substance called **saliva** that contains chemicals that begin to act on the food being chewed. During swallowing, the food moves in a moistened ball down the esophagus to the stomach. The stomach churns and mixes the food at the same time it is being broken down chemically. The most important area of digestion is the *duodenum*, the first loop of the *small intestine*, where **absorption** begins. It is here that the digestive juices, not only from the duodenum itself but also from the pancreas, finish the job of breaking down food into usable parts. In addition, bile, which has been stored in the gallbladder after being manufactured in the liver, also enters the duodenum and helps the reduction process.

A large amount of water is necessary for the chemical reduction of food into its end products. The food is moved by rhythmic contraction, called *peristalsis*, of the muscle walls of the organs of digestion. The next step is absorption.

Some of the final products of digestion are absorbed in the area of the duodenum. These end products are:

- Amino acids, the building blocks for all growth and repair of body tissue, which come from dietary proteins
- Fatty acids and glycerols, from fat
- Simple sugars, such as glucose, from carbohydrates
- Water and vitamins

The lining of the duodenum is composed of thousands of tiny finger-like projections called **villi** (singular, **villus**) (Figure 26-1). Each villus is

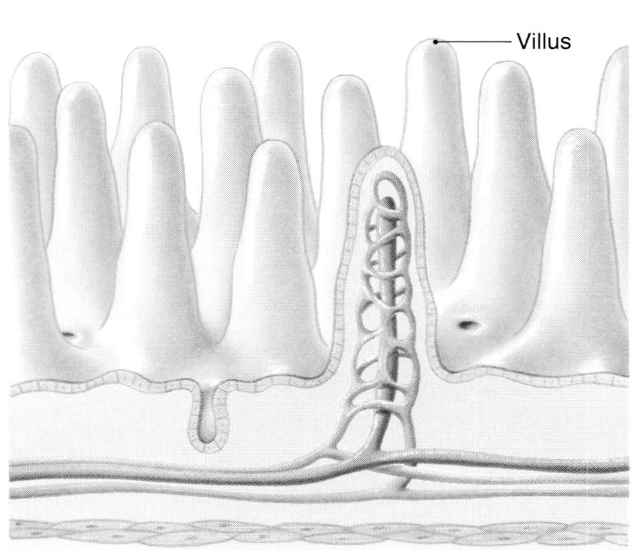

FIGURE 26-1 Internal view of the structure of the small intestine.

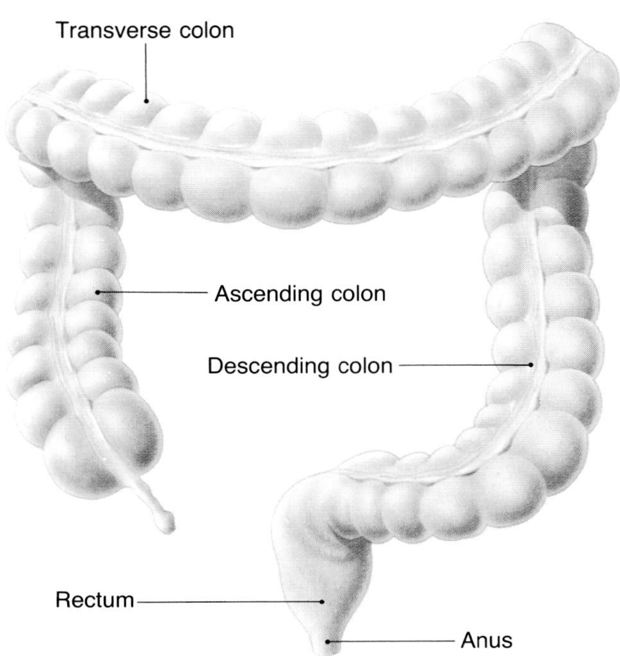

FIGURE 26-2 The large intestine.

Villus
A tiny, fingerlike projection in the lining of the small intestine into which the end products of digestion are absorbed and carried to the bloodstream and then to the individual cells.

Liver
The body's largest gland, located in the abdominal cavity. The liver has many functions in the chemistry and metabolism of the body and is essential to life.

Rectum
The lower 8 to 10 inches of the colon. The anus is the body opening from the rectum.

capable of absorbing these end products of digestion. The products are then moved into the bloodstream, where they are carried to individual cells.

Some digestion continues to take place in other parts of the small intestine. What is left of the food moves through the large intestine, where water is reabsorbed into the body. The material that cannot be used by the body is excreted from the rectum through the anus as feces.

The **liver** has important responsibilities aside from manufacturing bile. The liver is a storage area for glucose, a form of sugar released in large amounts when the cells need it for energy to carry on their activities. The liver also is the place where toxins, or poisons, are removed from the blood. Damage to the liver can be caused by drinking alcoholic beverages or taking drugs that are harmful to its tissues. The liver is also responsible for the production and storage of some proteins that are necessary for proper blood circulation and for blood clotting. Blood clots are not all bad. When a blood vessel has been injured, a clot may form that holds the blood within a closed tube (the blood vessel) until healing occurs.

On the lower right side of the colon, at the junction between the small intestine and the large intestine, known as the cecum, there is a pouch with a projection of tissue called the *appendix*. Because there is very little peristalsis in this area, the appendix has a tendency to become infected, in a condition known as appendicitis. Surgery is usually performed to correct this condition.

The lowest portion of the large intestine curves in an S-shape into the **rectum** (Figure 26-2). The rectum is made of very delicate tissue. It has an internal sphincter muscle and an external sphincter muscle. A sphincter is a ring-shaped muscle that surrounds and controls a natural opening in the body, such as the anus. Sometimes blood vessels that supply this area become enlarged and filled with blood clots, causing hemorrhoids.

Common Disorders and Diseases of the Gastrointestinal System

- *Malignancies:* cancerous tumors can occur anywhere and in any organ of the gastrointestinal system
- *Ulcers:* gastric (stomach) ulcers, duodenal ulcers, and ulcerative colitis; lesions of mucous membrane exposed to digestive juices
- *Hernias:* occur when there is a weakness in the walls of the muscle and underlying tissue pushes through
- *Gallbladder disorders*
    - *Cholecystitis:* inflammation of the gallbladder
    - *Cholelithiasis:* stones in the gallbladder
- *Constipation:* decrease in the frequency of bowel movements
- *Diarrhea:* increase in the frequency of bowel movements
- *Appendicitis:* inflammation of the appendix
- *Peritonitis:* inflammation of the peritoneal cavity
- *Intestinal obstruction:* interruption in the normal flow of intestinal contents along the gastrointestinal tract
- *Hemorrhoids:* varicose veins of the anal canal or outside the external sphincter
- *Hepatitis:* inflammation of the liver caused by viruses
- *Hepatic cirrhosis:* chronic disease of the liver
- *Jaundice:* abnormal high concentration of bilirubin in the blood, which is excreted by liver cells, causing a yellow discoloration of the skin, mucous membranes, and sclerae of the eyes

KEY QUESTIONS

1. Label a diagram showing the organs of the digestive system.
2. How does each organ help in the process of digestion?
3. What are the end products of digestion?
4. What are the responsibilities of the liver?
5. What are the common diseases and disorders of the gastrointestinal system?
6. Define: digestion, gastrointestinal system, liver, rectum, saliva, villus.

CHAPTER

27

Therapeutic Diets

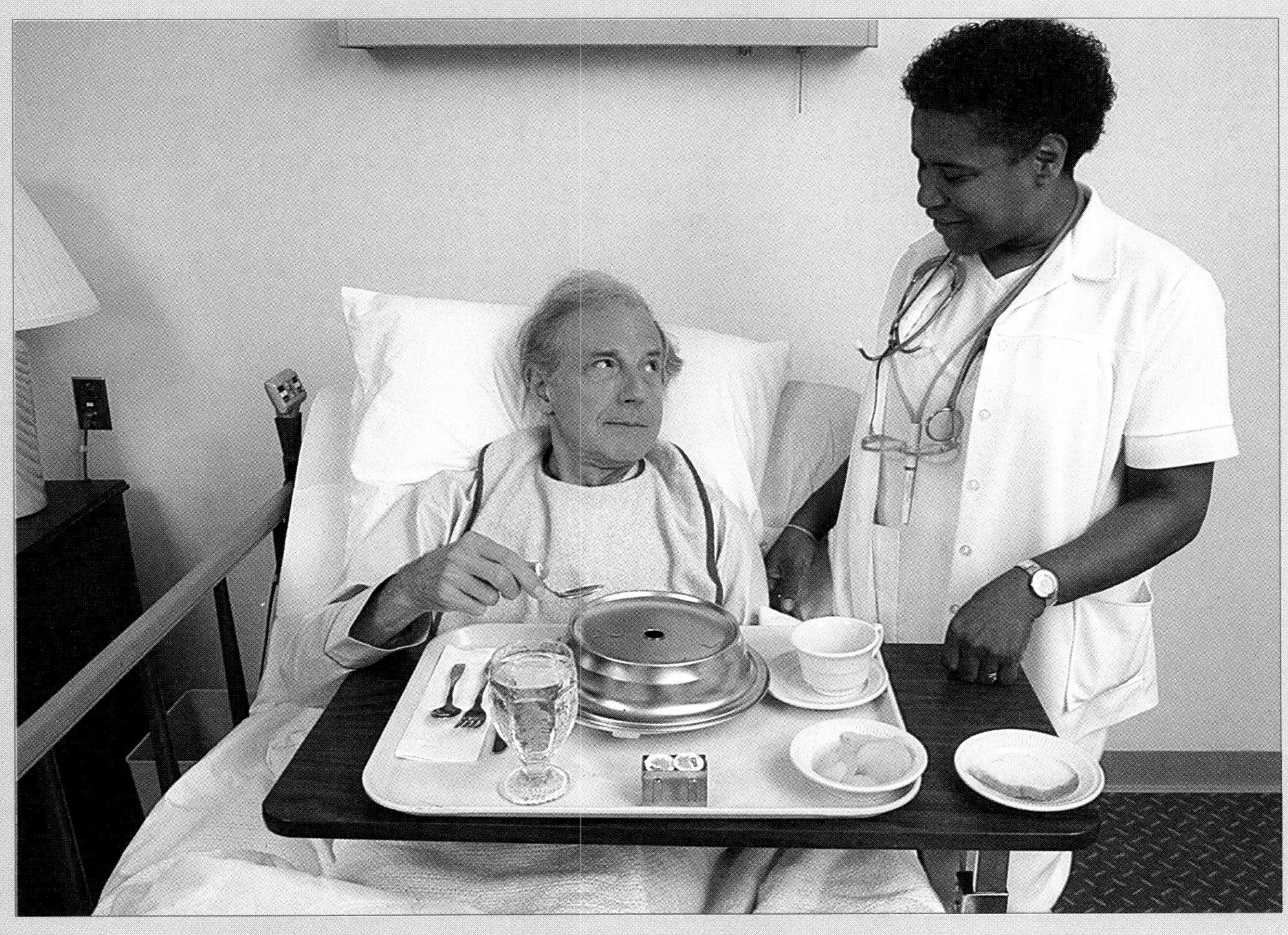

WARNING

For all patient contact, adhere to Universal Precautions (see page 91, 97, or the front cover flap). Wear protective equipment as indicated.

Objectives

What You Will Learn

When you have completed this chapter, you will be able to:

- Define a well-balanced diet.
- Name the basic food groups and give examples of some foods included in each group.
- Name the six classes of nutrients and give examples of the bodily function for which each is used.
- List food sources for each nutrient.
- List and describe the various types of therapeutic diets and explain the purpose of each type.
- Give some reasons the doctor may order changes in the regular diet.
- Define: calories, dietitian, nourishment, nutrients, restricted, therapeutic diet.

KEY IDEAS

A Well-Balanced Diet

THE KEY TO A HEALTHY, WELL-BALANCED diet lies in eating the correct amounts of a variety of foods. The foods that are essential for keeping the body well are divided into groups (Figure 27-1). If you eat the recommended number of portions of foods from each group on the pyramid every day, your diet will be adequate for good health. The number and size of portions will depend on the age, size, and activities of the individual.

- **Breads, cereals, rice, and pasta** provide carbohydrates for energy. One slice of bread, one-half cup of cooked rice or pasta, one-half cup of cooked cereal, or one ounce of ready-to-eat cereal constitutes one serving. The U.S. Department of Agriculture recommends six to eleven servings per day from this group.

- **Vegetables** supply vitamins, minerals, and roughage. One-half cup of chopped raw or cooked vegetables or one cup of leafy raw vegetables constitutes one serving. The U.S. Department of Agriculture recommends three to five servings per day from this group.

- **Fruits** also supply vitamins, minerals, and roughage. One piece of fruit or a melon wedge, three-quarters cup of juice, one-half cup of canned fruit, or one-quarter cup of dried fruit constitutes one serving. The U.S. Department of Agriculture recommends two to four servings per day from this group.

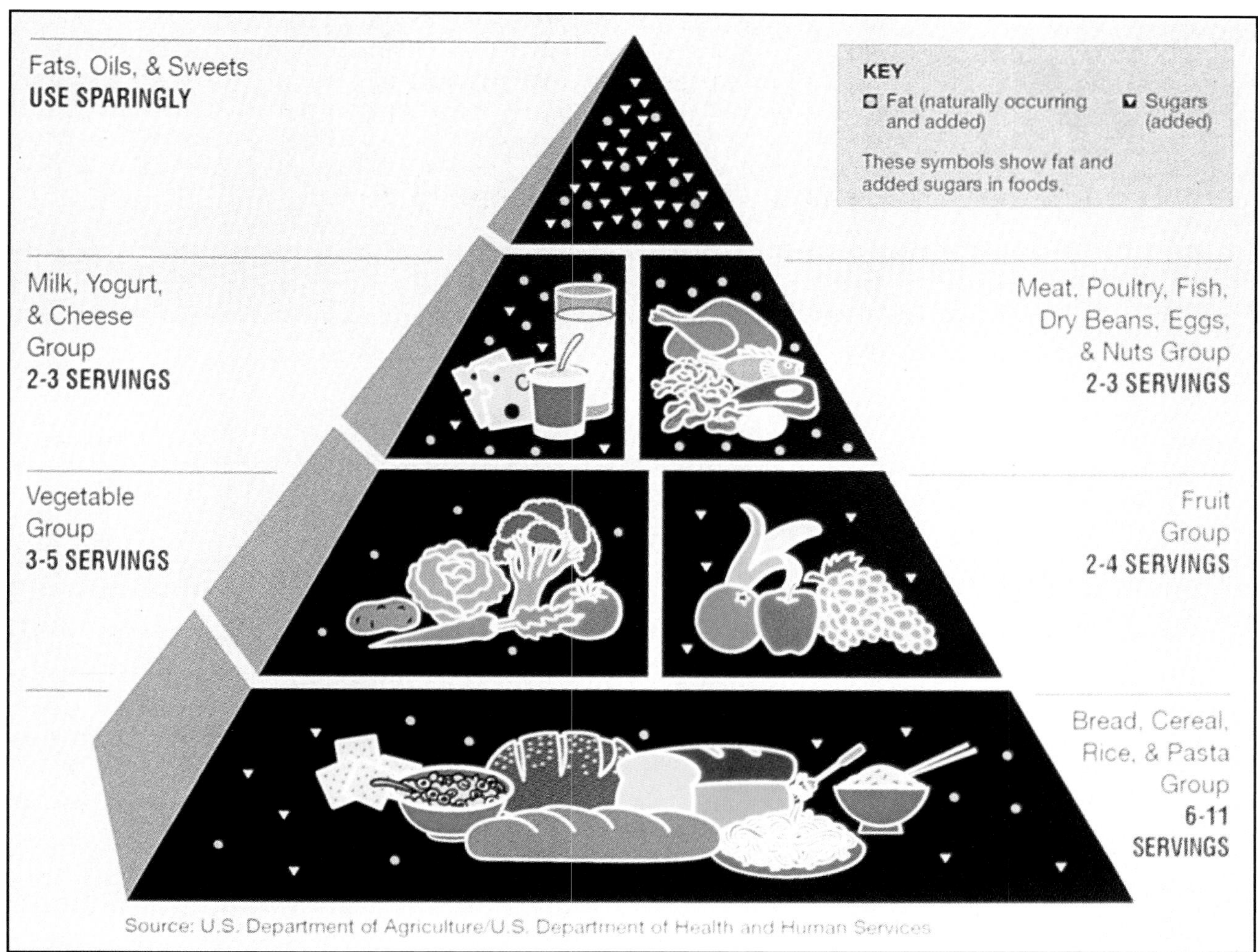

FIGURE 27-1 The food group pyramid.

- **Milk, yogurt, and cheese** provide protein, calcium, and other minerals plus vitamins and carbohydrates. One cup of milk or yogurt or one and a half to two ounces of cheese constitutes one serving. The U.S. Department of Agriculture recommends two to three servings per day from this group.

- **Meat, poultry, fish, dry beans, eggs, and nuts** provide proteins. Two and a half to three ounces of cooked lean meat, poultry, or fish; one-half cup of cooked beans; one egg; or two tablespoons of peanut butter constitutes one serving. The U.S. Department of Agriculture recommends two to three servings per day from this group.

- **Fats, oils, and sweets** should be eaten sparingly. These foods include salad dressings, cream, butter, margarine, sugars, soft drinks, candies, sweet desserts, and alcoholic beverages. When planning a healthful diet, determine the fat and sugar contents of your choices from all the food groups.

KEY IDEAS

What Are Nutrients?

Nourishment
The process of taking food into the body to maintain life.

Nutrients
Chemical substances found in food. Some 50 individual nutrients are needed to build the body. They work better together than alone. There are six classes of nutrients: carbohydrates, fats, minerals, proteins, vitamins, and water.

Food is able to give **nourishment** to the body because it contains various chemical substances called **nutrients**. Some 50 individual nutrients are needed to build the body. Many others are useful, although they may not be required. Scientists also have discovered that nutrients work better together than alone. For instance, you may get enough calcium from milk but it is wasted if you do not get enough vitamin C or D from other foods to help the calcium develop the bones.

Many foods we eat contain combinations of various nutrients that are responsible for body functions. For example, whole-grain cereals are high in carbohydrates, but they also contain some protein, minerals, and vitamins. Foods help the body perform its functions only if they contain the right nutrients.

NUTRIENT CLASS	BODILY FUNCTION	FOOD SOURCES
CARBOHYDRATES	Provides work energy for body activities, and heat energy for maintenance of body temperature.	Cereal grains and their products (bread, breakfast cereals, macaroni products), potatoes, sugar, syrups, fruits, milk, vegetables, nuts.
PROTEINS	Build and renew body tissues; regulate body functions and supply energy. Complete proteins: maintain life and provide growth. Incomplete proteins: maintain life but do not provide for growth.	Complete proteins: Derived from animal foods — meat, milk plus eggs, fish, cheese, poultry. Incomplete proteins: Derived from vegetable foods — soybeans, dry beans, peas, some nuts and whole-grain products.
FATS	Give work energy for body activities and heat energy for maintenance of body temperature. Carrier of vitamins A,D,E, and K, provide fatty acids necessary for growth and maintenance of body tissues.	Some foods are chiefly fat, such as lard, vegetable fats and oils, and butter. Many other foods contain variable proportions of fats — nuts, meats, fish, poultry, cream, whole milk.
MINERALS Calcium	Builds and renews bones, teeth, and other tissues; regulates the activity of the muscles, heart, nerves; and controls the clotting of blood.	Milk and milk products, except butter; most dark green vegetables; canned salmon.
Phosphorus	Associated with calcium in some functions needed to build and renew bones and teeth. Influences the oxidation of foods in the body cells; important in nerve tissue.	Widely distributed in foods; especially cheese, oat cereals, whole-wheat products, dry beans and peas, meat, fish, poultry, nuts.

FIGURE 27-2
Functions and sources of basic nutrients.

How Nutrients Are Made

The first step in making nutrients takes place in green plants. They take water and minerals from the soil and water and carbon dioxide from the air. With the help of the sun's energy, these substances are built into nutrients.

How Nutrients Are Used

When people eat plants, they get the nutrients from them. Also, when people eat meat, they get the nutrients that animals have taken from green plants.

FIGURE 27-2 (cont.)

NUTRIENT CLASS	BODILY FUNCTION	FOOD SOURCES
MINERALS (Continued) **Iron**	Builds and renews hemoglobin, the red pigment in blood which carries oxygen from the lungs to the cells.	Eggs, meat, especially liver and kidney; deep-yellow and dark green vegetables; potatoes, dried fruits, whole-grain products; enriched flour, bread, breakfast cereals.
Iodine	Enables the thyroid gland to perform its function of controlling the rate at which foods are oxidized in the cells.	Fish (obtained from the sea), some plant-foods grown in soils containing iodine; table salt fortified with iodine (iodized).
VITAMINS **A**	Necessary for normal functioning of the eyes, prevents night blindness. Ensures a healthy condition of the skin, hair, and mucous membranes. Maintains a state of resistance to infections of the eyes, mouth, and respiratory tract.	One form of Vitamin A is yellow and one form is colorless. Apricots, cantaloupe, milk, cheese, eggs, meat organs, (especially liver and kidney), fortified margarine, butter, fish-liver oils, dark green and deep yellow vegetables.
B Complex **B_1 (Thiamine)**	Maintains a healthy condition of the nerves. Fosters a good appetite. Helps the body cells use carbohydrates.	Whole-grain and enriched grain products; meats (especially pork, liver and kidney). Dry beans and peas.
B_2 (Riboflavin)	Keeps the skin, mouth, and eyes in a healthy condition. Acts with other nutrients to form enzymes and control oxidation in cells.	Milk, cheese, eggs, meat (especially liver and kidney), whole grain and enriched grain products, dark green vegetables.

NUTRIENT CLASS	BODILY FUNCTION	FOOD SOURCES
VITAMINS (Continued) Niacin B_3	Influences the oxidation of carbohydrates and proteins in the body cells.	Liver, meat, fish, poultry, eggs, peanuts; dark green vegetables, whole-grain and enriched cereal products.
B_6	Aids the body in absorbing and using proteins. Helps the body use fats. Assists in the formation of red blood cells.	Whole grain (not enriched) cereals and bread, liver, avocados, spinach, green beans, bananas, fish, poultry, meats, nuts, potatoes, green leafy vegetables
B_{12}	Regulates specific processes in digestion. Helps maintain normal functions of muscles, nerves, heart, blood — general body metabolism.	Liver, other organ meats, cheese, eggs, milk.
C (Ascorbic Acid)	Acts as a cement between body cells, and helps them work together to carry out their special functions. Maintains a sound condition of bones, teeth, and gums. Not stored in the body.	Fresh raw citrus fruits and vegetables — oranges, grapefruit, cantaloupe, strawberries, tomatoes, raw onions, cabbage, green and sweet red peppers, dark green vegetables.
D	Enables the growing body to use calcium and phosphorus in a normal way to build bones and teeth.	Provided by Vitamin D fortification of certain foods, such as milk and margarine. Also fish-liver oils and eggs. Sunshine is also a source of Vitamin D.
WATER	Regulates body processes. Aids in regulating body temperature. Carries nutrients to body cells and carries waste products away from them. Helps to lubricate joints. Water has no food value, although most water contains mineral elements. More immediately necessary to life than food — second only to oxygen.	Drinking water, and other beverages; all foods except those made up of a single nutrient, (sugar and some fats). Milk, milk drinks, soups, vegetables, fruit juices, ice cream, watermelon, strawberries, lettuce, tomatoes, cereals.

FIGURE 27-2 (cont.)

After food is eaten, it enters the digestive tract where the nutrients are changed into simple forms. These simple forms are then carried by the blood to the body cells, where the special functions of each are carried out.

There are six classes of nutrients: carbohydrates, fats, minerals, proteins, vitamins, and water. Because there are several kinds of each class of nutrients except water, it is clearer to speak of the classes instead of the individual nutrients. Figure 27-2 gives a brief description of each nutrient class and its bodily function.

KEY IDEAS

Regular and Special Diets

Eating properly is very important when you are healthy and feeling well. Good nourishment is even more important when a person is ill. The food service department or dietary department in your institution will be preparing a well-balanced diet of nourishing meals for many different patients. This basic balanced diet is often called by different names:

- Normal diet
- Regular diet
- House diet
- Full diet

A well-balanced diet is one that contains a variety of food from each of the four basic food groups at every meal.

The regular diet is sometimes changed to meet a patient's special nutritional needs. This modified diet is also known by several names:

Therapeutic Diet
A diet designed to meet a patient's special nutritional needs; also called special diet, restricted diet, modified diet.

Restricted
Not permitted.

- **Therapeutic diet**
- Special diet
- **Restricted diet**
- Modified diet

Dietitian
Plans well-balanced, nourishing diets, designed to meet the needs of individual patients.

Calories
Units for measuring the energy produced when food is oxidized in the body.

Therapeutic diets require the preparation of meals that differ from those prepared for patients on the regular diet. The special meals given to patients who cannot be on a normal diet are ordered by the doctor. They are worked out by the **dietitian** according to the patient's illness and what is needed for his or her recovery. These special meals help the doctor in treating a patient. For example, a man who has a disorder of his digestive system may be on a soft or high-fiber diet. A diabetic patient may be on a diet in which total **calories** are limited and the amounts of protein, fat, and carbohydrates are specified. A person with heart disease may be restricted to a low-salt (sodium) diet or a salt-free diet. The doctor may order changes in the regular diet for several reasons. These include:

- Changing the consistency of the patient's food, as in liquid or "soft" diets
- Changing the caloric intake, as in high- or low-calorie diets
- Changing the amounts of one or more nutrients, as in a high-protein, low-fat, or low-salt (sodium) diet
- Changing the amount of bulk, as in a low-residue diet
- Changing the seasonings in the patient's food, as in a bland diet
- Omitting foods that the patient is allergic to
- Changing the time and number of meals

Whenever the word salt is used, it means sodium and when sodium is used, it means salt. Therefore, when we refer to a salt-free diet, we mean a sodium-free diet, and when we refer to a low-sodium diet, we mean a low-salt diet.

Types of Diets Given to Patients; What They Are and Why They Are Used		
Type of Diet	Description	Common Purpose
Regular	Provides all essentials of good nourishment in normal forms	For patients who do not need special diets
Clear liquid	Broth, tea, ginger ale, gelatin	Usually for patients who have had surgery or are very ill
Full liquid	Broth, tea, coffee, ginger ale, gelatin, strained fruit juices, liquids, custard, ice cream, sherbet, pudding, soft-cooked eggs	For those unable to chew or swallow solid food
Light or soft	Foods soft in consistency; no rich or strongly flavored foods that could cause distress	Final stage for postoperative patient before resuming regular diet
Soft (mechanical)	Same foods as on a normal diet but chopped or strained	For patients who have difficulty in chewing or swallowing
Bland	Foods mild in flavor and easy to digest; omits spicy foods	Avoids irritation of the digestive tract, as with ulcer and colitis patients
Low residue	Foods low in fiber and bulk; omits foods difficult to digest	Spares the lower digestive tract, as with patients having rectal diseases
High residue/fiber		
High calorie	Foods high in protein, carbohydrates, minerals, and vitamins	For underweight or malnourished patients
Low calorie	Low in cream, butter, cereals, desserts, and fats	For patients who need to lose weight
Diabetic	Precise balance of carbohydrates, protein, and fats, devised according to the needs of the individual patients	For diabetic patients; matches food intake with the insulin nutritional requirements
High protein	Meals supplemented with high-protein foods, such as meat, fish, cheese, milk, and eggs	Assists in the growth and repair of tissues wasted by disease
Low fat	Limited amounts of butter, cream, fats, and eggs; no fried foods, less fatty meats, lowfat milk	For patients who have difficulty digesting fats, as in gallbladder, cardiovascular, and liver disturbances
Low cholesterol	Low in eggs, whole milk, and meats	Helps regulate the amount of cholesterol in the blood
Low sodium (low salt)	Limited amounts of foods containing sodium; no salt allowed on tray	For patients whose circulation would be impaired by fluid retention; patients with certain heart or kidney conditions
Salt-free (sodium-free)	Completely without salt	
Tube feeding	Specialized formulas or liquid forms of nutrients given to the patient through a tube; follow with a glass of water at room temperature	For patients who, because of a condition such as oral surgery or decreased level of consciousness, cannot eat normally

KEY QUESTIONS

1. What is meant by a well-balanced diet?
2. What are the basic food groups? Give examples of some foods included in each.
3. What are the six classes of nutrients? Give examples of bodily functions for which each is used.
4. Which foods are good sources for each nutrient?
5. List and describe the various types of therapeutic diets. Explain the purpose of each type.
6. Why might the doctor order changes in the regular diet?
7. Define: calories, dietitian, nourishment, nutrients, restricted, therapeutic diet.

CHAPTER

28 Nutrition for the Patient

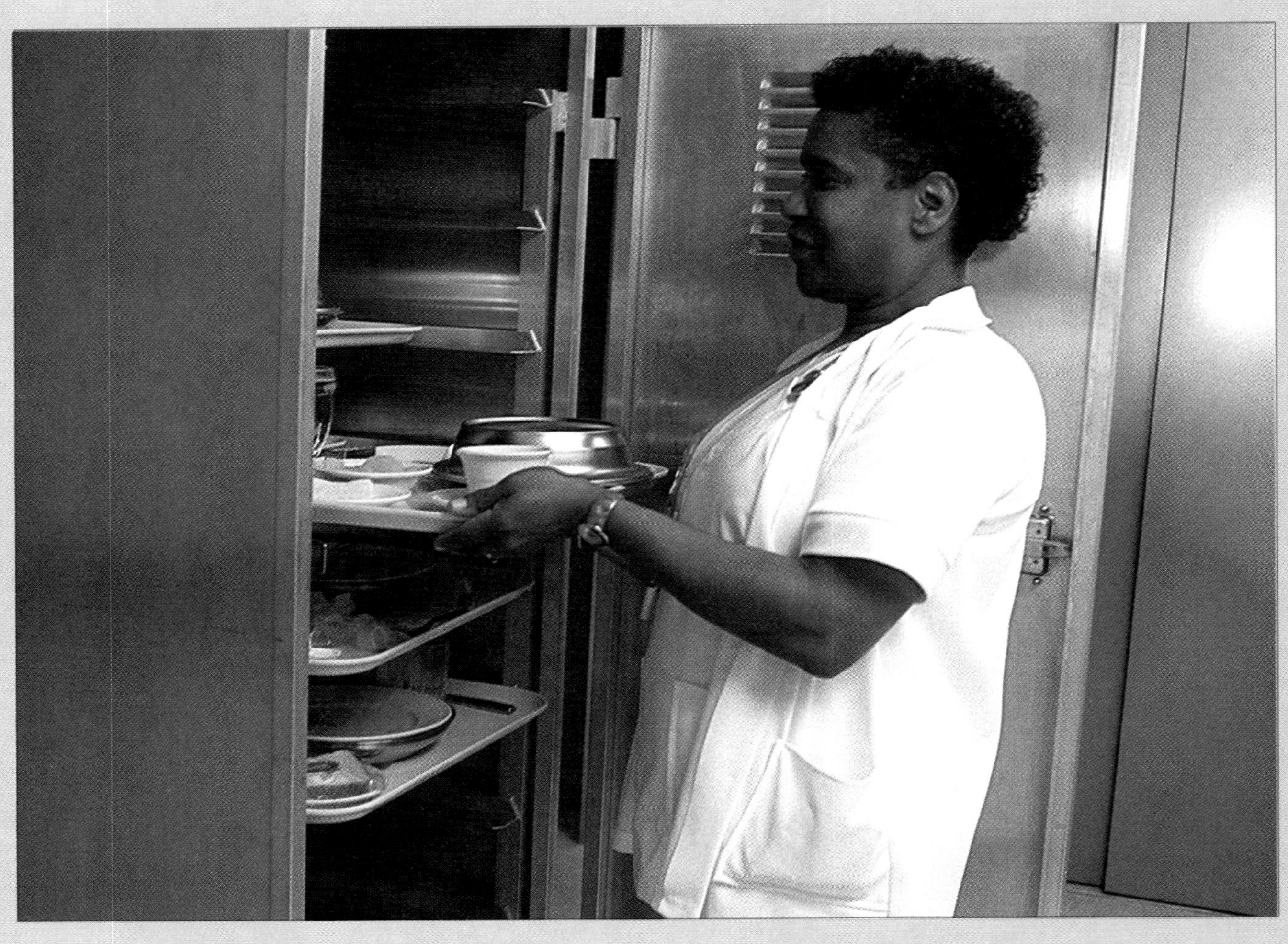

WARNING

For all patient contact, adhere to Universal Precautions (see page 91, 97, or the front cover flap). Wear protective equipment as indicated.

Objectives

What You Will Learn

When you have completed this chapter, you will be able to:

- Prepare the patient before mealtime.
- Serve the food tray.
- Observe and record information concerning meals.
- Feed the patient who is handicapped or unable to feed himself.
- Serve between-meal nourishment.
- Distribute drinking water.
- Define: appetite, discard, extra nourishment, omit.

KEY IDEAS

Preparing the Patient and Serving a Meal

Appetite
Desire for food or drink.

A POOR **APPETITE** DOES NOT MEAN that the body's need for food is lowered. The sick person's body is in a weakened condition. The patient needs as much food as ever, if not more, to return to health. The surroundings and the food served should be as cheerful, attractive, and appetizing as possible. The sight and aroma of food often make a person hungry. You often can increase a patient's appetite by showing him

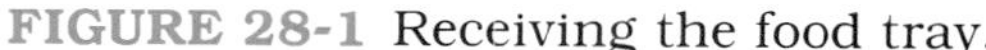

FIGURE 28-1 Receiving the food tray.

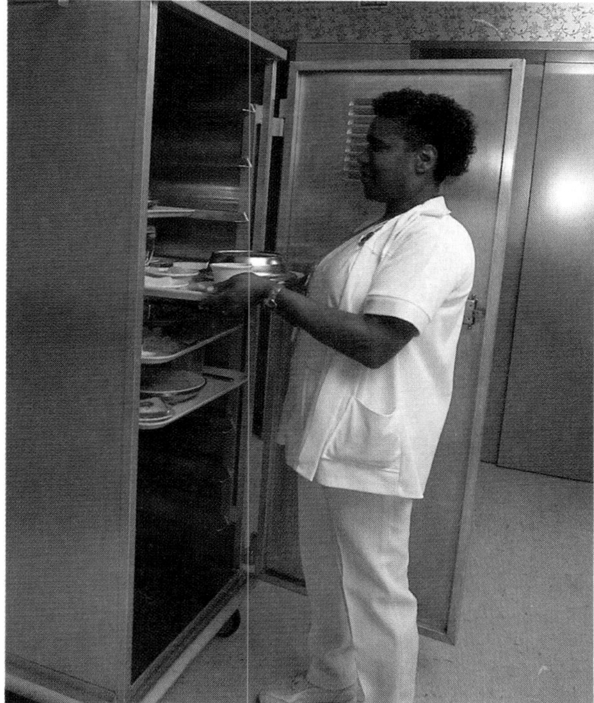

what he will be eating. People have a better appetite for foods they especially like; therefore, if a patient asks for a particular food (and if he is permitted to have it), you should try to arrange for that food to be served to him. You can do this by reporting the patient's request to your immediate supervisor.

Mealtime is often one of the highlights of the day for a convalescent patient or a patient who is not extremely sick. Mealtime is a break in the often boring routine and gives the patient something to look forward to. Many patients also enjoy making food selections from the menu, when choices are offered. This is another time when attitude is important. If the patient seems to want you to, look at the menu with her and make suggestions. When the food tray is delivered (Figure 28-1), do everything you can to make the patient's meal as pleasant and comfortable as possible.

As you know, eating in a pleasant, attractive place helps you enjoy your food. This is also true for the hospital patient. When a patient is going to have a meal, be sure the room is clean, quiet, free of unpleasant odors, and not too warm or cold. Take away things that might spoil the patient's appetite—items such as an emesis basin, urinal, or bedpan.

Procedure Preparing the Patient for a Meal

1. Assemble your equipment on the bedside table:
   a) Bedpan or urinal
   b) Basin of warm water at 115°F (46.1°C)
   c) Washcloth
   d) Towel
   e) Robe and slippers
2. Wash your hands.
3. Identify the patient by checking the identification bracelet.
4. Ask visitors to step out of the room, if this is your hospital's policy.
5. Tell the patient you are getting him ready for his next meal.
6. Pull the curtain around the bed for privacy.
7. Offer the bedpan or urinal or assist the patient to the bathroom.
8. Have the patient wash his hands or do this for him.
9. Raise the backrest so the patient is in a sitting position, if this is allowed. If not, you might prop up his head by using several pillows.
10. Clear the overbed table. Put it in a convenient position for the patient's meal.
11. If the patient wants to sit in a chair during his meal and if this is allowed, help him into his robe and slippers, and help him out of bed and to the chair.
12. Make the patient comfortable.
13. Lower the bed to a position of safety for the patient.
14. Pull the curtains back to the open position.
15. Raise the side rails where ordered, indicated, and appropriate for patient safety.
16. Place the call light within easy reach of the patient.
17. Wash your hands.
18. Report to your immediate supervisor:
    - That the patient is ready for his or her next meal
    - How the patient tolerated the procedure
    - Your observations of anything unusual.

Procedure Serving the Food

1. Wash your hands.
2. Check the tray before you give it to a patient. Is everything on it? All the silverware and a napkin? Does the tray look attractive? Was food spilled? Correct anything that is wrong.
3. Be sure you are giving the tray to the right patient. Check the menu card, which will have the patient's name on it, against the identification band to be sure they match (Figure 28-2).

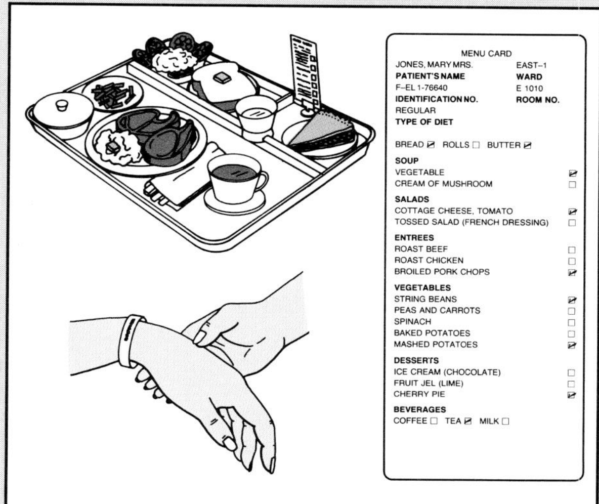

FIGURE 28-2

4. Put the tray on the overbed table. Adjust it to a height comfortable for the patient.
5. Arrange the dishes and silver so the patient can reach everything easily. Be sure drinking water is handy.
6. Help any patient who needs it (Figure 28-3). For example, if a patient seems to be weak or asks for help, you might offer to spread his napkin on his lap or tuck it under his chin. Spread butter on his or her bread. Cut up whatever needs cutting. Pour tea or coffee. Do not give any more help than he or she really needs. The more a patient can do for himself, the better.
7. A patient may discover that he cannot eat when he is served. If permitted, you may take his tray away and keep the hot food warm for him until he wants to eat.
8. When you are sure the patient can go on with his meal by himself, leave the room.

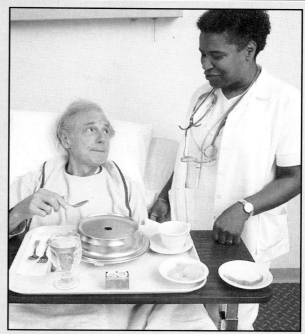

FIGURE 28-3

9. Go back for the food tray when the patient has finished eating.
10. Note how much the patient has eaten and how much he has had to drink.
11. Record the intake for those patients who are on intake and output on the intake and output sheet.
12. Record how the patient has eaten his meal on the daily activity flow sheet. Record this information separately for breakfast, lunch, and supper:
    a) Did the patient eat all the food served to him?
    b) Did the patient eat about half the food served?
    c) Did the patient eat very little food?
    d) Did the patient refuse to accept the tray and actually eat nothing?
13. Take the tray away and put it in its proper place.
14. If the patient ate sitting in a chair, help him back into bed.
15. Put the patient's personal articles back where he wants them.
16. If the patient ate in bed, brush crumbs from the bed, smooth out the sheets, and straighten the bedding.
17. Make the patient comfortable.

18. Lower the bed to a position of safety for the patient.
19. Pull the curtains back to the open position.
20. Raise the side rails where ordered, indicated, and appropriate for patient safety.
21. Place the call light within easy reach of the patient.
22. Wash your hands.
23. Report to your immediate supervisor:
    - That you have served the patient his or her food
    - The amount of food eaten (all, half, or refused to eat)
    - Your observations of anything unusual

KEY IDEAS

Feeding the Handicapped Patient

Some patients are incapable of feeding themselves and, therefore, will have to be fed. The reason might be:

- The patient cannot use his hands.
- The doctor wants the patient to save his strength and to be on "complete bed rest."
- The patient may be too weak to feed himself.
- The patient may have difficulties with swallowing (for example, due to a stroke or cleft palate) and may need assistance.

Usually, it is hard for an adult to accept the idea of not being able to feed himself. Because a patient is physically challenged or handicapped, he may feel resentful and depressed. Be friendly and natural. Help the patient by encouraging him to do as much as he can. Also, remember that because of medical reasons the patient may not always be allowed to help. You will learn how to judge the amount of help a patient can give you when he is being fed. For example, if a patient is strong enough, you might let him hold a piece of bread.

When feeding a challenged patient, the most important thing is not to rush him through the meal. The time he takes to chew his food, for example, may seem long to you, but he is probably very weak; otherwise, he would be feeding himself.

Remember that you should not bring the food tray or have it delivered until you have prepared the patient for his meal and are ready to feed him. Again, make sure you are serving the correct tray to the patient. Preparations before mealtime are the same for the challenged patient who cannot feed himself. Be observant throughout. Watch for signs of choking or anything unusual.

Procedure Feeding the Handicapped Patient or the Patient Who Is Unable to Feed Himself

1. Assemble your equipment on the overbed table:
   a) The patient's tray
2. Wash your hands.
3. Check the name on the card on the tray against the patient's identification bracelet.
4. Tell the patient you are going to feed him his meal.
5. If you plan to be seated while you feed the patient, bring a chair to a convenient position beside the bed.
6. Check the tray to make sure everything

is there. If anything is missing, have it brought in or get it yourself.

7. Tuck a napkin under the patient's chin.
8. Season the food the way the patient likes it. But do this only if his request agrees with the prescribed diet.
9. For most patients unable to feed themselves you will use a spoon. Fill the spoon only half-full. Give the food to the patient from the tip of the spoon, not the side. Put the food in one side of the patient's mouth so he can chew it more easily. If a patient is paralyzed on one side of his body, make sure you feed him on the side of his mouth that is not paralyzed.
10. If the patient cannot see the tray, name each mouthful of food as you offer it (Figure 28-4). Offer the different foods in a logical order, soup or juice before the main course. Alternate between liquids and solid foods throughout the meal. Feed the patient as you yourself would want to eat. Or follow the patient's suggestions about how he wants to alternate between various kinds of foods and a beverage.

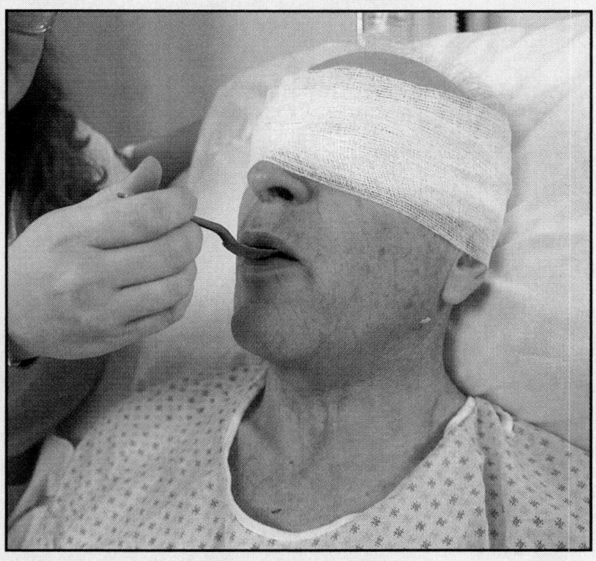

FIGURE 28-4

11. If the patient is unable to see and would like to feed himself, you can describe the position of the food on his tray. For example, cold liquids are in the left corner, hot liquids in the right corner. Tell him to picture his plate as the face of a clock, corn at the 3, mashed potatoes at the 6, roast beef at the 12. Try to maintain the patient's independence as much as possible.
12. Warn the patient if you are offering something hot. Use a straw for giving liquids (Figure 28-5). Use a new straw for each beverage.

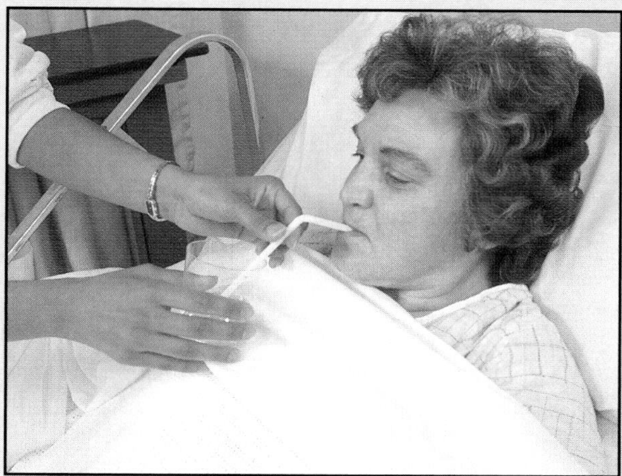

FIGURE 28-5

13. Feed the patient slowly. Remember that he may chew and swallow very slowly. Allow plenty of time between mouthfuls.
14. Encourage the patient to finish his meal, but do not force him.
15. When the patient has finished eating, help him to wipe his mouth with his napkin, or do this for him.
16. Note how much the patient has eaten and how much he has had to drink.
17. Record fluid intake on the intake and output sheet, when the patient is on intake and output.
18. Record how the patient has eaten his meal on the daily activity sheet. Record this information separately for breakfast, lunch, and supper:
    a) Did the patient eat all the food served to him?
    b) Did the patient eat about one-half the food served?
    c) Did the patient eat very little food?
    d) Did the patient refuse the tray and actually eat nothing?
19. As soon as you are sure the patient is finished with the tray, take it away. Put it in its proper place.

20. Adjust the backrest of the bed to make the patient comfortable, if this is allowed.
21. Brush crumbs from the bed, smooth the sheets, and straighten the bedding.
22. Make the patient comfortable.
23. Lower the bed to a position of safety for the patient.
24. Pull the curtains back to the open position.
25. Raise the side rails where ordered, indicated, and appropriate for patient safety.
26. Place the call light within easy reach of the patient.
27. Wash your hands.
28. Report to your immediate supervisor:
    - That you have fed the patient
    - Your observations of anything unusual

KEY IDEAS

Between-Meal Nourishments

Extra Nourishment
Snacks.

Extra nourishment in the form of food or drink is offered to patients during the day. This is a hospital "snack" given to patients to provide energy or to break the routine. Patients are often given extra nourishment as part of their medical care. The snack is usually a beverage such as white milk, chocolate milk, or fruit juice. Or it may be a portion of food such as gelatin, custard, crackers, or a sandwich. Some patients on special diets are allowed to have only certain kinds and amounts of extra nourishment. Other patients may not be allowed to have anything at all.

In some institutions, extra nourishment is passed out to patients by workers from the food service department. However, you may be assigned this responsibility. If you are, your immediate supervisor will give you a list of patients that will show:

- Those who are not to be given anything
- Those who are allowed to have certain nourishment, such as skim milk or tea
- Those who have no restrictions on their diet

A specific time for serving nourishments to patients on special diets may be given on the nourishment chart. Be sure to follow this time schedule carefully.

Discard
To throw away or get rid of something.

Procedure Serving Between-meal Nourishments

1. Wash your hands.
2. Assemble your equipment on a tray or a cart:
   a) Nourishment
   b) Cup, dish, and a spoon or straw
   c) Napkin
3. Identify the patient by checking the identification bracelet.
4. If the patient has a choice of items, ask her what she wants.
5. Prepare the nourishment.
6. Take the nourishment to the patient on a tray or cart.
7. Encourage the patient to take her nourishment. Help her if she needs it. Offer a straw if this is more convenient.
8. After the patient has finished, collect the tray.
9. **Discard** the disposable equipment.
10. Record the intake for those patients who are on intake and output (Figure 28-6).
11. Make the patient comfortable.
12. Lower the bed to a position of safety for the patient.
13. Pull the curtains back to the open position.

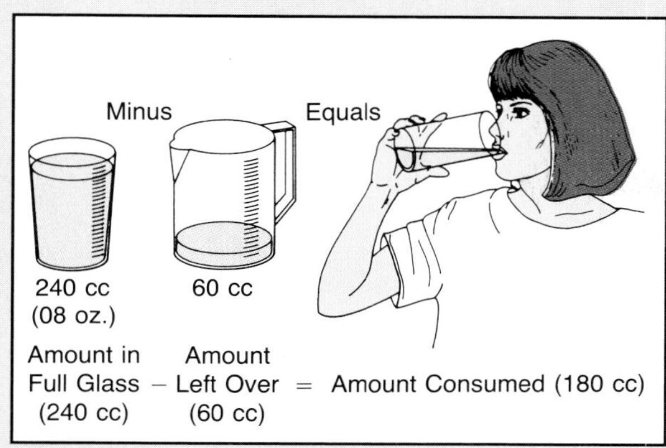

FIGURE 28-6 Determining amounts of liquid consumed.

14. Raise the side rails where ordered, indicated, and appropriate for patient safety.
15. Place the call light within easy reach of the patient.
16. Wash your hands.
17. Report to your immediate supervisor:
    - That you have served the between-meal nourishment
    - Your observations of anything unusual

KEY IDEAS

Passing Drinking Water

Part of your job as a nursing assistant will be to see that the patients you are caring for have plenty of fresh water at their bedsides, unless a doctor orders otherwise. Some patients are not allowed to have more than a certain amount of water. Some, for brief periods, may not have water at all.

Fresh ice water is passed to patients at regular intervals during the day. Your instructor will tell you the schedule of your institution. Disposable pitchers and cups are used everywhere.

Most patients like ice water. Others want water without ice, straight from the tap. You will be told which patients are allowed to have a choice. If a patient is not allowed to have ice, his water pitcher will be tagged **OMIT** ICE. Some patients are allowed ice chips only.

Omit
Leave out.

Procedure Passing Drinking Water

Note: In many institutions each water pitcher is taken individually to the clean kitchen or utility room, filled with clean water and ice, and then returned to each individual patient. When this is done, the following procedure is *not* used. Each water pitcher must be labeled with name and room number.

1. Assemble your equipment:
   a) Moving table (cart) with small Styrofoam ice chest and cover
   b) Ice cubes
   c) Scoop
   d) Paper or Styrofoam cups
   e) Disposable water pitchers
   f) Straws
   g) Paper towels
2. Wash your hands.
3. Fill the ice chest with ice cubes and cover it.
4. Put all the equipment on the table.
5. Before you pass drinking water, be sure you know:
   a) Which patients are NPO (nothing by mouth)
   b) Which patients are on restricted fluids and get only a measured amount of water
   c) Which patients get only tap water (omit ice)
   d) Which patients may have ice water
6. Roll the moving table into the hall outside the patient's room.
7. Go into the room and pick up one patient's water pitcher.
8. Empty it in the sink in the room. Fill it half full with tap water.
9. Walk to the water table in the hall. Fill the pitcher to the brim with ice cubes, being sure the scoop does not touch the water pitcher.

10. Replace the water pitcher on the same patient's table from which it was taken. If the pitcher is labeled with the patient's name, check it against the identification bracelet.
11. Throw away used paper cups.
12. Wipe the table with a clean paper towel. Discard the towel.
13. Place several clean paper cups next to the water pitcher.
14. Place several straws next to the water pitcher.
15. Be sure the patient can reach the water pitcher easily.
16. Offer to pour a fresh glass of water for the patient.
17. Wash your hands.
18. Report to your immediate supervisor:
    - That you have passed fresh drinking water to the patient
    - Your observations of anything unusual

KEY QUESTIONS

1. How can you prepare the patient for the meal?
2. How should the food tray be served?
3. Which information concerning meals should be observed and recorded?
4. How should the helpless or handicapped patient be fed?
5. When should between-meal nourishments be served?
6. How should drinking water be distributed?
7. Define: appetite, discard, extra nourishment, omit.

CHAPTER 29

Nasogastric Tubes and Feedings

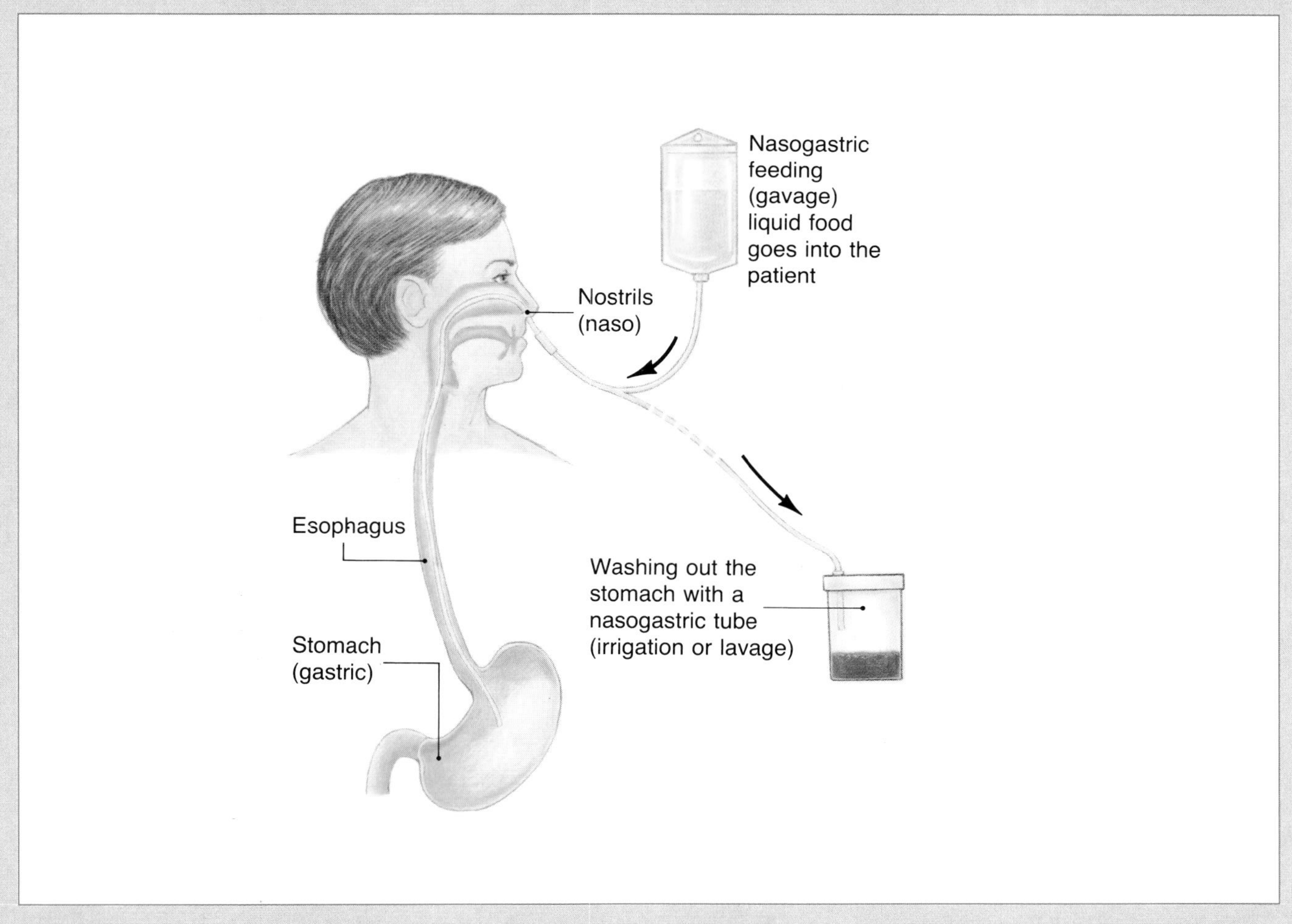

WARNING

For all patient contact, adhere to Universal Precautions (see page 91, 97, or the front cover flap). Wear protective equipment as indicated.

Objectives

What You Will Learn

When you have completed this chapter, you will be able to:

- Describe the uses for the nasogastric tube.
- List the rules to follow when caring for a patient with a nasogastric tube.
- Describe the uses for suction apparatus.
- List the rules to follow when suction is being used to remove fluids.
- List the rules to follow when feeding a patient through a nasogastric tube.
- Define: continuous, gavage, intermittent, lavage, nasogastric tube, suction.

KEY IDEAS

Nasogastric Tubes

Nasogastric Tube
Levine tube, n/g tube, stomach tube.

Gavage
Feeding a patient by putting a tube into his or her stomach. Nasogastric gavage is putting the tube through the patient's nostril and then through the esophagus into the stomach.

A NASOGASTRIC TUBE (ALSO CALLED A Levine tube or n/g tube) is inserted by a skilled nurse or a physician through one of the patient's nostrils, down the back of the throat, and through the esophagus until the end reaches the patient's stomach (gastric). These tubes may be used for nasogastric feedings. In such feedings, fluids or liquefied (blenderized) foods are given to a patient through the tube at regular times. Nasogastric feeding is also called **gavage**. (Figure 29-1).

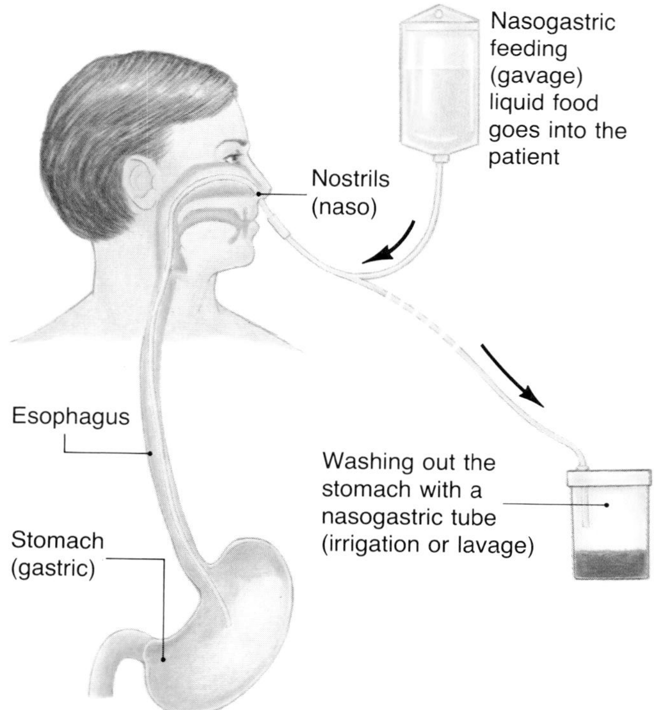

FIGURE 29-1 Nasogastric tubes (stomach tubes).

Lavage
Refers to the washing out of the stomach when drawing a specimen or draining fluids through a nasogastric tube.

Nasogastric tubes may also be used to drain fluids by suction from the patient's stomach. Sometimes a doctor wants to test a specimen of the contents of the stomach. Then the nasogastric tube is used to withdraw the specimen. This is called **lavage**. It refers to the washing out of the stomach through a nasogastric tube.

When a nasogastric tube is being used to drain substances out of the stomach or to collect a specimen, the patient is given nothing by mouth (NPO). The food would only be drawn back out through the tube.

Rules to Follow

CARING FOR THE PATIENT WITH A NASOGASTRIC TUBE

- Never pull on the tube when moving the patient or changing his or her position.
- Keep the tube clean and free from mucous deposits at the entrance to the nostril.
- Remember to fasten the connecting tubing to the patient's clean gown after you have finished bathing him or her. This eases the strain on the tube and prevents accidental withdrawal.
- If the patient begins to gag or vomit while the tube is in place, report this immediately to the registered nurse.

Suction
The action of, or capacity for, vacuuming up. This is accomplished by reducing the air pressure over part of the surface of a substance.

Suction

Fluids are removed from the patient's body through tubes by gravity or suction (Figure 29-2). When fluids are removed by gravity, the collecting container is placed near the patient at a level that is lower than his body. The fluid drips into the container. Low-level or intermittent suction is most often used. A suction cannister will be connected to wall suction or a suction machine. **Suction** is also used to remove thick secretions that cannot be drawn out easily by gravity.

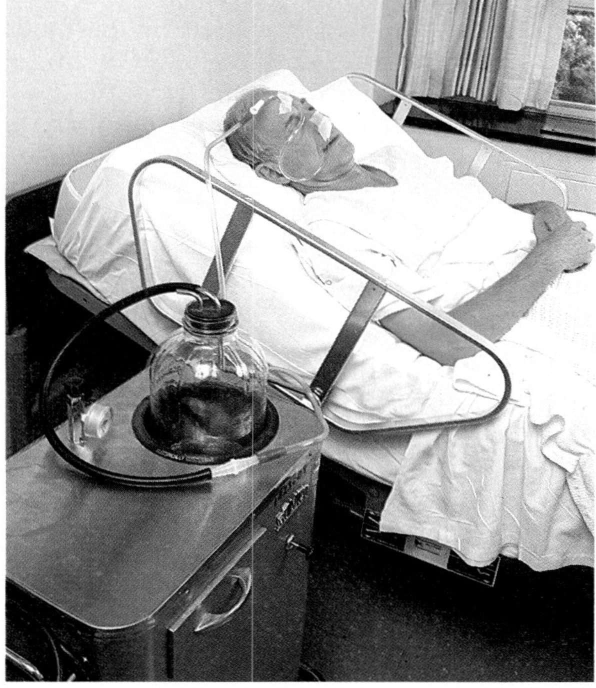

FIGURE 29-2 Portable suction (vacuum) apparatus for patient with a nasogastric tube. Suction is used to remove fluids from the body.

Rules to Follow

SUCTION (VACUUM DRAINAGE)

- Report immediately to your supervisor if you see what appears to be leakage in the tube or suction system.
- Never open the collecting containers to empty the drainage without instructions from the registered nurse.
- Never raise the drainage bottle.
- Never disconnect the tubing.
- Report to the registered nurse if the level of fluid in the container stops rising. The tubing may be blocked or drainage may be complete.
- The drainage collected through the tubes is measured at regular intervals. The color and kind of material being drained will have to be noted. You may be asked to take these measurements and record them on the output side of the intake and output sheet.
- If a specimen of the drainage is needed, collect the amount specified by the registered nurse.
- If there is a rapid increase in the amount of material being drained or any change in the material itself, report to the registered nurse.

Feeding a Patient through a Nasogastric Tube

Nasogastric feedings are done only on the order of a physician. The policy is different in every health care institution as to who is permitted to start a nasogastric feeding for a patient. The nursing assistant must follow the policy of the employing health care institution. Usually, the policy states that a nasogastric feeding is to be started by the registered nurse or the licensed practical nurse, and the nursing assistant is to watch the feeding and report anything unusual. When the policy states that the nursing assistant is to watch the feeding, it usually means the nursing assistant is to watch the level of the formula to be sure it is being fed slowly into the nasogastric tube and into the patient's stomach.

The formula may be prepared by the dietary department or may be bought ready to use, commercially. The ingredients of this type of formula contain all the nutrients required for a well-balanced diet. The formula is poured into a plastic container that is connected by a tube to the nasogastric tube. The rate of flow can be adjusted through the use of a special valve so the formula is fed into the patient's stomach very slowly. When the formula is completely drained into the patient's stomach, a glass of water at room temperature is then poured into the container and permitted to be fed into the nasogastric tube slowly. This serves two purposes:

- Gives the patient the required amount of daily water
- Prevents the nasogastric tube from clogging and keeps the tube open for the next feeding

If ordered by the physician, vitamins may be added to the formula by the skilled nurse. The formula is always administered at room temperature.

Rules to Follow

FEEDING A PATIENT THROUGH A NASOGASTRIC TUBE

Continuous
Uninterrupted, without a stop.

Intermittent
Alternating; stopping and beginning again.

- Nasogastric tube feedings are done by gravity and/or via pump. They may be **continuous** or **intermittent** feedings.
- Force is never used during the feeding as it may cause abdominal distress in the patient.
- Formula taken directly from a refrigerator is never used cold; it must return to room temperature before it is fed to the patient.
- If the nasogastric tube appears obstructed, stop the feeding and report to your immediate supervisor.
- Report to your immediate supervisor:
  - The time the feeding was started and the time the feeding was completed
  - If continuous feeding, the amount absorbed on your shift
  - The amount of water given at the end of the feeding
  - How the patient tolerated the procedure
  - Your observations of anything unusual

KEY QUESTIONS

1. Why is the nasogastric tube used?
2. Which rules should be followed when caring for a patient with a nasogastric tube?
3. Why is suction apparatus used?
4. Which rules should be followed when suction is being used to remove fluids?
5. Which rules should be followed when feeding a patient through a nasogastric tube?
6. Define: continuous, gavage, intermittent, lavage, nasogastric tube, suction.

CHAPTER

30 Rectal Treatments

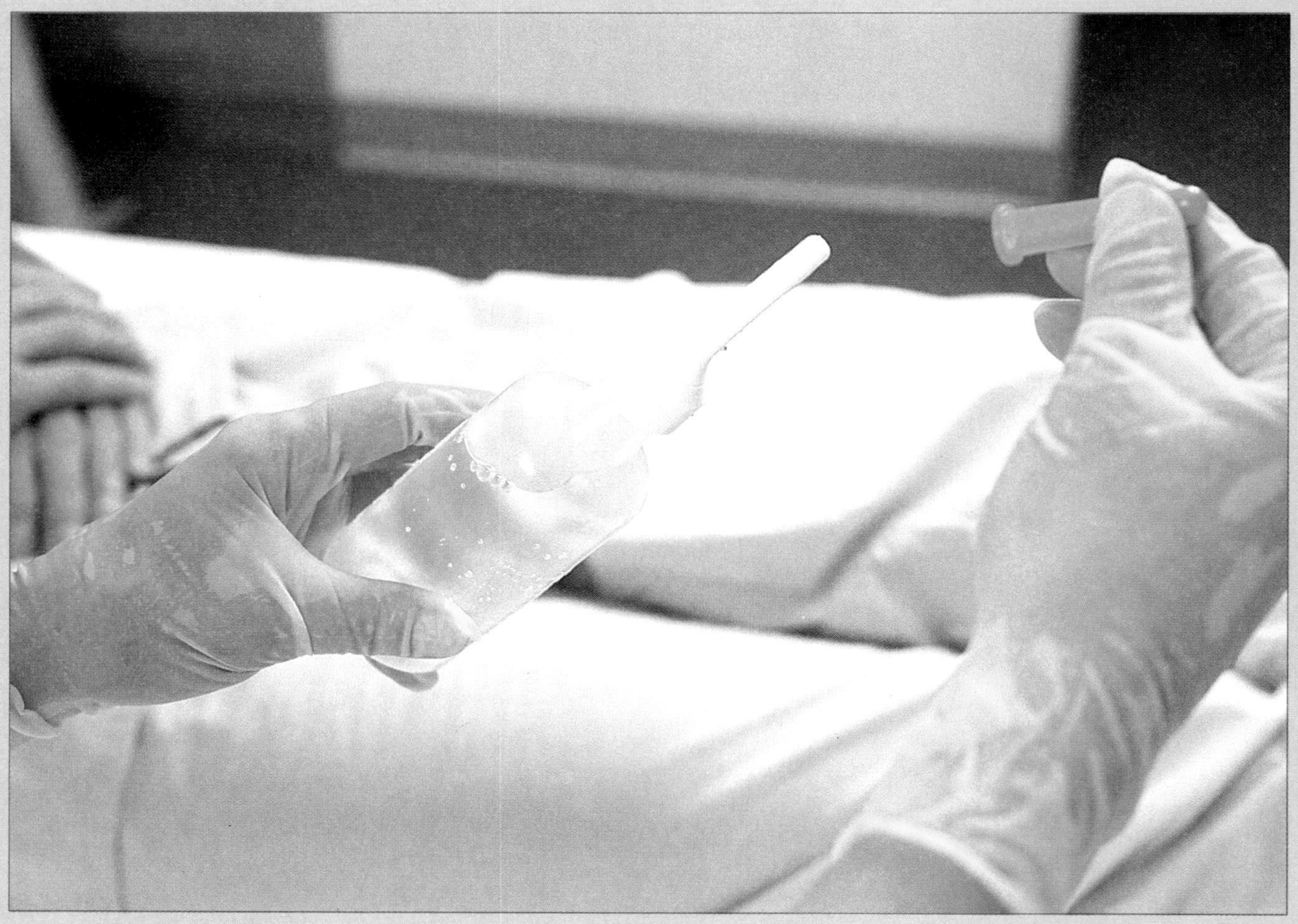

WARNING

For all patient contact, adhere to Universal Precautions (see page 91, 97, or the front cover flap). Wear protective equipment as indicated.

Objectives

What You Will Learn

When you have completed this section, you will be able to:

- Properly position a patient for an enema.
- Administer a cleansing enema.
- Administer a retention enema.
- Administer a Harris flush or return-flow enema.
- Use the disposable rectal tube with connected flatus bag.
- Define: anus, enema, evacuation, flatus, rectal irrigation, rectum, and retention.

KEY IDEAS

Rectal Treatments

Enema
A liquid that flows through a tube into the rectum to wash out its contents.

CLEANSING ENEMAS AND OIL RETENTION ENEMAS are administered to patients by nursing assistants. A **cleansing enema** washes out waste materials (feces or stool) from the person's lower bowel. An **oil retention enema** inserts oil into the rectum to soften the stool. Retention means that the patient keeps the fluid (oil) in his or her rectum for 20 minutes. Giving enemas has been made easier in recent years by the use of disposable, prepackaged enema kits. These plastic enema kits contain an enema bag, tubing, and a clamp. The kit should be used once and then thrown away.

If the patient has any complaints before you start giving the enema, report this to your immediate supervisor. Do not go ahead with the enema until you are told to do so.

Occasionally, a patient may complain of a cramplike pain after the enema has started. If this happens, stop the flow of solution until the pain goes away. If you stop the flow and then start again when the pain is gone, the full prescribed amount of solution can usually be given without causing the patient very much discomfort.

KEY IDEAS

Positioning the Patient for the Enema

Left Sim's Position

When the patient is on his or her left side with the right knee bent toward the chest, it is called *left Sim's position* (Figure 30-1). This is also called the enema position because most patients are given enemas in the left Sim's position.

Paraplegic Enema Position

Sometimes the patient cannot be on his side. He may be unconscious, paralyzed, mentally confused, unable to understand, or very uncooperative. He may be unable to retain the enema fluid. In these cases, the patient lies on his back. His buttocks are raised over the bedpan with

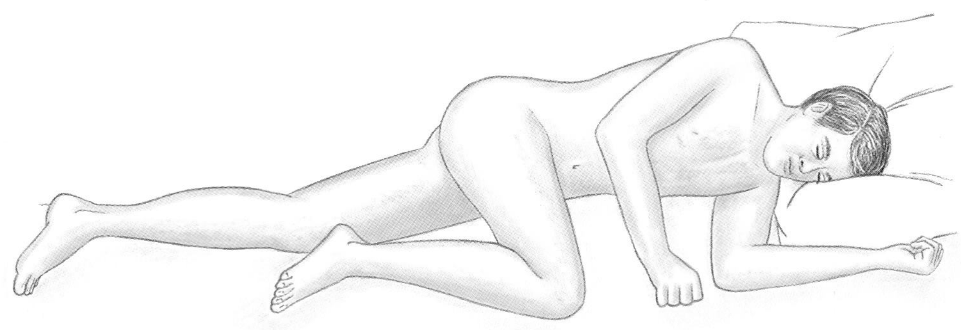

FIGURE 30-1 Left Sim's position.

the knees separated. The patient should be draped with a small sheet so as not to be exposed. The rectal tube is inserted into the patient's anus from between the legs. This is sometimes called the paraplegic method.

Rotating Enema Position

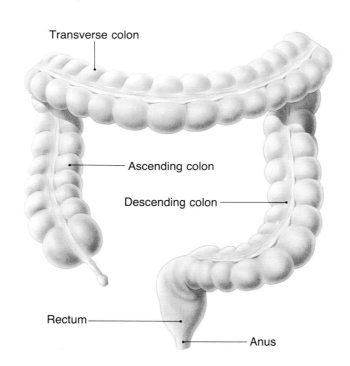

The patient is given one-third of the enema while lying on his or her left side. Then one-third more is given while the patient is lying on his or her abdomen (prone). The final one-third of the enema is given while the patient is lying on his or her right side. By this method, the enema solution first enters the descending colon, then enters the transverse colon, and last enters the ascending colon (Figure 30-2). This is called a rotating enema position.

FIGURE 30-2 The large intestine.

Evacuation
Emptying out.

Rectum
The lower 8 to 10 inches of the colon. The anus is the body opening from the rectum.

Anus
The posterior opening in the body through which feces is excreted.

KEY IDEAS

The Cleansing Enema

The cleansing enema is given only when it has been ordered by the patient's physician (Figure 30-3). This enema is used most often to promote evacuation of the lower bowel when this does not happen naturally. **Evacuation** means discharge of the contents of the lower bowel through the **rectum** and **anus**.

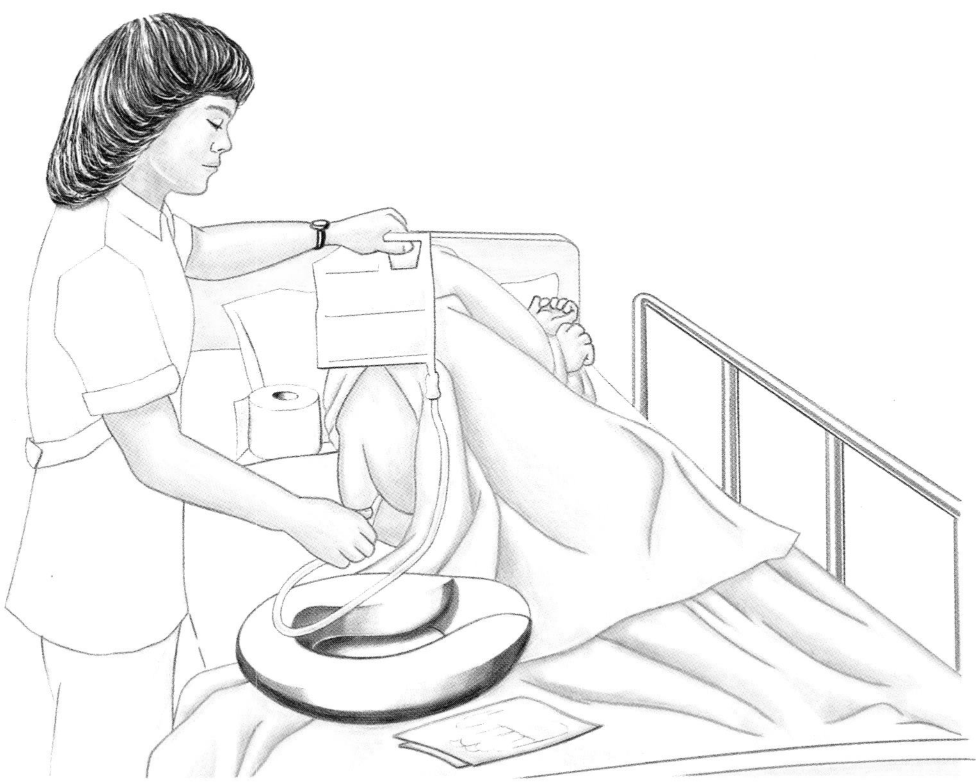

FIGURE 30-3
Administering the cleansing enema.

Cleansing enemas may also be given in preparation for certain diagnostic tests. They are frequently used in preparing a patient for procedures or surgery.

The solution used in the cleansing enema will vary. It may be a commercial preparation, a solution of salt and water (saline), a mixture of soap and water, or plain tap water.

Procedure The Cleansing Enema

1. Assemble your equipment:
   a) Disposable enema kit: enema container, tubing, and clamp (Figure 30-4)
   b) Lubricating jelly
   c) Graduated pitcher
   d) Bath thermometer (Figure 30-5).

FIGURE 30-4

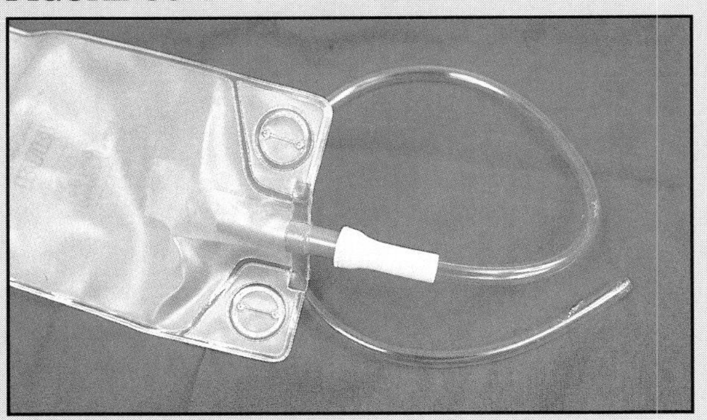

FIGURE 30-5

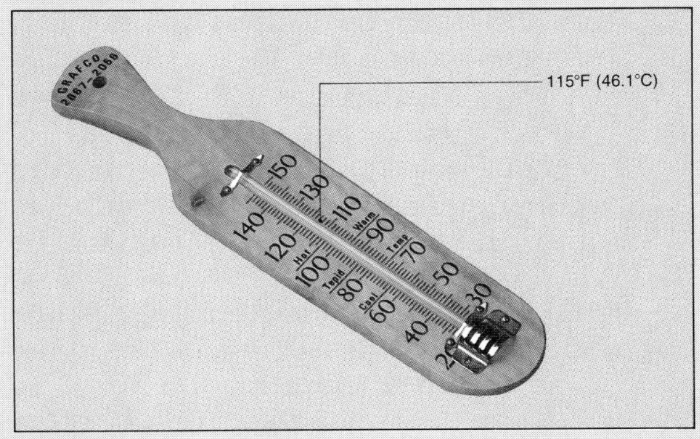

e) Solution as instructed by the registered nurse:
    - *Soapsuds:* 1 package of enema soap, 1000 cc of water, 105°F (40.5°C)
    - *Saline:* 2 teaspoons salt, 1000 cc of water, 105°F (40.5°C)
    - *Tap water:* 1000 cc of water, 105°F (40.5°C)

f) Bedpan and cover
g) Urinal, if necessary
h) Emesis basin
i) Toilet tissue
j) Disposable bed protector
k) Paper towel
l) Bath blanket
m) Disposable plastic gloves

2. Wash your hands.
3. Identify the patient by checking the identification bracelet.
4. Ask visitors to step out of the room, if this is your hospital's policy.
5. Tell the patient that you are going to give him an enema while he is in bed.
6. Pull the curtain around the bed for privacy.
7. Cover the patient with a bath blanket. Without exposing him, fan-fold the top sheets to the foot of the bed. Have the patient covered only with the bath blanket.
8. Place the disposable bed protector under the patient's hips and buttocks.
9. Turn the patient on his left side. Bend his right knee toward his chest. (This is the left Sim's position.)
10. Place the bedpan at the foot of the bed within easy reach.
11. Close the clamp on the enema tubing.
12. Fill the graduated pitcher with 1000 cc of water at 105°F (40.5°C).
13. Pour the water from the graduate into the enema container.
14. a) If your instructions call for a soapsuds enema, add one package of enema soap to the water in the container. Use the tip of the tubing to mix the solution gently so that no suds form.
    b) If your instructions call for a saline enema, add 2 teaspoons of salt to the water in the container.
    c) If your instructions call for a tap water enema, do not add anything to the water.
15. Open the clamp on the enema tubing. Let a little of the solution run through the tubing into the bedpan. This will eliminate any air in the tubing, warm the tube, and avoid giving the patient flatus. Then close the clamp.
16. Put the lubricating jelly on a piece of toilet tissue. Lubricate the enema tip by rubbing the jelly on it with the tissue, beginning at the end and going up the tube 2 to 4 inches. Be sure the tip is well lubricated and the opening is not plugged.
17. Expose the patient's buttocks by raising the blanket in a triangle over the anal area (Figure 30-6). Put on disposable gloves.

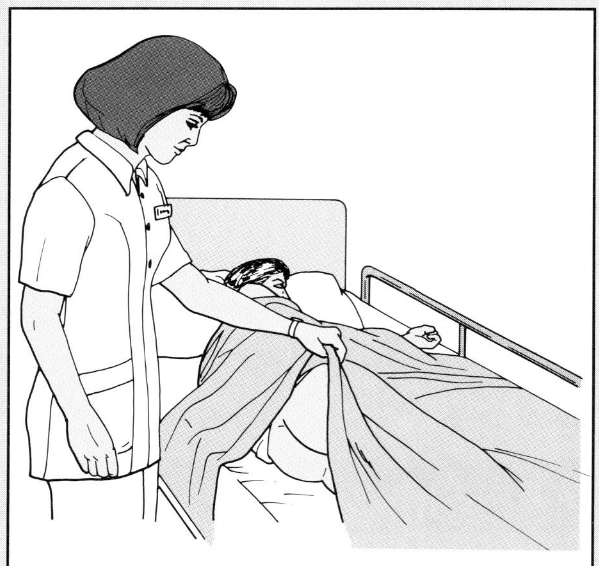

FIGURE 30-6

18. Raise the upper buttocks so you can see the anal area.
19. Gently insert the enema tip 2 to 4 inches through the anus into the rectum (Figure 30-7). If you feel resistance or if the patient complains of pain, stop and report this to your immediate supervisor.
20. Open the clamp and hold the enema container 12 inches above the anus or 18 inches above the mattress (Figure 30-8).
21. Tell the patient to take slow deep breaths. Explain that this will help relieve any cramps caused by the enema. It will also help the patient to relax.

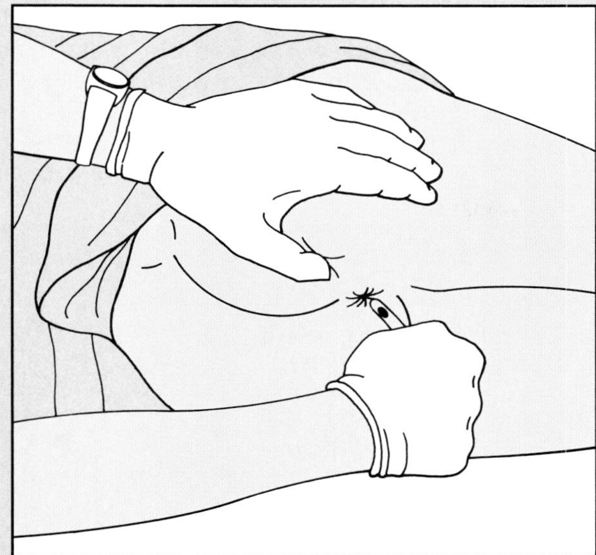

FIGURE 30-7

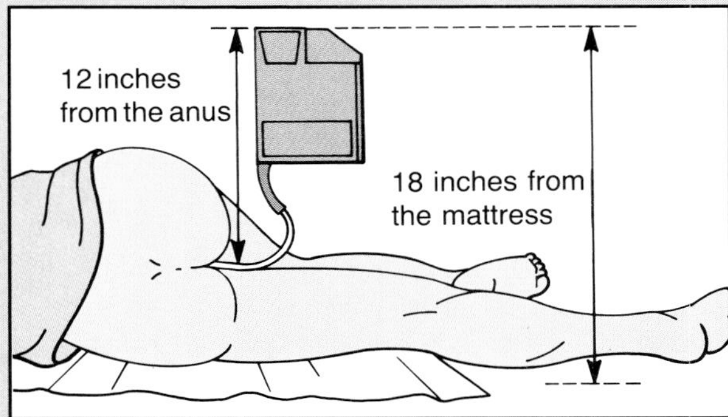

FIGURE 30-8

22. When most of the solution has flowed into the patient's rectum, close the clamp. Slowly withdraw the rectal tubing. Wrap it in the paper towel to avoid contamination, and place the tubing into the empty enema container. Encourage the patient to hold the solution for as long as possible.
23. Help the patient onto the bedpan. Raise the back of the bed, if allowed. Put the toilet tissue where the patient can reach it easily.
24. The patient may be allowed to go to the bathroom to expel the enema. If so, assist him to the bathroom and stay near the bathroom to assist the patient if he needs you. Tell the patient not to flush the toilet. This is so the results can be observed.
25. Give the patient the signal cord. Check on the patient every few minutes.
26. Dispose of the enema equipment while the patient is on the bedpan.
27. When observing the results of an enema, look for anything that does not appear normal. Check color, consistency, odor, and amount.
    a) Report to the registered nurse if the stool:
       - Is very hard
       - Is very soft
       - Is large in amount
       - Is small in amount
       - Is accompanied by flatus (gas).
    b) Collect a specimen and report to the registered nurse if the stool:
       - Is black (tarlike)
       - Is streaked with red, white, yellow, or gray
       - Has a very bad odor
       - Looks like perked coffee grounds
28. Empty the bedpan, clean it, and put it in its proper place.
29. Remove the disposable bed protector and discard.
30. Remove the bath blanket. At the same time, raise the top sheets to cover the patient.
31. Wash the patient's hands or have the patient wash his own hands.
32. Make the patient comfortable.
33. Lower the bed to a position of safety for the patient.
34. Pull the curtains back to the open position.
35. Raise the side rails where ordered, indicated, and appropriate for patient safety.
36. Place the call light within easy reach of the patient.
37. Wash your hands.
38. Report to your immediate supervisor:
    - That you have given the patient a cleansing enema
    - The time the enema was given
    - The type of solution used
    - The results, color of stool, consistency, flatus (gas) expelled, and unusual material noted
    - Whether or not a specimen was obtained
    - How the patient tolerated the procedure
    - Your observations of anything unusual

KEY IDEAS

The Prepackaged, Ready-to-Use Enema

The prepackaged, ready-to-use enema is an effective, easy to use enema. The physician must order this type before it can be administered. This enema is used frequently in the home as well as in the health care institution. It is completely disposable and can be purchased in any pharmacy or obtained from the central supply room in a health care institution. Many health care institutions have a policy of warming the prepackaged, ready-to-use enema. Follow your employing health care institution's policies.

Procedure Giving the Ready-to-Use Cleansing Enema

1. Assemble your equipment:
   a) Disposable prepackaged enema
   b) Bedpan and cover
   c) Urinal, if necessary
   d) Disposable bed protector
   e) Toilet tissue
   f) Disposable plastic gloves
2. Wash your hands.
3. Identify the patient by checking the identification bracelet.
4. Ask visitors to step out of the room, if this is your hospital's policy.
5. Tell the patient that you are going to give him an enema while he is in bed.
6. Pull the curtain around the bed for privacy. Ask patient if he needs to urinate. If so, provide equipment.
7. Cover the patient with a bath blanket. Without exposing him, fan-fold the top sheets to the foot of the bed. Have the patient covered only with the bath blanket.
8. Place the disposable bed protector under the patient's hips (buttocks). Warm the enema if this is the policy of your employing health care institution.
9. Turn the patient on his left side. Bend his right knee toward his chest. (This is the left Sim's position.)
10. Place the bedpan at the foot of the bed within easy reach.
11. Open the enema package. Take out the disposable enema. Remove the cap (Figure 30-9). Put on disposable plastic gloves now.
12. Expose the patient's buttocks by raising the blanket in a triangle over the anal area.
13. Raise the upper buttocks so you can see the anal area.

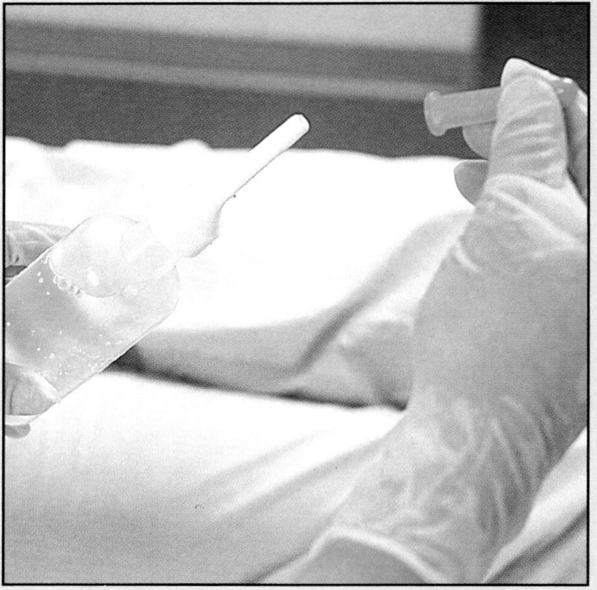

FIGURE 30-9

14. Gently insert the enema tip, which is prelubricated, 2 inches through the anus into the rectum (Figure 30-10).
15. Squeeze the plastic bottle gently until all the liquid goes into the patient's rectum.

FIGURE 30-10

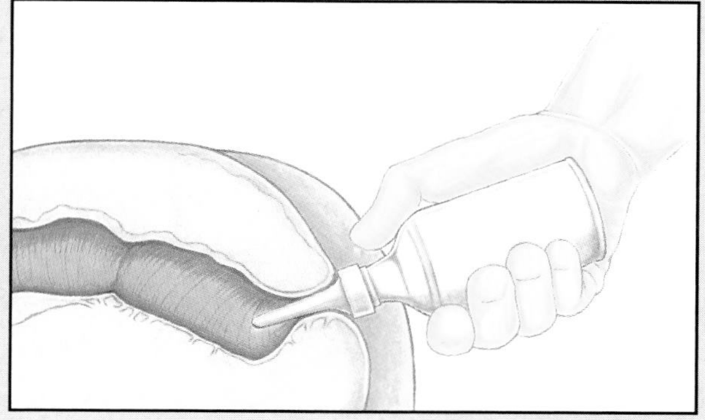

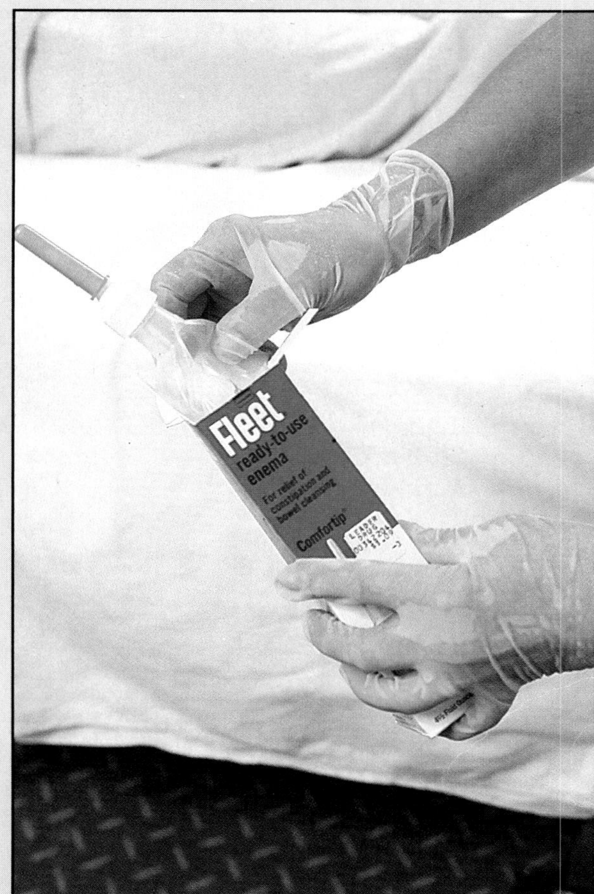

FIGURE 30-11

16. Remove the tube from the patient's anus. Put the empty plastic bottle back in the box (Figure 30-11). You will discard it later, in the dirty utility room. Encourage the patient to hold the solution as long as possible.
17. Help the patient onto the bedpan. Raise the back of the bed, if allowed. Put the toilet tissue where the patient can reach it easily.
18. The patient may be allowed to go to the bathroom to expel the enema. If so, assist him to the bathroom and stay near the bathroom to assist the patient if he needs you. Tell the patient not to flush the toilet. This is so the results can be observed.
19. Give the patient the signal cord. Check on the patient every few minutes.
20. Discard the disposable enema equipment. Return to the patient when he is finished using the bedpan. Check the contents for color of stool, consistency, amount, unusual material, or anything abnormal. If you observe anything unusual, collect a specimen.
21. Empty the bedpan. Clean it and put it in its proper place.
22. Remove the disposable bed protector and discard it.
23. Remove the bath blanket. At the same time, raise the top sheets to cover the patient.
24. Wash the patient's hands.
25. Make the patient comfortable.
26. Lower the bed to a position of safety for the patient.
27. Pull the curtains back to the open position.
28. Raise the side rails where ordered, indicated, and appropriate for patient safety.
29. Place the call light within easy reach of the patient.
30. Wash your hands.
31. Report to your immediate supervisor:
    - That you have given the patient a cleansing enema
    - The time the enema was given
    - The results, color of stool, consistency, flatus expelled, and unusual material noted
    - How the patient tolerated this procedure
    - Your observations of anything unusual

Retention
To hold in, retain.

KEY IDEAS

The Oil Retention Enema

The procedure for giving the **retention** enema is different from that for the cleansing enema. The patient is expected to retain (hold in) the enema solution for 10 to 20 minutes. Sometimes a soapsuds (cleansing) enema is given 20 minutes after the oil retention enema has been expelled.

Retention enemas are given:

- To help soften the feces and gently stimulate evacuation
- To lubricate the inside surface of the lower intestine
- To soften the stool, if necessary
- To ease the passage of feces without straining
- To provide laxative benefits when oral laxatives are not allowed
- To soften fecal impaction (hard stool retained in the lower bowel) when straining might be harmful or painful

Procedure Giving the Ready-to-Use Oil Retention Enema

1. Assemble your equipment:
   a) Disposable, prepackaged, ready-to-use enema kit
   b) Bedpan and cover
   c) Urinal, if necessary
   d) Disposable bed protector
   e) Equipment for soapsuds enema if ordered by the physician; give 20 minutes after oil retention enema
   f) Toilet tissue
   g) Disposable gloves
2. Wash your hands.
3. Identify the patient by checking the identification bracelet.
4. Ask visitors to step out of the room, if this is your hospital's policy.
5. Tell the patient that you are going to give him an oil retention enema while he is in bed.
6. Pull the curtain around the bed for privacy.
7. Cover the patient with a bath blanket. Without exposing him, fan-fold the top sheets to the foot of the bed. Have the patient covered only with the bath blanket.
8. Place the disposable bed protector under the patient's hips (buttocks).
9. Turn the patient on his left side. Bend his right knee toward his chest. (This is the left Sim's position.)
10. Place the bedpan at the foot of the bed within easy reach.
11. Open the package. Take out the disposable, prepackaged, ready-to-use enema bag filled with oil. Remove the cap. Put gloves on now. Warm the oil enema if this is the policy of your employing health care institution.
12. Expose the patient's buttocks by raising the blanket in a triangle over the anal area.
13. Raise the upper buttocks so you can see the anal area.
14. Gently insert the enema tip, which is prelubricated, 2 inches through the anus into the rectum.
15. Squeeze the plastic bottle gently until all the liquid goes into the patient's rectum.
16. Remove the tube from the patient's anus. Put the empty plastic bottle back in the box. You will discard it later.
17. Explain to the patient that he must retain (hold in) the oil for 20 minutes. Encourage the patient to stay in the Sims' position, if at all possible. Check on the patient every few minutes.
18. Your instructions may require you to give a soapsuds enema after the patient has retained the oil for 20 minutes. If so, give the soapsuds enema at that time.
19. Help the patient onto the bedpan. Raise the back of the bed, if allowed. Put the toilet tissue where the patient can reach it easily.
20. The patient may be allowed to go to the bathroom to expel the enema. If so, help him to the bathroom. Tell the patient not to flush the toilet. This is so the results can be observed.
21. Give the patient the signal cord. Check on the patient every few minutes.
22. Discard the disposable enema equipment.
23. Return to the patient when he is finished using the bedpan or bathroom. Check the contents for color of stool, consistency, amount, unusual material,

or anything abnormal. If you observe anything unusual, collect a specimen.

24. Empty the bedpan. Clean it and put it in its proper place.
25. Remove the disposable bed protector and discard it.
26. Remove the bath blanket. At the same time, raise the top sheets to cover the patient.
27. Wash the patient's hands.
28. Make the patient comfortable.
29. Lower the bed to a position of safety for the patient.
30. Pull the curtains back to the open position.
31. Raise the side rails where ordered, indicated, and appropriate for patient safety.
32. Place the call light within easy reach of the patient.
33. Wash your hands.
34. Report to your immediate supervisor:
    - That you have given the patient an oil retention enema
    - The time the oil retention enema was given
    - The results, color of stool, consistency, flatus expelled, and unusual material noted
    - How the patient tolerated this procedure

Rectal Irrigation
Washing out the rectum by injecting a stream of water;

Flatus
Intestinal gas.

KEY IDEAS

The Harris Flush (Return-Flow Enema)

The Harris flush is an irrigation of the rectum **(rectal irrigation)**. Irrigation means washing out. Clean water runs into the rectum. Gas **(flatus)** and water run out of the rectum. Again, clean water runs into the rectum. Flatus and water run out of the rectum in the return flow. The procedure is repeated for 10 minutes until the patient is relieved of excess gas.

Procedure Giving the Harris Flush (Return-Flow Enema)

1. Assemble your equipment:
    a) Disposable enema bag, tubing, and clamp
    b) Lubricating jelly
    c) Graduated pitcher
    d) Bath thermometer
    e) Urinal, if necessary
    f) Disposable plastic gloves
    g) Emesis basin
    h) Toilet tissue
    i) Disposable bed protector
    j) Paper towel
    k) Bath blanket
    l) Bedpan
2. Wash your hands.
3. Identify the patient by checking the identification bracelet.
4. Ask visitors to step out of the room, if this is your hospital's policy.
5. Tell the patient that you are going to give him a Harris flush, which is a rectal irrigation that will relieve him of gas.
6. Pull the curtain around the bed for privacy.
7. Cover the patient with a bath blanket. Without exposing him, fan-fold the top sheets to the foot of the bed. Have the patient covered only with the bath blanket.
8. Place the disposable bed protector under the patient's hips and buttocks.
9. Turn the patient on his left side. Bend his right knee toward his chest. (This is the left Sim's position.)
10. Put the bedpan at the foot of the bed within easy reach.
11. Close the clamp on the enema tubing.
12. Fill the graduated pitcher with 500 cc of water, 105°F (40.5°C). Measure the temperature of the water with the bath thermometer.

13. Pour the water from the graduated pitcher into the enema container.
14. Open the clamp on the enema tubing to let water run through the tubing into the bedpan. This will get rid of any air that may be in the tubing to avoid giving the patient flatus and will also warm the tube. Close the clamp.
15. Put the lubricating jelly on a piece of toilet tissue. Lubricate the enema tip by rubbing the jelly on it with the tissue. Be sure the tip is well lubricated and the opening is not plugged.
16. Expose the patient's buttocks by raising the blanket in a triangle over the anal area. Put gloves on now.
17. Raise the upper buttocks so you can see the anal area.
18. Gently insert the enema tip 2 inches through the anus into the rectum.
19. Open the clamp. Hold the enema container 12 inches above the anus. Allow about 200 cc of water to enter the rectum.
20. Lower the enema bag below the bed frame. Let the water run back into the enema bag without removing the tube from the patient's rectum.
21. Hold the enema bag 12 inches above the anus. Let 200 cc of water run into the patient's rectum; then lower the bag. Allow the water to run back into the enema bag. Keep the tube in the patient's rectum.
22. Continue letting water in and out of the rectum for 10 to 20 minutes, as you are instructed.
23. Tell the patient to take slow deep breaths. Explain that this kind of breathing will help relieve the pressure and cramps caused by the enema. It will also help him to relax.
24. Observe the amounts (large or small) of flatus the patient expels as the water runs out of the patient into the enema bag.
25. Remove the tubing when the treatment is finished. Wrap the enema tip in the paper towel. This is to avoid contamination. Place it in the disposable enema container.
26. Help the patient onto the bedpan. Raise the back of the bed, if allowed. Put the toilet tissue where the patient can reach it easily. Give the patient the signal cord. Check on the patient every few minutes.
27. The patient may be allowed by the nurse to go to the bathroom to expel more flatus. If so, help him to the bathroom. Tell the patient to notice the amount of flatus (large or small amounts) that he expels.
28. Discard the disposable enema equipment while the patient is on the bedpan.
29. Return to the patient when he is finished using the bedpan or bathroom. Check the contents for bowel movement, color of stool, consistency, amount, unusual material, or anything abnormal. If you observe anything unusual, collect a specimen. Ask the patient if flatus was expelled.
30. Empty the bedpan, clean it, and put it in its proper place.
31. Remove the disposable bed protector and discard it.
32. Remove the bath blanket. At the same time, raise the top sheets to cover the patient.
33. Wash the patient's hands.
34. Make the patient comfortable.
35. Lower the bed to a position of safety for the patient.
36. Pull the curtains back to the open position.
37. Raise the side rails where ordered, indicated, and appropriate for patient safety.
38. Place the call light within easy reach of the patient.
39. Wash your hands.
40. Report to your immediate supervisor:
    - That you have given the patient a Harris flush
    - The time the Harris flush was given and how long it was continued
    - The results, amount of flatus expelled, and unusual material noted
    - Whether or not a specimen was obtained
    - How the patient tolerated the procedure
    - Your observations of anything unusual

KEY IDEAS

Disposable Rectal Tube with Connected Flatus Bag

A rectal tube with connected bag is used to relieve intestinal gas (flatus) that often accumulates in the patient's lower bowel (Figure 30-12). You will use the rectal tube only once a day for 20 minutes, unless otherwise instructed. The whole kit—tube and bag—is discarded after one use.

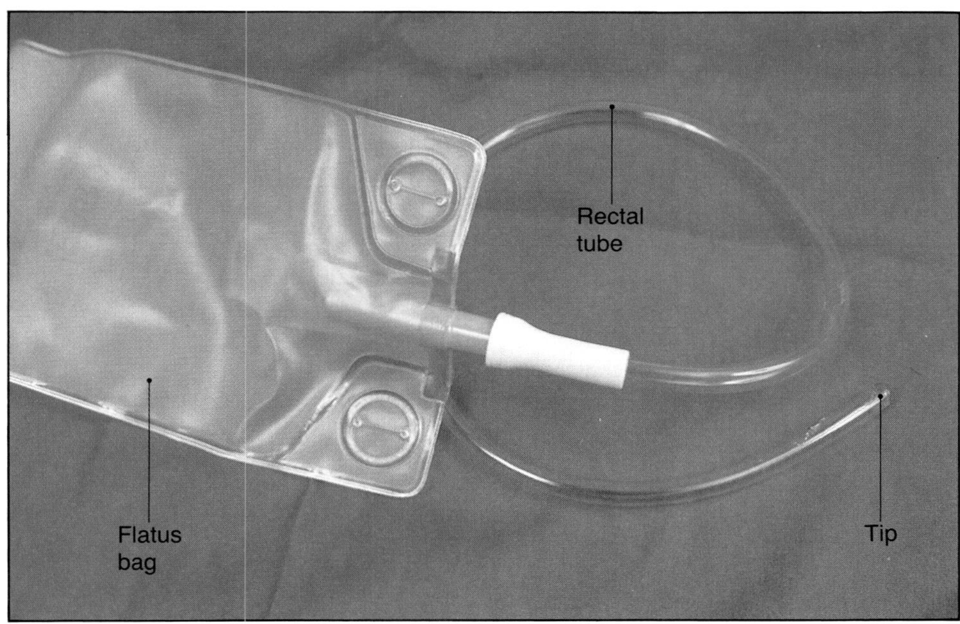

FIGURE 30-12 Disposable rectal tube with flatus bag.

Procedure Using the Disposable Rectal Tube with Connected Flatus Bag

1. Assemble your equipment:
   a) Disposable rectal tube with connected flatus bag
   b) Small piece of adhesive tape
   c) Tissue
   d) Lubricating jelly
   e) Disposable gloves
2. Wash your hands.
3. Identify the patient by checking the identification bracelet.
4. Ask visitors to step out of the room, if this is your hospital's policy.
5. Tell the patient that you are going to insert a rectal tube for the purpose of relieving her of gas (flatus).
6. Pull the curtain around the bed for privacy.
7. Turn the patient on her left side. Bend her right knee toward her chest. (This is the left Sim's position.)
8. Expose the patient's buttocks by raising the blanket in a triangle over the anal area. Put on the disposable plastic gloves.
9. Lubricate the tip of the rectal tube. Do this by squeezing lubricating jelly onto the tissue and rubbing the jelly on the tip. Be sure the opening at the end of the tube is not clogged. (If the rectal tube is prelubricated, this step is not necessary.)
10. Raise the upper buttocks so you can see the anal area.
11. Gently insert the rectal tube 2 to 4 inches through the anus into the rectum.
12. Use a small piece of adhesive tape to attach the tube to the patient's buttocks in order to hold the tube in place.
13. Let the tube remain in place for 20 minutes. Then remove and discard the equipment. (Usually this procedure is done once in a 24-hour period.)
14. Make the patient comfortable.

15. Lower the bed to a position of safety for the patient.
16. Pull the curtains back to the open position.
17. Raise the side rails where ordered, indicated, and appropriate for patient safety.
18. Place the call light within easy reach of the patient.
19. Wash your hands.
20. Report to your immediate supervisor:
    - The time the rectal tube was inserted and the time it was removed
    - The patient's comments about the amount (small or large) of flatus that she expelled through the tube
    - How the patient tolerated the procedure
    - Your observations of anything unusual.

KEY QUESTIONS

1. What are the three positions used for administering enemas? Describe each.
2. How should a cleansing enema be administered?
3. How should a retention enema be administered?
4. How should a Harris flush or return flow enema be administered?
5. How should you use a disposable rectal tube with connected flatus bag?
6. Define: anus, enema, evacuation, flatus, rectal irrigation, rectum, retention.

CHAPTER

31

Anatomy and Physiology of the Excretory System and Fluid Balance

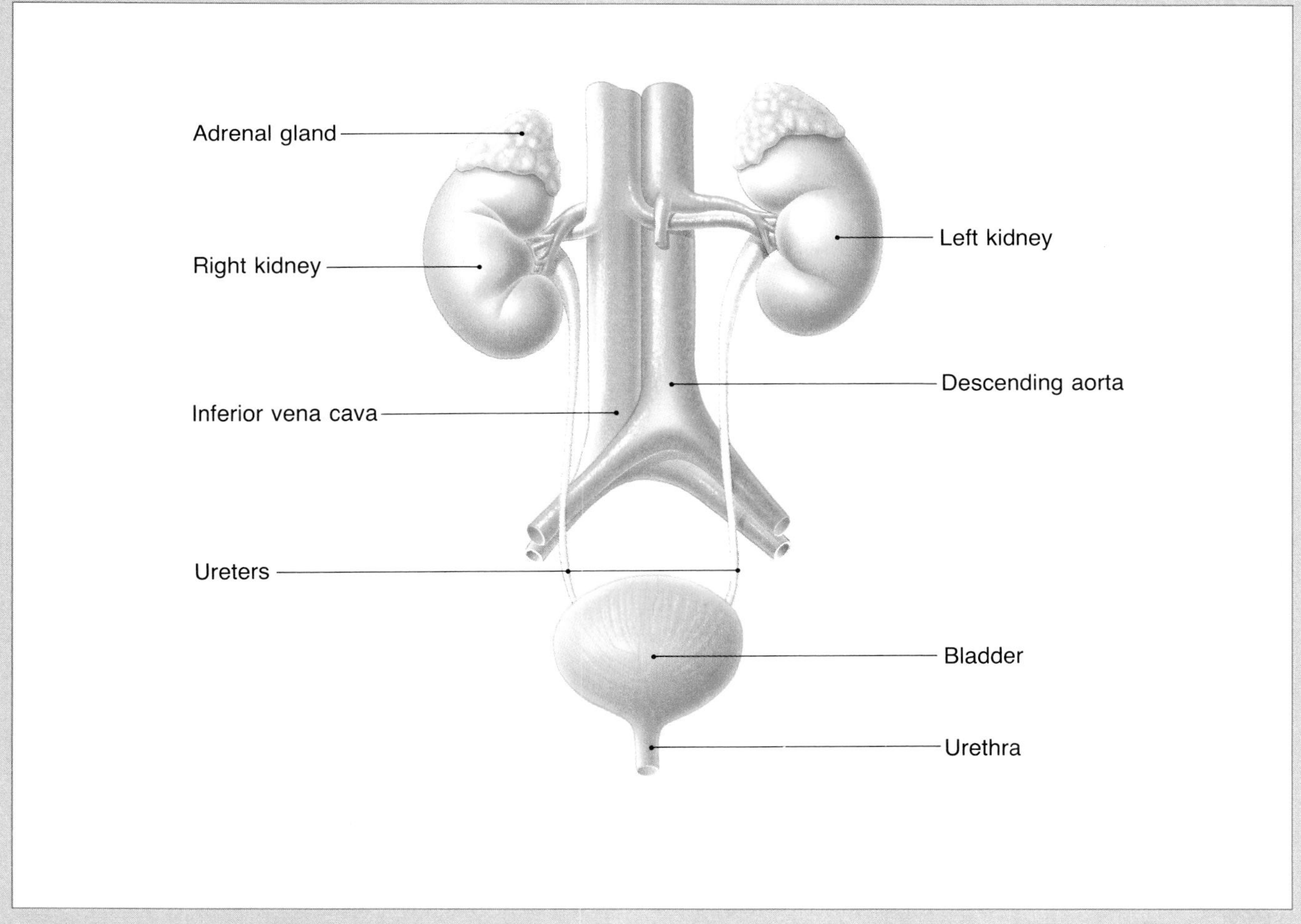

WARNING

For all patient contact, adhere to Universal Precautions (see page 91, 97, or the front cover flap). Wear protective equipment as indicated.

Objectives

What You Will Learn

When you have completed this chapter, you will be able to:

- Label a diagram with the organs of the excretory system.
- Explain the process by which urine is formed.
- List common diseases and conditions of the excretory system.
- Explain the importance of water to life.
- Explain fluid balance and imbalance.
- List the reasons for making accurate records of fluid intake and output.
- List the ways of producing fluid output.
- Define: absorb, discharge, edema, eliminate, evaporate, excretory system (urinary system), fluid, fluid balance, fluid imbalance, fluid intake, fluid output, homeostasis, perspiration, retain, tissue fluid, urinate, urine, void.

KEY IDEAS

The Excretory System

Homeostasis
Stability of all body functions at normal levels.

Excretory System (urinary system)
The group of body organs including the kidneys, ureters, bladder, and urethra that remove wastes from the blood and produce and eliminate urine.

Urine
The fluid secreted by the kidneys, stored in the bladder, and excreted through the urethra.

A VITAL BODY SYSTEM IN MAINTAINING **homeostasis** (a relative constancy in the internal environment of the body) is the **excretory system**, which eliminates waste products. The organs that make up this system include:

- Kidneys
- Ureters, tubes leading from the kidneys to the bladder
- Urinary bladder
- Urethra, tube leading from the bladder to the outside of the body

The other organs that help rid the body of waste material include the lungs, which get rid of carbon dioxide by exhalation (breathing out); the skin, which not only is protective but contains glands that secrete moisture and so help maintain body temperature; and, of course, the large intestine.

The functional unit of the kidneys is called a *nephron*. An exchange of substances takes place between the blood capillaries and a part of the nephron. A network of capillaries, called the glomerulus, lies within a cupping of a tube, known as Bowman's capsule. Materials from the blood are filtered into Bowman's capsule. They are then carried through a series of tubules, which help make up the nephron. As the filtered material flows through these tubules, the blood vessels surrounding them reabsorb those materials still needed by the body, particularly the water. Near the end of the winding tubules, substances from the blood, such as toxins and some drugs, pass into the **urine**. The fluid left (called filtrate) is collected in a larger tube. This tube joins those of all the other nephrons in a basinlike portion of the kidney. From here it drips steadily through the ureter, helped by a peristaltic motion very similar to that

Urinate
To discharge urine from the body. Other words for this function are void, micturate, and pass water.

Void
To urinate, pass water.

of the gastrointestinal tract, to the urinary bladder. The bladder is capable of expanding greatly. There are stretch receptors in the muscular wall of the bladder. When these receptors are stimulated by a full bladder, messages are sent to the brain that cause the person to **urinate** or **void**.

Because the urethra is open to the outside of the body, it may also provide a passageway for disease-causing organisms. These organisms may go up to the bladder, causing a bladder infection (cystitis). The infection may also spread through the ureters to the kidney, causing a kidney infection (nephritis). Cystitis and nephritis are often called urinary-tract infections. Long-term nephritis may lead to kidney damage.

Homeostasis

Tissue fluid
A watery environment around each cell that acts as a place of exchange for gases, food, and waste products between the cells and the blood.

Homeostasis is the body's attempt to keep its internal environment stable or in balance. The urinary system is perhaps the most important system for maintaining homeostasis. This is because the system determines the content (water and chemical) of the blood. The blood content, in turn, determines the content of the **tissue fluid,** which is the immediate environment of the cells. Many changes in kidney function, some normal, can be found in urine samples. Such changes are also revealed in accurate measurement of intake and output. Sometimes in illness, especially after surgery, the patient is unable to void (urinate). Examples of the body's ability to maintain homeostasis are:

- The body temperature stays constant.
- The blood pressure stays within specific limits.
- The chemistry of the blood stays within certain normal limits.

KEY IDEAS

Fluid Balance and Fluid Imbalance

Water is essential to human life (Figure 31-1). Next to oxygen, water is the most important thing the body takes in. A starving person can lose half of his body protein and almost half his body weight and still live. But losing only one-fifth of the body's fluid will result in death.

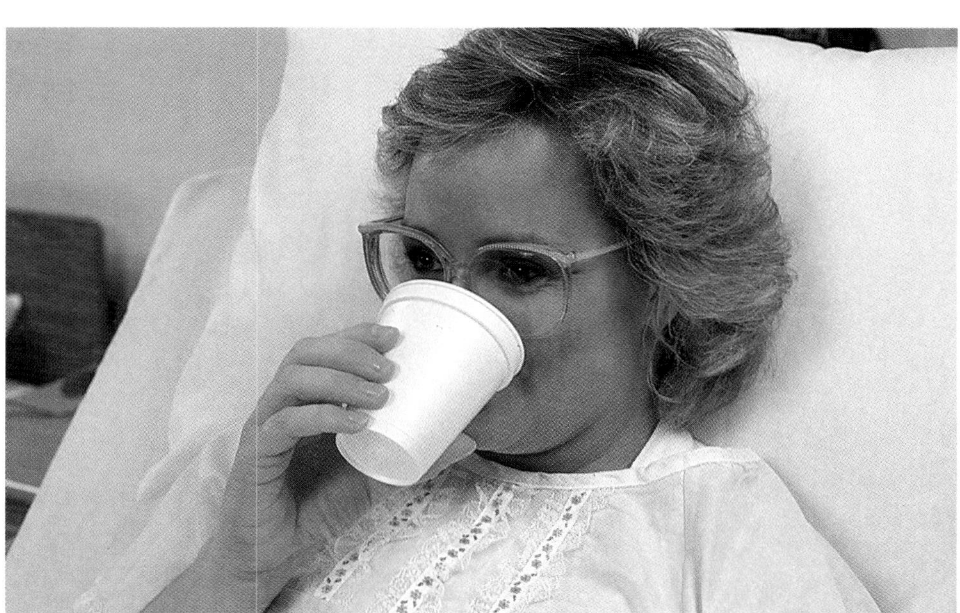

FIGURE 31-1 Water is essential to human life. Next to oxygen, water is the most important substance the body must have.

Fluid Balance
The same amount of fluid that is taken in by the body is given out by the body.

Eliminate
To rid the body of waste products, to excrete, expel, remove, put out.

Evaporate
To pass off as vapor, as water evaporating into the air.

Absorb
To take or soak in, up, or through.

Discharge
Flowing out of material (secretion or excretion) from any part of the body such as pus, feces, urine, or drainage from a wound.

Fluid Balance

Through eating and drinking, the average health adult will take in about 3½ (3,312 cc) quarts of fluid every day. This is his fluid intake. The same adult also will **eliminate** about 3½ quarts (3,312 cc) of fluid every day. This is his fluid output. Fluid is discharged from the body of a healthy person in several ways.

- Most of the fluid passes through the kidneys and is discharged as urine.
- Some of the fluid is lost from the body through perspiration.
- Some fluid is **evaporated** from the lungs in breathing.
- The rest is **absorbed** and **discharged** through the intestinal system.

It is difficult to measure accurately the amount of fluid discharged through evaporation and breathing. Therefore, a person may seem to have a greater fluid intake than output. There is, however, a fluid balance in the normally functioning body. Fluid balance means that the body eliminates just about the same amount of fluid that it takes in.

Fluid Imbalance
When too much fluid is kept in the body or when too much fluid is lost.

Fluid
Applies to both liquid and gaseous substances.

Edema
Abnormal swelling of a part of the body caused by fluid collecting in that area. Usually the swelling is in the ankles, legs, hands, or abdomen.

Perspiration
Sweat.

Fluid Imbalance

An imbalance of **fluid** in the body occurs when too much fluid is kept in the body or when too much fluid is lost (Figure 31-2). In some medical conditions, fluid may be held in the body tissues and make them swell. This is called **edema**. In other conditions, much fluid may be lost by vomiting, bleeding, severe diarrhea, or excessive sweating **(perspiration)**.

FIGURE 31-2 Fluid intake and output.

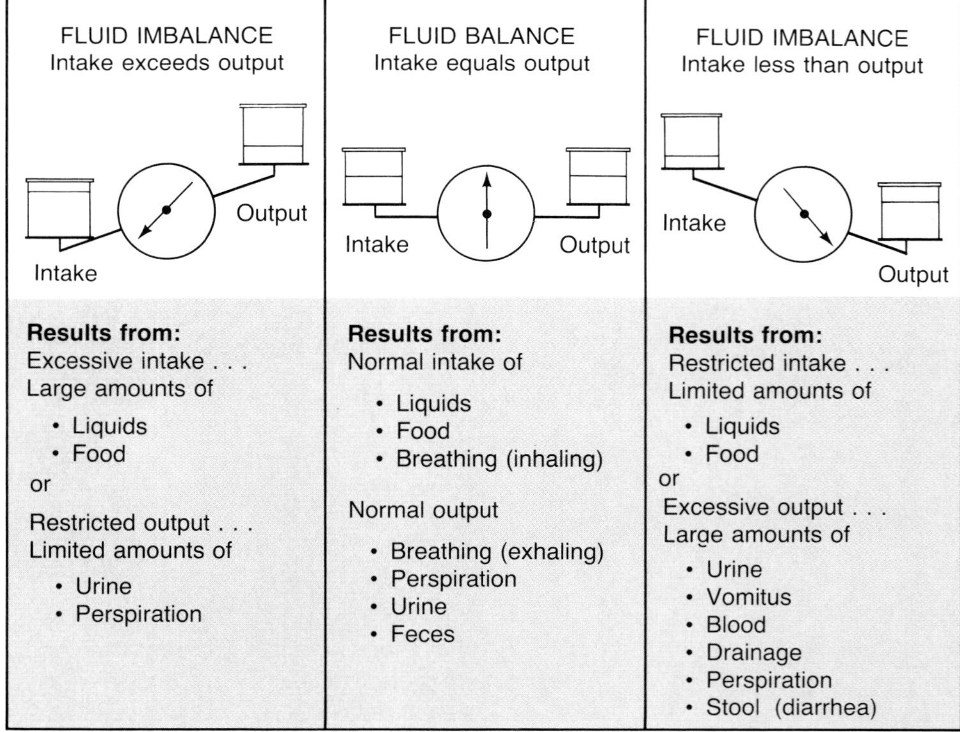

Retain
To keep or hold in.

When a patient's body loses more fluid than he is taking in or **retains** more than he is putting out, his doctor can treat the condition in various ways. A specific method is prescribed to meet the needs of the individual patient. The only way a doctor can know when a patient's balance of fluids is not right is by knowing the patient's measurable intake and output. Therefore, it is very important for members of the nursing staff to keep accurate records of fluid intake and output. The record of the patient's intake and output is kept for a full 24-hour period.

Fluid Intake
The fluid taken into the body, from whatever source.

Fluid Output
The fluid passed or excreted out of the body, no matter how.

The amounts of **fluid intake** and **fluid output** are written on a special record form. It is called the intake and output (I&O) sheet and is kept in the patient's records (Figure 31-3). The patient's name, room number, the institution identification number, and date are recorded on the page. The intake and output sheet is divided into two parts, with intake on the left side and output on the right side. After measuring intake or output, you record the amount and time in the proper columns. At the end of each 8-hour shift, the amounts in each column are totaled and recorded and/or reported.

INTAKE AND OUTPUT SHEET

Hospital # ____________ Patient Name ____________

Date ____________ Room # ____________

INTAKE				OUTPUT			
				URINE		GASTRIC	
Time 11-7	BY MOUTH	TUBE	PARENTERAL	VOIDED	CATHETER	EMESIS	SUCTION
TOTAL							
Time 7-3							
TOTAL							
Time 3-11							
TOTAL							
24 HOUR TOTAL							
24 Hour Grand Total • Intake				24 Hour Grand Total • Output			

FIGURE 31-3 Intake and output sheet.

Diseases and Disorders of the Excretory System

- *Pain:* due to renal colic (sharp, severe pain in lower back over kidney that accompanies forcible dilation of a ureter due to a stone or urinary calculus) or urinary tract infections
- *Urinary retention:* inability to urinate
- *Hematuria:* blood in the urine
- *Dysuria:* painful voiding
- *Acute renal failure:* loss of kidney function

- *Chronic renal failure:* progressive deterioration of renal function
- *Urinary tract infections:* presence of pathogenic microorganisms in the urinary tract
- *Cystitis:* inflammation of the urinary bladder
- *Pyelonephritis:* infection of the kidney (acute or chronic)
- *Tuberculosis of the kidney:* caused by *Mycobacterium tuberculosis* in the kidney
- *Hydronephrosis:* distention of the pelvis of one or both kidneys (urine being made but cannot be excreted)
- *Urolithiasis* (renal calculi): presence of stones in the urinary excretory system
- *Tumors of the kidney:* are considered malignant until proved otherwise
- *Injury* to the bladder due to trauma
- *Cancer of the urinary bladder:* malignant tumor
- *Urinary diversion:* changing the urinary stream to exit the body through a new avenue
- *Urethral stricture:* narrowing of the urethra
- *Urethritis:* Inflammation of the urethra, often by sexually transmitted diseases such as chlamydia or gonorrhea.

KEY QUESTIONS

1. Where is urine formed? Label a diagram with the organs of the excretory system.
2. How is urine formed?
3. Name and describe common diseases and conditions of the excretory system.
4. Why is water important to human life?
5. What is the difference between fluid balance and imbalance?
6. Why should accurate records of fluid intake and output be made?
7. How is fluid output produced?
8. Define: absorb, discharge, edema, eliminate, evaporate, excretory system (urinary system), fluid, fluid balance, fluid imbalance, fluid intake, fluid output, homeostasis, perspiration, retain, tissue fluid, urinate, urine, void.

CHAPTER 32

Fluid Intake and Output

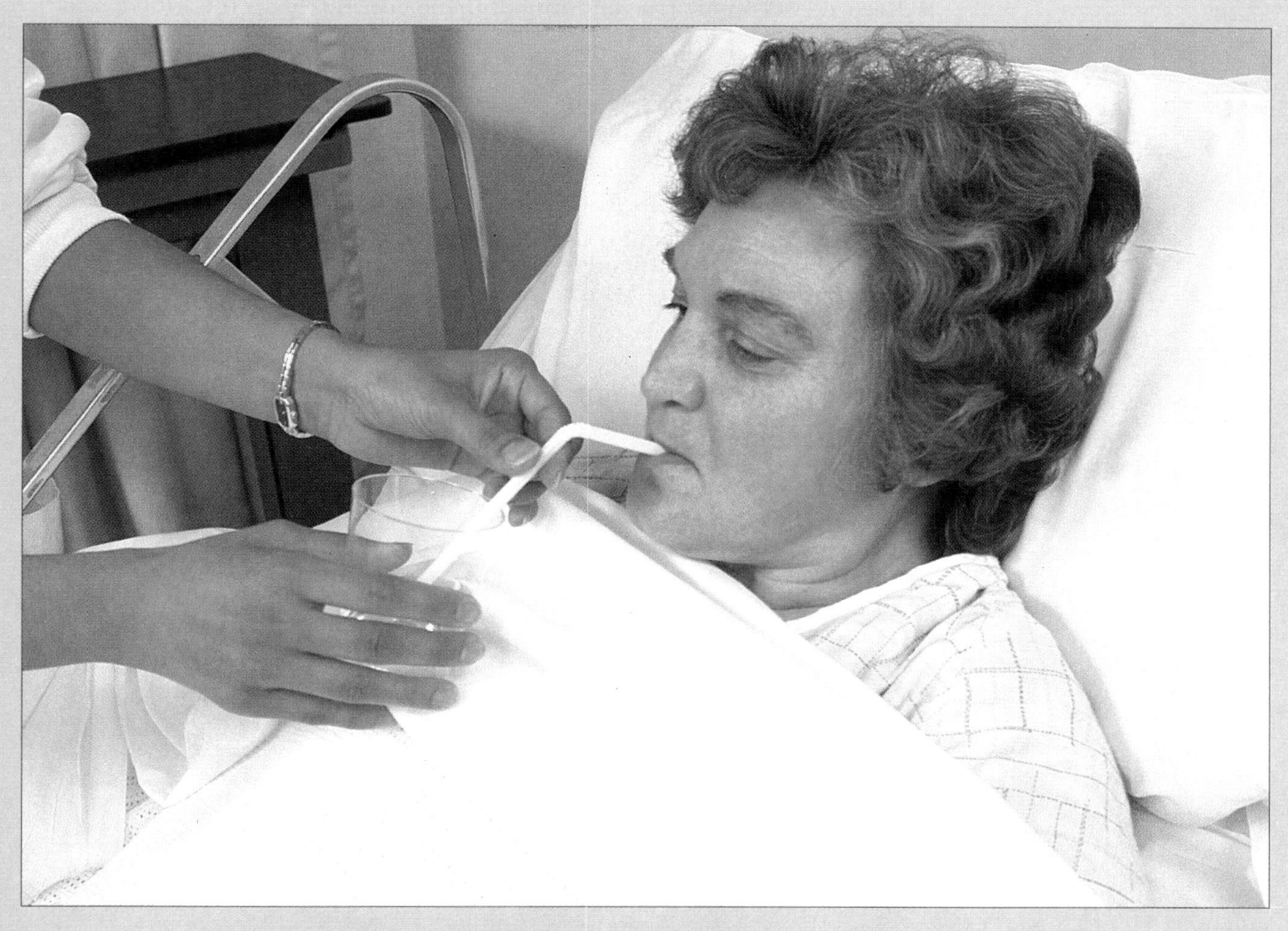

WARNING

For all patient contact, adhere to Universal Precautions (see page 91, 97, or the front cover flap). Wear protective equipment as indicated.

Objectives

What You Will Learn

When you have completed this chapter, you will be able to:

- Identify the measurement cc.
- Accurately measure fluids using the metric system.
- Measure the capacity of serving containers.
- Determine the amounts of fluids consumed by the patient.
- Accurately record the amounts of fluids consumed by the patient on the intake and output sheet.
- List ways to encourage a patient to increase fluid intake.
- Explain ways to restrict the patient's intake of fluid.
- Demonstrate the nursing assistant's role when a patient is on nothing by mouth.
- List the ways in which the body loses fluid.
- Use the metric system accurately to measure urinary output.
- Record and report the amounts of urine accurately on the intake and output sheet.
- Explain the function of urinary cathethers.
- Check catheters, urine containers (drainage bags), and tubing.
- Empty urine from an indwelling catheter container.
- Give daily indwelling catheter care.
- Record fluid output for the incontinent patient.
- Define: calibrated, convert, cubic centimeter, force fluids, graduate, incontinent, indwelling urinary catheter, insensible fluid loss, nothing by mouth, parenteral intake, restrict fluids.

KEY IDEAS

Fluid Intake

A DOCTOR MUST KNOW EXACTLY HOW much liquid is taken in every day by certain patients. Although solid foods also contain some liquid, most of the fluids in the body are taken in when a person drinks liquids (Figure 32-1). Therefore, a patient's *fluid intake* includes everything he or she drinks: water, milk, milk drinks, fruit juices, soup, tea, coffee, or anything liquid. Ice cream and gelatin also are counted as liquids. Fluid taken in through an intravenous tube and tube feedings are also included in the patient's total fluid intake.

You probably have already noticed that many quantities used in the health care field are measured in cubic centimeters or milliliters. Because most institutions use these terms for measuring intake and output, you should understand what they mean.

Cubic Centimeter
Having a volume equal to a cube whose edges are 1 centimeter long.

The term cc is an abbreviation for **cubic centimeter**, a unit of measurement in the metric system (Figure 32-2). The metric system of measurement is used in many countries of the world. In the United States, we normally use one system for measuring liquids (ounces,

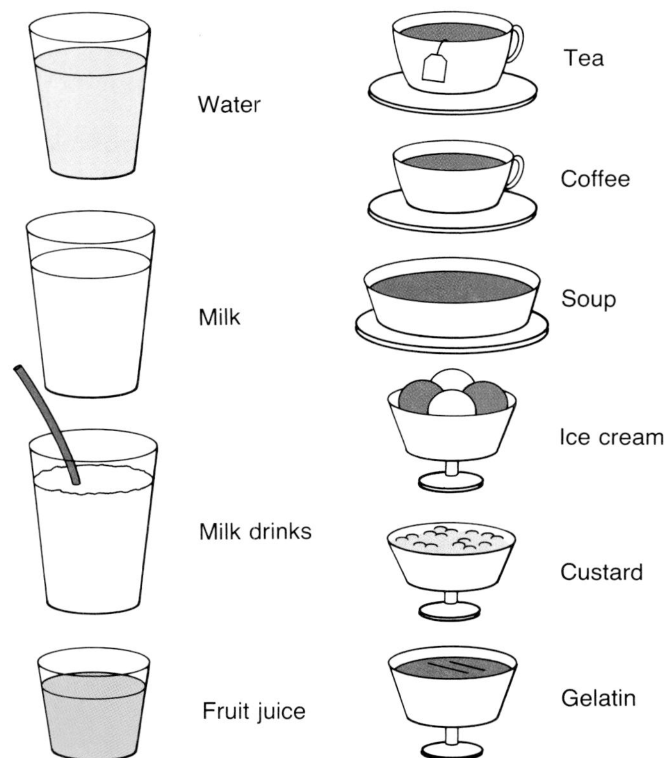

FIGURE 32-1 Fluid intake. The main source of fluids for the body is liquids taken by mouth.

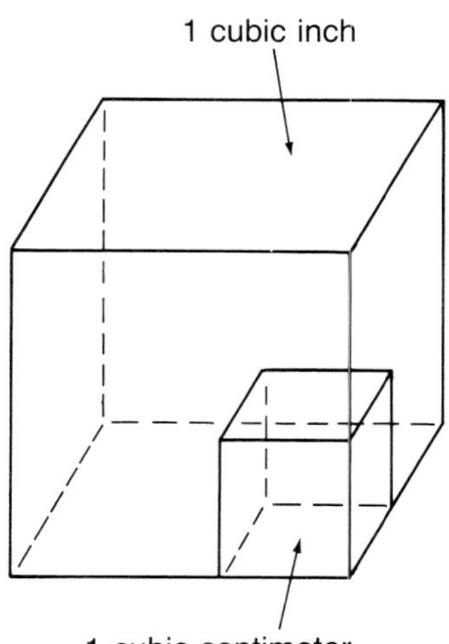

FIGURE 32-2 Actual size of cubic inch and cubic centimeter.

pints, quarts) and a different system for measuring lengths (inches, feet, yards, miles). Scientists, engineers, and many health care institution personnel use the metric system for measuring liquids, lengths, and weight, as well. The basic metric unit of measurement of length is the meter, which is a little longer than the yard. A centimeter [one one-hundredth ($1/100$) of a meter] is about four-tenths ($4/10$) of an inch long.

A cubic centimeter can be thought of as a square block with each edge of the block 1 centimeter long. If we filled this block with water, we would have 1 cubic centimeter (1 cc) of water. The accompanying list gives liquid amounts in cubic centimeters.

Graduate
A measuring cup marked along its side to show various amounts so that the material placed in the cup can be measured accurately. The marks are called *calibrations.*

Calibrated
Marked with lines and numbers for measuring.

The liter is the basic unit of liquid measure in the metric system. It is approximately the same as a quart. A milliliter (1/1000 liter) is the amount that would fill a cubic centimeter. Therefore the two units are often used interchangeably. The patient's liquid intake is measured in cubic centimeters (cc) or milliliters (ml). A container called a **graduate** (Figure 32-3) or a measuring cup is used to measure intake and output (I&O). The side of the graduate is marked **(calibrated)** with a row of short lines and numbers. These show the amount of liquid in both milliliters and ounces. This graduate is like the measuring cup you use at home to measure ingredients for cooking, only larger. Another calibrated graduate used in the home is a baby's milk bottle. This, too, is marked with a row of short lines and numbers. They show the amount of milk in both ounces and milliliters. When full, most baby's bottles contain 8 ounces, or 240 cubic centimeters (cc). To give the baby 4 ounces of milk, or 120 cc, you would fill it half-full or to the 4-ounce line.

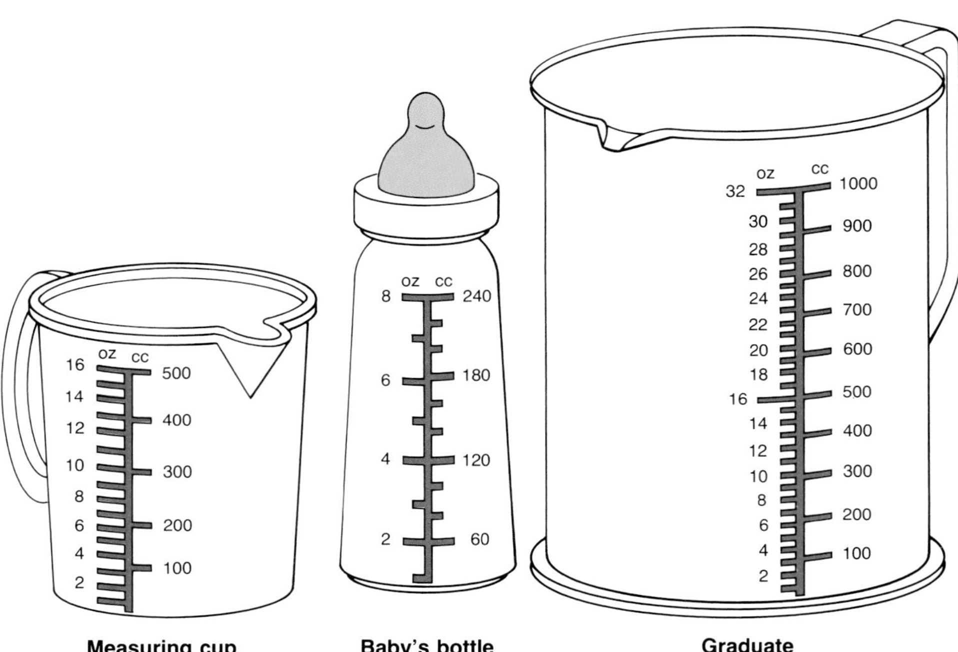

- They are all calibrated
- They are made of metal, glass, or plastic
- They are used for measuring liquids in cubic centimeters (cc)
- They are used for measuring liquids in ounces (oz)
- The measuring cup is used to measure liquids in the home
- The baby's bottle is used to measure liquids in the home
- The calibrated graduate is used to measure fluid in the health care institution

FIGURE 32-3 Three containers for measuring.

It is very important that you observe the exact amounts of fluids taken in by the patient and that you record them accurately. You will have to measure the amount of liquid contained in each serving container, bowl, glass, or cup used by the patient. If your institution does not have a list of the amounts contained in each container, bowl, glass, or cup, you will find it helpful to make such a list yourself.

U.S. Customary Liquid Measure with Approximate Equivalent Apothecary and Metric Measurements	
cc = cubic centimeter	150 cc = 5 oz
ml = milliliter	180 cc = 6 oz
oz = ounce	210 cc = 7 oz
1 cc = 1 ml	240 cc = 8 oz
¼ teaspoon = 1 cc	270 cc = 9 oz
1 teaspoon = 4 cc	300 cc = 10 oz
30 cc = 1 oz	500 cc = 1 pint
60 cc = 2 oz	1000 cc = 1 quart
90 cc = 3 oz	4000 cc = 1 gallon
120 cc = 4 oz	

Examples of Capacities of Serving Containers	
4-oz juice cup	120 cc
6-oz cup	180 cc
8-oz cup	240 cc
12-oz cup	360 cc
1-cup milk carton	240 cc
4-oz ice cream cup	120 cc
6-oz jello cup	120 cc
6-oz coffee cup	180 cc
1-qt water pitcher	1000 cc

KEY IDEAS

Measuring Fluid Intake

Parenteral Intake
Fluids taken in intravenously.

Convert
Change.

Tell the patient that his intake is being measured and recorded. You can encourage him to help you, if he is not too ill, by asking him to keep track of how much liquid he drinks. *This is not his responsibility, however, it is yours.*

Fluids taken in by patients intravenously are recorded by the registered nurse. This record may also be kept on the intake and output sheet in a special column headed **Parenteral Intake**. Regardless of how fluids are consumed by a patient, the important thing is that the doctor must know as accurately as possible how much fluid the patient has taken.

The proper time for the nursing assistant to record the patient's fluids on the intake and output sheet is as soon as the patient has consumed the fluids. Before the end of each shift, the complete amount of intake should be totaled (added). Your task will be to remember to record all fluid taken each time the patient eats or drinks. Think about fluid intake every time you remove a tray, water pitcher, glass, or cup from a patient's bedside. Remember especially to check the water pitcher.

When measuring fluid intake, you will have to note the difference between the amount the patient actually drinks and the amount he leaves in the serving container. You will be required to **convert** (change) amounts such as ½ bowl of soup, ½ glass of orange juice, or ¼ cup of tea into cc (cubic centimeters) when recording them.

Procedure Measuring the Capacity of Serving Containers

1. Assemble your equipment in the utility room:
   a) Complete set of dishes, bowls, cups, and glasses used by the patients
   b) Graduate (measuring cup)
   c) Water
   d) Pen and paper
2. Fill the first container with water.
3. Pour this water into the graduate.
4. Place the graduate on a flat surface for accuracy in measurement.
5. At eye level, carefully look at the level of the water and determine the amount in cc (cubic centimeters).
6. Write this information on the paper. For example, carton of milk = 240 cc.
7. Repeat these steps for each dish, glass, bowl, or cup used by the patients.
8. You will have a complete list to use when measuring intake.

Procedure Determining the Amounts Consumed

1. Assemble your equipment on the bedside table:
   a) Graduate
   b) Pen and paper
   c) Leftover liquids in their serving containers
2. Pour the leftover liquid into the graduate.
3. Look at the level and determine the amount in cc.
4. From your list, determine the amount in the full serving container.
5. Subtract the leftover amount from the full-container amount. This figure is the amount the patient actually drank.
6. Immediately record this amount on the intake side of the intake and output sheet.

Example

1. Assemble equipment.
2. Pour the leftover orange juice into the graduate.
3. Look at the level of the juice. There are 60 cc in the graduate (Figure 32-4).
4. Look at the list. A full glass of juice = 240 cc.

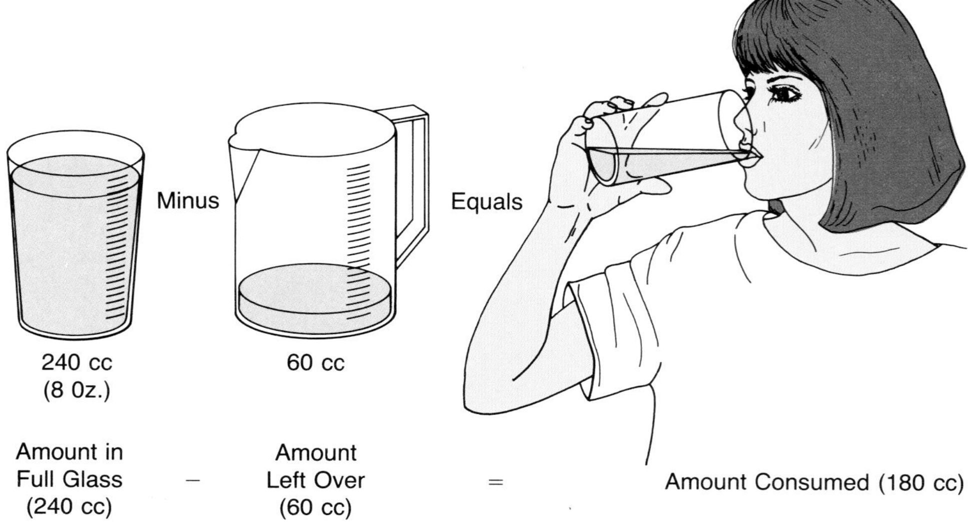

FIGURE 32-4
Determining amount of fluid consumed.

5. Subtract: 240 cc = full glass
   − 60 cc = leftover amount
   180 cc = amount the patient actually drank
6. Record: 180 cc on the intake side of the I&O sheet.

KEY IDEAS

Force Fluids

Force Fluids
Extra fluids to be taken in by a patient according to the doctor's orders (FF).

Patients who need to have more fluids added to their normal intake are put on **force fluids** and often need encouragement to drink more. FF is the abbreviation for force fluids. Some ways you can persuade the patient to drink more fluids are by:

- Showing enthusiasm and being cheerful
- Providing different kinds of liquids that the patient prefers as permitted on his or her therapeutic diet
- Offering hot or cold drinks
- Offering liquids without being asked
- Reminding patient of the importance of fluids in getting better

Rules to Follow

FORCE FLUIDS

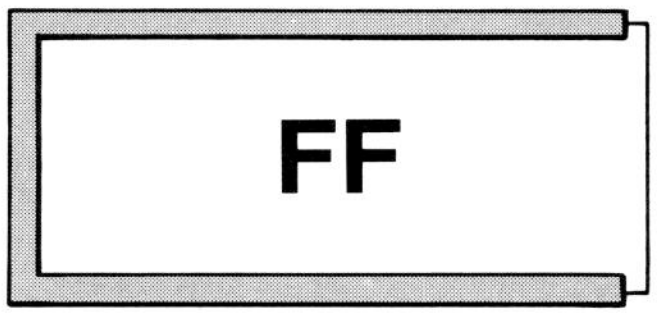

FF

FIGURE 32-5 Sign placed on door or bed of patient who is on forced fluids.

- Check your assignment sheet or card to see if patient is on force fluids.
- Place a sign on the bed or door (Figure 32-5).
- If the patient is on force fluids, encourage him to drink the amount required. For example, 800 cc every 8 hours means the patient would have to drink 100 cc every hour. At the end of the 8-hour shift, he would have taken in 800 cc of fluids.
- Use different kinds of fluids as permitted by the patient's therapeutic diet. Examples are hot tea, gelatin, soda, ice cream, milk, juice, broth, coffee, custard, and water.
- Record the amount taken in by the patient in cc's on the intake side of the intake and output sheet.

KEY IDEAS

Restrict Fluids

Restrict Fluids
Fluids that are limited to certain amounts.

For some patients, the doctor writes orders to **restrict fluids**. This means that fluids may be limited to certain amounts. When you are caring for a patient on restrict fluids, it is important to follow orders exactly and to measure accurately. Your calm and reassuring attitude can make a big difference in how the patient feels and reacts.

Rules to Follow

RESTRICT FLUIDS

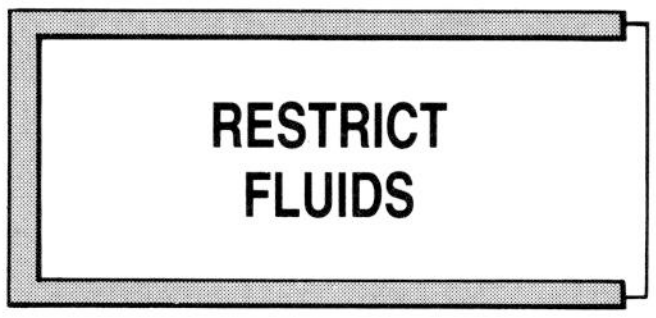

RESTRICT
FLUIDS

FIGURE 32-6 Sign placed on door or bed of patient who is on restricted fluids.

- Check your assignment sheet to see if the patient is on restrict fluids.
- If he is, the patient must stay within the limits stated by your immediate supervisor.
- Place a sign stating restrict fluids on the bed or door (Figure 32-6).
- Alternate different fluids as permitted by the therapeutic diet. Be sure to limit the patient to the correct amount.
- Record the amount on the intake side of the intake and output sheet.
- Usually, the water pitcher is removed from the bedside.
- Frequent oral hygiene is often necessary.

KEY IDEAS

Nothing by Mouth

Nothing by Mouth
Cannot eat or drink anything at all (NPO).

For some patients, the doctor writes orders that the patient is to have **nothing by mouth**. This means that the patient cannot eat or drink anything at all. You may be asked to take away the patient's water pitcher and glass at midnight. You will post a sign saying NPO (Figure 32-7). NPO is taken from the Latin *nils per os*, which means nothing by mouth. An NPO sign is put at the foot or the head of the bed or on the door of the patient's room. Some institutions do not allow a patient on NPO to have oral hygiene.

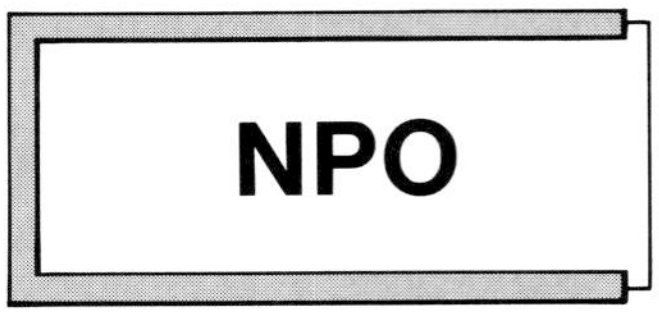

FIGURE 32-7 Sign placed on door or bed of patient who is on nothing by mouth restriction.

NPO

Patients often become very irritable when they are not allowed to have anything to eat or drink. They may, therefore, be hard for you to deal with. Calm and reassuring behavior on your part can help the patient go through a very uncomfortable period. A smile and a few kind words will go a long way here.

Rules to Follow

NOTHING BY MOUTH

- Check the assignment sheet to see if the patient is on NPO.
- Explain to the patient that she or he is now on nothing by mouth.
- Remove the water pitcher and anything else with which the patient could take a drink or eat.
- Place a sign stating NPO on the bed or door.
- Do not give any liquids or food to this patient.
- Make a note on the intake side of the intake and output sheet that the patient is NPO.

KEY IDEAS

Measuring Fluid Output

Fluid output is the sum total of liquids that come out of the body. To urinate means to discharge urine from the body. Other terms for this body function are:

- To void
- To pass water

Insensible Fluid Loss
Fluid that is lost from the body without being noticed, such as in perspiration or air breathed out.

The rest of the fluid that is discharged goes out of the body by a process called **insensible fluid loss**. This means that the fluid is lost in the air breathed out and perspiration. Approximately 100 to 200 cc of fluid is discharged from the body in feces. Output also includes emesis (vomitus), drainage from a wound or from the stomach, and loss of blood.

A patient who is on intake and output must have his or her output as well as intake measured and recorded. This means that every time the patient uses the urinal, emesis basin, or bedpan, the urine and other liquids must be measured (Figure 32-8).

You should tell the patient his output is being measured and ask him to cooperate. A female patient must urinate in a bedpan or specipan. The specipan is a disposable container that fits into the toilet bowl under the seat. The specipan can be placed in the patient's toilet bowl, if the patient is allowed out of bed. This pan covers only the front of the toilet, so stool can be expelled through the back of the toilet and toilet paper can be tossed. Ask the patient not to place toilet paper in the

INTAKE AND OUTPUT SHEET

Hospital # 125689400-2 Patient Name Mary Smith Jones

Date 1-2-88 Room # 4011A

INTAKE				OUTPUT			
				URINE		GASTRIC	
Time 11-7	BY MOUTH	TUBE	PARENTERAL	VOIDED	CATHETER	EMESIS	SUCTION
7:30a	120cc			250cc			
9:45	240cc						
10:30	60cc						
11:00				350cc			
11:20						200cc	
12:Noon	N.P.O.						
TOTAL	420cc	----	----	600c	----	200c	----
Time 7-3	NPO						
2:50p				450cc			
3:00			1000cc	200cc			300cc
TOTAL	----	----	1000cc	650cc	----	----	300cc
Time 3-11	NPO						
5:00p				200cc			
11:00			1000cc	480cc			
							250cc
TOTAL	----	----	1000cc	680cc	----	----	250cc
24 HOUR TOTAL	320cc	----	2000cc	1930cc	----	----	550cc
24 Hour Grand Total • Intake 2320cc				24 Hour Grand Total • Output 2480cc			

FIGURE 32-8 Intake and output sheet.

bedpan. Provide a wastepaper basket for her. Then discard tissue into the toilet or hopper. Female patients must also be asked not to let their bowels move while urinating into a bedpan. Male patients on output must be instructed to use a urinal.

Each patient on output should have his or her own bedpan, specipan, urinal, etc. Any device used for measuring a patient's output must be used for that patient only and disposed of or sterilized when the patient is discharged.

Procedure Measuring Urinary Output

1. Assemble your equipment in the patient's bathroom:
   a) Bedpan, cover, urinal, or specipan
   b) Graduate (measuring container or calibrated container)
   c) Intake and output sheet
   d) Pencil or pen
2. Wash your hands and put on gloves.
3. Pour the urine from the bedpan or urinal into a graduate.
4. Place the graduate on a flat surface for accuracy in measurement.
5. At eye level, carefully look at the level of urine in the graduate to see the number reached by the level of the urine.
6. Record this amount on the output side of the intake and output sheet.
7. Write down the time and record the amount in cc.
8. Wash, rinse, and return the graduate to its proper place.
9. Wash, rinse, and return the urinal or bedpan to its proper place.
10. Dispose of gloves and wash your hands.
11. Report to your immediate supervisor:
    - That you have measured the output for the patient
    - Your observations of anything unusual

Urinary Catheters

The urinary catheter is the most common kind of catheter used for draining urine out of the body (Figure 32-9). This catheter is made of plastic and inserted through the patient's urethra into the bladder. This catheter may also be used when a patient is unable to void (urinate) naturally, or it may be used to measure the amount of urine left in the bladder after a patient has voided naturally.

Sometimes a urinary catheter is used for only one withdrawal of urine. Sometimes, however, it is kept in place in the bladder for a number of days or even weeks. In health care institutions, only a doctor or a nurse can insert or withdraw a catheter.

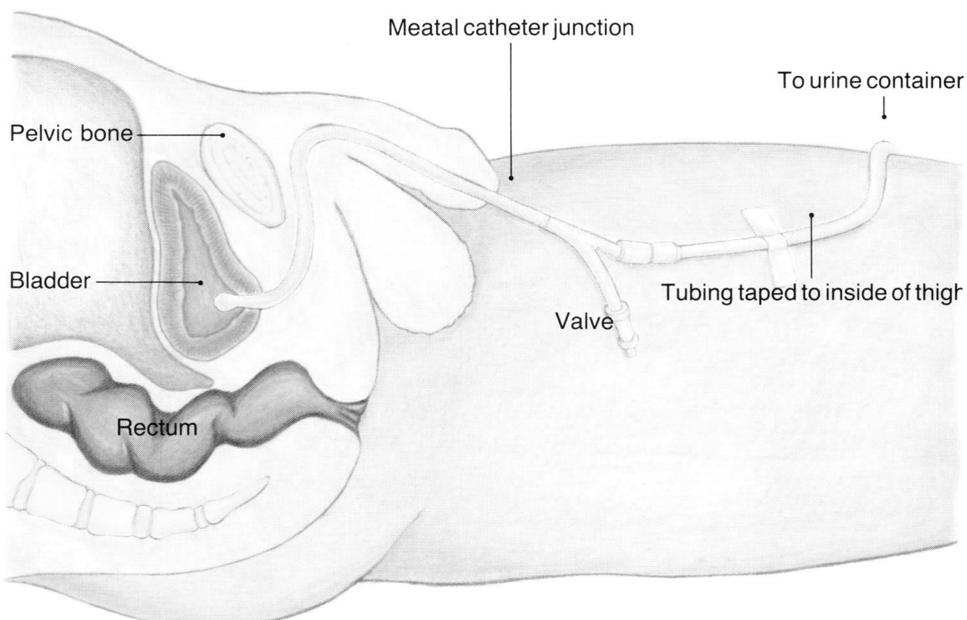

FIGURE 32-9 Urinary catheter in the male.

Incontinent
Unable to control urine or feces.

Indwelling Urinary Catheter
A bladder drainage tube that is allowed to remain in place within the bladder.

Sometimes the bladder-drainage catheter is used to help keep an incontinent patient dry. An **incontinent** patient is one who cannot control his urine or feces. An **indwelling catheter** is a tube inserted through the patient's urethra into the bladder to allow for urinary drainage. It really is two tubes, one inside the other. The inside tube is connected at one end to a kind of balloon. After the catheter has been inserted, the balloon is filled with water or air so the catheter will not slip out through the urethra. Urine drains out of the bladder through the outer tube. The urine collects in a container attached to the bed frame lower than the patient's urinary bladder. This is always maintained as a closed system, which means it is never opened except when emptying the urine collecting bag. A commercially prepared condom catheter is sometimes used for external drainage of urine from a male incontinent patient.

You will empty this container, measure the urine, and record the amount. This will always be done whenever it is full and always before the end of your working shift. The measurement is not taken from the soft expandable plastic urine container. A hard plastic graduate is always used as it is more accurate.

Rules to Follow

INDWELLING URINARY CATHETER

- Check from time to time to make sure the level of urine has increased. If the level stays the same, report this to your immediate supervisor.
- If the patient says he feels that his bladder is full or that he needs to urinate, report this to your immediate supervisor.
- If the patient is allowed to get out of bed for short periods, the bag goes with the patient. It must be held lower than the patient's urinary bladder (below hip level) at all times to prevent the urine in the tubing and bag from draining back into the urinary bladder.
- Check to make sure there are no kinks in the catheter and tubing.
- Be sure the patient is not lying on the catheter or the tubing. This would stop the flow of urine.
- The catheter may be loosely taped at all times to the patient's inner thigh. This keeps it from being pulled on or being pulled out of the bladder.
- All patients with urinary drainage through a catheter are on output. You must keep a careful record of urinary output.
- Keep tubing and drainage bag from touching the floor.
- Catheter care should be done as ordered for these patients.
- Report to your immediate supervisor any complaints the patient may have of burning, tenderness, or pain in the urethral area or any changes in the appearance of the urine.

Figure 32-10 shows a drainage bag used for ambulatory patients and Figure 32-11 shows the plastic urine container for the nonambulatory patient.

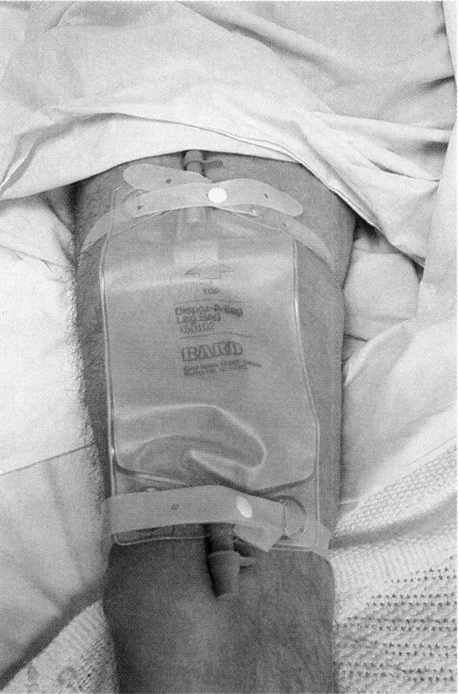

FIGURE 32-10 Leg drainage bag for ambulatory patient.

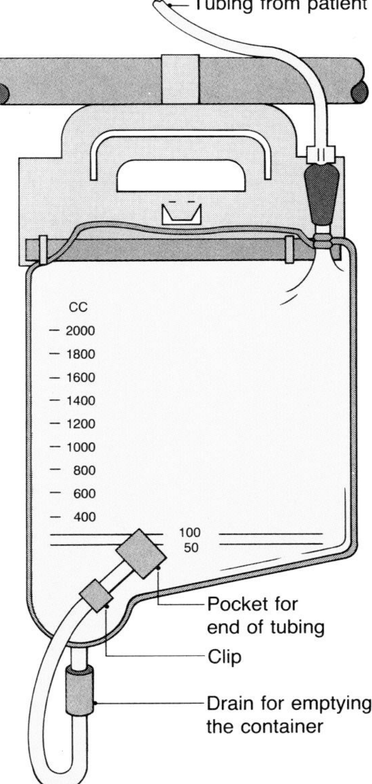

FIGURE 32-11 Plastic urine container for nonambulatory patient.

Rules to Follow
CHECKING CATHETERS AND CONTAINERS

- Check tubing for kinks.
- Be sure patient is not lying on tubing.
- If level remains the same or increases rapidly, report to your immediate supervisor.
- Check level in container for increase in level. If level remains the same or increases rapidly, report to your immediate supervisor.
- The plastic urine container is hung on bed frame below the level of the patient's urinary bladder.

Procedure Emptying Urine from an Indwelling Catheter Container

1. Assemble your equipment:
   a) Calibrated graduate
   b) Alcohol swab
2. Wash your hands and put on gloves.
3. Open the drain at the bottom of the plastic urine container and let the urine run into the graduate; then close the drain, wipe with alcohol swab, and replace in the holder on the bag.
4. Measure the amount of urinary output.
5. Record the amount immediately on the output side of the intake and output sheet.
6. Wash and rinse the graduate and put it in its proper place.
7. Remove gloves and wash your hands.
8. Report to your immediate supervisor:
   - That you have emptied the urine container (drainage bag) and measured the amount of output
   - That you have recorded the amount on the output side of the intake and output sheet
   - Your observations of anything unusual

KEY IDEAS
Daily Indwelling Catheter Care

Daily catheter care is very important to prevent infection. Aseptic technique should be used at all times when you are handling and caring for the equipment.

The catheter is attached to tubing that should be taped loosely to the inner side of the patient's thigh. This is so it does not pull and irritate the bladder. This tubing leads to a plastic urine container. The container is attached to the bed frame. It is kept lower than the level of the urinary bladder so that there is a constant downhill flow from the patient caused by gravity. The urine collects in the plastic container.

This is a *closed* drainage system. The system must never be opened. If the patient is allowed to get out of bed, the container is carried at a lower level than the patient's bladder. A careful record of urinary output is kept for all patients who have indwelling catheters in place.

Many health care institutions have discontinued daily indwelling catheter care. They consider daily washing of the genital area with soap and water as sufficient to maintain cleanliness. Follow the policy of your employing health care institution and the instructions of your immediate supervisor with regard to indwelling catheter care.

Note: In most health care institutions the nursing assistant does not discontinue an indwelling catheter. However, if the health care institution where you are employed has a policy to this effect and it is on your job description that you are expected to discontinue indwelling catheters, follow these rules:

- Cut the end of the indwelling catheter off with a bandage scissors (Figure 32-12), which will deflate the balloon inside the patient, or use a syringe to remove contents of inflated balloon, if permitted by your employing health care institution.
- Gently pull the catheter out.
- If you meet any resistance, do *not* apply force.
- Wait a minute; then gently pull the catheter out. It should come out easily.

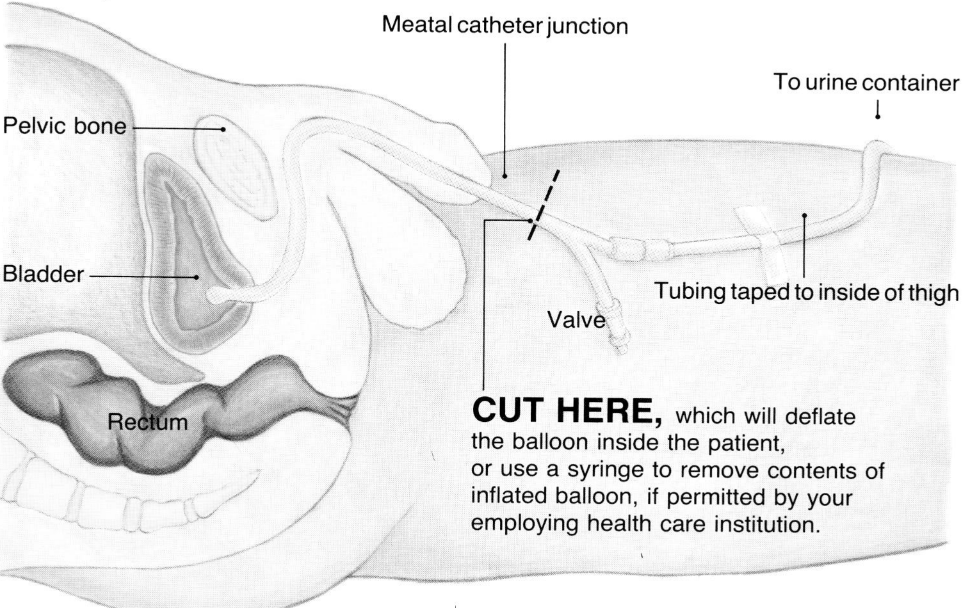

Meatal catheter junction
To urine container
Pelvic bone
Bladder
Tubing taped to inside of thigh
Valve
Rectum
CUT HERE, which will deflate the balloon inside the patient, or use a syringe to remove contents of inflated balloon, if permitted by your employing health care institution.

FIGURE 32-12 Removing the urinary catheter.

Procedure Giving Daily Indwelling Catheter Care

1. Assemble your equipment:
   a) Disposable catheter care kit
   b) Disposable gloves
   c) Disposable bed protector
2. Wash your hands.
3. Identify the patient by checking the identification bracelet.
4. Ask visitors to step out of the room.
5. Tell the patient you are going to clean the area around his catheter tube. Make sure the patient's genital area has already been washed or that perineal care has been done.
6. Pull the curtain around the bed for privacy.
7. Raise bed to a comfortable working position.
8. Make sure there is plenty of light. Observe for crusting, lesions, or anything else abnormal.
9. Cover the patient with a bath blanket. Without exposing him, fan-fold the top sheets to the foot of the bed. Have the patient covered with only the blanket.
10. Open the catheter kit. Place the disposable bed protector under the patient's buttocks.
11. Put on the disposable gloves.
12. Take the applicators from the kit. The applicators are covered with antiseptic solution. With your gloved thumb and forefinger (index finger), gently separate the labia on female patients. If the male patient has a foreskin, gently pull it back to apply antiseptic solution to the entire area. Apply antiseptic solution on the entire area where the catheter enters the patient's body.
13. Check the tape to be sure the tubing is taped correctly in place.
14. Cover the patient with the top sheets. Remove the bath blanket.
15. Make the patient comfortable.

16. Lower the bed to a position of safety for the patient.
17. Pull the curtains back to the open position.
18. Raise the side rails where ordered, indicated, and appropriate for patient safety.
19. Place the call light within easy reach of the patient.
20. Remove the disposable bed protector.
21. Discard disposable equipment.
22. Wash your hands.
23. Report to your immediate supervisor:
    - That catheter care has been given
    - The time it was given
    - How the patient tolerated the procedure
    - Your observations of anything unusual

KEY IDEAS

Fluid Output and the Incontinent Patient

If a patient is incontinent of urine, record this on the output side of the I&O sheet each time the patient wets the bed. Even though the urine cannot be measured, the doctor at least knows that the patient's kidney's are functioning.

KEY QUESTIONS

1. In what ways can fluid be taken into the human body?
2. What is a cc?
3. What equipment do you need to measure fluids using the metric system?
4. Demonstrate the procedure for measuring the capacity of serving containers.
5. If a patient ate half a bowl of chicken soup, how would you determine the amount actually consumed?
6. When and where would you record the amount of soup the patient consumed?
7. How can you encourage a patient to increase fluid intake?
8. When caring for a patient who is on restricted fluids, what is your role?
9. What are your responsibilities when a patient is on nothing by mouth?
10. How does the body lose fluid?
11. Demonstrate the use of the metric system to measure urinary output accurately.
12. Where should you record the amount of urinary output you have measured?
13. Explain the functions of urinary catheters.
14. What are your responsibilities when checking catheters, urine containers (drainage bags), and tubing?
15. How should urine be emptied from an indwelling catheter container?
16. How should indwelling catheter care be given?
17. How should fluid output be recorded for the incontinent patient?
18. Define: calibrated, convert, cubic centimeter, force fluids, graduate, incontinent, indwelling urinary catheter, insensible fluid loss, nothing by mouth, parenteral intake, restrict fluids.

CHAPTER

33

Specimen Collection

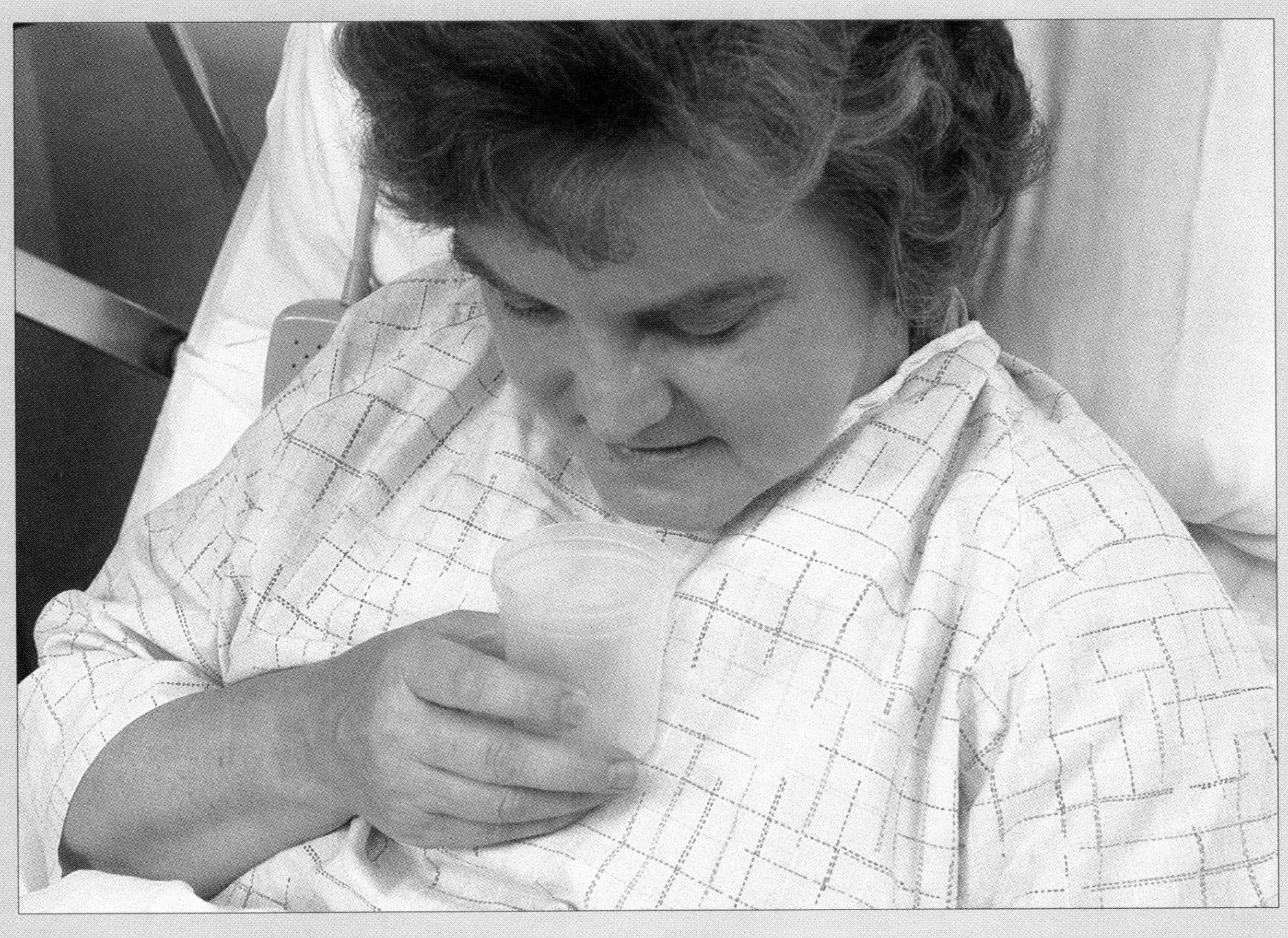

WARNING

For all patient contact, adhere to Universal Precautions (see page 91, 97, or the front cover flap). Wear protective equipment as indicated.

Objectives

What You Will Learn

When you have completed this chapter, you will be able to:

- List the types of specimens nursing assistants are expected to collect.
- Label specimens properly.
- Explain the need for accuracy in specimen collection.
- Explain the need for asepsis in specimen collection.
- Collect a routine urine specimen.
- Collect a routine urine specimen from an infant.
- Collect a midstream, clean-catch urine specimen.
- Collect a 24-hour urine specimen.
- Strain the urine.
- Collect a sputum specimen.
- Collect a stool specimen.
- Define: asepsis, clean catch, expectorate, feces, genital, medical asepsis, midstream, saliva, specimen, sputum, stool.

KEY IDEAS

Specimen Collection

Expectorate
To cough up matter from the lungs, trachea, or bronchial tubes and spit it out.

Specimen
A sample of material taken from the patient's body. Examples are urine specimens, feces specimens, and sputum specimens.

AS ONE OF ITS NATURAL LIVING functions, the human body regularly gets rid of various waste materials. Most of the body's waste materials are discharged in the urine and feces. The body also gets rid of wastes in the material coughed up and spit out of the mouth (**expectorated**). This material is called sputum.

These body waste materials, when tested in the laboratory, often show changes in the sick person's body. By examining the results of laboratory tests, doctors get information that can help them make their diagnosis and decide on appropriate treatment for the patient.

For these reasons, the doctor will sometimes need **specimens** (samples) of these waste products: urine, feces, and sputum. Members of the health care institution nursing staff are responsible for collecting such specimens. Figure 33-1 shows equipment used in collecting specimens.

When you are collecting specimens, you must be very accurate in following the procedure and labeling the specimen. You have to collect the specimen at the exact time that is indicated. You must look at the patient's identification bracelet for the correct name, identification number, and room number when filling out the cover or label on the specimen container (Figure 33-2). The time and date the specimen was obtained should be printed on the label. The label must be printed clearly so that it can be read easily. It must be attached to the container immediately after the specimen has been collected. Unlabeled specimens should be thrown away so that mistakes will not be made.

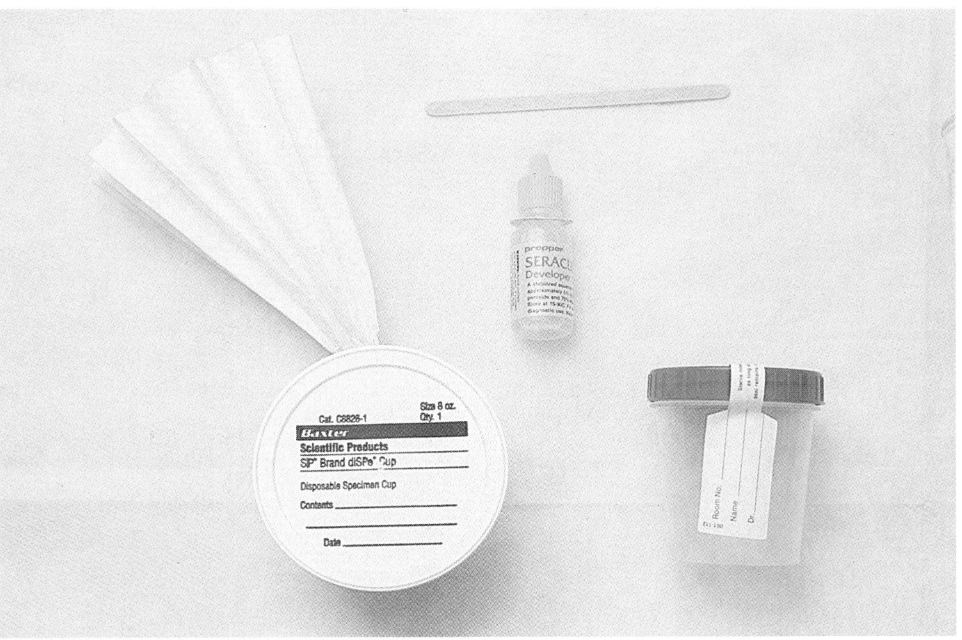

FIGURE 33-1 Equipment used in collecting specimens.

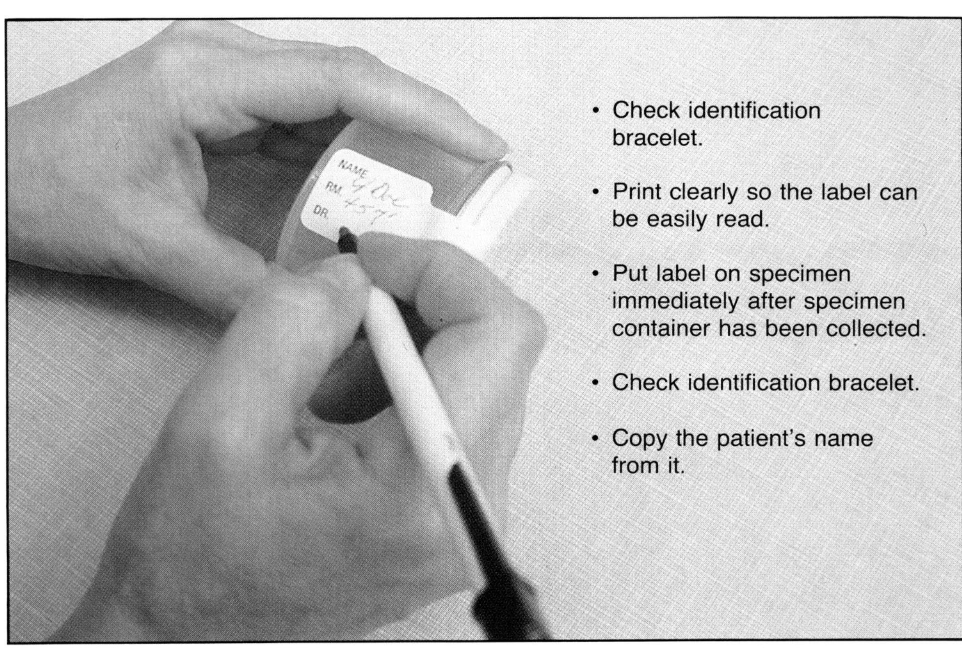

NAME
RM
DR.
• Check identification bracelet.
• Print clearly so the label can be easily read.
• Put label on specimen immediately after specimen container has been collected.
• Check identification bracelet.
• Copy the patient's name from it.

FIGURE 33-2 Be accurate when filling out the specimen label.

Need for Accuracy

Be sure you follow all the "rights" listed here:

- Right patient—from whom the specimen is to be collected.
- Right specimen—as ordered by the doctor.
- Right time—when the specimen is to be collected.
- Right amount—measured exactly for each specimen.
- Right container—the cup that is correct for each specimen.

- Right label—filled out properly from the patient's identification bracelet.
- Right requisition or laboratory slip—lists the kind of laboratory examination or test to be done.
- Right method—procedure by which you collect the specimen.
- Right asepsis—washing your hands before and after collecting the specimen.
- Right attitude—how you approach and speak to the patient.

KEY IDEAS
Asepsis in Specimen Collection

Asepsis
Free of disease-causing organisms.

As you learned from the chapter on infection control, **asepsis** means free of disease-causing organisms. When collecting specimens, it is very important to use good asepsis technique. You must wash your hands very carefully before and after collecting each specimen to prevent spreading bacteria (Figure 33-3).

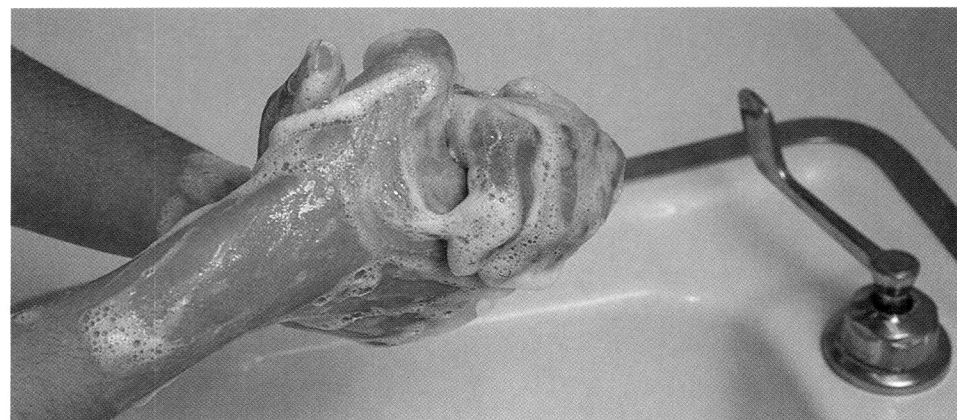

FIGURE 33-3 Wash your hands very carefully before and after collecting a specimen.

Medical Asepsis
Special practices and procedures for preventing the conditions that allow disease-producing bacteria to live, multiply, and spread.

Medical asepsis means preventing the conditions that allow disease-producing bacteria to live, multiply, and spread. As a nursing assistant, you will share the responsibility for preventing the spread of disease and infection by using aseptic technique. Remember especially to wash your hands before and after collecting specimens.

KEY IDEAS
Routine Urine Specimen

The usual single urine specimen collected is called the routine urine specimen. This is the specimen that is taken routinely on admission, daily, or preoperatively by the nursing assistant and sent to the laboratory.

Procedure Collecting a Routine Urine Specimen

1. Assemble your equipment:
   a) Patient's bedpan and cover, or urinal, or specipan.
   b) Graduate used for measuring output.
   c) Urine specimen container and lid
   d) Label, if your institution's procedure is not to write on the lid
   e) Laboratory requisition or request slip, which should be filled out by the head nurse, team leader, or ward clerk
   f) Disposable gloves
2. Wash your hands.
3. Identify the patient by checking the identification bracelet.

4. Ask visitors to step out of the room, if this is your hospital's policy.
5. Tell the patient a urine specimen is needed.
6. Pull the curtains around the bed for privacy and explain the procedure to the patient. If he is able, he may collect the specimen himself.
7. Have the patient urinate into a clean bedpan, urinal, or specipan, or directly into a specimen cup if you are not measuring output.
8. Ask the patient not to put toilet tissue into the bedpan or specipan, but to use the plastic lined wastebasket temporarily. You will then discard the tissue in the toilet or hopper.
9. Prepare the label immediately by copying all necessary information from the patient's identification bracelet or using the addressograph. Record the time and date.

FIGURE 33-4 Collecting a urine specimen, pour the urine into a clean, graduated container, if the patient's intake and output are being recorded. Note the amount of urine and time of collection. Then pour the urine into a specimen container.

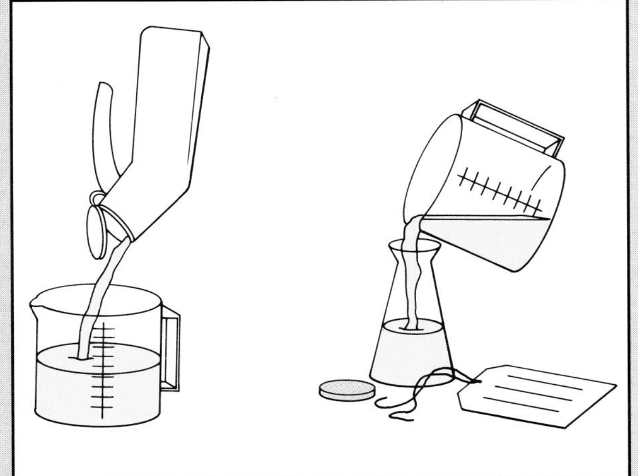

10. Take the bedpan or urinal to the patient's bathroom or to the dirty utility room.
11. Pour the urine into a clean graduated container that is used for that patient only (Figure 33-4).
12. If the patient is on output, note the amount of the urine and record it on the intake and output sheet.
13. Pour urine from the graduate into a specimen container and fill it three-fourths full, if possible.
14. Put the lid on the specimen container. Place the correct label on the container for the correct patient.
15. Pour the leftover urine into the toilet or hopper.
16. Clean and rinse out the graduate. Put it in its proper place in the patient's bathroom.
17. Clean the bedpan or urinal and put it in its proper place.
18. Make the patient comfortable. (If patient collected the specimen, wash his hands.)
19. Lower the bed to a position of safety for the patient.
20. Pull the curtains back to the open position.
21. Raise the side rails where ordered, indicated, and appropriate for patient safety.
22. Place the call light within easy reach of the patient.
23. Wash your hands.
24. Send or take the labeled specimen container to the laboratory with a requisition or laboratory request slip.
25. Report to your immediate supervisor:
    - That a routine urine specimen has been obtained
    - That the specimen has been sent to the laboratory
    - The date and time of collection
    - Your observations of anything unusual

Genital
Refers to the external reproductive organs.

Procedure Collecting a Routine Urine Specimen from an Infant

1. Assemble your equipment on the bedside table:
   a) Urine specimen bottle or container
   b) Plastic disposable urine collector
   c) Label, if your institution's procedure is not to write on the lid

d) Laboratory request slip, which should be filled out by the head nurse, team leader, or ward clerk
e) Disposable gloves

2. Wash your hands.
3. Identify the patient by checking the identification bracelet.
4. Ask visitors except parents or guardian to step out of the room.
5. Tell the parents or guardian and the patient that you want to collect a urine specimen (children who are not yet toilet trained can understand language and are more likely to cooperate if told).
6. Pull the curtains around the bed (even a 2-year-old may be shy about having his pants pulled down in front of the strangers who may be visiting the child in the next bed).
7. Take off the child's diaper.
8. Make sure the child's skin is clean and dry in the **genital** area. This is where you are going to apply the urine collector, which is a small plastic bag.
9. Remove the outside piece that surrounds the opening of the plastic urine collector. This leaves a sticky area, which is placed around the baby boy's penis or the baby girl's vulva (Figures 33-5 and 33-6). Do not cover the baby's rectum.
10. Put the child's diaper on as usual.
11. Return and check every half hour to see if the infant has voided. You cannot feel the diaper to find out. You must open the diaper and look at the urine collector.
12. When the infant has voided, put on gloves, then remove the plastic urine collector. It comes off easily. Wash off any sticky residue, rinse, and pat dry.
13. Replace the child's diaper.
14. Put the specimen in the specimen container and cover it immediately.
15. Label the container properly by checking the patient's identification bracelet.
16. The labeled specimen container must be sent or taken to the laboratory with the requisition or laboratory request slip, which is usually filled out by the ward clerk.
17. Make the baby comfortable.
18. Lower the crib to a position of safety for the patient.
19. Pull the curtains back to the open position.
20. Raise the crib side rails to assure patient safety.
21. Wash your hands.
22. Report to your immediate supervisor:
    - That a routine urine specimen has been obtained
    - That the specimen has been sent to the laboratory
    - The date and time of collection
    - Your observations of anything unusual

FIGURE 33-5 Collecting a urine sample from a male infant.

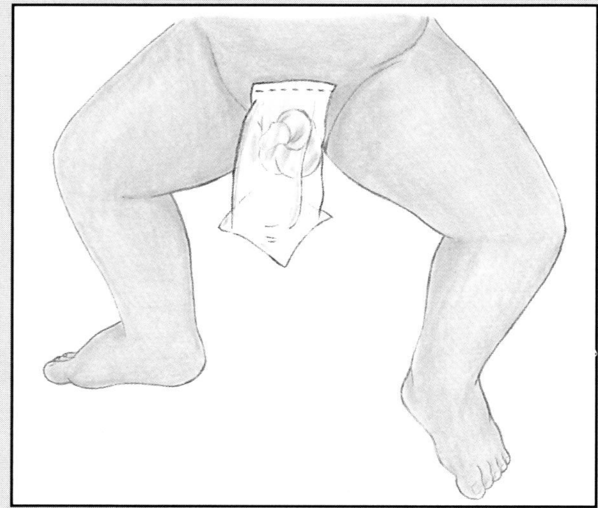

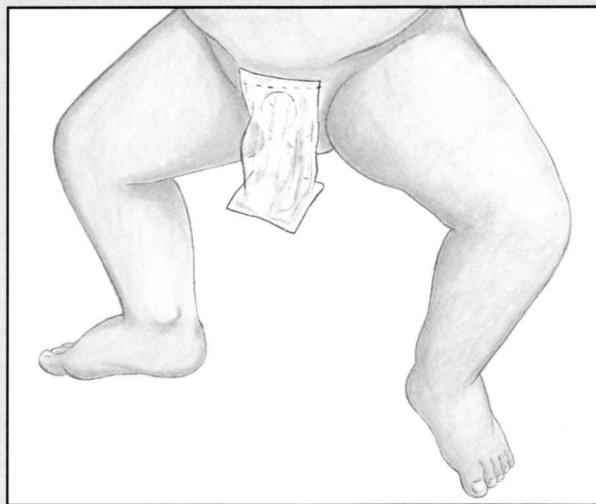

FIGURE 33-6 Collecting a urine sample from a female infant.

KEY IDEAS

Midstream, Clean-Catch Urine Specimen

Midstream
Catching the urine specimen between the time the patient begins to void and the time he stops.

Clean Catch
Refers to the fact that the urine for this specimen is not contaminated by anything outside the patient's body.

A special method is used to collect a patient's urine when the specimen must be free from contamination. This special kind of specimen is called a midstream, **clean-catch** urine specimen. In some health care facilities, a disposable midstream, clean-catch package can be obtained from the central supply room.

All the equipment and supplies necessary for this specimen are in the kit. **Midstream** means catching the urine specimen between the time the patient begins to void and the time he stops. **Clean catch** refers to the fact that the urine is not contaminated by anything outside the patient's body. The procedure requires careful washing of the genital area. This ensures a clean catch, as the urine itself washes off the body opening.

Procedure Collecting a Midstream Clean-Catch Urine Specimen

1. Assemble your equipment (Figure 33-7):
   a) Obtain a requisition slip from the ward clerk or your supervisor for a disposable collection kit for this specimen, or go to the CSR exchange cart, if used in your institution, and get the kit. If your institution does not use disposable equipment, CSR will supply the cotton balls and solution to be used for the cleansing process according to your institution's policy.
   b) Label, if your institution's procedure does not call for writing directly on the cover of the urine container
   c) Disposable gloves
   d) Laboratory request slip, which should be filled out by the nurse, team leader, or ward clerk
   e) Patient's bedpan or urinal, if the patient is unable to go to the bathroom

FIGURE 33-7 Equipment for collecting a midstream, clean-catch urine specimen.

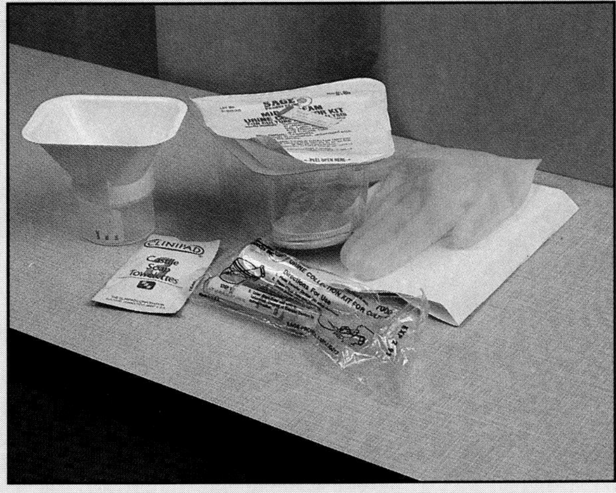

2. Wash your hands.
3. Identify the patient by checking the identification bracelet.
4. Ask visitors to step out of the room, if this is your hospital's policy.
5. Tell the patient you need a midstream, clean-catch urine specimen.
6. Pull the curtain around the bed for privacy.
7. Explain the procedure. If the patient is able, he may collect this specimen on his own in his bathroom.
8. If the patient is not able to collect the specimen himself, help him with the procedure.
9. Open the disposable kit.
10. Remove the towelettes and the urine specimen container from the kit.
11. For female patients:
    a) Put on the disposable gloves.
    b) Use all three towelettes to clean the perineal area.
    c) Separate the folds of the labia (lips) and wipe with one towelette from the front to the back (anterior to posterior) on one side. Then throw away the towelette.
    d) Wipe the other side with a second towelette, again from front to back. Discard the towelette.
    e) Wipe down the middle from front to back, using the third towelette, and discard it.
12. For male patients:
    a) Put on gloves.
    b) If the patient is not circumcised, pull the foreskin back (retract foreskin) on

the penis to clean, and hold it back during urination.

c) Use a circular motion to clean the head of the penis. Discard each towelette after each use.

13. Ask the patient to start to urinate into bedpan, urinal, or the toilet. After the flow of urine has started, ask the patient to stop urinating. Place the urine specimen container under the patient and ask the patient to start urinating again, directly into the urine specimen container. If the patient cannot stop urinating, once having started, move the container into the stream of urine to collect the middle of the stream specimen directly into the urine specimen container. Remove the container with the specimen before the flow of urine stops.
14. If a funnel type of container is used, remove the funnel and discard it.
15. Cover the urine container immediately with the lid from the kit. Be careful not to touch the inside of the container or the inside of the lid.
16. Label the container right away. Copy all needed information from the patient's identification bracelet. Record the date and time of collection.
17. Clean the bedpan or urinal. Put it in its proper place. Remove gloves.
18. Discard all used disposable equipment.
19. Make the patient comfortable.
20. Lower the bed to a position of safety for the patient.
21. Pull the curtains back to the open position.
22. Raise the side rails where ordered, indicated, and appropriate for patient safety.
23. Place the call light within easy reach of the patient.
24. Wash your hands.
25. The labeled specimen container must be sent or taken to the laboratory with a requisition or laboratory request slip, which is usually filled out by the head nurse, team leader, or ward clerk.
26. Report to your immediate supervisor:
    - That a midstream, clean-catch urine specimen has been obtained
    - That it has been sent or taken to the laboratory
    - The date and time of collection
    - Your observations of anything unusual

KEY IDEAS

24-Hour Urine Specimen

A 24-hour urine specimen is a collection of all urine voided by a patient over a 24-hour period. All the urine is collected for 24 hours (Figure 33-8).

When you are to obtain a 24-hour urine specimen, it is necessary to ask the patient to void and discard the first voided urine in the morning.

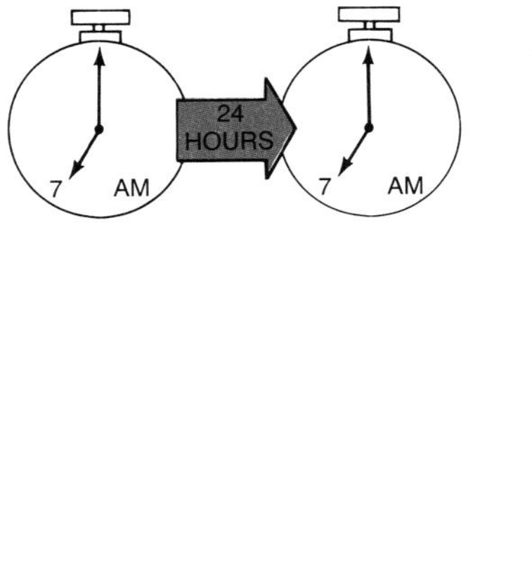

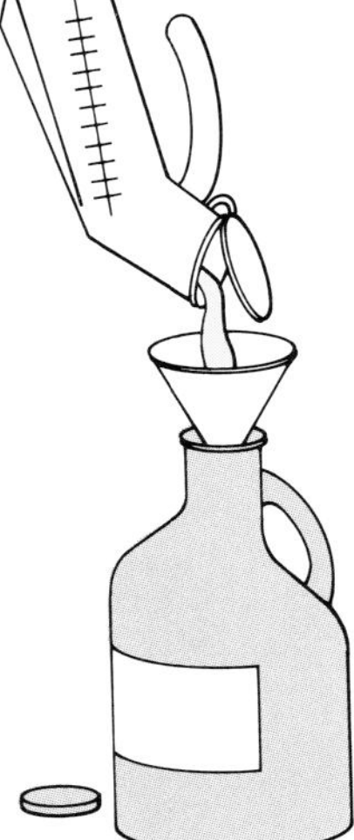

FIGURE 33-8 Collecting a 24-hour urine specimen.

This is because this urine has remained in the bladder an unknown length of time. The test should begin with the bladder empty. For the next 24 hours, save all the urine voided by the patient. On the following day at the same time, ask the patient to void and add this specimen to the previous collection. In this way the doctor can be sure that all the urine for the test came from the urinary bladder during the 24 hours of the test period.

Procedure Collecting a 24-Hour Urine Specimen

1. Assemble your equipment:
   a) Large container, usually a 1-liter plastic disposable bottle
   b) Funnel, if the neck of the bottle is small
   c) Graduate, used for measuring output, if the patient is on intake and output
   d) Patient's bedpan, urinal, or specipan
   e) Label for the container
   f) Laboratory request slip, which should be filled out by the nurse, team leader, or ward clerk
   g) Tag, to be placed over or on the patient's bed, and in the patient's bathroom to indicate that a 24-hour urine specimen is being collected
   h) Disposable gloves
2. Wash your hands.
3. Identify the patient by checking the identification bracelet.
4. Ask visitors to step out of the room, if this is your hospital's policy.
5. Tell the patient that a 24-hour urine specimen is needed.
6. Explain the procedure. Tell the patient you will be placing the large container in her bathroom.
7. Fill in the label for the large container. Copy all needed information from the patient's identification bracelet. Record the date and time of the first collection. Attach the label to the urine specimen container (the large, 1-liter, plastic disposable bottle). Place the container in the patient's bathroom. In many institutions specimens are refrigerated or kept on ice to control odor and the growth of bacteria.
8. Post the tag over or on the patient's bed and in the patient's bathroom. This is so all personnel will be aware that a 24-hour specimen is being collected.
9. Pull the curtain around the bed for privacy each time the patient voids, if she uses a bedpan or urinal at bedside rather than a specipan or urinal in the bathroom. Ask the patient to avoid placing tissue in the bedpan with the specimen, as tissue absorbs urine needed for testing. Provide the patient with a plastic-lined wastepaper basket to temporarily dispose of the toilet tissue. Then discard it in the toilet or hopper.
10. If the patient is on intake and output, measure all the urine each time the patient voids. Write the amount on the intake and output sheet.
11. When the collection starts, have the patient void. Throw away (discard) this first amount of urine. This is to be sure that the bladder is completely empty. This first voiding should not be included in the specimen. This is usually done at 7 A.M. The test will continue until the next day at 7 A.M.
12. You may be instructed to refrigerate the urine or put it on ice. If so, fill a large bucket with ice cubes. Keep the large urine container in the ice in the patient's bathroom. All nursing assistants caring for this patient for the next 24 hours will be responsible for keeping the bucket filled with ice.
13. For the next 24 hours, save all urine voided by the patient. Pour the urine from each voiding into the large container.
14. At the end of the 24-hour period, have the patient void at 7 A.M. Add this to the collection of urine in the large container. This will be the last time you will collect the urine for this test.
15. The large labeled container with the 24-hour collection of urine is taken to the laboratory with a requisition or laboratory request slip that is made out by the head nurse, team leader, or ward clerk.

16. Clean the equipment and put it in its proper place. Discard disposable equipment.
17. Remove the 24-hour specimen tag from the patient's bed.
18. Make the patient comfortable.
19. Lower the bed to a position of safety for the patient.
20. Pull the curtains back to the open position.
21. Raise the side rails where ordered, indicated, and appropriate for patient safety.
22. Place the call light within easy reach of the patient.
23. Wash your hands.
24. Report to your immediate supervisor:
    - That a 24-hour urine specimen has been obtained
    - That the specimen has been sent to the laboratory
    - The date and time of collection
    - Your observations of anything unusual

KEY IDEAS

Straining the Urine

The urine is strained to determine if a patient has passed stones (calculi) or other matter from the kidneys. The doctor may order that all urine passed by the patient is to be strained.

Procedure Straining the Urine

1. Assemble your equipment in the patient's bathroom:
    a) Disposable paper strainers or gauze squares
    b) Specimen container with cover or a small plastic bag to be used as a specimen container
    c) Label, if your institution's procedure is not to write on the cover
    d) Patient's bedpan and cover, urinal, or specipan
    e) Laboratory request slip, which should be filled out by the nurse, team leader, or ward clerk
    f) Tag, to be placed over or on the patient's bed indicating that all urine must be strained
    g) Disposable gloves
2. Wash your hands.
3. Identify the patient by checking the identification bracelet.
4. Ask visitors to step out of the room, if this is your hospital's policy.
5. Tell the patient that each time she urinates it must be into a urinal, bedpan, or specipan, as all urine must be strained. Caution the patient not to put any tissue into the container. Provide the patient with a plastic-lined wastepaper basket to temporarily dispose of the toilet tissue. Then discard it in the toilet or hopper.
6. Pull the curtain around the bed for privacy whenever the patient voids.
7. Put on gloves.

FIGURE 33-9 Filtering urine.

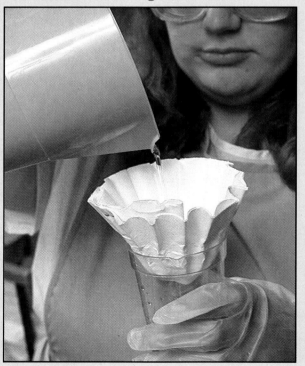

8. When the patient voids, take the bedpan or urinal to the patient's bathroom. Pour the urine through the strainer or gauze into the measuring container (Figure 39-9).
9. If any particles show up on the gauze or the paper strainer, place the gauze or paper strainer with particles in a plastic bag or specimen container. Do not attempt to remove the particles, because they may be lost or damaged.
10. Label the specimen container immediately. Copy all needed information from the patient's identification bracelet. Record the date and time of collection.
11. Measure the amount of the voiding and record it on the intake and output sheet, if the patient is on intake and output.
12. Discard the urine.
13. Clean and rinse the bedpan and graduate and put them in their proper places.
14. Remove gloves.
15. Make the patient comfortable.
16. Lower the bed to a position of safety for the patient.
17. Pull the curtains back to the open position.
18. Raise the side rails where ordered, indicated, and appropriate for patient safety.
19. Place the call light within easy reach of the patient.
20. Wash your hands.
21. Report at once to your immediate supervisor:
    - That, in straining the urine, particles were obtained
    - That a specimen was collected
    - The date and time of collection
    - Your observations of anything unusual

The labeled specimen container must be taken to the laboratory with a requisition or laboratory request slip at the nurse's request.

KEY IDEAS

Sputum Specimen

Sputum
Waste material coughed up from the lungs or trachea.

Saliva
The secretion of the salivary glands into the mouth. Saliva moistens food and helps in swallowing. It also contains an enzyme (protein) that helps digest starches.

Sputum is a substance collected from a patient's lungs that contains saliva, mucus, and sometimes pus or blood. It is thicker than ordinary **saliva** (spit). Most of it is coughed up from the lungs and bronchial tubes. In some health care facilities, this procedure is carried out by the Respiratory Therapy Department (Pulmonary Medicine).

Usually, early morning is the best time to obtain this specimen.

Procedure Collecting a Sputum Specimen

1. Assemble your equipment:
   a) Sputum container with cover and tissues
   b) Label, if your institution's procedure is not to write on the cover
   c) Laboratory request slip, which should be filled out by the nurse, team leader, or ward clerk
   d) Disposable gloves
2. Wash your hands.
3. Identify the patient by checking the identification bracelet.
4. Tell the patient that a sputum specimen is needed.
5. If the patient has eaten recently, have him rinse out his mouth. If he wants to have oral hygiene at this time, help him as necessary.
6. Put on gloves.
7. Give the patient a sputum container (Figure 33-10). Ask him to take three consecutive deep breaths and on the third exhalation to cough deep from within the lungs to bring up the thick

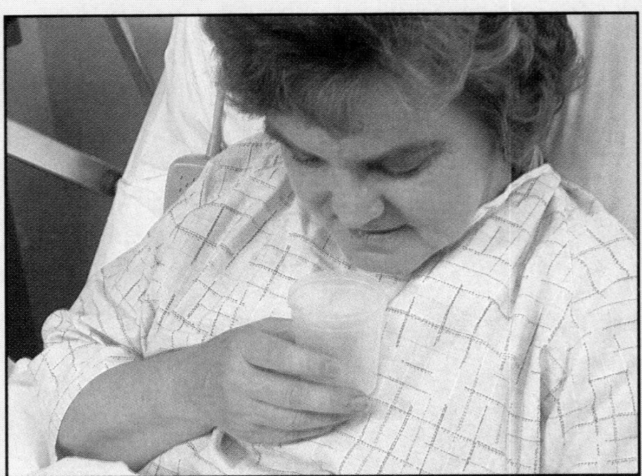
FIGURE 33-10 Collecting the sputum specimen.

sputum. Explain that saliva (spit) and nose secretions are not adequate for this test.

8. The patient may have to cough several times to bring up enough sputum for the specimen. One to two tablespoons is usually the required amount.
9. Cover the container immediately. Be careful not to touch the inside of either the container or the cover to avoid contamination.
10. Label the container right away. Copy all needed information from the patient's identification bracelet. Record the time of collection and the date.
11. The labeled specimen container must be sent or taken immediately to the laboratory with a requisition or laboratory request slip. This should be filled out by the nurse or ward clerk. The test must be done in the laboratory before the sputum begins to dry.
12. Make the patient comfortable.
13. Lower the bed to a position of safety for the patient.
14. Pull the curtains back to the open position.
15. Raise the side rails where ordered, indicated, and appropriate for patient safety.
16. Place the call light within easy reach of the patient.
17. Wash your hands.
18. Report at once to your immediate supervisor:
    - That a sputum specimen has been obtained
    - The color, amount, odor, and consistency of the specimen
    - That the specimen has been sent to the laboratory
    - The date and time of collection
    - How the patient tolerated the procedure
    - Your observations of anything unusual

KEY IDEAS

Stool Specimen

Feces, Stool
Solid waste material discharged from the body through the rectum and anus. Other names include excreta, excrement, bowel movement, and fecal matter.

Feces, **stool**, b.m., bowel movement, and fecal matter all mean the same thing, the solid waste from a patient's body. The doctor sometimes orders a stool specimen to help him in the diagnosis of a patient's illness. Sometimes a warm specimen is ordered. This means that the specimen must be tested in the laboratory while the specimen is still warm from the patient's body. You will be told whether the specimen is to be warm or cold.

Procedure Collecting a Stool Specimen

1. Assemble your equipment (Figure 33-11):
    a) Patient's bedpan and cover
    b) Stool specimen container
    c) Wooden tongue depressor
    d) Label, if your institution's procedure is not to write on the cover
    e) Laboratory request slip, which should be filled out by the nurse, team leader, or ward clerk

f) Plastic bag for warm specimen, if used by your institution
g) Disposable gloves

2. Wash your hands.

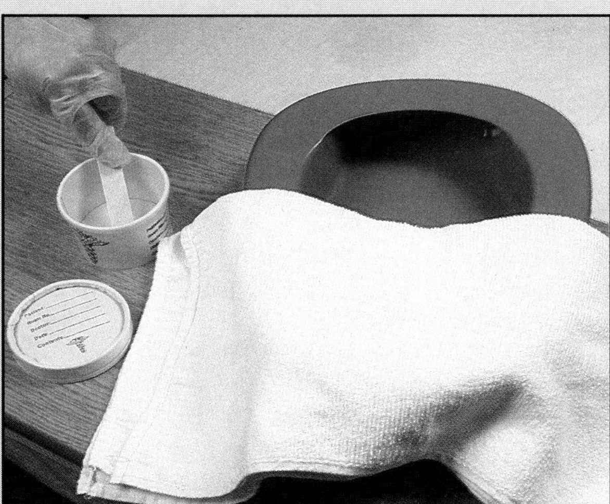

FIGURE 33-11 Equipment for collecting a stool specimen.

3. Identify the patient by checking the identification bracelet.
4. Ask visitors to step out of the room, if this is your hospital's policy.
5. Tell the patient that a stool specimen is needed. Explain that whenever he can move his bowels he is to call you so the specimen can be collected.
6. Pull the curtain around the bed for privacy while the patient is on the bedpan.
7. Have the patient move his bowels into the bedpan or into a specipan placed in the back half of the toilet.
8. Ask the patient not to urinate into the bedpan and not to put toilet tissue in the bedpan. Provide the patient with a plastic-lined wastepaper basket to temporarily dispose of the toilet tissue. Then discard it in the toilet or hopper.
9. Prepare the label immediately by copying all needed information from the patient's identification bracelet. Record the time of collection and the date.
10. Put on gloves.
11. After the patient has had a bowel movement, take the covered bedpan to the patient's bathroom or to the dirty utility room.
12. Using the wooden tongue depressor, take about 1 to 2 tablespoons of feces from the bedpan and place them in the stool specimen container. Label the specimen container.
13. Cover the container immediately. Be careful not to touch the inside of either the container or the cover to avoid contamination.
14. Wrap the tongue depressor in a paper towel and discard it.
15. Empty the remaining feces into the toilet or hopper.
16. Clean the bedpan and return it to its proper place.
17. Remove and discard gloves.
18. Wash your hands.
19. If your head nurse or team leader told you this is a warm specimen, it must be taken to the laboratory for examination while it is still warm from the patient's body. Place the stool specimen container, fully labeled, in the plastic bag (if used by your institution). Attach the laboratory request slip to the bag. Carry it immediately to the laboratory.
20. Make the patient comfortable.
21. Lower the bed to a position of safety for the patient.
22. Pull the curtains back to the open position.
23. Raise the side rails where ordered, indicated, and appropriate for patient safety.
24. Place the call light within easy reach of the patient.
25. Wash your hands.
26. Report at once to your immediate supervisor:
    - That a stool specimen has been obtained
    - That the specimen has been sent to the laboratory
    - The date and time of collection
    - Your observations of anything unusual

In some institutions, you may be requested to prepare Hemoccult slides. The correct procedure is as follows:

Procedure Preparing a Hemoccult Slide

Note: Some states require that Hemoccult slides be collected by a nurse.

1. Ask the patient to move his or her bowels into a bedpan or specipan, whenever this is possible.
2. Wash your hands.
3. Put on gloves.
4. Check the patient's identification bracelet.
5. Label the outside of the Hemoccult slide with the patient's name, address, hospital number, and the date this specimen is collected.
6. Collect a small amount of stool on a depressor.
7. Apply small amount in box A on Hemoccult slide.
8. Open side 1.
9. Collect a small amount of stool on depressor.
10. Apply small amount in box B.
11. Close cover of slide card and secure.
12. Check information with patient identification bracelet.
13. Send to the laboratory.
14. Report to your immediate supervisor:
    - That the Hemoccult specimen has been collected and sent to the laboratory
    - The time and date it was collected
    - Your observations of anything unusual

KEY QUESTIONS

1. List the types of specimens nursing assistants are expected to collect.
2. What information must be written on the specimen label?
3. What are ten things you should do to ensure accuracy when collecting specimens?
4. Why is it important to use good medical asepsis when collecting specimens?
5. How should a routine urine specimen be collected?
6. What is the difference between collecting a routine urine specimen from an infant and from an adult?
7. What is the difference between collecting a routine urine specimen and a midstream clean-catch urine specimen?
8. Why should the first urine voided at 7 A.M. be discarded when collecting a 24-hour urine specimen?
9. How should urine be strained?
10. Usually, when is the best time to collect a sputum specimen?
11. How should a stool specimen be collected?
12. Define: asepsis, clean catch, expectorate, feces, genital medical asepsis, midstream, saliva, specimen, sputum, stool.

CHAPTER

34

Anatomy and Physiology of the Endocrine System

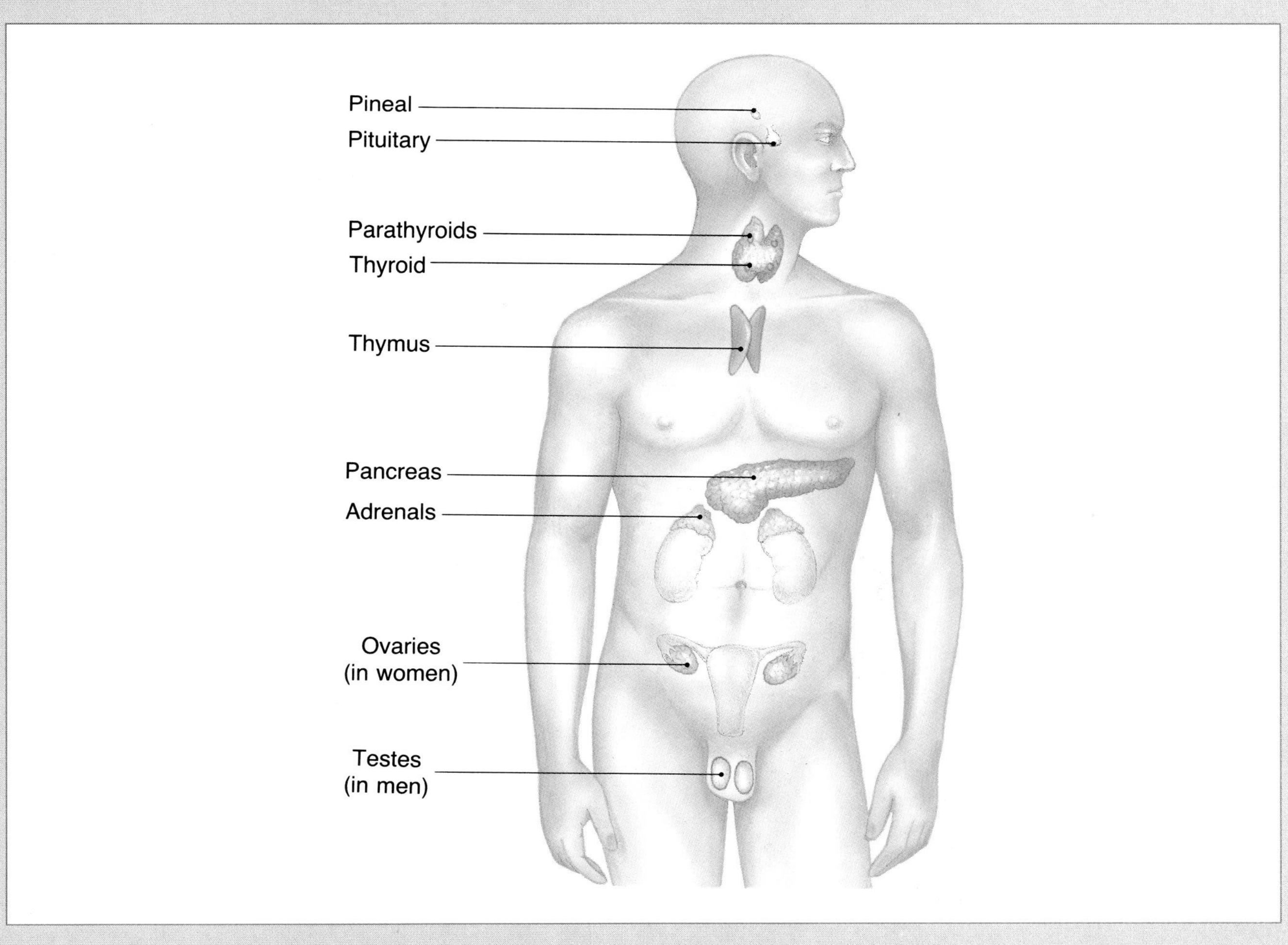

WARNING

For all patient contact, adhere to Universal Precautions (see page 91, 97, or the front cover flap). Wear protective equipment as indicated.

Objectives

What You Will Learn

When you have completed this chapter, you will be able to:

- Label a diagram of the body with the endocrine glands.
- Describe the function of each gland.
- List the common diseases and disorders of the endocrine system.
- Define: endocrine glands, endocrine system, exocrine glands, gland, hormones, insulin, secrete.

KEY IDEAS

Hormones and the Endocrine System

Hormones
Protein substances secreted by endocrine glands directly into the blood, to be circulated to another part of the body where they stimulate increased activity by chemical action.

Endocrine System
The system composed of the endocrine glands, which regulates body function by secreting hormones into the blood or lymph to be circulated to all parts of the body.

Endocrine Glands
Ductless glands that produce hormones and secrete them directly into the blood or lymph.

Secrete
To produce a special substance and expel or discharge it. The salivary glands secrete saliva. The pancreas secretes insulin.

Exocrine Glands
Glands that produce hormones and secrete them either directly or through a duct to epithelial tissue, such as a body cavity or the skin surface.

THE **ENDOCRINE GLANDS** SECRETE LIQUIDS CALLED hormones. These help the nervous system organize and direct the activities of the body. The endocrine hormones are **secreted** directly into the bloodstream from the organ that makes them. **Exocrine glands**, such as the salivary glands, deliver their products through ducts into a body cavity or to the skin surface, as from sweat glands.

The hormones from the pituitary gland, both the anterior and posterior portions, regulate the metabolism of our billions of cells. The anterior portion manufactures and releases seven hormones.

The pituitary gland is the master **gland**. Its hormones directly affect the other endocrine glands, stimulating them to produce their hormones. Its hormones are especially important in reproduction and in all functions leading to puberty. This is the time at which a child takes on the physical characteristics of an adult man or woman. Hormones from the pituitary gland regulate the menstrual cycle in the female and sperm production in the male. Without these hormones, it would not be possible for us to reproduce.

The pituitary gland and all these important hormones are under the direct control of the hypothalamus, a tiny piece of tissue lying near the base of the brain. This structure seems to be the real link between our thinking, our emotions, and our body functions.

The thyroid gland produces a hormone that regulates growth and general metabolism. The thymus gets smaller after puberty, but it plays an important part in the body's immune system. The immune system prevents us from getting many diseases.

The parathyroids are located within the capsule of the thyroid. They produce a hormone that, along with one of the hormones in the thyroid gland, regulates the level of calcium and potassium in the blood. Calcium is important for many functions of the body, such as muscle contraction and conduction of nerve impulses.

The pancreas is both an endocrine gland and an exocrine gland, or a gland that has a duct. Its endocrine portion produces the hormone insulin. **Insulin** regulates the sugar content of the blood. If the body does not have enough insulin, the person develops hyperglycemia (high blood

Gland
An organ that is able to manufacture and discharge a chemical that will be used elsewhere in the body.

Insulin
A hormone produced naturally by the pancreas that helps the body change sugar into energy. Insulin can be produced from an animal pancreas for use in the treatment of diabetes.

sugar) and becomes diabetic. He or she must be treated by reducing the carbohydrate or sugar intake and by regulating the balance between insulin and blood sugar.

The adrenal glands lie on top of the kidneys. They are very important in helping the body adapt to stress conditions by stimulating the autonomic nervous system.

The ovaries in the female are responsible for secreting the hormones estrogen and progesterone. The rise and fall of the levels of these hormones in the blood determine the menstrual cycle. The hormones are also important in causing an ovum, or egg, to develop and in maintaining a pregnancy.

The testes in the male produce testosterone, the primary sex hormone of the male, which also causes the production of sperm.

Common Diseases and Disorders of the Endocrine System

- *Hypothyroidism:* the thyroid gland does not secrete enough hormone.
- *Hyperthyroidism:* the thyroid gland secretes too much hormone.
- *Hyperparathyroidism:* overactivity of the parathyroid glands.
- *Hypoparathyroidism:* absence of activity of the parathyroid glands.
- *Diabetes mellitus:* abnormality of the endocrine secretions of the pancreas, which results in metabolic abnormalities.
- *Cushing's syndrome:* hyperactivity of the adrenal glands.
- *Addison's disease:* hypo(less) function of the adrenal glands.
- *Hyperpituitarism:* excessive amount of growth hormone is secreted from the pituitary gland.
- *Hypopituitarism:* pituitary insufficiency; not enough hormone is secreted.
- *Pituitary tumors:* causes changes in normal growth.

KEY QUESTIONS

1. List the endocrine glands.
2. What does each gland do?
3. What are the common diseases and disorders of the endocrine system?
4. Define: endocrine glands, endocrine system, exocrine glands, gland, hormones, insulin, secrete.

CHAPTER

35 Care of the Diabetic Patient

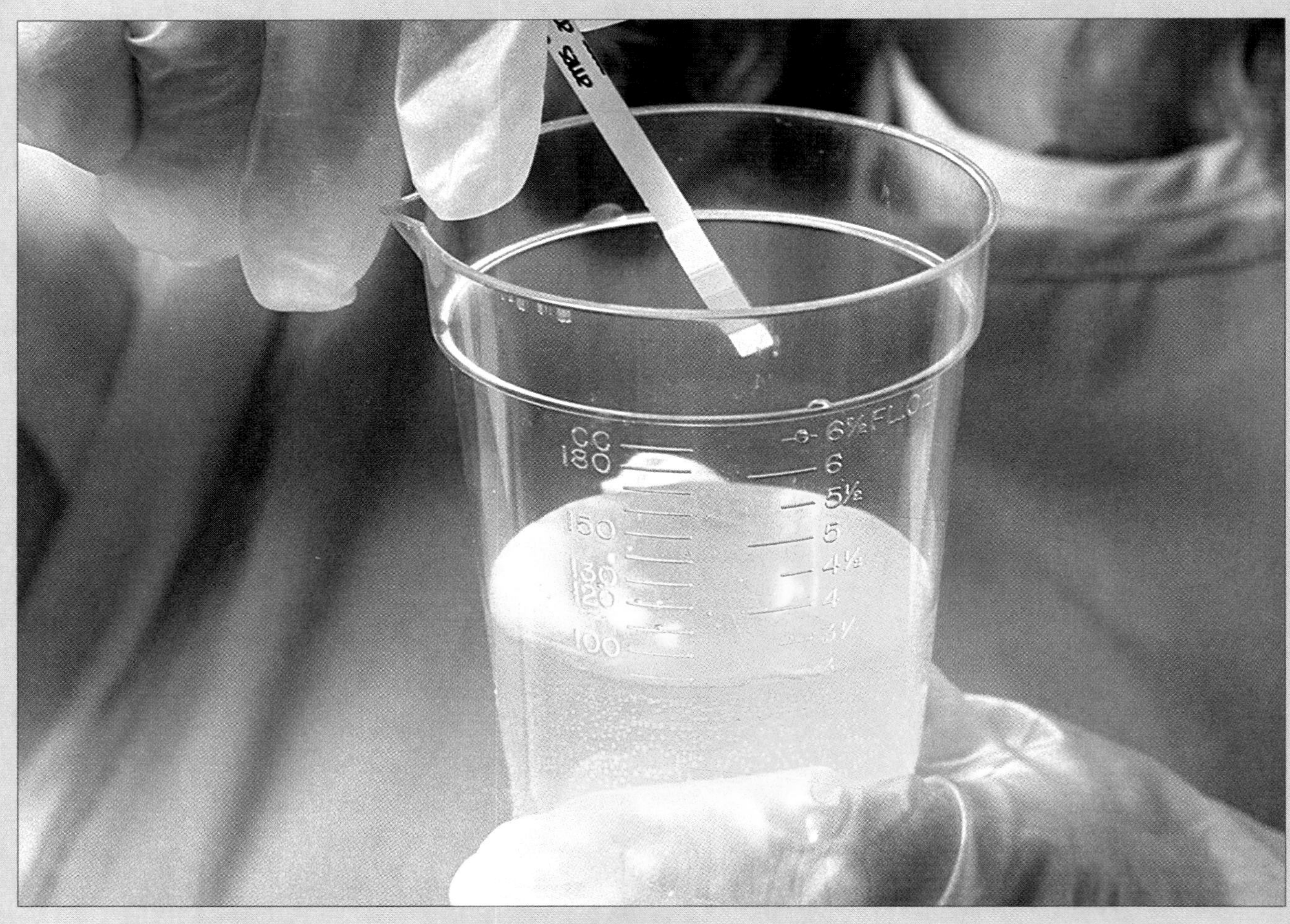

WARNING

For all patient contact, adhere to Universal Precautions (see page 91, 97, or the front cover flap). Wear protective equipment as indicated.

Objectives

What You Will Learn

When you have completed this chapter, you will be able to:

- Recognize the signs and symptoms of diabetes mellitus, insulin shock, and diabetic coma.
- Collect a fresh urine specimen.
- Test urine for sugar, acetone, and ketones.
- Teach the patient with diabetes how to avoid pressure points and skin problems.
- Describe testing the blood glucose level via a finger stick using a blood glucose meter.
- Define: Acetest, acetone, carbohydrate, Clinitest, diabetes mellitus, diabetic coma, fresh urine, glucose, hyperglycemia, hypoglycemia, insulin shock, ketones, metabolism, reagent.

SOMETIMES THE BODY CANNOT CHANGE STARCHES and sugar into energy and cannot store them because of an imbalance of the hormone insulin. The result is the chronic disease known as **diabetes mellitus**, which is a disturbance of **carbohydrate metabolism**.

There are two types of diabetes:

- Insulin-dependent Diabetes Mellitus (IDDM), also known as Type I or Juvenile-Onset Diabetes
- Non-Insulin-Dependent Diabetes Mellitus (NIDDM), also known as Type II or Adult-Onset Diabetes

Insulin shock is a condition that occurs in patients with diabetes when they receive too much insulin or when they miss a meal or have too much physical activity. It has a sudden onset.

Diabetic coma may occur when the diabetic patient does not receive enough insulin to metabolize carbohydrates or when there is increased stress or infection. It may have a gradual onset.

Terms Often Used with Diabetes Mellitus

- FBS: fasting blood sugar
- GTT: glucose tolerance test
- **Hypoglycemia**
- **Hyperglycemia**
- Ketone bodies
- Gangrene: necrosis
- S&A test: sugar and acetone test
- Pancreas (organ that produces insulin) and islands of Langerhans (part of pancreas that produces insulin): endocrine and exocrine glands

KEY IDEAS

Diabetes Mellitus

Diabetes Mellitus
A disorder of carbohydrate metabolism that develops when the body cannot change sugar into energy due to inadequate production or utilization of insulin. When this sugar collects in the blood, the patient needs a special diet and may have to be given medications.

Carbohydrate
One of the basic food elements used by the body; composed of carbon, hydrogen, and oxygen (includes sugars and starches).

Metabolism
The total of all the physical and chemical changes that take place in living organisms and cells, including all the processes involved in the use of substances taken into the body.

Insulin Shock
A condition that can occur in a diabetic patient with too much insulin, which results in very low blood sugar.

Diabetic Coma
A coma (abnormal deep stupor) that can occur in a diabetic patient from lack of insulin.

Hypoglycemia
Abnormally low blood sugar.

Hyperglycemia
Abnormally high blood sugar.

- PPBS: postprandial blood sugar
- Fresh urine specimen

Signs and Symptoms of Diabetes Mellitus

- Fatigue, tiredness
- Loss of weight
- Vaginitis: inflammation of the vagina
- Skin erosions (lesions); sores heal poorly and slowly (a late sign)
- Hyperglycemia: high blood sugar
- Glycosuria: sugar in the urine
- Polyuria: frequent and large amounts of urine
- Polydipsia: excessive thirst
- Poor vision: eyesight affected

Signs and Symptoms of Insulin Shock (Hypoglycemia, Low Blood Sugar, or Insulin Reaction)

- Excessive sweating, perspiration
- Faintness, dizziness, weakness
- Hunger (polyphagia)
- Irritability, personality change, nervousness
- Numbness of tongue and lips
- Not able to awaken, coma, unconsciousness, stupor
- Headache
- Tremors, trembling
- Blurred or impaired vision
- Upon examination: low blood sugar or no sugar in the urine

Signs and Symptoms of Diabetic Coma (Hyperglycemia, High Blood Sugar, or Diabetic Acidosis)

- Air hunger, heavy labored breathing, increased respirations
- Loss of appetite
- Nausea and/or vomiting
- Weakness
- Abdominal pains or discomfort
- Generalized aches
- Increased thirst and parched tongue
- Sweet or fruity odor of the breath
- Flushed skin
- Dry skin
- Increased urination
- Dulled senses
- Loss of consciousness
- Upon examination: large amounts of sugar and ketones in the urine or high blood sugar

KEY IDEAS

Testing Urine for Sugar/Glucose and Acetone/Ketones

When caring for a patient with diabetes, you may be asked to perform certain tests on the patient's urine. There are two basic tests: one for sugar (the Clinitest) and one for acetone (the Acetest). In your work you will collect the fresh urine specimen (specimen collected for both sugar and acetone tests). However, the actual test may be done in a laboratory or by the nurse. In certain situations you may do the tests. The results of these tests are needed by the doctor and the nurse to determine changes that must be made in the diabetic patient's diet and medications.

These tests are usually done four times a day: one-half hour before breakfast, lunch, and supper, and at bedtime.

Reagent
A substance used in a chemical reaction to determine the presence of another substance.

For each test you will be using either a reagent strip or a reagent tablet. A **reagent** is a substance in a chemical reaction that indicates the presence of another substance. The names for these tablets or strips vary. When testing for sugar (doing the Clinitest®) you will be using Clinitest® tablets, Tes-tape®, or Clinistix® strips. When testing for acetone (doing the Acetest®), you will be using Ketostix® or Acetone® tablets. Keto-Diastix® is a multiuse reagent strip that tests for both sugar/glucose and acetone/ketones. This multiuse strip is simply dipped into a fresh urine specimen and then compared to the color charts on the container according to the manufacturer's directions.

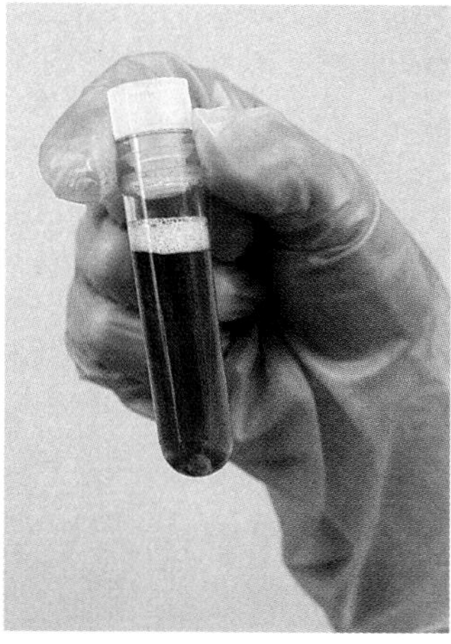

FIGURE 35-1 Heat is generated during the Clinitest. Hold the test tube by its top and do not touch the bottom.

Some institutions have a small, individual disposable kit for these tests, which is ordered for each patient. The patient's name should be written on the container. It should be kept in the patient's bathroom or in a designated place in the dirty utility room.

Instructions for these tests are usually posted in the dirty utility room or on the package of reagent strips or reagent tablets. All tablets and strips used for these tests are poisonous. Always put equipment in a safe place where children cannot reach it. Heat is generated during the Clinitest®. Do not touch the bottom of the glass test tube while doing the tests as it will be hot and you could burn yourself (Figure 35-1). Do not touch the tablet with your fingers, because it can burn your skin.

Fresh Specimens

Fresh Urine
Urine that has been accumulated recently in the patient's urinary bladder.

A fresh specimen is needed for each testing. However, since the sugar test and the acetone test are done at the same time, only one specimen is needed. The term **fresh urine** is used to refer to urine that has been accumulated recently in the patient's urinary bladder. To obtain fresh urine, it is necessary to discard the first urine voided in the morning because this urine has remained in the urinary bladder for an unknown length of time. One-half hour after discarding the urine, collect a fresh urine specimen for the test. This will be urine recently accumulated in the urinary bladder. Only a very small amount of urine is needed for these tests.

Procedure Collecting a Fresh Urine Specimen

1. Assemble your equipment:
   a) Bedpan and cover, urinal, or specipan and cover
   b) Urine specimen container with cover
   c) Graduate, to measure output if the patient is on intake and output
   d) Label, if necessary. You will write on the label or on the cover of the container depending on the policy of the institution.
   e) Disposable gloves
2. Wash your hands and put on gloves.
3. Identify the patient by checking the identification bracelet.
4. Ask visitors to step out of the room.
5. Tell the patient you need some urine for a urine test.
6. Pull the curtain around the bed for privacy.
7. Ask the patient to urinate into a clean bedpan, urinal, or specipan one-half

hour before the test is to be done, in order to empty the bladder if this is the first void of the day. If the patient is unable to void at this time, report this to your immediate supervisor.

8. If the patient is on intake and output, measure the urine and record the amount on the intake and output sheet.
9. Throw away this urine.
10. Have the patient void again at the correct time for the test so that fresh urine is used for the test.
11. Take the covered bedpan or urinal to the patient's bathroom or to the dirty utility room.
12. If the patient is on intake and output, measure and record the amount on the intake and output sheet.
13. Label the specimen container with the patient's name copied from the patient's identification bracelet. Record the time and date of collection.
14. If the urine is to be tested on the patient care unit, test it at this time. If the specimen is to be tested in the laboratory, send or take the specimen with a requisition or laboratory request slip to the laboratory immediately.
15. Discard the remaining urine. Wash the bedpan or urinal and put it in its proper place.
16. Wash the patient's hands and make him comfortable.
17. Lower the bed to a position of safety for the patient.
18. Pull the curtains back to the open position.
19. Raise the side rails where ordered, indicated, and appropriate for patient safety.
20. Place the call light within easy reach of the patient.
21. Remove gloves and wash your hands.
22. Report to your immediate supervisor:
    - That the fresh urine specimen has been obtained.
    - The result of the test or that the specimen has been sent to the laboratory or that it is in the proper place for testing
    - The date and time of collection
    - Your observations of anything unusual

Procedure Collecting a Fresh Urine Specimen from a Closed Urinary Drainage System through a Collection/Puncture/Speci-port

1. Assemble your equipment:
    a) Alcohol sponge or the disinfectant of choice at your institution
    b) Syringe with attached needle
    c) Urine specimen container with cover
    d) Label, if necessary. You will write on the label or on the cover of the container depending on the policy of the institution.
    e) Disposable gloves
2. Wash your hands.
3. Identify the patient by checking the identification bracelet.
4. Ask visitors to step out of the room, if this is your hospital's policy.
5. Tell the patient you need some urine for a urine test.
6. Pull the curtain around the bed for privacy.
7. Close clamp on drainage tubing below the collection/puncture/speci-port. *Do not* leave the bedside at this time for any reason, as the clamp cannot be left on the tubing for more than the time it takes to collect the fresh urine specimen from a closed urinary drainage system.
8. Cleanse the collection/puncture/speci-port with the alcohol sponge or the disinfectant used in your institution (may be Betadine®, Hibiclens®, and so on) (Figure 35.2).
9. Put on gloves. Remove the needle cover from the syringe.
10. Insert the needle into the collection/puncture/speci-port and pull gently back on the plunger to obtain the amount required by your employing institution (often approximately 2 cc).

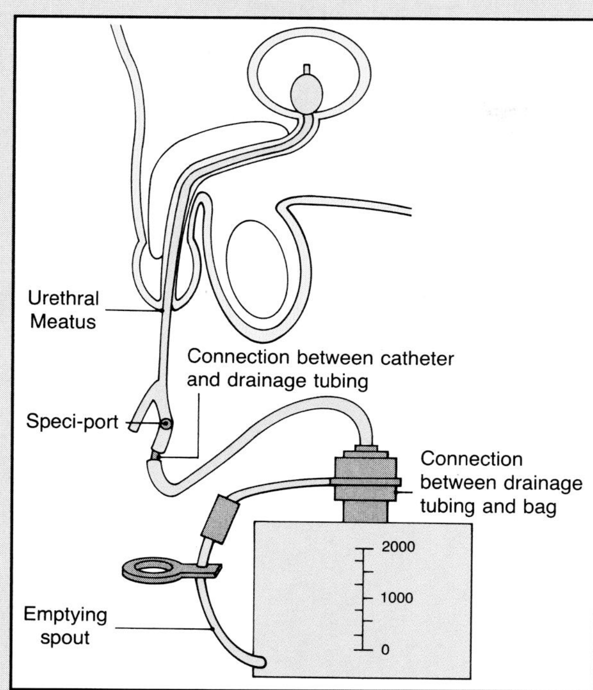

FIGURE 35-2 Sites where bacteria enter the urinary drainage system.

11. Remove the needle and syringe from the collection/puncture/speci-port. Cleanse the collection/puncture/speci-port with an alcohol sponge.
12. Open the clamp from the drainage tubing. Be sure the urine is now running freely down the tubing into the collection bag.
13. Place the needle of the syringe into the specimen container and push the plunger to expel the urine into the specimen container.
14. Cover the specimen container and label with the patient's name copied from the patient's identification bracelet. Record the time and date of collection.
15. Take the syringe with needle and cover to the proper container and dispose of them in accordance with your institution's policies. Do not recover the needle as this can cause an accident or needle stick.
16. Take the urine specimen to the testing area. If in your institution you test urine, do so at this time. However, if in your institution the urine is sent to the laboratory, get a laboratory request slip or requisition slip from the ward clerk and send to the laboratory.
17. Make the patient comfortable.
18. Lower the bed to a position of safety for the patient.
19. Pull the curtains back to the open position.
20. Raise the side rails where ordered, indicated, and appropriate for patient safety.
21. Place the call light within easy reach of the patient.
22. Remove gloves.
23. Wash your hands.
24. Report immediately to your supervisor:
    - That the fresh urine specimen has been obtained from the closed urinary drainage system
    - The result of the test or that the specimen has been sent to the laboratory or that it is in the proper place for testing
    - The date and time of collection
    - Your observations of anything unusual

KEY IDEAS
The Clinitest and Clinistix Test

The **Clinitest** and Clinistix tests are done to determine the amount of **glucose** (sugar) in the patient's urine. Urine glucose level refers to the amount of sugar in the urine.

Procedure The Clinitest

1. Assemble your equipment:
    a) Fresh urine specimen labeled with the patient's name
    b) Clean and dry test tube
    c) Color chart
    d) Medicine dropper
    e) Clinitest reagent tablets
    f) Paper cup of water for rinsing dropper

g) Paper cup of clean water for test
h) Paper towel
i) Disposable gloves

2. Wash your hands and put on gloves.
3. Place the paper towel on the countertop that will be your working area.
4. Rinse the dropper in the paper cup of water that is used for rinsing only.
5. With the dropper in the upright position, place 5 drops of urine in the center of the test tube.
6. Rinse the dropper.
7. Place 10 drops of clean water in the center of the test tube.
8. Place one Clinitest tablet in the test tube by first dropping the tablet into the cover of the bottle and then dropping the tablet into the test tube from the cover (Figure 35-3). Never touch the tablet with your hands. (If your hands are wet and you touch the tablet, the moisture will activate the reaction and you will be burned.) Cap the bottle immediately. If the tablets are individually wrapped, open the foil carefully and drop the tablet into the test tube without touching the tablet. Monitor the entire reaction.

FIGURE 35-3

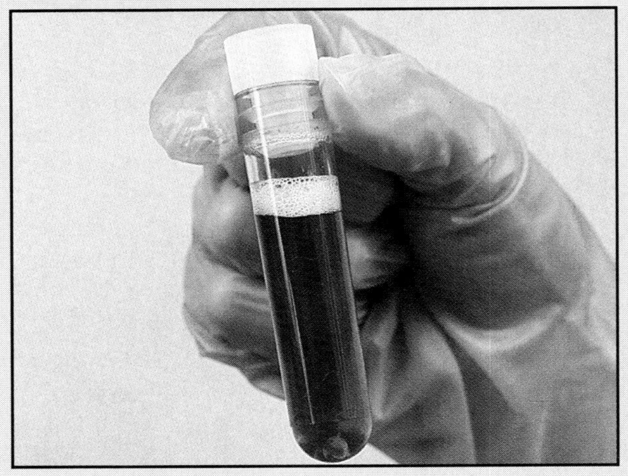

9. Wait 15 seconds after the reaction (boiling) has stopped. Then gently shake the test tube. Remember not to touch the bottom of the test tube; it will be hot.
10. Match the color of the liquid in the test tube to the nearest matching color on the chart. Be sure to use the color chart that goes with the tablets you have used for the test. If the color is questionable, or moves to a bright orange 2 percent, then changes back to one of the other colors at the time you are to read the test, consult your immediate supervisor.
11. Read the number inside the matching color box. For example, if the color is bright orange, it will say 2% or 4^{++++} (plus) inside the orange-colored box.
12. Throw away the used disposable equipment. Wash the test tube with cold water. Replace it upside down so that any remaining water will drain out. The test tube will then be ready for the next test. Rinse the medicine dropper with cold water. Put it in the rack in the upright position.
13. Remove gloves and wash your hands.
14. Report immediately to your supervisor:
    - That you have completed the Clinitest
    - Your findings (the number from the matching color box) so that she or he can enter the information on the patient's chart or designated form
    - Your observations of anything unusual

Procedure The Clinistix Test

1. Assemble your equipment:
    a) Fresh urine specimen labeled with the patient's name
    b) Clinistix reagent strips
    c) Disposable gloves
2. Wash your hands and put on gloves.
3. Dip the reagent strip into the urine in the specimen container (Figure 35-4).
4. Remove it immediately.
5. Tap the edge of the strip against the side of the urine container to remove excess urine.
6. Hold the strip in a horizontal position to prevent the mixing of the chemical from the adjacent reagent area.
7. Read the results 10 seconds (or at the

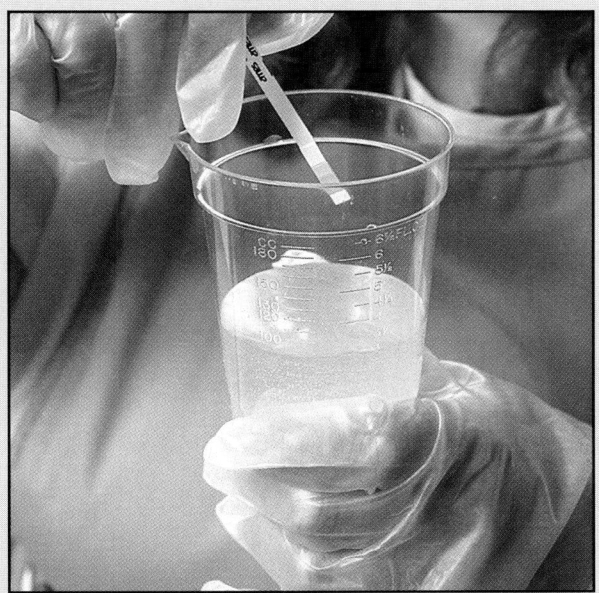
FIGURE 35-4

manufacturer's specified time) after removing the strip from the urine. Clinistix reagent strips are used for the glucose level and should be read at the proper time for qualitative results.

8. Read the results from the color chart, matching the color carefully. The color chart is on the bottle label that holds the Clinistix.
9. Discard disposable equipment.
10. Remove gloves and wash your hands.
11. Report immediately to your supervisor:
    - That you have completed the Clinistix test
    - Your findings (the number from the matching color box) so that she or he can enter the information on the patient's chart or designated form
    - Your observations of anything unusual

KEY IDEAS

The Acetest and Ketostix Reagent Strip Test

The **Acetest** and Ketostix reagent strip tests determine the amount of acetone or ketones in the patient's urine. **Acetone** level refers to the amount of acetone in the urine. **Ketone** level refers to the amount of ketones in the urine.

Acetest®
A test used to measure the amount of acetone in the patient's urine.

Acetone
A chemical compound found in the blood and urine of diabetic patients.

Ketones
Organic chemical substances that are produced when fatty acids combine with oxygen.

Procedure The Acetest

1. Assemble your equipment:
    a) Fresh urine specimen labeled with the patient's name
    b) Color chart
    c) Medicine dropper
    d) Acetest reagent tablets
    e) Paper cup of water for rinsing dropper
    f) Paper towel
    g) Disposable gloves
2. Wash your hands and put on gloves.
3. Place the paper towel on the countertop that will be your working area.
4. Place one Acetest tablet on the paper towel.
5. Never touch the tablet, but drop it into the cover of its container. Then place it on the paper towel from the cover.
6. Rinse the medicine dropper with water from the paper cup.
7. Drop one drop of urine on the tablet. Wait 30 seconds.
8. Compare it to the color chart.
9. Match the tablet color to the closest matching color on the chart.
10. Read the results from the chart. For example, if the color is dark purple, it will say "Large Quantity."
11. Throw away the used disposable equipment and rinse the medicine dropper with clean water.
12. Remove gloves and wash your hands.
13. Report immediately to your supervisor:
    - That you have completed the Acetest
    - Your findings so that she or he can enter the information on the patient's chart or designated form
    - Your observations of anything unusual

Procedure The Ketostix Reagent Strip Test

1. Assemble your equipment:
   a) Fresh urine specimen labeled with the patient's name
   b) Ketostix reagent strips
   c) Disposable gloves
2. Wash your hands and put on gloves.
3. Dip the Ketostix strip into the urine in the container.
4. Remove it immediately.
5. Tap the edge of the strip against the side of the urine container to remove excess urine.
6. Hold the strip in a horizontal position to prevent the mixing of the chemical from the adjacent reagent area.
7. Read the results 15 seconds after removing the strip from the urine. The Ketone test is read at 15 seconds.
8. Read the results from the color chart, in good lighting, matching the color carefully. The color chart is on the Ketostix bottle label.
9. Throw away used disposable equipment.
10. Remove gloves and wash your hands.
11. Report immediately to your supervisor:
    - That you have completed the Ketostix test
    - Your findings so that she or he can enter the information on the patient's chart or designated form
    - Your observations of anything unusual

KEY IDEAS

Reducing Pressure Points for the Diabetic Patient

All patients with diabetes must be taught to reduce pressure points to avoid skin irritation. The person with diabetes is more susceptible to a condition called arteriosclerosis in which the arteries are narrow. This condition results in less blood flowing to the extremities, especially the legs and feet. Changes also may occur in the nerves of the feet, which cause less nerve sensation, called neuropathy. When a person with diabetes has neuropathy, they are not aware when a pressure point is causing skin irritation. One extreme complication of such skin irritations is gangrene (no blood passes to a toe or to the foot). The body part with gangrene dies, which results in surgical amputation. The patient with diabetes should be taught the following to avoid pressure points and the problems that follow:

- Avoid standing or lying in one position for a long period of time. Change from sitting to walking or lying to sitting and walking.
- Never walk barefoot or in stocking feet. Always wear shoes for protection. A cut will have difficulty healing.
- Never cross knees. This stops circulation in the lower extremities.
- Never wear rubber or elastic bands for garters and never roll stockings or socks.
- Bathe every day, washing the feet very well.
- Never use very hot water for a shower or bath as a burn will not heal readily.
- When drying the body after a shower or bath, do not rub hard; pat dry, especially between the toes.
- Use skin cream to prevent hard, dry skin areas.
- Follow the instructions of the physician for cutting toe nails.
- Do not use any nonprescription drugs, internally or externally, without your physician's permission.
- Tell every physician, dentist, eye doctor, and podiatrist that you have diabetes.
- Wear shoes and stockings that fit so that movement is not restricted in the toes to cause pressure points.

- If you see any open skin, red area, scratched skin, sores, blisters, or any area of skin that looks different than normal, call and report this to your physician.

KEY IDEAS

Testing of Blood Glucose (Sugar) via a Finger Stick Using a Blood Glucose Meter

Self-monitoring of blood glucose using meters can greatly improve the home patient's quality of life, as it allows the patient to know whether or not his or her diet, exercise, and medication protocol are working. This home testing of blood glucose enables patients to have some control of their diabetes rather than feeling that diabetes is controlling their lives. There are many types of meters, each having different features. Each patient must use the type of meter recommended by his or her physician.

Patients can easily monitor their blood glucose by performing a simple finger stick and using chemically treated plastic strips that are inserted into the meter. The results are then read. This method eliminates the high cost of laboratories, and the results are immediate.

There are many manufacturers of battery-operated blood glucose meters. Scientists are currently developing noninvasive methods of blood glucose monitoring that are not yet available.

KEY QUESTIONS

1. What are the signs and symptoms of diabetes mellitus, insulin shock, and diabetic coma?
2. How should a fresh fractional urine specimen be collected?
3. Which tests are done to determine the level of glucose in the patient's urine? Which tests are done to determine the amount of acetone or ketones in the patient's urine?
4. How can a diabetic patient avoid pressure points and skin problems?
5. What is the method of reading the blood glucose via a finger stick?
6. Define: Acetest, acetone, carbohydrate, Clinitest, diabetes mellitus, diabetic coma, fresh urine, glucose, hyperglycemia, hypoglycemia, insulin shock, ketones, metabolism, reagent.

CHAPTER 36

Anatomy and Physiology of the Reproductive System and Sexuality

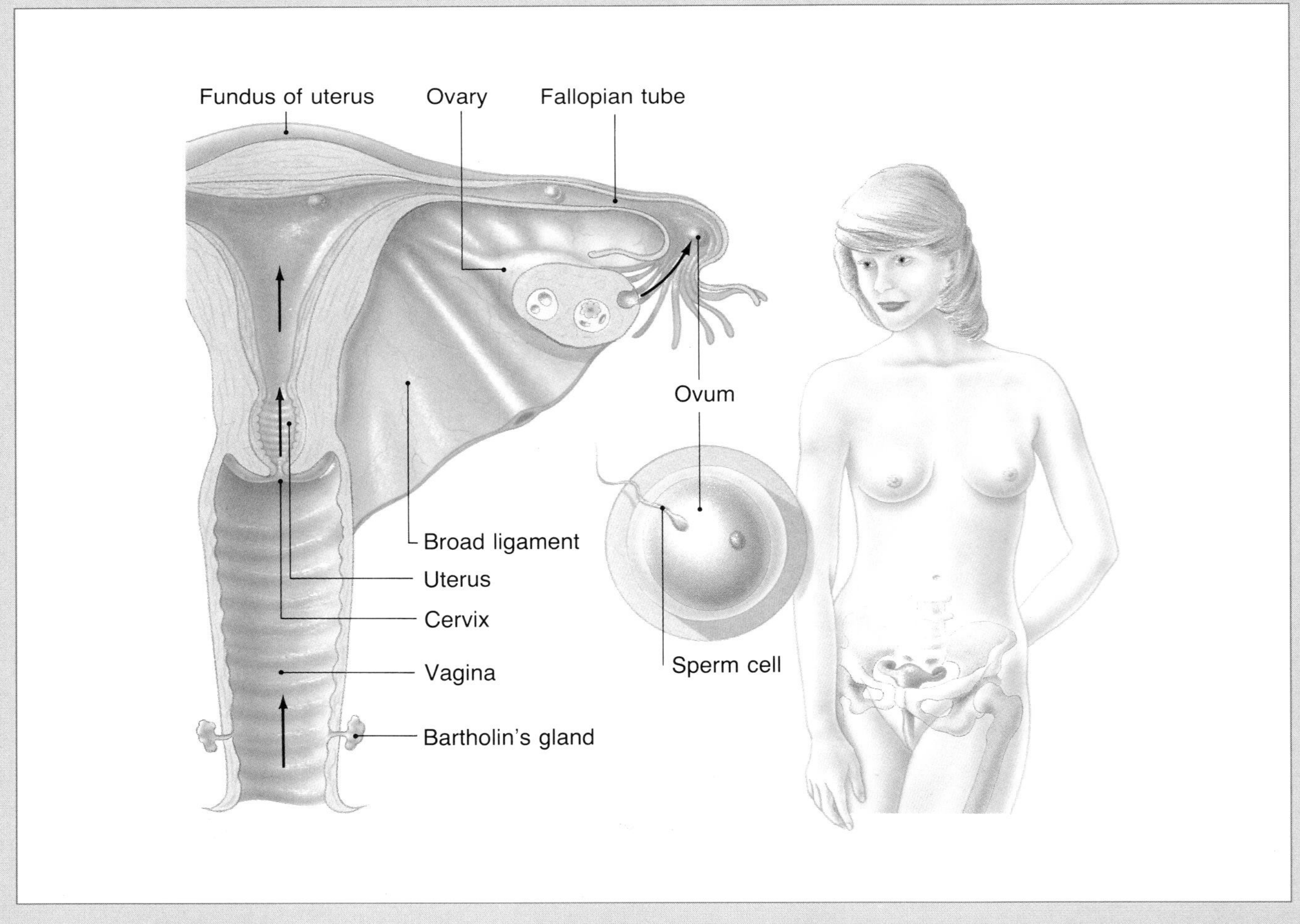

WARNING

For all patient contact, adhere to Universal Precautions (see page 91, 97, or the front cover flap). Wear protective equipment as indicated.

Objectives

What You Will Learn

When you have completed this chapter, you will be able to:

- Label a diagram with the female organs of the reproductive system and explain how each organ helps in the process of reproduction.
- Label a diagram with the male organs of the reproductive system and explain how each organ helps in the process of reproduction.
- Explain the meaning of sexuality.
- List the common diseases and disorders of the reproductive system.
- Define: AIDS, estrogen, fertile, fertilization, menstruation, ovulation, ovum, reproductive system, sperm, testosterone, venereal diseases.

FIGURE 36-1 Female reproductive organs.

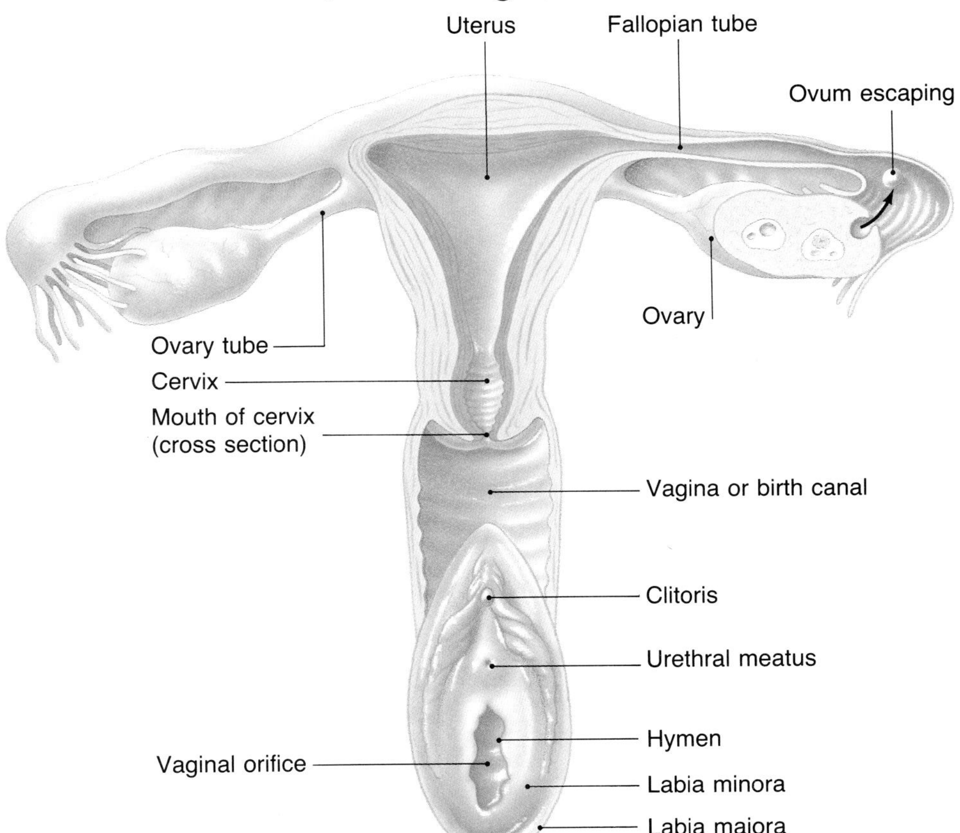

KEY IDEAS

The Reproductive System

Reproductive System
The group of body organs that makes possible the creation of a new human life.

Sperm
The male reproductive cell produced in the testes, which is capable of uniting with an ovum and developing into a new organism.

Fertilization
When the sperm and ovum join to form a new cell.

Estrogen
A female hormone produced by the ovaries that causes a buildup of the lining of the uterus. It prepares the uterus for possible pregnancy, and is responsible for the development of secondary sexual characteristics (for example, pubic hair).

Ovulation
The process whereby an ovum is released from one ovary into the opening of the Fallopian tube and moves to the uterus.

Fertile
Capable of reproduction.

Menstruation
The periodic (monthly) loss of some blood and a small part of the lining of the uterus.

Ovum
The female reproductive cell produced in the ovaries, which is capable of uniting with a sperm cell and developing into a new organism.

IN THE FEMALE, THE PRIMARY REPRODUCTIVE organs are the two ovaries (Figure 36-1). The main task of the ovaries is the production of ova (eggs) and female hormones. The ovaries are the major sites of production of **estrogen** and progesterone in the amounts required for normal female growth, development, and function. Ova are specialized cells that unite with a **sperm** cell released from the male during intercourse **(fertilization)** and then grow over a period of 40 weeks into a new human being (Figure 36-2). **Ovulation** is the process whereby an ovum is released from one ovary into the opening of the Fallopian tube and moves to the uterus (womb). This usually occurs once each month, usually 14 days before the onset of the next menstrual period. During this time, a woman is **fertile** (able to become pregnant). During ovulation, the release of estrogen causes a buildup of the lining of the uterus (endometrium), preparing it for a possible pregnancy. The process of ovulation is controlled by hormones from the pituitary gland, under the control of the hypothalamus. The hormones from the pituitary gland are involved in the development of the **ovum** and in maintaining pregnancy.

Menstruation is the periodic (monthly) loss of some blood and a small part of the lining of the uterus (Figure 36-3). The discharge flows out of the vagina for a period of 8 or 9 days.

In the human female there are three openings in the perineal area.

1. The external urinary meatus, the end of the urethra
2. The vagina, which is not only the organ for intercourse but also the birth canal
3. The anus, the last portion of the gastrointestinal tract

In the male, the primary reproductive organs are the testes, which produce sperm (Figure 36-4). Testicles, or testes, are paired glands that lie in the sac called the scrotum outside the body, posterior to the penis, which is the primary male sex organ. During intercourse, sperm travel up the vas deferens, or sperm duct, to a point where they enter the urethra. The entrance is made along with secretions from other glands in the male reproductive system. These glands (the seminal vesicles, the prostate gland, the Cowper's glands) contribute water, nutrients, and vitamins, which, when added to the sperm, make up the semen, a fluid

FIGURE 36-2 Fertilization and cell division.

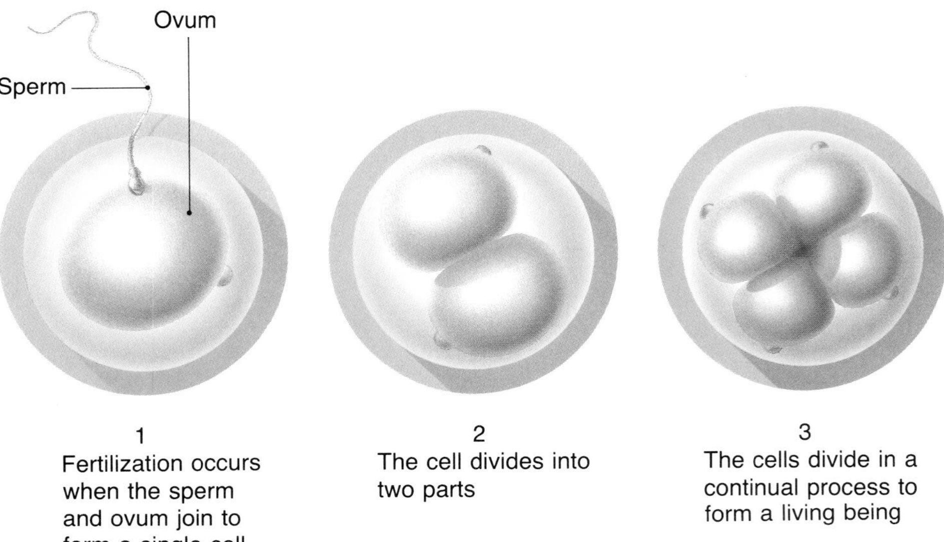
Ovum
Sperm
1
Fertilization occurs when the sperm and ovum join to form a single cell
2
The cell divides into two parts
3
The cells divide in a continual process to form a living being

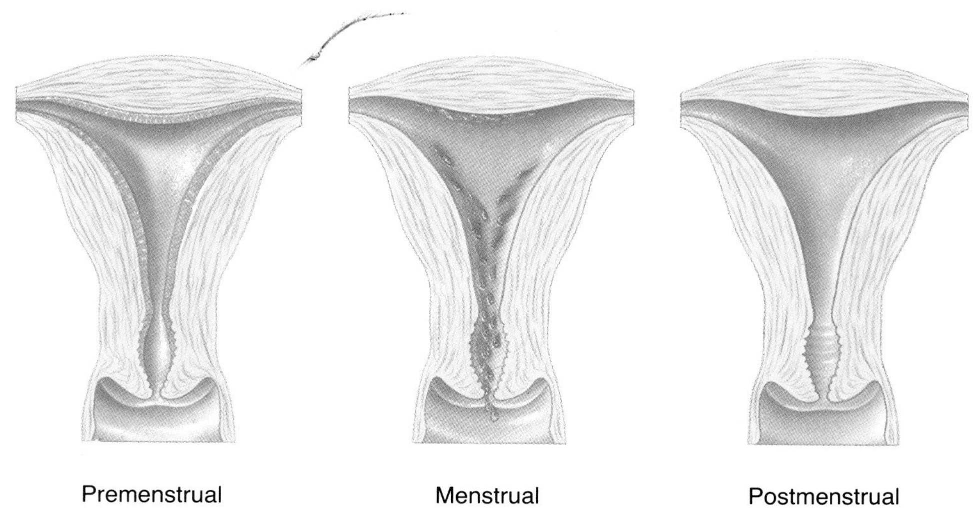

FIGURE 36-3 The menstrual cycle, a physiological process in women of childbearing age.

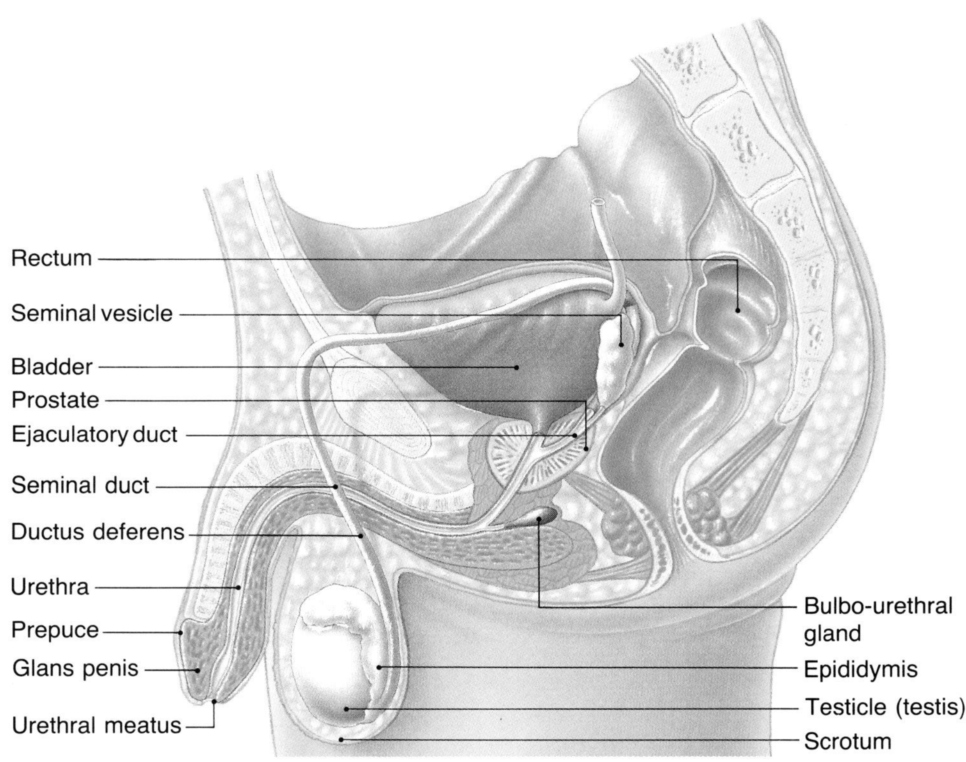

FIGURE 36-4 Male reproductive organs.

that is ejaculated (expelled) at the same time the male has an orgasm. There is only one duct in the penis. It is used for the flow of urine and for the ejaculation of sperm in the semen. During intercourse, the internal sphincter of the male's urinary bladder closes tightly, so urine does not become mixed with the semen. The penis has three columns of spongy or cavernous tissue. During sexual excitement, blood rushes in through the penile artery and the veins constrict, trapping the blood so it fills these spaces. Then the penis becomes erect. This activity oc-

Testosterone
The primary male sex hormone manufactured in the testes, which is essential for normal sexual behavior and the development of secondary sexual characteristics.

curs under the influence of **testosterone**, the primary male sex hormone, which is also manufactured in the testes. It is secreted into the blood through the influence of the hormones from the anterior pituitary, which is under the control of the hypothalamus.

Sometimes during the aging process the prostate gland, which encircles the urethra like a doughnut, becomes enlarged. When the prostate expands, it squeezes the urethra and causes painful urination. Many men fear surgery on their prostate glands, because they believe it will end their sex lives. The amount of semen ejaculated will be less, but, otherwise, men who have had a prostatectomy are almost always capable of having the same sexual relations as before surgery.

KEY IDEAS
Sexuality

Sexuality means the group of characteristics that identify the differences between male and female. During all the stages of growth and development, emotions, thoughts, and experiences that are related to warm, loving, and caring feelings shared between people, whether associated with the sex organs or not, are all part of sexuality. Sexuality stems from sexual instincts as they are developed in individual behavior patterns.

Society has attitudes that regulate sexual practices. For example, some societies prohibit incest and punish anyone who engages in this type of sexual gratification. These attitudes are reflected in stereotypes and myths that assign varying levels of status and acceptability to sexual behavior, depending on the age, sex, or actions of the person. Behavior within the confines of these prohibitions has the potential to bring love, joy, and comfort to the individual, but guilt and shame are often imposed on those who deviate from prescribed norms.

Double standards based on sex and age are often present. The stereotype is that vigorous interest in sex is expected in a 25-year-old but is shocking in an 80-year-old. Our language reflects these prejudices in such expressions as "swinger," "playboy," or "dirty old man," which are used in reference to men of different ages who behave similarly. There is a need for awareness, acceptance, and respect of the older person's sexuality in our society. Just as sexual behavior is discouraged in the elderly, younger people may feel pressured into sexual activity before they are ready for it.

Diseases and Disorders of the Reproductive System

Sexually Transmitted Diseases
Diseases acquired as a result of sexual intercourse with a person who is infected.

AIDS (Acquired Immune Deficiency Syndrome)
A viral infection characterized by decreased immunity to opportunistic infections. It is a group of signs and symptoms that characterize a lethal disorder in T-cell immunity.

- **Sexually transmitted diseases:** acquired as a result of sexual intercourse with a person who is infected:
  - *Chlamydia:* a sexually transmitted disease caused by chlamydia (rickettsia) whose incidence is on the rise
  - *Gonorrhea:* contagious infection caused by gonococcus bacteria
  - *Herpes simplex genitalis:* viral lesions on the male or female genitalia
  - **AIDS** (acquired immune deficiency syndrome): group of signs and symptoms that characterizes a lethal disorder in T-cell immunity associated with either Karposi's sarcoma or opportunistic infections. Acquired immune deficiency syndrome results from a virus that impairs immune function. This virus attacks white blood cells and impairs their response to infection. Current AIDS research supports the value of preventive measures because at present this is a fatal syndrome. The groups most commonly afflicted by AIDS

are IV drug users, homosexuals, and people who have received contaminated blood. Tests are available that indicate exposure to the virus, but don't confirm a diagnosis. To prevent transmission of AIDS, safe sexual practices, including the use of condoms, are recommended.

  - *Syphilis:* an infectious, chronic, venereal disease characterized by lesions that may involve any organ or tissue. Caused by *Treponema pallidum,* a spirochete.
- *Dysmenorrhea:* painful menstruation
- *Amenorrhea:* absence of menstruation
- *Menorrhagia:* excessive bleeding during menstruation
- *Pelvic Inflammatory Disease (PID):* infection which spreads to all structures in the pelvic cavity
- *Tumors of the breast:* may be benign or malignant
- *Vaginitis:* inflammation of the vagina
- *Cystocele:* downward protrusion of the urinary bladder into the vagina
- *Rectocele:* protrusion of the rectum into the vagina
- *Cancer of the uterus:* malignancy of the uterus
- *Fibroids:* benign tumors of the uterus
- *Benign prostatic hyperplasia:* enlargement of the prostate gland
- *Cancer of the prostate gland:* malignant tumor
- *Prostatitis:* inflammation of the prostate gland
- *Hydrocele:* abnormal accumulation of fluid within the scrotum
- *Varicocele:* enlargement of the veins within the scrotum
- *Tumors of the testicle:* may be benign or malignant

KEY QUESTIONS

1. How does each organ of the reproductive system help in the process of reproduction?
2. Label diagrams with the female and male organs of the reproductive system.
3. Discuss sexuality in various stages of growth and development in our society.
4. Describe 15 common diseases and disorders of the reproductive system.
5. Define: AIDS, estrogen, fertile, fertilization, menstruation, ovulation, ovum, reproductive system, sperm, testosterone, venereal diseases.

CHAPTER

37 Care of the Gynecological Patient

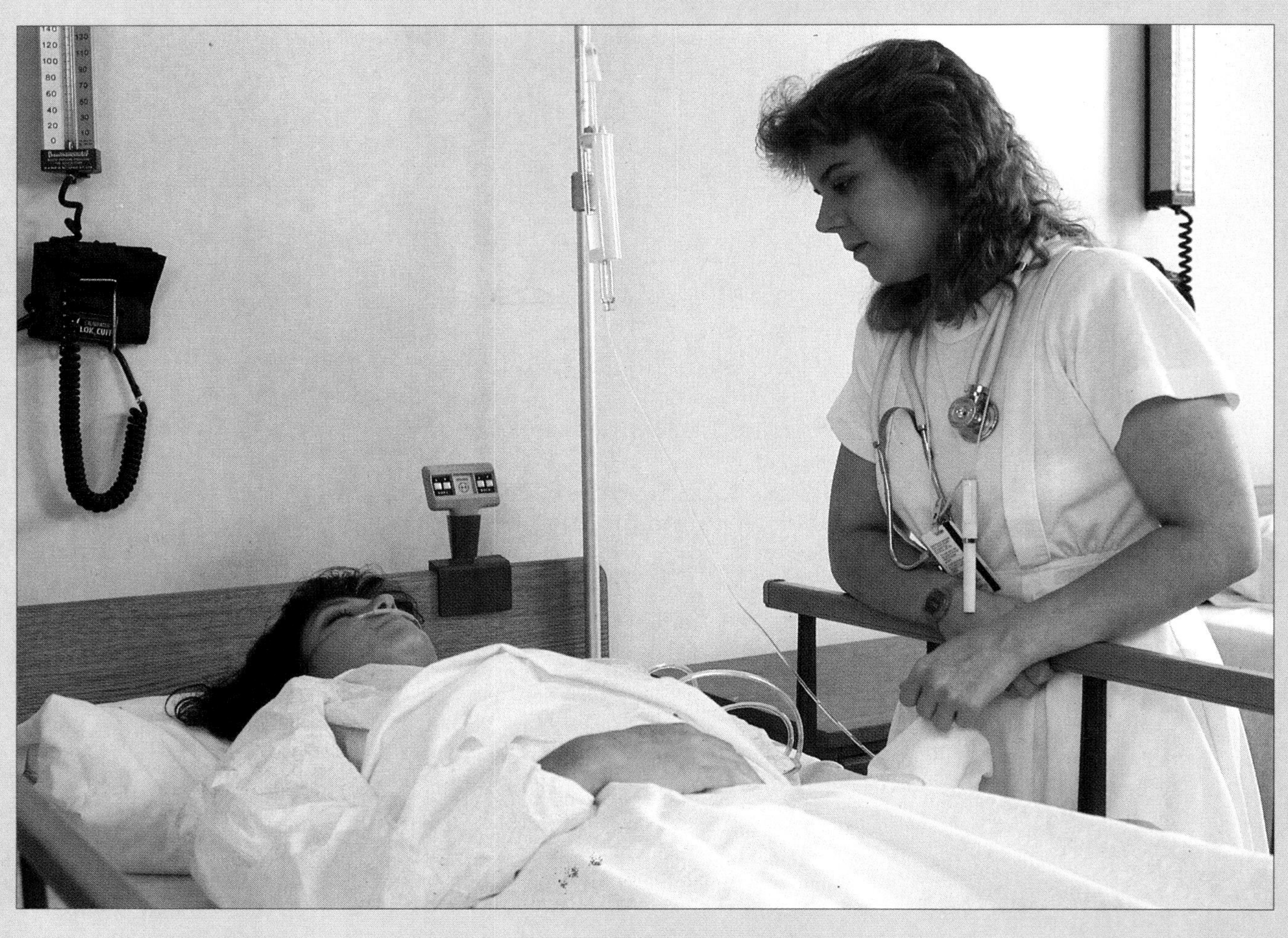

WARNING

For all patient contact, adhere to Universal Precautions (see page 91, 97, or the front cover flap). Wear protective equipment as indicated.

Objectives

What You Will Learn

When you have completed this chapter, you will be able to:

- Give perineal care.
- Give the vaginal douche or irrigation.
- Define: douche, gynecological patient, perineum (perineal area), vagina (vaginal canal, vaginal tract), vaginal irrigation or douche.

KEY IDEAS

Perineal Care

Gynecological Patient
Patients being treated for diseases or conditions of the female reproductive organs, including the breasts.

Perineum (perineal area)
The body area between the thighs. It includes the area of the anus and the external genital organs.

PERINEAL CARE IS SPECIFIC CARE GIVEN to the **perineum** or perineal area (the external genitalia and rectal area) during the daily bath and after voiding or defecating. Cleansing is always done anterior to posterior (front to back).

Perineal care provides cleanliness and comfort for the patient. It helps to prevent irritation and infection. Perineal care is also given following childbirth. Follow the instructions of your immediate supervisor in your institution. In some institutions this procedure is done in the bathroom while the patient is on the toilet. In this case you will use a squirt bottle and toilet paper. Follow the instructions of your immediate supervisor.

Procedure Perineal Care

1. Assemble your equipment:
   a) Disposable bed protector
   b) Bedpan and cover
   c) Squirt bottle (peri bottle)
   d) Toilet paper
   e) Disposable gloves
2. Wash your hands.
3. Identify the patient by checking the identification bracelet.
4. Ask visitors to leave the room, if this is your hospital's policy.
5. Tell the patient you are going to clean the genital area.
6. Pull the curtain around the bed for privacy.
7. Be sure there is plenty of light. Raise the bed to a comfortable working position.
8. Cover the patient with a bath blanket. Without exposing her, fanfold the top sheets to the foot of the bed. Have the patient covered only with the blanket. Put on gloves.
9. Fill the squirt bottle with warm water at 100°F (37.7°C) or use the solution provided in your institution.

10. Place the disposable bed protector under the patient's hips (buttocks).
11. Help the patient to get on the bedpan.
12. Put on disposable gloves.
13. Spray the perineum with solution, working from anterior to posterior.
14. Dry the patient gently with the toilet paper. Remove and discard the disposable gloves.
15. Remove the bedpan and disposable bed protector. Place them on a chair.
16. Cover the patient with the top sheets. Remove the bath blanket.
17. Make the patient comfortable.
18. Lower the bed to a position of safety for the patient.
19. Pull the curtains back to the open position.
20. Raise the side rails where ordered, indicated, and appropriate for patient safety.
21. Place the call light within easy reach of the patient.
22. Empty, rinse, and put the equipment back where it belongs.
23. Discard disposable equipment.
24. Wash your hands.
25. Report to your immediate supervisor:
    - That you have given the patient perineal care
    - The time it was given
    - Your observations of anything unusual

KEY IDEAS

Vaginal Douche or Nonsterile Irrigation

Vagina
In the female, the birth canal leading from the vulva to the cervix of the uterus (vaginal canal, vaginal tract).

Vaginal Irrigation or Douche
A procedure by which a stream of water is sent into the patient's vaginal opening. The water may be plain or it may contain medication.

The introduction of solution into the **vagina** or vaginal canal with an immediate return of the solution by gravity is called the **vaginal irrigation** or **douche**. This type of irrigation is usually used for cleansing the vaginal canal (vaginal tract) or relieving inflammation of the vaginal tract. When used to excess, it can wash away normal protective secretions and never should be done without a physician's order. A doctor may order this treatment to cleanse before surgery, before an examination, in cases of severe discharge, to treat an inflammation, or to neutralize secretions in the vaginal canal. The rules of medical asepsis must be followed for this treatment.

In some institutions this procedure is done while the patient is on the toilet. Prepackaged douche bottles are often used. If a douche kit is used you might not be instructed to prep with cotton balls and cleaning solution. Follow the instructions of your immediate supervisor.

Douche
A stream of water or air applied to a part or cavity of the body for cleansing or for the treatment of a localized condition.

Procedure The Vaginal Douche/Nonsterile Irrigation

1. Assemble your equipment:
   a) Disposable douche kit (irrigation container with tubing, clamp, and douche nozzle)
   b) Graduated pitcher
   c) Bath thermometer
   d) Bedpan and cover
   e) Bath blanket
   f) Disposable waterproof bed protector
   g) Solution as instructed by immediate supervisor, usually 1000 cc of tap water at 105°F (40.5°C)
   h) Disposable gloves
   i) Emesis basin
   j) Cotton balls and cleansing solution in small disposable container, as ordered by your immediate supervisor
2. Wash your hands.

3. Identify the patient by checking the identification bracelet.
4. Ask visitors to step out of the room, if this is your hospital's policy.
5. Tell the patient you are going to give her a vaginal douche.
6. Pull the curtains around the bed for privacy.
7. Offer the patient the bedpan, explaining that her bladder must be empty to ensure the desired results from the douche.
8. Remove the bedpan. Measure output if the patient is on intake and output. Record on the I&O sheet. Empty the contents of the bedpan; wash it and place it on a chair nearby.
9. Wash the patient's hands.
10. Wash your hands.
11. Cover the patient with a bath blanket. Without exposing her, fanfold the top sheets to the foot of the bed. The patient holds the bath blanket while you do this. Leave the patient covered with only the bath blanket.
12. Place the disposable bed protector under the patient's hips (buttocks).
13. Raise the bed to a comfortable working position.
14. Open the douche kit; close the clamp on the tubing.
15. Fill the graduated pitcher with 1000 cc of water or solution as ordered at 105°F (40.5°C). Test the temperature of the water with the bath thermometer. Then pour the water into the irrigating douche container.
16. Pour the cleansing solution over cotton balls in a small disposable container to saturate them with the solution.
17. Place the patient into the dorsal recumbent position. The head of the bed should be flat. Drape the patient with a small sheet.
18. Place the bedpan under the patient's hips (buttocks).
19. Place the emesis basin on the bed to receive the used cotton balls.
20. Put on disposable gloves.
21. To cleanse the vulva using cotton balls saturated with cleansing solution:
    a) Wipe from the front to the back over the large outside lips (labia majora) on one side. Discard in the emesis basin.
    b) Wipe from the front to the back over the large outside lips (labia majora) on the other side. Discard in the emesis basin.
    c) Wipe from the front to the back over the midline of the large outside lips (labia majora). Discard in the emesis basin.
    d) Expose the small inside lips (labia minora) by using the thumb and forefinger to separate the large outside lips (labia majora) and clean as follows:
    e) Wipe from front to back on the far side of the small lips (labia minora). Discard cotton ball.
    f) Wipe from front to back on the near side of the small lips (labia minora). Discard cotton ball.
    g) Wipe from front to back in the center (midline) over the vaginal orifice (opening).
    h) Repeat until the entire area is clean, always using new cotton balls.
22. Open the clamp to expel air and allow the solution to flow over the vulva. Do not touch the vulva with the nozzle.
23. With solution flowing, insert the douche nozzle tip into the vagina from 2 to 3 inches with an upward and then downward and backward gentle movement.
24. Allow the solution to flow, holding the douche container no more than 12 inches above the vulva or 18 inches above the mattress.
25. Rotate the nozzle until all the solution has been given. This will ensure cleansing of the vagina.
26. Clamp the tubing and remove the douche nozzle gently. Wrap in paper towel to prevent contamination. Put the tubing into the douche container. Remove and discard the disposable gloves.
27. Help the patient to sit up on the bedpan by raising the back of the bed, if allowed (Fowler's position). This will help the solution to drain from the vagina.
28. Dry the perineum with toilet tissue and discard into the bedpan.
29. Remove the bedpan and place on the chair.

30. Help the patient to turn on her side and dry the buttocks with toilet tissue.
31. Remove the bed protector.
32. Lower the bed to its lowest horizontal position.
33. Change any linen that has become damp.
34. Raise the top sheets over the bath blanket and then remove the bath blanket from under the top sheets.
35. Make the patient comfortable.
36. Lower the bed to a position of safety for the patient.
37. Pull the curtains back to the open position.
38. Raise the side rails where ordered, indicated, and appropriate for patient safety.
39. Place the call light within easy reach of the patient.
40. Observe the contents of the bedpan. Collect a specimen if the returned solution is not as clear as when it was inserted.
41. Clean the bedpan and emesis basin and return to their proper place.
42. Discard disposable supplies.
43. Wash the patient's hands.
44. Wash your hands.
45. Report to your immediate supervisor:
    - That you have given the patient a vaginal douche
    - The time the douche was given
    - The type of solution used
    - That a specimen was collected and why
    - How the patient tolerated the procedure
    - Your observation of the returned solution and any unusual material noted
    - Your observations of anything unusual

KEY QUESTIONS

1. How should perineal care be given?
2. How should a vaginal douche be given?
3. Define: douche, gynecological patient, perineum (perineal area), vagina (vaginal canal, vaginal tract), vaginal irrigation or douche.

CHAPTER

38

Anatomy and Physiology of the Nervous System

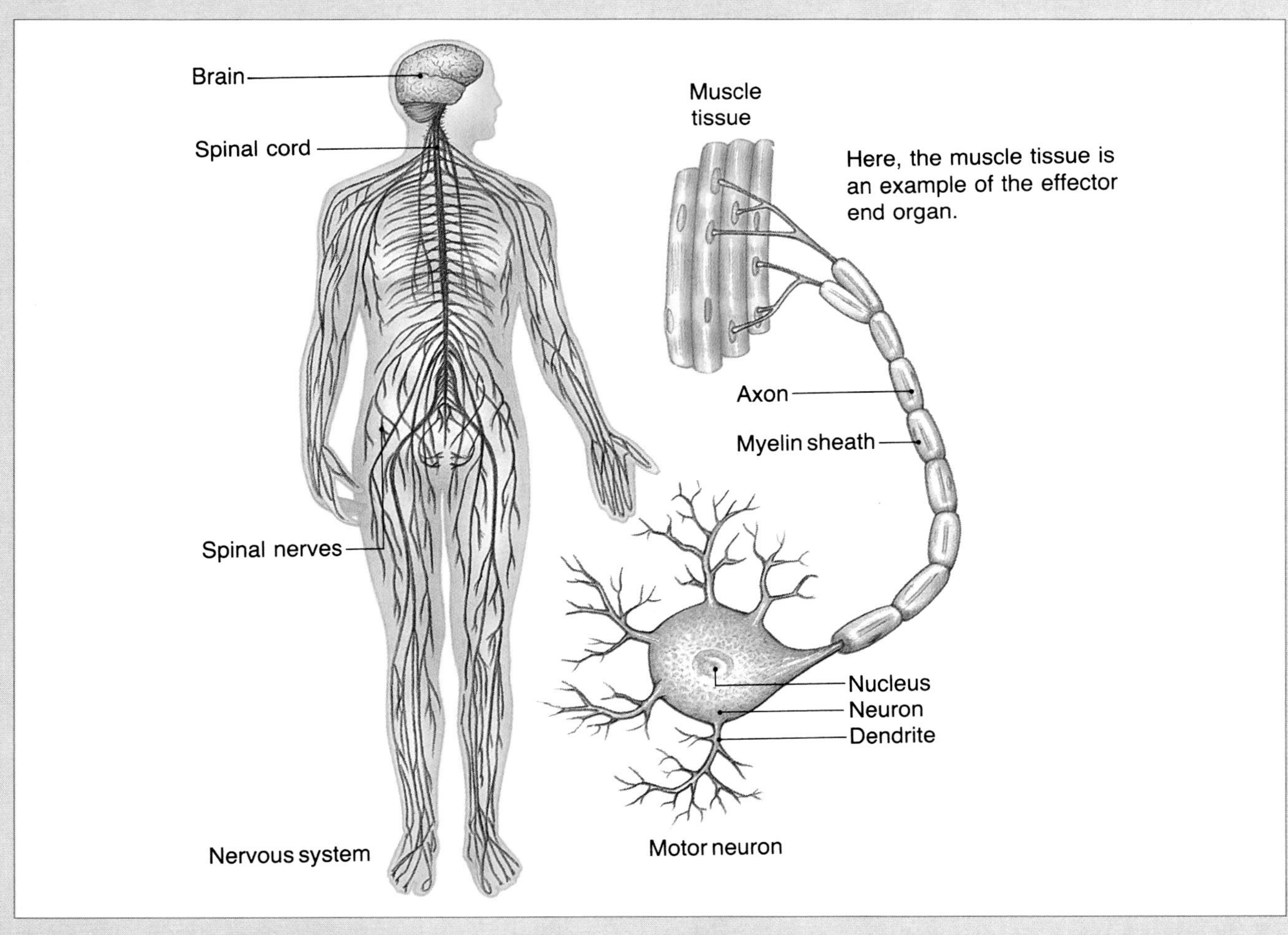

WARNING

For all patient contact, adhere to Universal Precautions (see page 91, 97, or the front cover flap). Wear protective equipment as indicated.

Objectives

What You Will Learn

When you have completed this chapter, you will be able to:

- Label a diagram of the body with the organs of the nervous system.
- Explain the function of each organ.
- Describe the functions of the two divisions of the autonomic nervous system.
- List the five sense organs.
- List the common diseases and disorders of the nervous system.
- Define: autonomic nervous system, environment, hemisphere, impulse, involuntary, nervous system, respond, stimuli, vascular, voluntary.

KEY IDEAS

The Nervous System

Nervous System
The group of body organs consisting of the brain, spinal cord, and nerves that controls and regulates the activities of the body and the functions of the other body systems.

Voluntary
Under control of the will; with conscious decision.

Environment
All the surrounding conditions and influences affecting the life and development of an organism.

Impulse
An electrical or chemical charge transmitted through certain tissues, especially nerve fibers and muscles.

Respond
To react; to begin, end, or change activity in reaction to stimulation.

Vascular
Pertaining to blood vessels.

THE NERVOUS SYSTEM CONTROLS AND ORGANIZES all body activity, both **voluntary** and involuntary. The nervous system is made up of the brain, the spinal cord, and the nerves. The nerves are spread throughout all areas of the body in an orderly way.

Nervous tissue is made up of cells called neurons and other supporting cells called neuroglia. A typical neuron is made up of a cell body with one long column called the axon and many small outbranchings called dendrites. Nerve impulses move from the dendrites through the cell body along the axon. Inside and outside our bodies, we have structures called receptor-end organs. Any change in our external or internal **environment** that is strong enough will set up a nervous **impulse** in these receptor-end organs. This impulse is carried by a sensory neuron to some part of the brain or spinal cord where it connects with an interneuron. The connection is called a synapse (Figure 38-1). This interneuron often makes hundreds of synapses (particularly in the cerebrum, the part of the brain in which we think) before a decision is made. Once that happens, the proper impulses are sent down a motor neuron to the effector-end organs, those organs that are going to **respond** to the nerve impulse.

Most nerve cells outside the brain and spinal cord have a protective covering known as the myelin sheath. The task of the myelin sheath is to insulate the nerve cell. The nerve cell can be compared to an electrical wire that requires insulation to keep the current in the correct pathway. This insulation sheath helps prevent damage to the cells and often helps the nerve return to healthy function, or regenerate, if it has been injured. Nerve cells with a myelin sheath also carry an impulse faster than those without myelin. The neurons in the brain and spinal cord do not have this kind of protection. When nerve cells are injured, as they are by a stroke or cerebral **vascular** accident (CVA), it is necessary for another part of the brain to take over the function of the part that has been damaged. The rehabilitation department in your health care in-

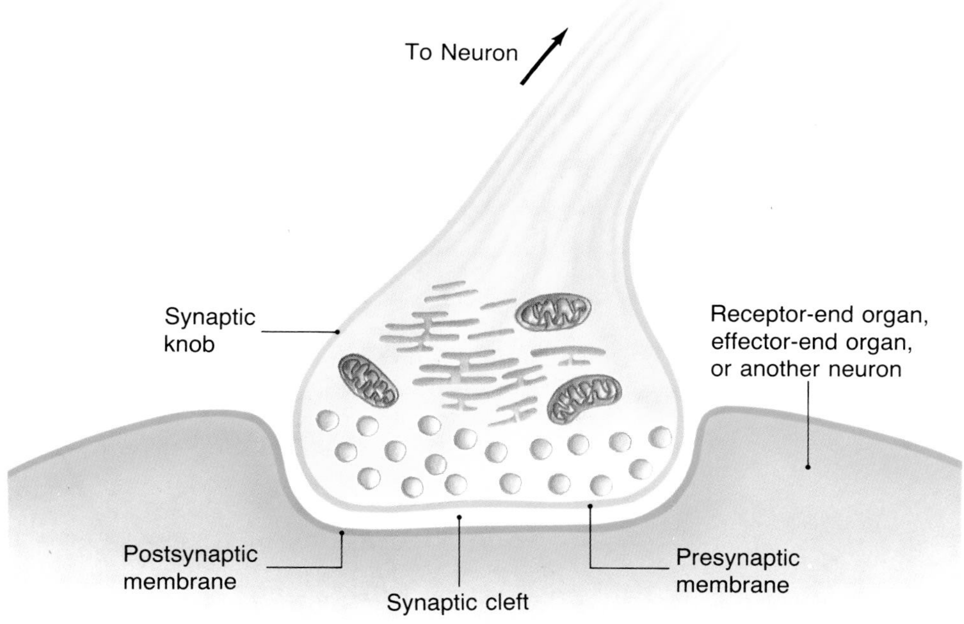

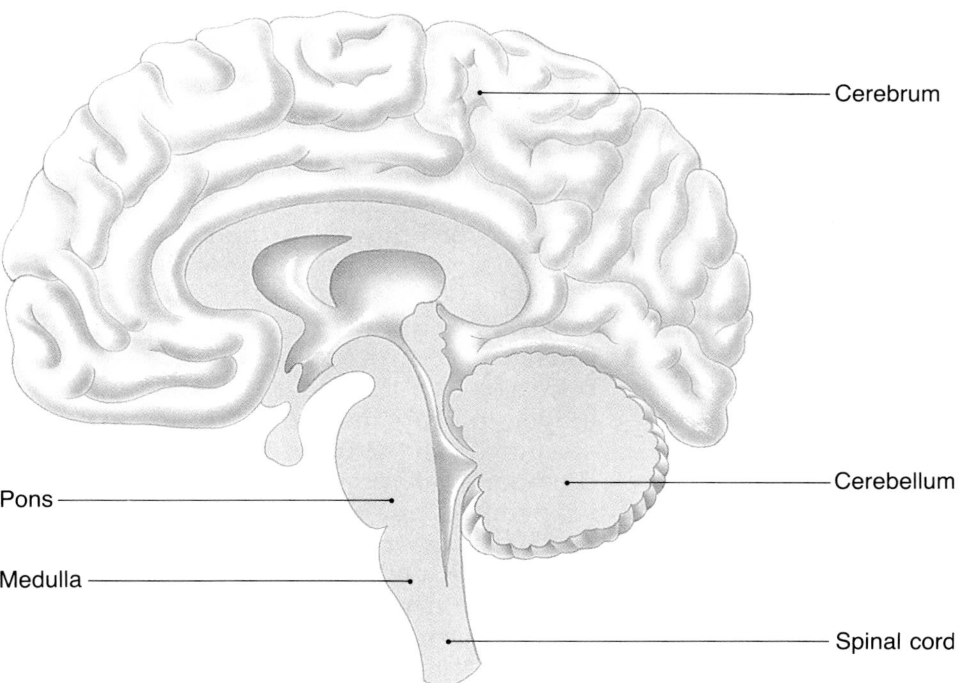

FIGURE 38-2 The brain.

stitution helps patients learn to do things again after such damage has been done.

Hemisphere
Half of a sphere. In the nervous system it refers to one half of the brain.

The brain (Figure 38-2) is well protected by bones, membranes, the meninges, and a cushion of fluid called cerebral spinal fluid. This fluid circulates outside of and within the brain, as well as around the spinal cord. The brain is a very complicated organ made up of five portions. The cerebrum is divided into two halves, called **hemispheres**. They are connected to one another by white material known as corpus callosum. The right hemisphere controls most of the activity on the left side of the body. And the left hemisphere of the cerebrum controls activity on the right side of the body. The cerebrum has many indentations known as convolutions. It is here that all learning, memory, and associations are stored so that thought is possible. Also, decisions are made for voluntary action. Certain areas of the cerebrum seem to perform special organizing activities. For example, the occipital lobe is the place where what you see is interpreted. The frontal lobe is the primary area of thought and reason. The cerebellum is the part of the brain that coordinates voluntary motion. It works with part of the inner ear, the semicircular canals, to enable us to walk and move smoothly through our world. The midbrain, pons, and medulla are primarily pathways through which nervous impulses reach the brain from the spinal cord.

Nerves throughout the body send messages into the tracts of white matter in the spinal cord, from which they rise to higher centers in the brain. There are 12 pairs of cranial nerves and 32 pairs of spinal nerves. These have many branches that go to all parts of the body.

One of the most important areas of the brain is an area called the diencephelon. It is here that small structures surround one of the ventricles of the brain. These structures help circulate cerebral spinal fluid and exercise an almost dictatorial control over the body's activities. They screen all nervous impulses going to the brain, either getting them there faster or slowing them down. One of these tiny structures is the hypothalamus, which in times of stress, emergency, excitement, or danger actually takes control of the body by controlling the pituitary gland, the body's master gland. Although the pituitary gland can be mapped, like the subways of a great city, we still know very little about its activity. We do know that it has tremendous control over most body activities. The hypothalmus seems to be the link between the mind and the body. It receives messages from the cerebrum, from the cerebellum, and from impulses coming up the spinal cord, and it has direct control over all the endocrine glands.

Involuntary
Without conscious will, control, or decision.

Autonomic Nervous System
The part of the nervous system that carries messages without conscious thought.

Much of the activity of the organs of the body is **involuntary**. In other words, we do not think about it. Or, for the most part, we have no conscious control over this activity. The part of the nervous system that controls such things as digestion and the functions of other visceral (abdominal) organs is the **autonomic nervous system**. This is really not separate from the brain and the spinal cord. The neurons that make up the autonomic nervous system use the same pathways as the neurons that control our voluntary actions. However, the two divisions of this part of the nervous system direct and control the activity of our internal organs. Each organ is supplied with neurons from each division of the autonomic nervous system.

One division is called the *sympathetic division.* The neurons that make up this division become active during stress, danger, excitement, or illness. These neurons cause the pupils of our eyes to become larger so that we can see more clearly and can see better at a distance. They also cause the heart to beat more strongly and to send more oxygen to the large muscles of the body in case it is necessary to fight or run. In today's fast-paced world, we are all subject to stress and sometimes we cannot run away from it or fight it. The action of the neurons from the sympathetic system then causes changes in the shape or activity of some of our organs. This action may also cause illness.

The *parasympathetic division* of the autonomic nervous system is in control when we are relaxed. It is known to conserve our energy. Fortunately, there is a checks and balances system between the two divisions. When one has been in action too long, the other automatically switches on. We have all had the experience of eating a large meal after being emotionally upset and feeling as if we had lead in our stomach. This is because of the sympathetic division of the autonomic nervous system. Peristalsis (which is movement of the intestines) lessens and digestion slows.

The Sense Organs

Stimuli
Changes in the external or internal environment strong enough to set up a nervous impulse or other responses in an organism.

We are aware of our environment through our eyes, ears, nose, tongue, and skin. These sense organs contain specialized endings of the sensory neurons that are excited by sudden changes in the outside environment called **stimuli** (Figure 38-3).

- Eyes respond to visual stimuli (what we see) (Figure 38-4).
- Ears respond mainly to sound stimuli (what we hear) and one's position in space (Figure 38-5).
- Membranes of the nose respond to smell.
- Taste buds, located chiefly on the tongue, respond to taste sensations.
- Skin responds to touch, pressure, heat, cold, and pain (Figure 38-6).

FIGURE 38-3 Sensory and motor processes.

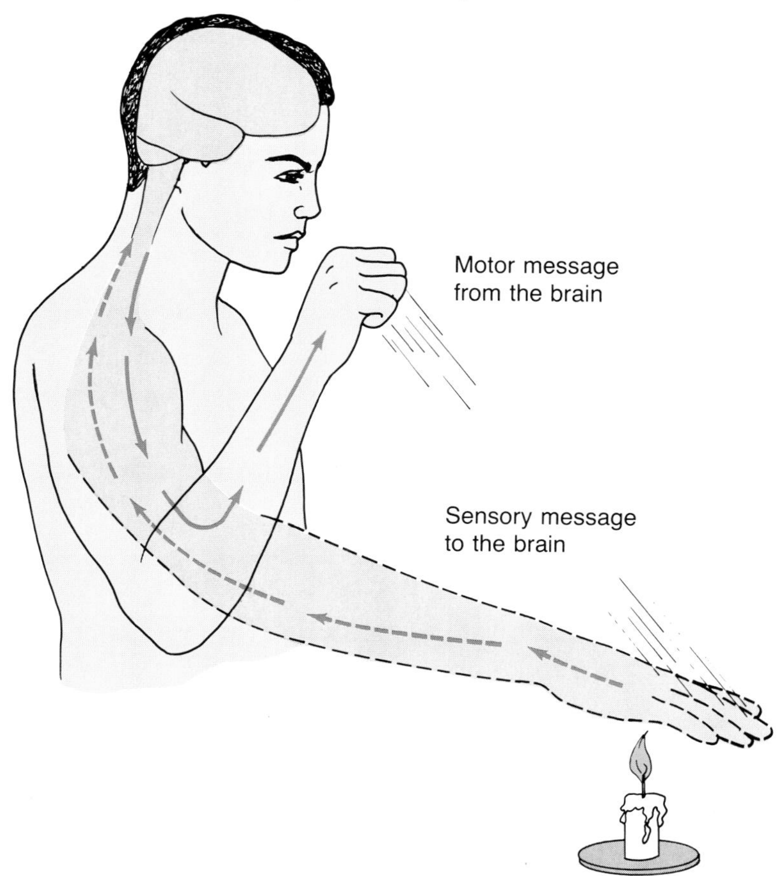

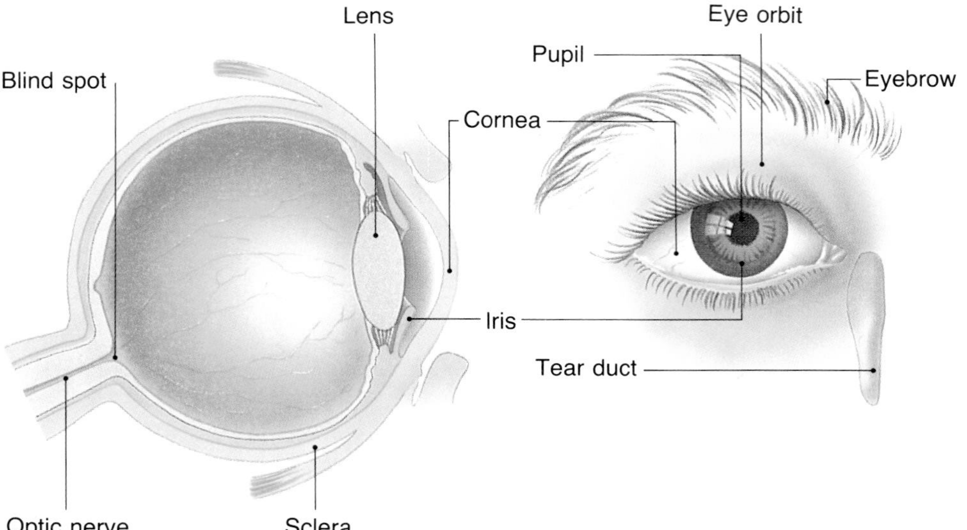

FIGURE 38-4 The eye.

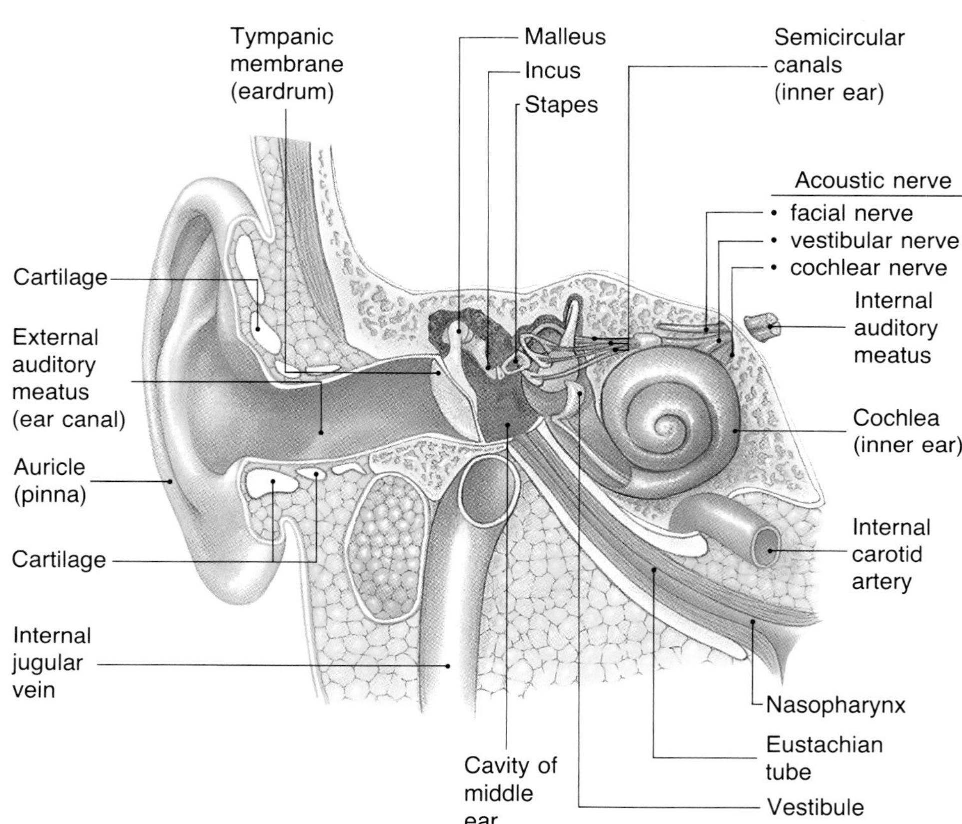

FIGURE 38-5 The outer, middle, and inner ear.

Common Diseases and Disorders of the Nervous System

- *Bell's palsy:* paralysis or weakness of one side of the face
- *Stroke or cerebral vascular accident* (CVA): blood supply is reduced to the brain due to cerebral thrombosis, cerebral embolism, or intracerebral hemorrhage
- *Aphasia:* impairment of the ability to speak, and sometimes listen, read, comprehend
- *Brain tumor:* may be benign or malignant
- *Epilepsy:* a group of neurological disorders with recurrent episodes of convulsions or seizures; an electrical dysfunction of the nerve cells

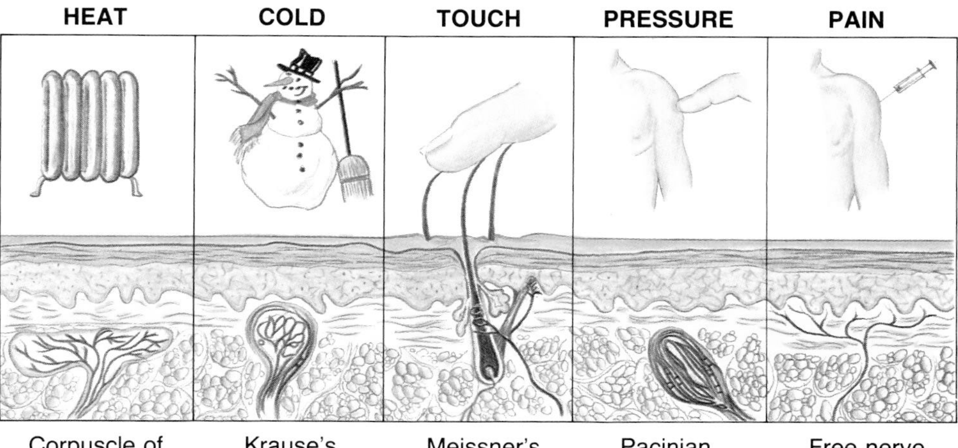

FIGURE 38-6 The skin responds to heat, cold, touch, pressure, and pain.

of the brain; may be related to cerebral trauma, infection, tumor, vascular disturbances, chemical imbalance, or unknown causes

- *Parkinson's disease:* progressive disorders with loss of control of movement
- *Multiple sclerosis:* chronic progressive disease, which begins slowly and progresses throughout the life span, but which may have periods of remission
- *Shingles* (Herpes zoster): characterized by blisters along the (path) course of certain nerves
- *Hemiplegia:* paralyzed on one side of the body; loss of motion and sensation
- *Paraplegia:* paralyzed on lower part of the body; loss of motion and sensation
- *Quadriplegia:* all four extremities are paralyzed; loss of motion and sensation
- *Detached retina:* the sensory retina detaches from the pigment epithelium
- *Cataracts:* the crystalline lens becomes opaque
- *Glaucoma:* increase of pressure within the eye
- *Chronic otitis media:* caused by breaks in the eardrum
- *Meniere's disease:* inner ear is involved and causes dizziness

KEY QUESTIONS

1. List the organs of the nervous system.
2. What does each organ do?
3. What are the two divisions of the autonomic nervous system called and what does each division do?
4. What are the five sense organs?
5. What are the common diseases and disorders of the nervous system?
6. Define: autonomic nervous system, environment, hemisphere, impulse, involuntary, nervous system, respond, stimuli, vascular, voluntary.

CHAPTER

39

Health Problems of the Nervous System

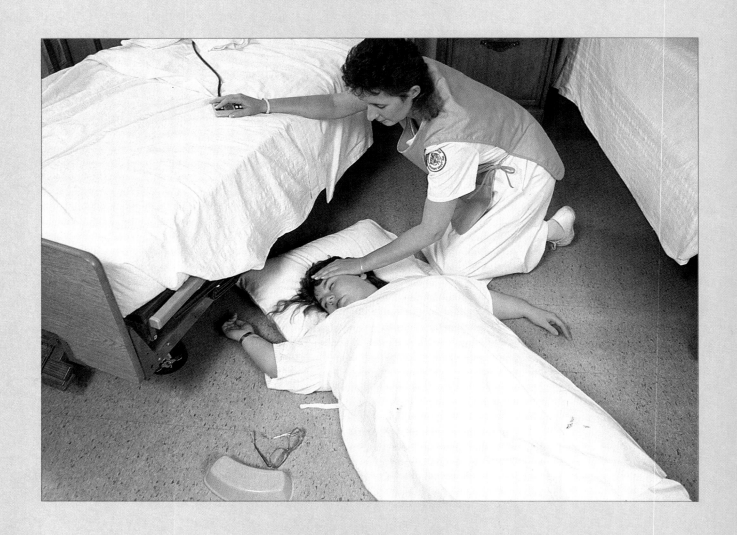

WARNING

For all patient contact, adhere to Universal Precautions (see page 91, 97, or the front cover flap). Wear protective equipment as indicated.

Objectives

What You Will Learn

When you have completed this chapter, you will be able to:

- Describe a grand mal and a petit mal seizure.
- Demonstrate safety measures for the patient having a seizure.
- Care for a patient's artificial eye.
- Care for a patient's hearing aid.
- List the causes of cerebrovascular accidents.
- Describe some common results of cerebrovascular accidents.
- Assist in the care of the cerebrovascular accident patient.
- Describe the psychological aspects of caring for a cerebrovascular accident patient.
- Talk to an aphasic patient using correct technique.
- Define: aphasia, cerebrovascular accident, contracture, embolus, hemiplegia, hemorrhage, plaque, rupture, seizure, spasm, thrombus.

KEY IDEAS

Care of the Seizure Patient

Seizure
An episode, either partial or generalized, which may include altered consciousness, motor activity, or sensory phenomena or convulsions.

A **seizure** is caused by an abnormality within the central nervous system thought to be an electrical problem or disturbance in the nerve cells or activity of the brain. Seizures can occur from the time of birth or may be the result of cancer (tumor), cerebral trauma (head injury), infection, vascular disturbances, imbalance or abnormality in brain chemistry, cerebrovascular accident (stroke), or unknown causes.

There are several types of seizures, ranging from the total body seizures known as the *grand mal* (also known as *generalized tonic-clonic* seizure), to the partial small seizure, known as the *petit mal* (also known as *absence*) seizure. In the grand mal seizure, there may be stiffness of the total body followed by a jerking action of the muscles. Sometimes the patient's tongue may be bitten and usually the patient becomes unconscious. In the petit mal seizure, the patient may appear to be daydreaming, his eyes may roll back, and there may be some quivering of the body muscles. The petit mal seizure usually lasts less than 30 seconds. The grand mal seizure may last for several minutes and varies greatly. The terms *grand mal, petit mal,* and *psychomotor* are generally used to describe types of seizures. The most recently developed system describes them as partial or generalized.

The major role of the nursing assistant in caring for a patient having a seizure is to prevent the patient from injuring herself. Wherever you are, help the patient to lie down (Figure 39-1). If she is not in bed, carefully help her to the floor. Loosen her clothing and move any equipment or furniture that she might bump. Place a pillow or something soft under her head. *Turn her head to the side to promote drainage of saliva or vomitus. Never place anything in the mouth of a patient having a seizure. Objects can break and obstruct the patient's airway. Never try to move or restrain the patient.* Stay with the patient and pull

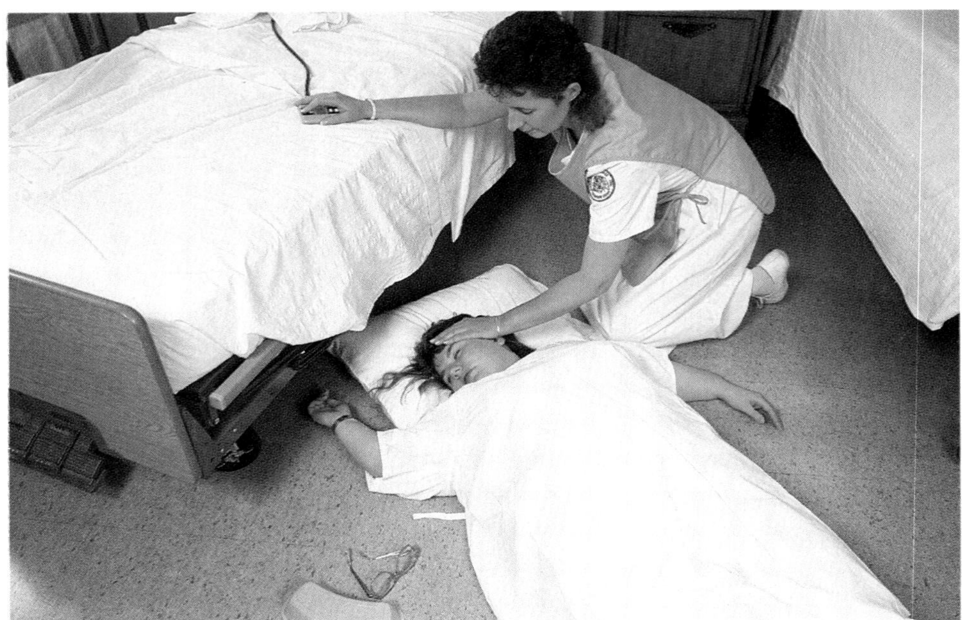

FIGURE 39-1 Stay with the seizure victim and call for help.

the emergency signal cord for help. Observe carefully what the seizure looked like. Give this information to the nurse.

KEY IDEAS

Care of the Artificial Eye

Cleaning the patient's artificial eye is part of daily personal hygiene. Often a patient cannot care for it himself. If he has an artificial eye, it must be cared for properly to prevent infection and encrustation (formation of dried mucous material in the eye socket and around the artificial eye). Assist the patient, but permit him to do as much as he is able.

Procedure Caring for the Artificial Eye

1. Assemble your equipment on the bedside table:
   a) An eyecup half-filled with lukewarm water at 98° to 100°F (36.6° to 37.7°C) and labeled with the patient's name and room number (if no eyecup is available, use a clean denture cup)
   b) Gauze, 4 × 4 (2 pieces), for the bottom of the cup
   c) Small basin with lukewarm water
   d) Four cotton balls
   e) Optional: any special cleansing solution the doctor orders
2. Wash your hands.
3. Ask visitors to step out of the room, if this is your hospital's policy.
4. Identify the patient by checking the identification bracelet.
5. Tell the patient you are going to take care of his eye.
6. Pull the curtain around the bed for privacy.
7. Help the patient to lie down on the bed. This is to prevent accidental dropping of the artificial eye. Put on gloves.
8. Have the patient close his eyes. Clean any external secretions from the patient's upper eyelid. Use cotton balls and warm water from the basin. Clean from the inner canthus to the outside of the eye area. This means you move from the nose to the outside of the eye. If you need

to wipe more than once, use a clean (new) cotton ball each time. Use gentle strokes.

9. Remove the artificial eye. To do this, carefully depress the lower eyelid with your thumb. Lift the upper lid gently with your forefinger. The eye should slide out and down, into your hand. Have the patient do this, if he is able.
10. Place the eye in the cup on the 4 × 4 gauze. Let it soak in the water.
11. Wash off external matter and encrustations from the outside of the eye socket with cotton balls and warm water. Using gentle strokes, clean from the inner canthus to the outside of the eye.
12. Take the eyecup to the patient's bathroom. Close the drain in the sink. Fill the sink one-half full with water to prevent breakage if the eye is dropped.
13. Take the eye in your hand and wash with running lukewarm water 98° to 100°F (36.6° to 37.7°C). Use plain water unless the doctor orders a special solution. Place the eye in the gauze and rub gently between your thumb and forefinger. *Do not use alcohol, ether, or acetone. These may dissolve the plastic of the artificial eye or may dull the luster.*
14. Rinse the eye under running lukewarm water at 98° to 100°F (36.6° to 37.7°C); then dry it using the second 4 × 4 gauze. Discard the water from the eyecup. Place the slightly moistened eye on dry gauze in the eyecup. A slightly moistened eye is easier to insert. Return to the patient's bedside.
15. If the patient cannot wear the eye, store it in the eyecup with water and place in bedside table drawer. Label the cup with the patient's name and room number.
16. Wash your hands thoroughly a second time before inserting the artificial eye. If the patient is to insert the eye, have him wash his hands.
17. Insert the eye in the patient's eye socket. Have the notched edge toward the nose. Raise the upper lid with your forefinger. With your other hand, insert the eye. Place the eye under the upper lid. Then depress the lower lid. The eye should settle in place.
18. Make the patient comfortable.
19. Lower the bed to a position of safety for the patient.
20. Pull the curtains back to the open position.
21. Raise the side rails where ordered, indicated, and appropriate for patient safety.
22. Place the call light within easy reach of the patient.
23. Wash your hands.
24. Report at once to your immediate supervisor:
    - That you have completed care of the artificial eye
    - The time the procedure was done
    - How the patient tolerated the procedure
    - Your observations of anything unusual

KEY IDEAS

Hearing Aids

Remember, even the best hearing aid cannot restore full, normal hearing ability. The patient may still have trouble hearing. Always face the patient when talking to him or her and speak clearly.

Parts of the Hearing Aid

- *Microphone:* changes sound waves into electric signals and transmits sound.
- *Amplifier:* uses battery energy to make the sound signals strong.
- *Earmold:* channels the sound through the external ear canal to the ear drum (tympanic membrane).
- *Cord:* connects the amplifier to the earmold.
- *On/off switch:* controls volume.

Placement of the Hearing Aid

- Turn down the volume before placing the hearing aid in the external ear canal. It should fit tightly but comfortably. After the hearing aid is in place, turn it on and adjust the volume so the patient can hear in a normal tone. The patient will tell you when he or she can hear comfortably.
- If the patient complains of an unpleasant whistle or squeal, check the placement in the ear and for a crack or break.

Checking the Batteries

- Before applying a hearing aid, check the batteries. Be sure they are the right size for the hearing aid. The battery case must close easily or something is wrong.
- To test the batteries, place the control switch to on and turn up the volume control. Cup your hand over the hearing aid and you should hear a whistle. If you do not hear the whistle, change the batteries.
- If the patient complains that he or she cannot hear any sound, remove the hearing aid and check the batteries and that the appliance is not broken.
- If the patient complains of hearing only intermittent sound, remove and check the batteries.

Caring for the Hearing Aid

- Caution: *Never wash a hearing aid: you will ruin it.* When the hearing aid needs cleaning, it must go back to the dealer to be cleaned properly.
- Never drop the hearing aid.
- Do not expose the hearing aid to heat.
- Do not let moisture get into the hearing aid.
- Do not use any kind of hair spray or medical spray on patients while their hearing aids are in place. The spray can clog the microphone opening.

Storage of a Hearing Aid

- Turn the hearing aid off when it is not in use.
- Remove the battery from the battery case when not in use and leave the case open.
- Store a hearing aid in a well-marked container with the patient's name and room number.

KEY IDEAS

The Cerebrovascular Accident (CVA) Stroke Patient

Cerebrovascular Accident (CVA)
Stroke; blood vessels in the brain become blocked or bleed, interrupting the blood supply to that part of the brain and damaging the surrounding area of the brain.

The **cerebrovascular accident** (CVA) or stroke is a disease or disorder of the circulatory system, but the results affect the nervous system. The term is defined as follows:

- Cerebro—dealing with the brain
- Vascular—dealing with the blood vessels
- Accident—an unpredictable and unexpected occurrence

A cerebrovascular accident occurs when the blood supply to a part of the brain is interrupted due to a blocked blood vessel. When the tissue of the brain is not supplied with blood, which carries oxygen and nutrients, it dies. The blood supply may be interrupted due to a blood clot or rupture of a blood vessel in the brain. The results of a cerebrovascular accident depend on which blood vessel is blocked and where it is located in the brain. Sometimes blood vessels surrounding the damaged area of the brain take over to supply the injured tissues. This is called collateral circulation. High blood pressure and atherosclerosis increase the risk of cerebrovascular accidents.

The four main causes of CVA are:

Plaque
Fatty deposits within blood vessels attached to vessel walls.

Rupture
Break open.

Hemorrhage
Excessive bleeding.

Embolus
A blood clot or mass of other undissolved matter that travels through the circulatory system from its place of formation to another site, lodges in a small blood vessel, and causes an obstruction.

Thrombus
A blood clot that remains at its site of formation.

Hemiplegia
Paralysis of only one-half of the body.

- *Plaque:* accumulates in a blood vessel and eventually closes it so that no blood can pass through.
- *Rupture:* breaks open a blood vessel and causes a **hemorrhage** into the brain tissue.
- *Embolus:* a clot that forms elsewhere in the body, travels to the brain through the circulatory system, lodges in a small blood vessel, and causes an obstruction.
- *Thrombus:* a blood clot that remains at the site of its formation.

Common Results of Cerebrovascular Accidents

Frequently, following the stroke, the patient remains paralyzed on one side of the body. This is called **hemiplegia**. The term left hemiplegia or right hemiplegia is used to describe the side of the body that is paralyzed. Loss of sensation may also be a result of the cerebrovascular accident. This includes loss of the ability to feel heat, cold, pressure, and pain in the affected areas.

When the face is involved, there may be a drooping of the eyelid or an inability to close the eyelid. The eye may become dry and irritated, because of decreased or absent tearing. The patient may have difficulty chewing and swallowing. There is often an inability to feel the food on the paralyzed side, increasing the risk of burns, choking, and accumulating food inside the cheek. Drooping of the muscles on one side of the face may cause drooling.

Spasm
An involuntary sudden movement or convulsive muscular contraction.

Contracture
When muscle tissue becomes drawn together, bunched up, or shortened because of spasm or paralysis, either permanently or temporarily.

Spasm, an involuntary contraction of muscles, may occur in paralyzed limbs. The stimulation of exercise, bathing, or dressing may cause the muscles to spasm into a position of flexion or extension. Spasms are increased by nervous tension, cold temperature, and pain. This greatly increases the risk of **contractures,** if the limb remains fixed in one position.

Paralysis of the arm and leg interferes with the ability to perform all activities of daily living. The inability to move increases the risk of contractures, pressure sores, pneumonia, constipation, blood clots, and urinary retention.

Rules to Follow

WHEN CARING FOR A CEREBROVASCULAR ACCIDENT PATIENT

- Encourage the patient. Point out the positive aspects of his or her progress.
- Always show patience and understanding.
- Use techniques that provide a safe and secure environment.
- To prevent disability:
  - Position the patient in proper alignment.
  - Provide good skin care and repositioning to prevent pressure areas that contribute to the cause of pressure ulcers.
  - Do complete, passive range-of-motion exercises to strengthen muscles and prevent contractures, or assist the patient as he is able with active range-of-motion exercises.

- Encourage a well-balanced diet.
- Prevent withdrawal by treating the patient as a unique person with potential to improve.
- When feeding, place food on the unaffected side of the mouth (side not paralyzed).
- Assist with ambulation to prevent falls.
- To move the patient from the bed to the wheelchair when one side of the body has been affected by the stroke, position the wheelchair on the unaffected side of the patient's body. This permits the patient to see the wheelchair and lead with the stronger leg.
- Encourage involvement in self-care.
- Provide a climate or environment where independence is praised and encouraged.

Psychological Aspects of Caring for a Cerebrovascular Accident Patient

When individuals experience a cerebrovascular accident, their lives change suddenly and drastically. The patient may grieve for the lost functions of paralyzed limbs, loss of ability to communicate, loss of independence, loss of control over his or her life, and lost hopes and dreams for the future.

Multiple emotions, possibly including denial, anger, depression, acceptance, emotional instability, or overreaction to a stimulus may be experienced. The patient may burst into tears or laughter for no apparent reason. This is frightening to both the patient and the family.

The loss of the ability to communicate also has multiple effects on the patient. Anger, fear, frustration, depression, and withdrawal may be common responses.

Aphasia

Aphasia
Loss of language or speech.

Many patients who have a cerebrovascular accident experience aphasia. The term **aphasia** refers to a loss of language. Aphasia occurs most commonly with the right hemiplegic, as the language area of the brain is on the left in most people. The patient may have difficulties in understanding what is heard, using numbers, reading, writing, or speaking. Some have difficulty in all these areas. Usually, automatic speech is retained. This means the patient may sing, swear, or use common phrases like "yes" or "no," even though not used correctly. These words or phrases are said automatically.

The most important aspect of caring for the aphasic patient is patience. Do not avoid the patient or attempt to anticipate all her needs. Speech may return completely or partially. You can help most by using the following techniques for talking with an aphasic patient:

- If the patient is able to read, communicate through writing.
- Allow enough time for a response.
- Trigger the word by saying the first sound. For example, "Do you want cr—— in your coffee?" If the patient cannot find the word, tell him.

With patience and cooperation, communication may be established. Keys to communication with the aphasic patient should be written into the nursing plan of care so that continuity of care continues on all shifts.

KEY QUESTIONS

1. What are the differences between grand mal and petit mal seizures?
2. What should you do to maintain the safety of a patient who is having a seizure?
3. How should an artificial eye be cared for?
4. How should a hearing aid be cared for?
5. What are the causes of cerebrovascular accidents?
6. What are some common results of cerebrovascular accidents?
7. List the rules to follow when caring for a cerebrovascular accident patient.
8. What are some common psychological responses to a cerebrovascular accident?
9. Describe the correct technique for talking to the aphasic patient.
10. Define: aphasia, cerebrovascular accident, contracture, embolus, hemiplegia, hemorrhage, plaque, rupture, seizure, spasm, thrombus.

CHAPTER

40 Warm and Cold Applications

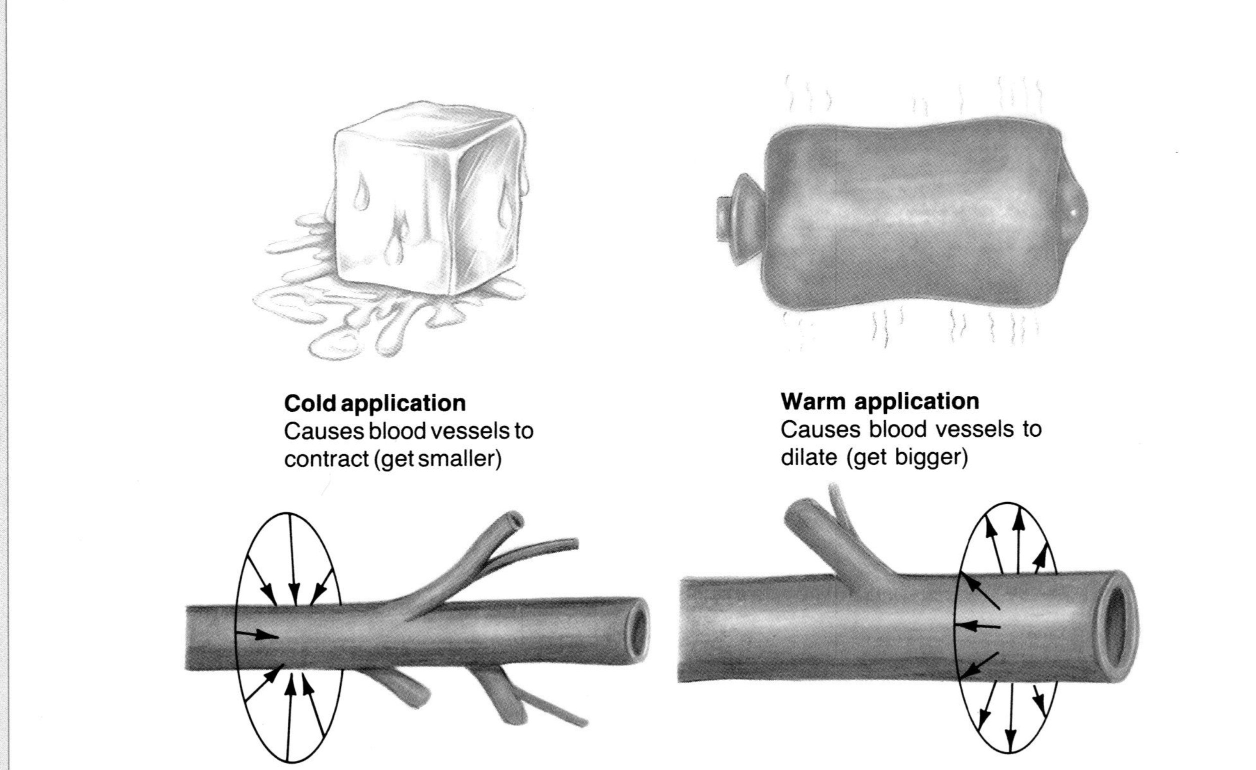
Cold application
Causes blood vessels to contract (get smaller)
Warm application
Causes blood vessels to dilate (get bigger)

WARNING

For all patient contact, adhere to Universal Precautions (see page 91, 97, or the front cover flap). Wear protective equipment as indicated.

Objectives

What You Will Learn

When you have completed this chapter, you will be able to:

- Explain the principles of warm and cold applications.
- Explain the reasons warm and cold applications are used.
- Explain the difference between generalized and localized applications.
- Explain the difference between moist and dry applications.
- Demonstrate safe, correct, and comfortable applications.
- Demonstrate the application of the warm compress.
- Demonstrate the application of the cold soak.
- Demonstrate the application of the cold compress.
- Demonstrate the application of the warm soak.
- Demonstrate the application of the warm-water bottle.
- Demonstrate the application of the ice bag, ice cap, or ice collar.
- Demonstrate the application of the commercial unit cold pack.
- Demonstrate the application of the commercial unit heat pack.
- Demonstrate the application of the heat lamp.
- Demonstrate the application of the perineal heat lamp.
- Demonstrate the application of the Aquamatic K-pad.
- Use the disposable, portable, or built-in sitz bath.
- Define: compress, continuous, contract, cyanosis, dilate, dry application, generalized, generalized application, inflammation, intermittent, localized, localized application, moist application, sitz bath, soak.

KEY IDEAS

Principles for Warm and Cold Applications

Dilate
Get bigger; expand.

Sitz Bath
A bath in which the patient sits in a specially designed chairtub or a regular bathtub with his hips and buttocks in water.

Inflammation
A reaction of the tissues to disease or injury. There is usually pain, heat, redness, and swelling of the body part.

HEAT MAY BE APPLIED TO AN area of the body to speed up the healing process. Heat **dilates** (expands) the blood vessels in the body and causes more blood to circulate to the injured tissues nearby (Figure 40-1). Increased circulation can provide the body tissue with more food and oxygen. These are needed for the repair (healing) of body tissue. Warm tub baths, sometimes with medication in the water, are often prescribed for this reason. A **sitz bath** is another example. In this procedure, warm water is applied to the patient's perineal or rectal area to speed healing after childbirth or surgery.

Heat may also be applied to an area of the body to ease the pain caused by **inflammation** and congestion. When the blood vessels become dilated, the increased supply of blood may absorb and carry away the fluids that are causing the inflammation and pain. For example, people with certain bone and joint conditions often get relief from pain and can increase the movement of their body parts because of exercises in warm water.

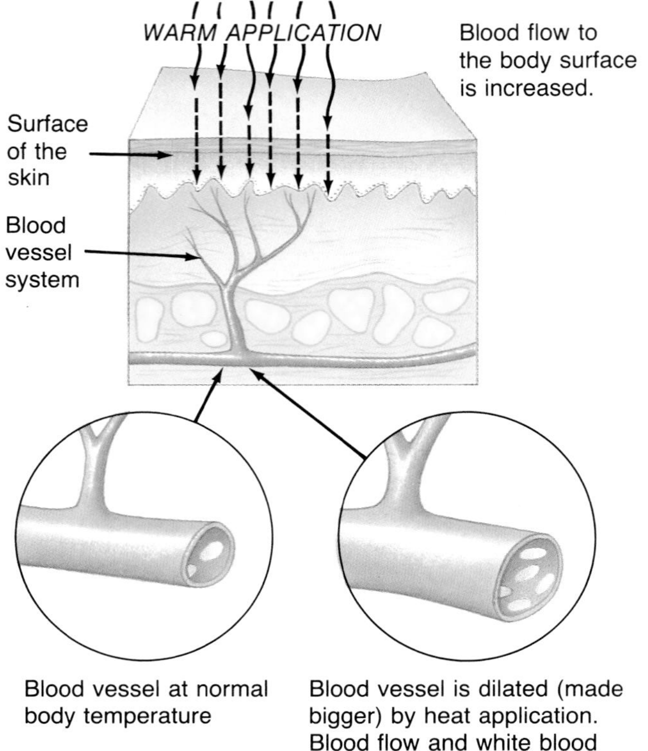
WARM APPLICATION
Blood flow to the body surface is increased.
Surface of the skin
Blood vessel system
Blood vessel at normal body temperature
Blood vessel is dilated (made bigger) by heat application. Blood flow and white blood cells are increased in area of application.

FIGURE 40-1 Principle of warm application.

FIGURE 40-2 Principle of cold application.

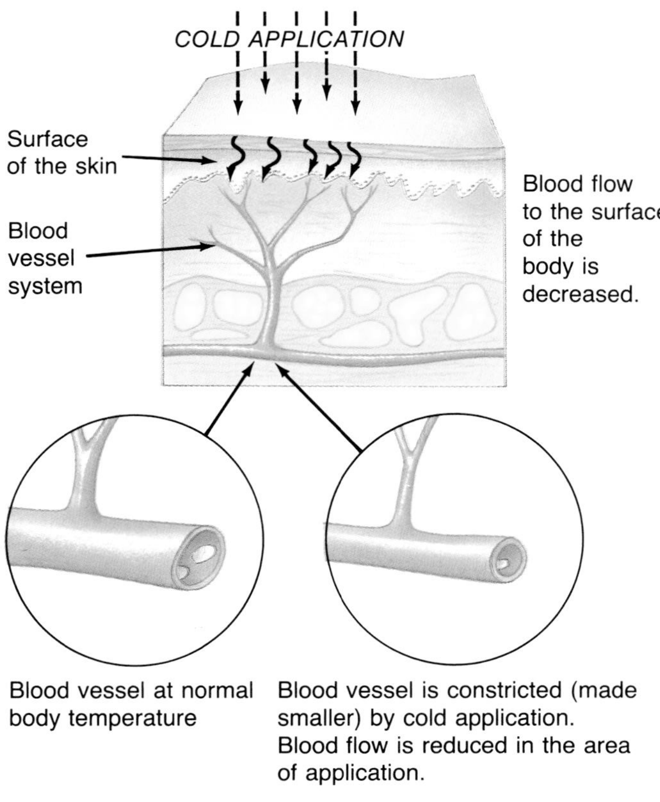
COLD APPLICATION
Surface of the skin
Blood vessel system
Blood flow to the surface of the body is decreased.
Blood vessel at normal body temperature
Blood vessel is constricted (made smaller) by cold application. Blood flow is reduced in the area of application.

Contract
Get smaller.

Cold applications cause the blood vessels to **contract** (Figure 40-2). This contraction may help to prevent or reduce swelling, as in the case of a sprained ankle or the beginning of a black eye. The contraction slows down the flow of blood, thereby reducing the amount of body fluids that are carried into the injured area. This may also reduce the pain that usually goes along with the swelling. Cold applications may be applied to control bleeding. When cold is applied, the blood flow becomes slower and less blood is able to seep out through a cut or other wound. For example, when a patient has had a tonsillectomy, an ice collar or ice pack may be applied to the neck region.

Cold may be applied to a patient's entire body. This is usually done to lower a patient's body temperature when he or she has a fever. Special equipment such as a hypothermia blanket is used to help lower the body temperature.

Localized
Limited to one place or part; affecting, involving, or pertaining to a definite area.

Localized Application
One in which warmth or coldness is applied to a specific area or small part of the body.

Generalized Application
One in which warmth or cold is applied to the entire body.

Generalized
Affecting, involving, or pertaining to the whole body.

Localized and Generalized Applications

Be sure you know exactly where on the patient's body the warmth or cold is to be applied. A **generalized application** is one in which a warm or cold application is applied to a patient's whole body. A **localized application** is one that is applied to a specific part or area of a patient's body.

Moist Application
An application of warmth or cold in which water touches the skin.

Dry Application
An application of warmth or cold in which no water touches the skin.

Moist and Dry Applications

All applications are either moist or dry (Figure 40-3). A **moist application** is one in which water touches the skin. A **dry application** is one

FIGURE 40-3 (a) Moist and (b) dry applications.

(a)

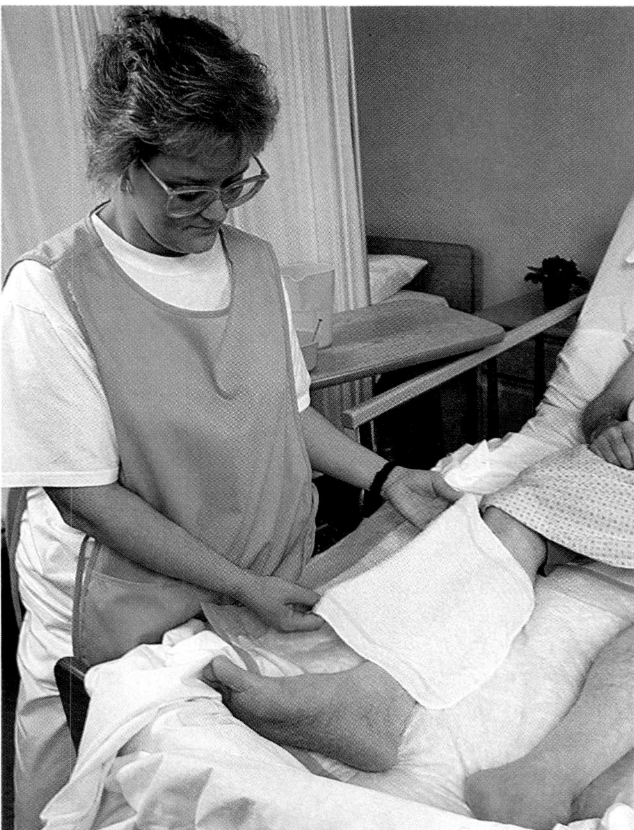

(b)

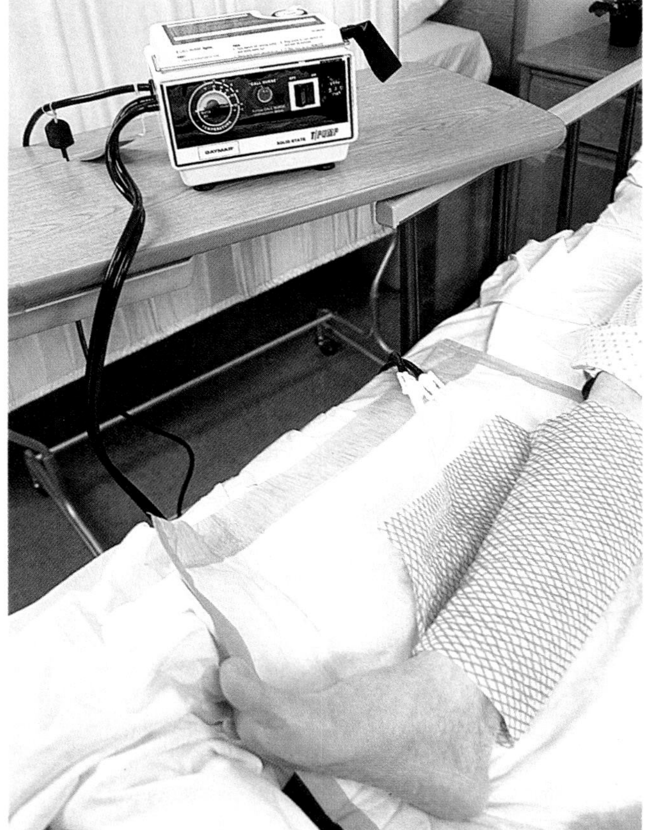

in which no water touches the skin. There are several types of both moist and dry applications:

Moist	**Dry**
Soak: warm or cold	Ice cap and ice collar
Compress: warm or cold	Warm-water bottle
Tub	Heat lamp
Sitz bath	Aquamatic K-pad
Cool wet packs	Hypothermia blankets
Commercial unit warm pack	Electric heat cradle
	Commercial unit cold pack

Compress
Folded piece of cloth used to apply pressure, moisture, heat, cold, or medication to a specific part of the body.

Soak
Immerse the body or body part completely in water.

Compresses and soaks are both moist applications and can be either warm or cold. A **compress** is a localized application. A **soak** can be either localized or generalized. In applying a compress, a cloth is dipped into water, wrung out, and applied to the skin. To apply a soak, you immerse the body or body part completely in water. Warm-water bottles, ice caps, and Aquamatic K-pads are considered dry applications because they have a dry surface. Water is used only inside the equipment and never touches the skin. Warm dry applications are sometimes used to keep warm moist applications at the correct temperature.

Length of Applications

Follow the instructions given to you by your immediate supervisor for the exact time to begin the application. Also follow his or her instructions about how long the application is to stay in place.

Checking the Application

Check the application often to keep it at the right temperature throughout the treatment. Suggested times for checking the temperatures of different kinds of applications are:

Intermittent
Alternating; stopping and beginning again.

- Soaks and **intermittent** compresses: every 5 minutes
- Heat lamps: every 5 minutes

Keeping the Patient Safe

Avoid accidents. Be careful not to spill any water. Be sure electrical equipment does not come in contact with water. Be sure your hands are dry before touching electrical equipment. Be sure the bed is properly protected. Put the side rails in the upright position if needed.

Check the patient's skin under warm applications (Figure 40-4). Watch for too much redness. Look for a darker discoloration that might mean the patient is being burned. Listen when the patient complains. If you think a patient is being burned, remove the heat application and report to your immediate supervisor at once.

Cyanosis
When the skin looks blue or has a darkened appearance because there is not enough oxygen in the blood; often seen in the patient's lips and nailbeds and in the skin under the fingernails.

Check the patient's skin where cold is being applied (Figure 40-5). If the area appears to be blanched, very pale, white, or bluish, tell your immediate supervisor at once. Watch for changes in the color of parts of the patient's body. For example, if the patient's lips, fingernails, and eyelids look blue or turn a dark color, this is **cyanosis**, which is a sign of less oxygen getting to that part of the body. Stop the treatment immediately and report to your immediate supervisor.

FIGURE 40-4 Check the skin under the application for discoloration (red or white). If you think the patient is being burned or frozen, discontinue treatment and report to the nurse immediately.

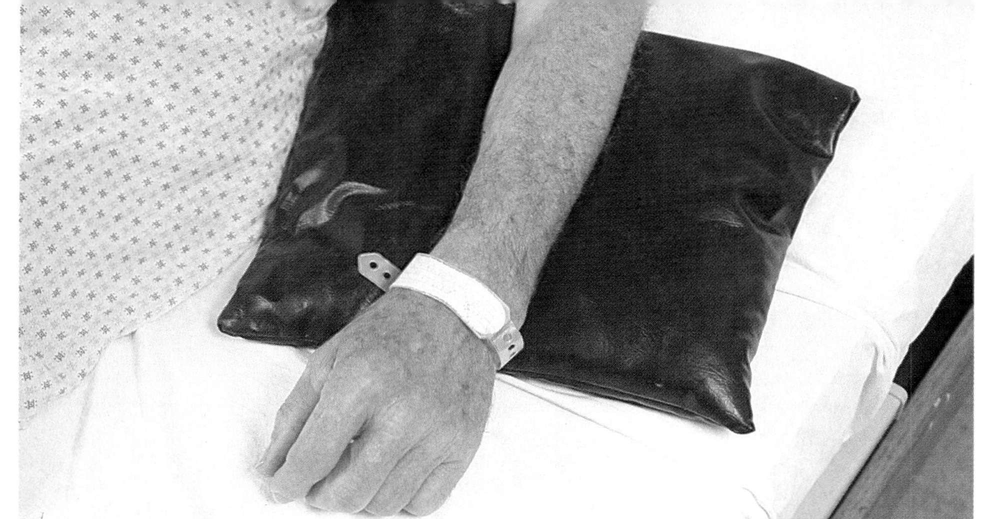

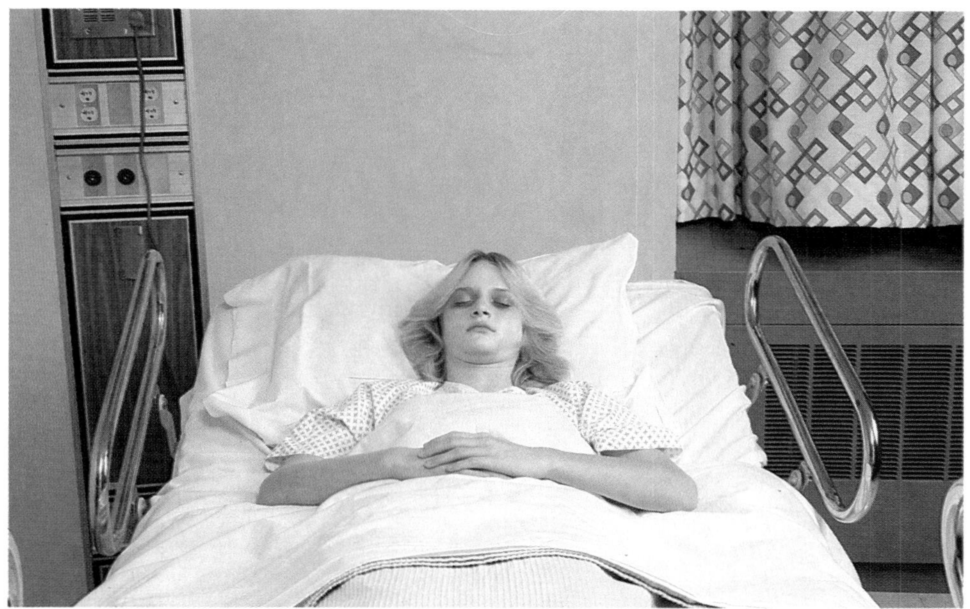

FIGURE 40-5 Observe the patient for signs of cyanosis. Watch for blueness or darkening of the lips, fingernails, or eyelids.

Always apply the ice cap and warm-water bottle with its metal or plastic stopper away from the patient's body. The stopper should never touch the patient's skin. It will be much warmer or colder than the application and could burn or freeze the patient's skin. You may be working with an unconscious patient. If so, you may be directed to protect him from a burn by putting a blanket between the skin and the warm water bottle or ice cap.

Keeping the Patient Comfortable

Make sure the patient is in a position that is comfortable for him and convenient for your work. Keep the patient covered and warm during the treatment. Otherwise, the patient might become chilled and uncomfortable. If a patient shivers during the cold application, stop the treatment. Cover him with a blanket. Then report this at once to your immediate supervisor. She or he will tell you what to do.

Never put the warm-water bottle or ice bag on top of a painful area. The weight may increase the pain. Never fill a warm-water bottle or ice bag more than half full. It gets too heavy.

Always dry the bottle or bag. Check it for leaks by turning it upside down. Place it in a flannel cover or the case used by your hospital. Never let the patient lie on an uncovered warm-water bottle or ice bag.

Procedure Applying the Warm Compress (Moist Heat Applications)

☐ In some institutions warm compresses are made by holding a cloth under running warm water or by microwaving a wet cloth. If you are instructed to do this be careful to prevent too much heat. Follow the instructions of your immediate supervisor.

1. Assemble your equipment:
   a) Disposable bed protector
   b) Basin
   c) Pitcher of water at 115°F (46.1°C)
   d) Washcloth, towel, or gauze pads (compress)
   e) Bath thermometer
   f) Large sheet of plastic
   g) Bath towel
   h) Bath blanket
2. Wash your hands.
3. Identify the patient by checking the identification bracelet.
4. Ask visitors to step out of the room, if this is your hospital's policy.
5. Tell the patient you are going to apply a warm compress.
6. Pull the curtain around the bed for privacy.
7. Raise the bed to a comfortable working position.
8. Help the patient into a comfortable, safe position. Have the body area exposed for application of a warm compress.
9. Place a disposable bed protector under the body area that is to be given the warm compress.
10. Fill the pitcher with warm water. Check the temperature of the water with a bath thermometer (115°F or 46.1°C). Then pour the water into the basin.
11. Dip the compress into the water and wring it out thoroughly.
12. Apply the compress gently to the proper area (Figure 40-6).
13. Wrap the entire area with a large towel or a blue pad, covering the wet compress. Cover the entire area, compress, and towel with a plastic sheet (Figure 40-7). Be sure the plastic does not touch the patient's skin. This will keep the compress warm.
14. If the patient is cold or chilly, cover him with a blanket.
15. Change the compress and remoisten it, as necessary, to keep it warm. Sometimes a patient is able to apply the compress himself. If your immediate supervisor gives permission for this, position and assist the patient as necessary.

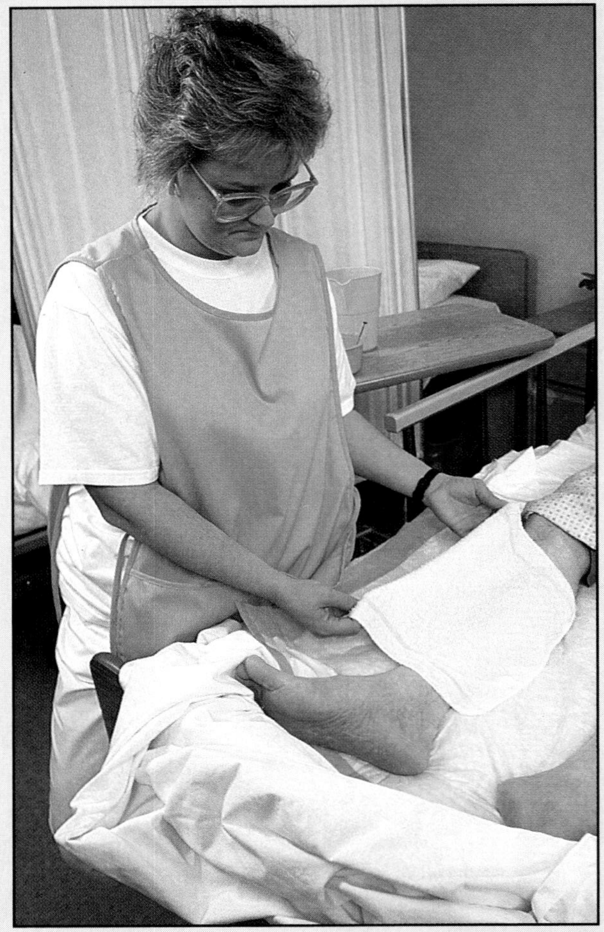

FIGURE 40-6 Applying the warm compress.

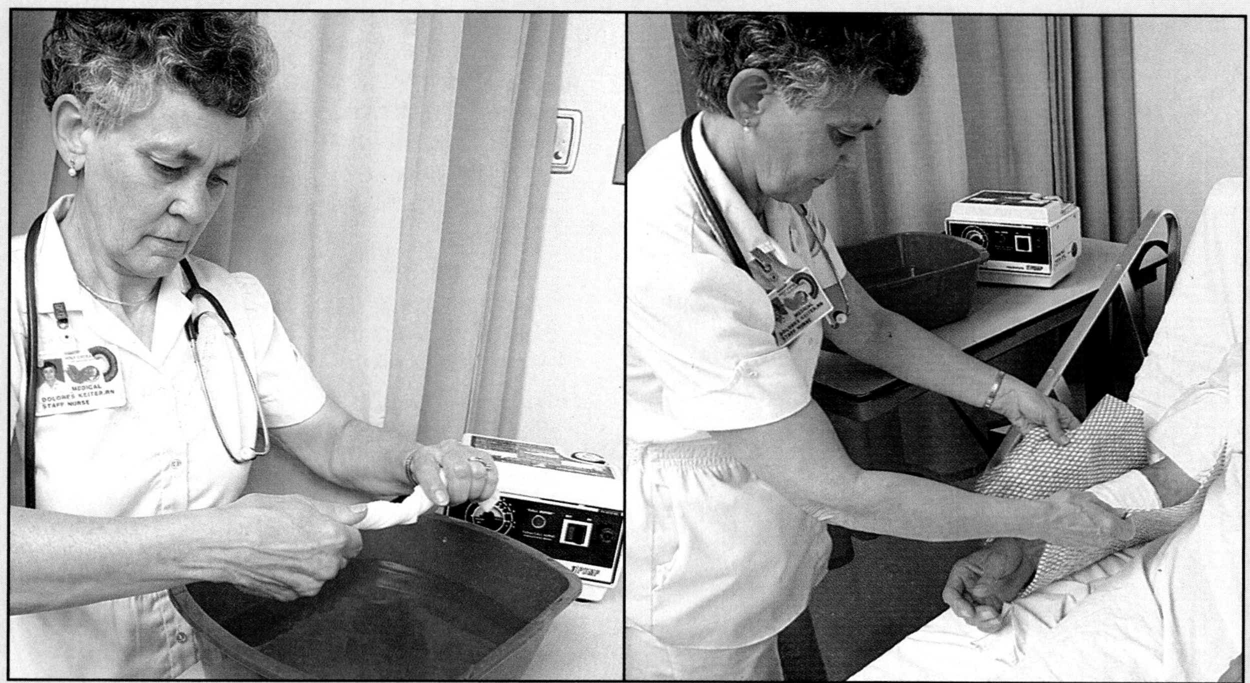

FIGURE 40-7

16. Check the skin under the application every 5 minutes. If the skin appears red, remove the compress. Cover the area with a towel or blanket. Report this to your immediate supervisor.
17. A warm compress is usually applied for 15 to 20 minutes. However, follow the instructions given to you by your immediate supervisor as to how long the warm compress is to be applied.
18. After the treatment is completed, remove the compress and gently pat the area dry with a towel.
19. Make the patient comfortable.
20. Lower the bed to a position of safety for the patient.
21. Pull the curtains back to the open position.
22. Raise the side where ordered, indicated, and appropriate for patient safety.
23. Place the call light within easy reach of the patient.
24. Clean standard equipment and put it in its proper place. Discard disposable equipment.
25. Wash your hands.
26. Report to your immediate supervisor:
    - The time the warm compress was started
    - How long the compress was in place
    - The area of application
    - How the patient tolerated the procedure
    - Your observations of anything unusual

Procedure Applying the Cold Compress (Moist Cold Application)

1. Assemble your equipment:
    a) Disposable bed protector
    b) Basin
    c) Washcloth, towel, or gauze pads (compress)
    d) Bath towel
    e) Bath blanket
    f) Pitcher of cold water (ice cubes, if ordered by your immediate supervisor)
2. Wash your hands.
3. Identify the patient by checking the identification bracelet.

4. Ask visitors to step out of the room, if this is your hospital's policy.
5. Tell the patient you are going to apply a cold compress.
6. Pull the curtain around the bed for privacy.
7. Raise the bed to a comfortable working position.
8. Help the patient into a comfortable, safe position. Expose the area to be treated.
9. Place a disposable bed protector under the body area that is to be given the cold compress.
10. Put cold water in the basin (ice cubes only if ordered).
11. Dip the compress into the water and wring it out thoroughly.
12. Apply the compress gently to the proper area of the patient's body as quickly as possible. If you are slow, the compress will absorb heat from your hands and the air (Figure 40-8).
13. If the patient is cold or chilly, cover him with a blanket. Do not cover the compress or the area being treated.

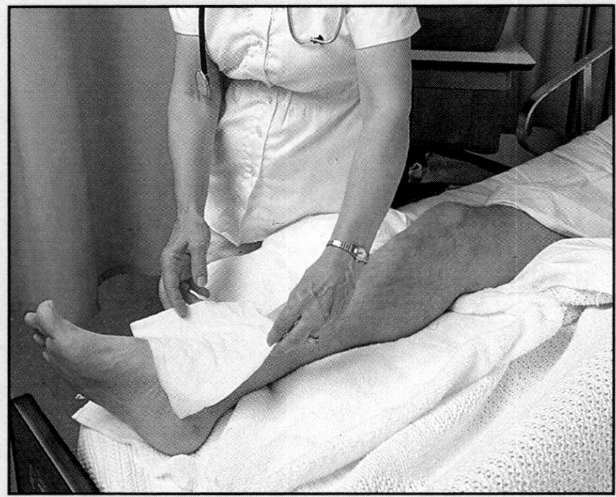

FIGURE 40-8

14. Change the compress and remoisten it, as necessary, to keep it cold. Sometimes a patient is able to apply the compress himself. If your immediate supervisor gives permission for this, position and assist the patient as necessary.
15. Check the skin under the application every 5 minutes. If the skin appears to be blanched or white, remove the compress. Cover the area with a towel or blanket. Report this to your head nurse or team leader.
16. A cold compress is usually applied for 15 to 20 minutes. However, follow the instructions of your immediate supervisor.
17. When the treatment is finished, remove the compress and gently pat the area dry with a towel.
18. Make the patient comfortable.
19. Lower the bed to a position of safety for the patient.
20. Pull the curtains back to the open position.
21. Raise the side rails where ordered, indicated, and appropriate for patient safety.
22. Place the call light within easy reach of the patient.
23. Clean your standard equipment and put it in its proper place.
24. Discard disposable equipment.
25. Wash your hands.
26. Report to your immediate supervisor:
    - The time the cold compress was started
    - How long it remained in place
    - The area of application
    - How the patient tolerated the procedure
    - Your observations of anything unusual

Procedure Applying the Cold Soak (Moist Cold Applications)

1. Assemble your equipment:
    a) Basin, foot tub, or arm basin
    b) Disposable bed protector
    c) Washcloth, towel, or gauze pads (compress)
    d) Bath towel
    e) Bath blanket
2. Wash your hands.
3. Identify the patient by checking the identification bracelet.

4. Ask visitors to step out of the room, if this is your hospital's policy.
5. Tell the patient you are going to apply a cold soak.
6. Pull the curtain around the bed for privacy.
7. Raise the bed to a comfortable working position.
8. Help the patient into a safe, comfortable position. Expose the area to be treated.
9. Fill the basin half full with cold water (Figure 40-9).

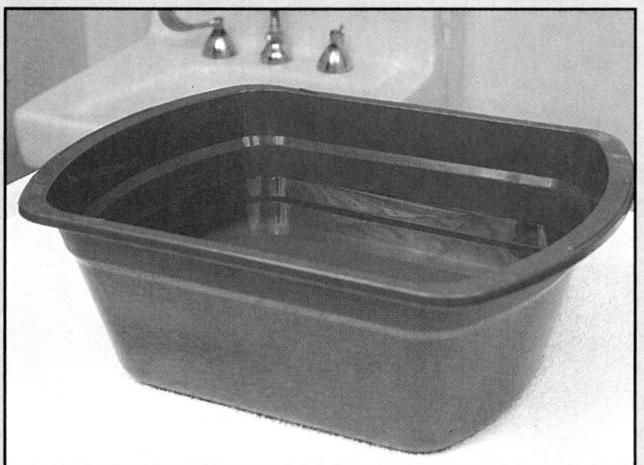

FIGURE 40-9

10. Place a disposable bed protector under the body area that is to receive the cold soak.
11. Place the basin in a position so that the patient's arm, leg, foot, or hand can be dipped into the basin easily (Figure 40-10).
12. Place the patient's arm or leg into the water gradually.
13. When you have to change the water, take the patient's arm or leg out of the basin. Wrap it with a bath towel or bath blanket to keep it warm.
14. If the patient says he feels weak or cold, stop the treatment. Cover the patient with extra blankets and report this to your immediate supervisor.
15. Check the skin every 5 minutes. If the skin is blanched or white, stop the treatment. Report to your immediate supervisor.
16. When the treatment is finished, dry the patient's arm or leg by gently patting with a towel.
17. Make the patient comfortable.

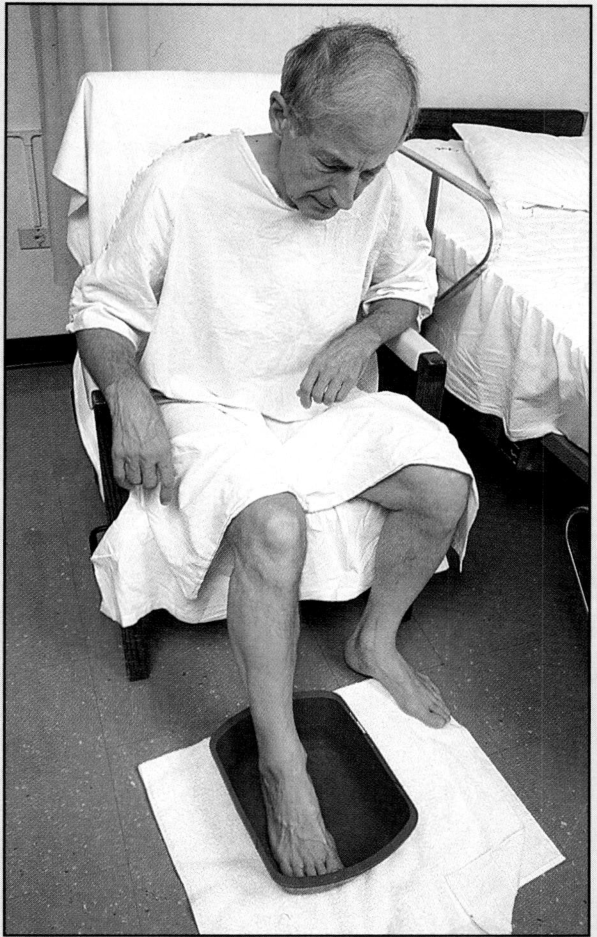

FIGURE 40-10

18. Lower the bed to a position of safety for the patient.
19. Pull the curtains back to the open position.
20. Raise the side rails where ordered, indicated, and appropriate for patient safety.
21. Place the call light within easy reach of the patient.
22. Clean standard equipment and put it in its proper place. Discard disposable equipment.
23. Wash your hands.
24. Report to your immediate supervisor:
    - The time the cold soak was started
    - The length of treatment
    - The area of application
    - How the patient tolerated the procedure
    - Your observations of anything unusual

Procedure Applying the Warm Soak (Moist Warm Application)

1. Assemble your equipment:
   a) Basin, foot tub, or arm basin
   b) Bath thermometer
   c) Disposable bed protector
   d) Bath towel
   e) Bath blanket
2. Wash your hands.
3. Identify the patient by checking the identification bracelet.
4. Ask visitors to step out of the room, if this is your hospital's policy.
5. Tell the patient you are going to apply a warm soak.
6. Pull the curtain around the bed for privacy.
7. Raise the bed to a comfortable working position.
8. Help the patient into a safe, comfortable position. Expose the area to be treated.
9. Fill the basin one-half full with warm water at 100°F (37.8°C). Check the temperature with a bath thermometer.
10. Place a disposable bed protector under the body area that is to receive the soak.
11. Place the basin in a position so the patient's arm, leg, foot, or hand can be dipped into the basin easily (Figure 40-11).
12. Place the patient's arm or leg into the water gradually.
13. Check the temperature of the water every 5 minutes. When you need to change the water, take the patient's arm, foot, or leg out of the basin. Wrap it with a bath blanket or bath towel to keep it warm.
14. If the patient says he feels weak or cold, stop the treatment. Cover the patient with extra blankets and report this to your immediate supervisor.
15. Check the skin every 5 minutes. If the skin is red, stop the treatment. Report this to your immediate supervisor.
16. When the treatment is finished, dry the patient's arm or leg by patting gently with a towel.
17. Make the patient comfortable.
18. Lower the bed to a position of safety for the patient.
19. Pull the curtains back to the open position.
20. Raise the side rails where ordered, indicated, and appropriate for patient safety.
21. Place the call light within easy reach of the patient.
22. Clean standard equipment and put it in its proper place. Discard disposable equipment.
23. Wash your hands.
24. Report to your immediate supervisor:
    - The time the warm soak was started
    - The length of treatment
    - The area of application
    - How the patient tolerated the procedure
    - Your observations of anything unusual

FIGURE 40-11
(a) (b)

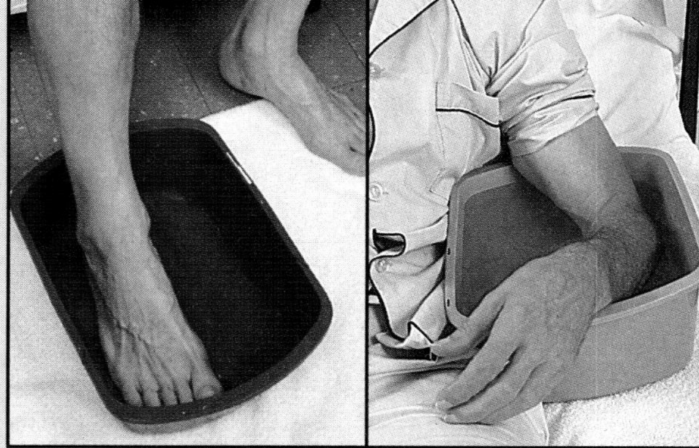

Procedure Applying the Warm-water Bottle (Dry Heat Application)

1. Assemble your equipment:
   a) Warm-water bottle (may be disposable)
   b) Pitcher of water at 120°F (48.9°C). If warm-water bottle is disposable, follow your institution's policies for the correct temperature of the water.
   c) Bath thermometer

d) Flannel cover (or whatever type of cover is used in your institution)

2. Wash your hands.
3. Identify the patient by checking the identification bracelet.
4. Ask visitors to step out of the room, if this is your hospital's policy.
5. Tell the patient you are going to apply a warm-water bottle.
6. Pull the curtain around the bed for privacy.
7. Raise the bed to a comfortable working position.
8. Fill the pitcher with water at 120°F (48.9°C). Check the temperature with a bath thermometer.
9. Fill the warm-water bottle half full of water (Figure 40-12).

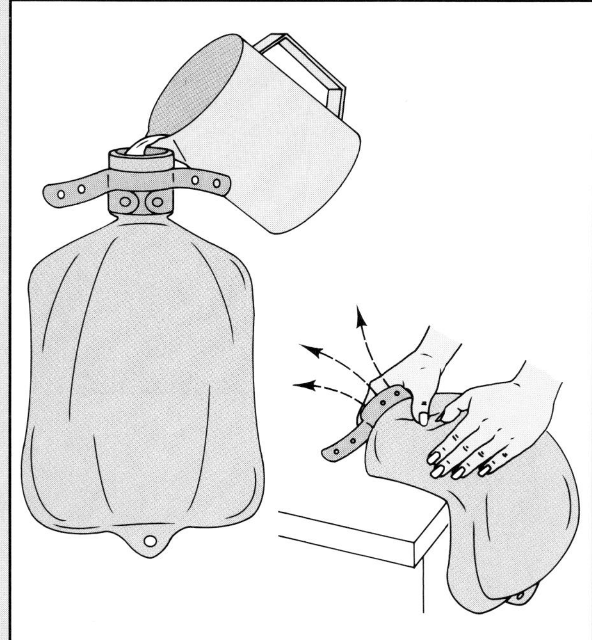

FIGURE 40-12 Filling the warm-water bottle.

10. Two methods of squeezing the air out of the bottle are:

Method A. Place the bag on the edge of a counter. Have the part of the bag containing the water hanging down. Place the part of the bag without the water lying on the counter top. Put your hand on the top of the bag at the edge of the counter. Move your hand slowly toward the opening of the bag, pressing out the air. With the other hand, close the bag.

Method B. Place the warm-water bottle in a horizontal position on a flat surface. Hold the neck of the warm-water bottle upright until you can see water in the neck of the bottle. The water squeezes out the air.

11. Fasten the top tightly.
12. Dry the warm-water bottle. Check for leaks by turning it upside down.
13. Place the warm-water bottle in the type of cover used in your institution (Figure 40-13).

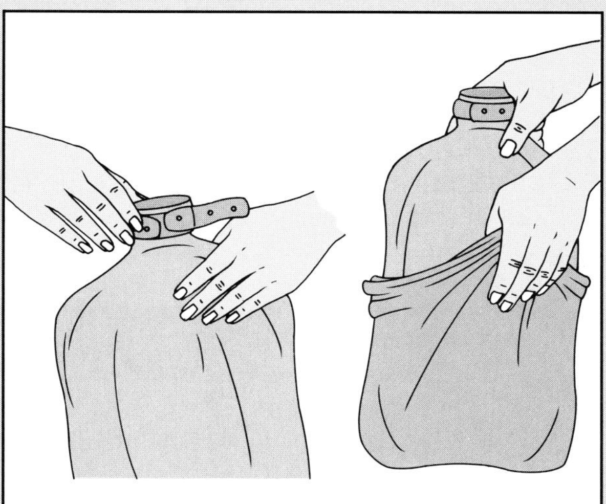

FIGURE 40-13 Placing the water bottle in a cover.

14. Help the patient into a safe, comfortable position. Expose the area to be treated. Apply the bottle gently to the proper body area (Figure 40-14).

FIGURE 40-14 Warm-water bottle inside cover being used on patient.

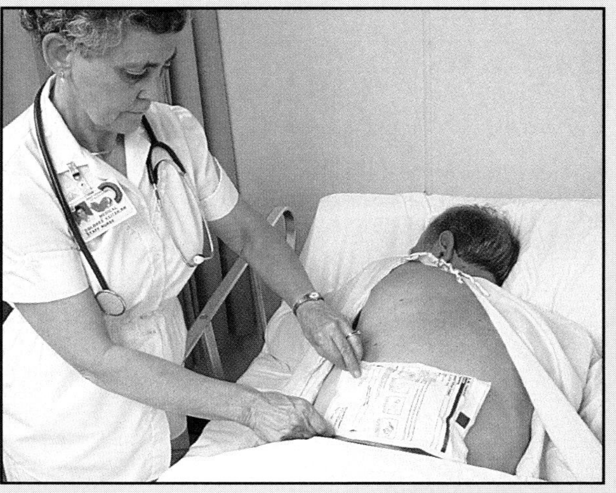

15. Never place the warm-water bottle on top of a painful area. The weight will increase the pain. Place it on the side.
16. Check the warm-water bottle every hour to be sure the temperature is correct. Change the water in the bottle, when necessary, to continue the treatment at the same temperature.
17. Check the skin under the warm-water bottle after the first five minutes and then every hour. If the skin is red, remove the warm-water bottle and report to your immediate supervisor.
18. Clean standard equipment and put it in its proper place. Discard disposable equipment.
19. Make the patient comfortable.
20. Lower the bed to a position of safety for the patient.
21. Pull the curtains back to the open position.
22. Raise the side rails where ordered, indicated, and appropriate for patient safety.
23. Place the call light within easy reach of the patient.
24. Wash your hands.
25. Report to your immediate supervisor:
    - The time the warm-water bottle was applied
    - The length of treatment
    - The area of application
    - How the patient tolerated the procedure
    - Your observations of anything unusual

Procedure Applying the Ice Bag, Ice Cap, or Ice Collar (Dry Cold Application)

1. Assemble your equipment:
   a) Ice bag, ice cap, or ice collar (may be disposable); Figure 40-15
   b) Flannel cover (whatever type of cover is used in your institution)
   c) Ice in a clean container
   d) Bath blanket

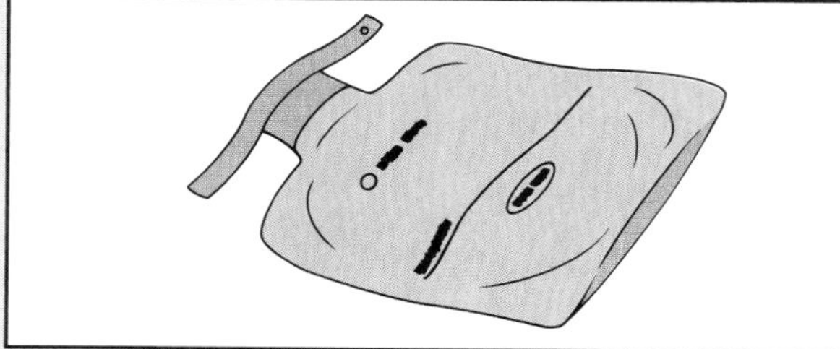

FIGURE 40-15 Disposable ice bag.

2. Wash your hands.
3. Identify the patient by checking the identification bracelet.
4. Ask visitors to step out of the room, if this is your hospital's policy.
5. Tell the patient you are going to apply the ice bag, ice cap, or ice collar.
6. Pull the curtain around the bed for privacy.
7. Raise the bed to a comfortable working position.
8. Help the patient into a safe, comfortable position. Expose the area to be treated.
9. Pour cold water over the ice to melt the sharp edges.
10. Fill the ice collar, ice bag, or ice cap one-half full of ice (Figure 40-16).

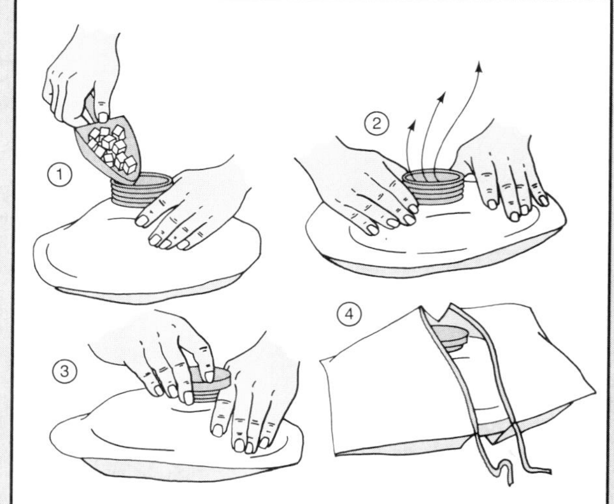

FIGURE 40-16

11. Squeeze the sides of the ice bag to force the air out of it.
12. Fasten the stopper tightly.

13. Dry the outside of the ice bag with a paper towel.
14. Invert the ice bag to test for leaking.
15. Place the ice bag into the type of cover used in your institution.
16. Apply the ice bag to the proper area of the patient's body.
17. If the patient is cold or chilly, cover him with a blanket. Do not cover the ice bag or the area being treated.
18. Follow the instructions of your immediate supervisor as to the length of application. Replace the ice as necessary.
19. Check the skin under the application every 10 minutes. If the skin appears to be blanched or white, remove the ice bag. Cover the area with a towel and report to your head nurse or team leader.
20. Clean standard equipment and put it in its proper place. Discard disposable equipment.
21. Make the patient comfortable.
22. Lower the bed to a position of safety for the patient.
23. Pull the curtains back to the open position.
24. Raise the side rails where ordered, indicated, and appropriate for patient safety.
25. Place the call light within easy reach of the patient.
26. Wash your hands.
27. Report to your immediate supervisor:
    - The time the ice bag was applied
    - The length of treatment
    - The area of application
    - How the patient tolerated the procedure
    - Your observations of anything unusual

Procedure Applying the Commercial Unit Cold Pack (Dry Cold Application)

1. Assemble your equipment:
   a) Commercial unit, single-use cold pack
   b) Cover used in your institution
   c) Bath blanket
2. Wash your hands.
3. Identify the patient by checking the identification bracelet.
4. Ask visitors to step out of the room, if this is your hospital's policy.
5. Tell the patient you are going to apply a cold pack.
6. Pull the curtain around the bed for privacy.
7. Raise the bed to a comfortable working position.
8. Help the patient into a safe, comfortable position. Expose the area to be treated.
9. Place the flannel cover on the cold pack (or whatever type of cover is used by your institution).
10. Hit or squeeze the cold pack to activate it according to the manufacturer's directions (Figure 40-17).

FIGURE 40-17

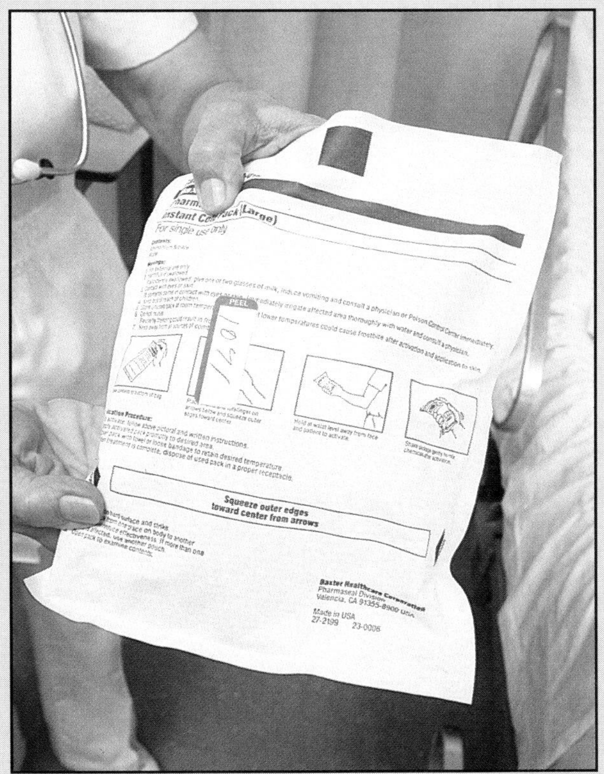

11. Apply the pack to the proper area of the patient's body.
12. Check the skin under the application every 10 minutes. If the skin appears blanched or white, remove the pack and cover the area with a blanket. Report this to your immediate supervisor.
13. Follow the instructions of your immediate supervisor as to the length of application. Replace with a new cold pack as necessary.
14. Discard disposable equipment.
15. Make the patient comfortable.
16. Lower the bed to a position of safety for the patient.
17. Pull the curtains back to the open position.
18. Raise the side rails where ordered, indicated, and appropriate for patient safety.
19. Place the call light within easy reach of the patient.
20. Wash your hands.
21. Report to your immediate supervisor:
    - The time the cold pack was applied
    - The length of treatment
    - The area of application
    - How the patient tolerated the procedure
    - Your observations of anything unusual

Procedure Applying the Commercial Unit Heat Pack (Moist Warm Application)

1. Assemble your equipment:
    a) Commercial unit, single-use heat pack that has been warmed in the heating lamp unit
    b) Disposable bed protectors
    c) Large sheet of plastic or disposable bed protector
    d) Bath blanket
2. Wash your hands.
3. Identify the patient by checking the identification bracelet.
4. Ask visitors to step out of the room, if this is your hospital's policy.
5. Tell the patient you are going to apply a warm pack.
6. Pull the curtain around the bed for privacy.
7. Raise the bed to a comfortable working position.
8. Help the patient into a safe, comfortable position. Expose the area to be treated.
9. Place the bed protector under the body part that is to receive the warm pack.
10. Tear the foil covering from the warm pack.
11. Place the moist warm pack on the proper body area.
12. Cover the pack with the sheet of plastic or the disposable bed protector. This will keep the pack warm.
13. Check the skin under the application every five minutes. If the skin appears red, remove the pack and cover the area with a blanket. Report this to your immediate supervisor.
14. Follow the instructions of your immediate supervisor as to the length of application. Replace with a new warm pack as necessary.
15. When the treatment is finished, discard disposable equipment.
16. Make the patient comfortable.
17. Lower the bed to a position of safety for the patient.
18. Pull the curtains back to the open position.
19. Raise the side rails where ordered, indicated, and appropriate for patient safety.
20. Place the call light within easy reach of the patient.
21. Wash your hands.
22. Report to your immediate supervisor:
    - The time the warm pack was applied
    - The length of treatment
    - The area of application
    - How the patient tolerated the procedure
    - Your observations of anything unusual

Procedure Applying a Heat Lamp (Dry Warm Application)

1. Assemble your equipment:
   a) Heat lamp
   b) Bath blanket
   c) Bath towel
   d) Tape measure
2. Wash your hands.
3. Identify the patient by checking the identification bracelet.
4. Ask visitors to step out of the room, if this is your hospital's policy.
5. Tell the patient you are going to apply heat with a heat lamp.
6. Pull the curtain around the bed for privacy.
7. Raise the bed to a comfortable working position.
8. Help the patient into a safe, comfortable position.
9. Expose only the body area that is to receive the heat. Drape the patient so that heat is directed to the proper area of the skin (Figure 40-18). Cover the rest of the patient's body with a bath blanket, sheet or towel.
10. Check the electric cord to be sure it is in good condition and there are no frayed areas.
11. Plug in the lamp.
12. Position the lamp so that heat will be directed to the proper skin area.
13. The part of the patient's body that is being treated should be at least 18 inches away from the heat lamp. Use a tape measure to check the distance.
14. Turn on the lamp. Be sure it is working properly.
15. Check the skin after 3 minutes. If the patient's skin becomes red, stop the treatment and report to your immediate supervisor.
16. There is a danger of fire when a heat lamp is being used. Therefore, keep all linen away from the lamp.
17. Leave the heat lamp on the patient from 5 to no more than 10 minutes, unless you have other instructions from your immediate supervisor.
18. After treatment is completed, unplug and remove the lamp.
19. Make the patient comfortable.
20. Lower the bed to a position of safety for the patient.
21. Pull the curtains back to the open position.
22. Raise the side rails where ordered, indicated, and appropriate for patient safety.
23. Place the call light within easy reach of the patient.
24. Wipe the lamp with disinfectant solution and put it back in its proper place.
25. Wash your hands.
26. Report to your immediate supervisor:
    - The time the heat was applied
    - The length of treatment
    - The area of application
    - How the patient tolerated the procedure
    - Your observations of anything unusual

FIGURE 40-18 Applying the heat lamp. Drape the patient so that heat is directed to the proper skin area. The heat lamp should be at least 18 inches from the surface of the patient's skin. Check frequently for redness of skin.

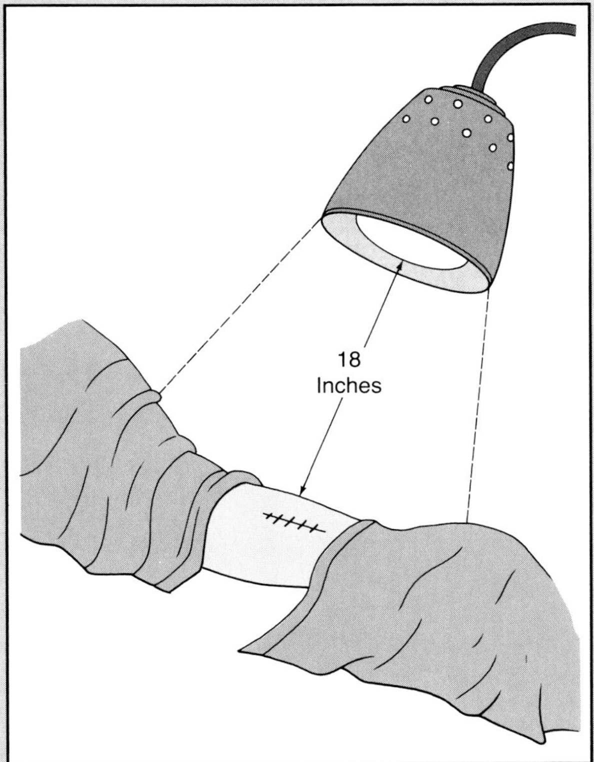

KEY IDEAS

Perineal Heat Lamp

When you are using the heat lamp as a perineal, or "peri" lamp, help the patient into the lithotomy position. Place her feet on the mattress. Bend the knees and separate them. Place the lamp 18 inches away from the perineum. Remove the peripad to expose the perineal area. Remove the patient's pillow. Instruct the patient to keep her head flat, exposing more of the perineum. Watch for excessive heat. The light should be on from 5 to 10 minutes. When the treatment is finished, remove the lamp. Put a new peripad in place and make the patient more comfortable.

Procedure Applying the Aquamatic Hydro-Thermal (K-Pad) (Dry Heat Application)

1. Assemble your equipment (Figure 40-19):
   a) Aquamatic Hydro-Thermal (K-pad) and control unit. (The temperature is preset by the central supply room. The container is filled with distilled water by central supply.)
   b) Cover for pad (pillowcase, flannel cover or cover from manufacturer)

FIGURE 40-19

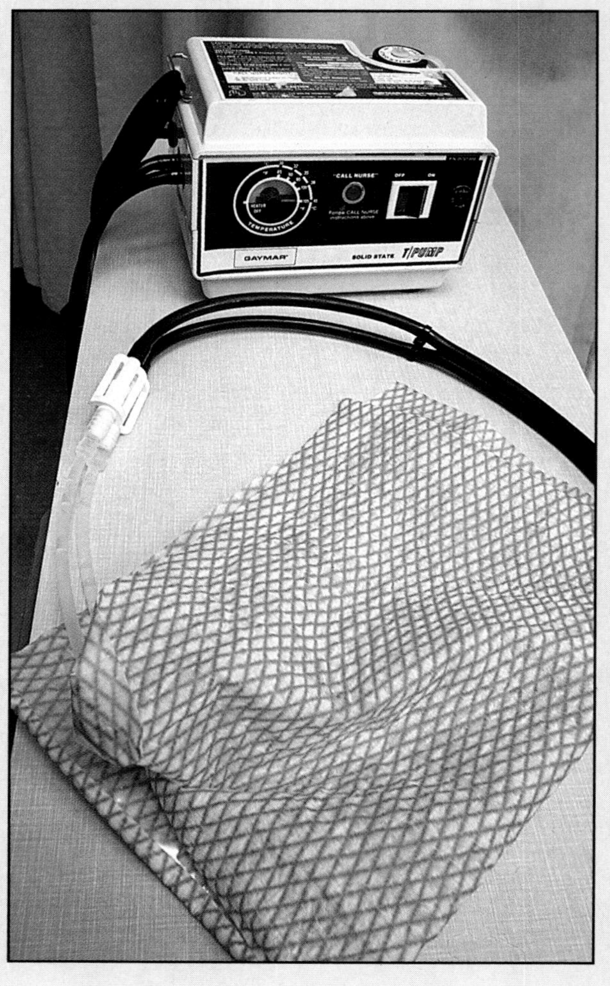

2. Wash your hands.
3. Identify the patient by checking the identification bracelet.
4. Ask visitors to step out of the room, if this is your hospital's policy.
5. Tell the patient you are going to apply the K-pad.
6. Pull the curtain around the bed for privacy.
7. Raise the bed to a comfortable working position.
8. Help the patient into a safe, comfortable position. Expose the area to be treated.
9. Inspect the K-pad for leaks and make sure the cord and plug are in good condition.
10. Plug the cord into an electrical outlet.
11. Place the pad in the cover. *Do not use any pins!*
12. Place the container on the bedside table. Arrange the tubing at the level of the pad. Do not allow the tubing to hang below the level of the bed.
13. Gently apply the pad in its cover to the proper body area.
14. Check the skin under the pad. Follow the instructions of your immediate supervisor as to how frequently to check the skin and the length of the application.
15. When the treatment is finished, return the equipment to its proper place.
16. Make the patient comfortable.
17. Lower the bed to a position of safety for the patient.
18. Pull the curtains back to the open position.
19. Raise the side rails where ordered, indicated, and appropriate for patient safety.

20. Place the call light within easy reach of the patient.
21. Wash your hands.
22. Report to your immediate supervisor:
    - The time the K-pad was applied
    - The length of treatment
    - The area of application
    - How the patient tolerated the procedure
    - Your observations of anything unusual

Procedure Using the Disposable Sitz Bath (Moist Warm Application)

1. Assemble your equipment:
   a) Disposable sitz bath kit (Figure 40-20):
      - Plastic bowl with a large brim
      - Water bag
      - Tubing and stopcock (clamp)
   b) Plastic laundry bag
   c) Bath thermometer
   d) Bath towels
   e) Pitcher of water at 105°F (40.5°C)

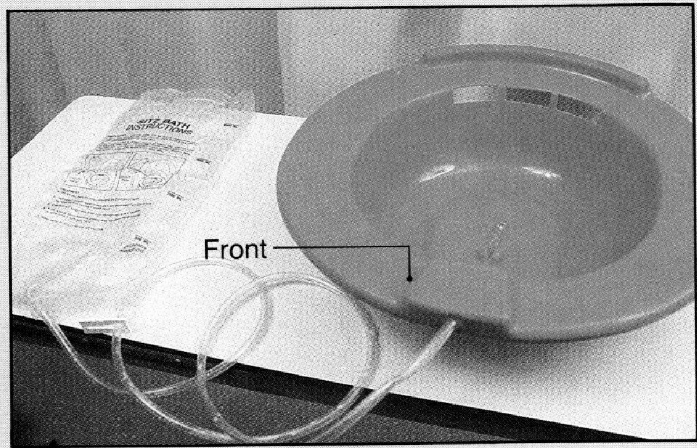

FIGURE 40-20 Disposable sitz bath kit.

2. Wash your hands.
3. Identify the patient by checking the identification bracelet.
4. Ask visitors to step out of the room, if this is your hospital's policy.
5. Tell the patient you are going to give him a sitz bath.
6. Pull the curtain around the bed for privacy.
7. Help the patient to put on his slippers and robe.
8. Help the patient into the bathroom.
9. Raise the toilet seat.
10. Check the temperature of the water with the bath thermometer. It should be 105°F (40.5°C).
11. Put the plastic bowl into the toilet bowl. Be sure that the opening for overflow is toward the front of the toilet.
12. Pour the water into the bowl, filling it half full.
13. Close the stopcock on the tubing. Fill the water bag with water (105°F, 40.5°C) from the pitcher. Close the bag.
14. Hang the container for water 12 inches higher than the bowl.
15. Help the patient remove his robe and pajamas and sit down into the sitz bath. Be sure the patient can reach the signal cord.
16. Place the tubing inside the bowl with the opening of the tube under the water level. The tube fits into a little groove in the front of the basin.
17. Open the stopcock and adjust the flow if necessary.
18. Have the patient sit in the sitz bath with water running in for from 10 to 20 minutes, as instructed by your immediate supervisor.
19. If the patient says he feels weak or faint, stop the treatment. Turn on the signal light if you need help getting the patient out of the bathroom.
20. When the treatment is finished, remove the tubing. Help the patient out of the sitz bath.
21. Pat the patient's body gently with a towel to dry.
22. Help the patient back into bed. Make him comfortable.
23. Lower the bed to a position of safety for the patient.
24. Pull the curtains back to the open position.
25. Raise the side rails where ordered, in-

dicated, and appropriate for patient safety.

26. Place the call light within easy reach of the patient.
27. Clean your equipment and return it to its proper place. If it is not to be used again, discard the disposable equipment.
28. Put the dirty towels in the plastic laundry bag. Bring the bag to the dirty linen hamper in the dirty utility room.
29. Wash your hands.
30. Report to your immediate supervisor:
    - The time the sitz bath was started
    - The length of time the patient was in the sitz bath
    - How the patient tolerated the procedure
    - Your observations of anything unusual

Procedure Using the Portable Chair-type or Built-in Sitz Bath (Moist Warm Application)

1. Assemble your equipment:
    a) Portable chair or built-in sitz bath (Figure 40-21):
    b) Disinfectant cleaner
    c) Bath towels
    d) Bath blanket
    e) Bath thermometer
    f) Plastic laundry bag

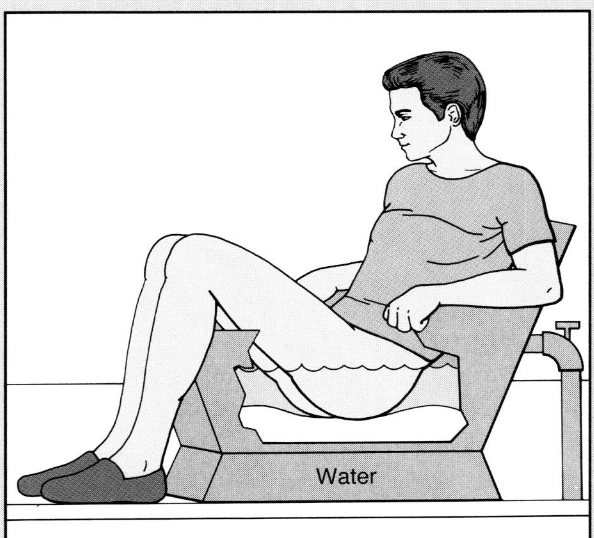

FIGURE 40-21

2. Wash your hands.
3. Identify the patient by checking the identification bracelet.
4. Ask visitors to step out of the room, if this is your hospital's policy.
5. Tell the patient you are going to give him a sitz bath.
6. Pull the curtain around the bed for privacy.
7. Clean the sitz bath with disinfectant cleanser.
8. Rinse it well.
9. Bring the portable, chair-type sitz bath into the patient's room. Or help the patient (using a wheelchair if necessary) into the bathroom with the built-in chair-type sitz bath.
10. Fill it half full with water at 105°F (40.5°C).
11. Place a towel on the seat and on the front edge of the sitz bath.
12. Help the patient undress, except for his gown and slippers.
13. Help the patient to sit down in the tub. Hold his gown up so it does not get wet.
14. Cover the patient's shoulders with a bath blanket if he complains of being cold.
15. Continue the treatment for 10 to 20 minutes, unless you have other instructions from your immediate supervisor.
16. Check the patient every 5 minutes.
17. If the patient feels weak or faint, stop the treatment. Turn on the signal light for help in getting the patient out of the tub. Let the water out of the tub.
18. When the treatment is finished, help the patient out of the tub.
19. Pat his body gently with a towel to dry.
20. Help the patient back into bed. Make him comfortable.

21. Lower the bed to a position of safety for the patient.
22. Pull the curtains back to the open position.
23. Raise the side rails where ordered, indicated, and appropriate for patient safety.
24. Place the call light within easy reach of the patient.
25. Clean the sitz tub with disinfectant cleanser.
26. Put the portable, chair-type tub back in its proper place.
27. Put the dirty towels in the plastic laundry bag. Bring the bag to the dirty linen hamper in the dirty utility room.
28. Wash your hands.
29. Report to your immediate supervisor:
    - The time the sitz bath was started
    - The length of time the patient was in the sitz bath
    - How the patient tolerated the procedure
    - Your observations of anything unusual

KEY QUESTIONS

1. What are the principles of warm and cold applications?
2. Why are warm and cold applications used?
3. What is the difference between a generalized and localized application?
4. What is the difference between a moist and dry application?
5. How can you keep the patient safe and comfortable during these applications?
6. How should a warm compress be applied?
7. How should a cold compress be applied?
8. Explain how to apply a cold soak.
9. Explain how to apply a warm soak.
10. Describe the method for applying the warm-water bottle.
11. Describe the method for applying the ice bag, cap, or collar.
12. How should the commercial unit cold pack be applied?
13. How should the commercial unit heat pack be applied?
14. Explain how to apply the heat lamp.
15. Describe the method for applying the perineal heat lamp.
16. Explain how to apply the Aquamatic K-pad.
17. Describe the methods for using the disposable, portable, or built-in sitz bath.
18. Define: compress, continuous, contract, cyanosis, dilate, dry application, generalized, generalized application, inflammation, intermittent, localized, localized application, moist application, sitz bath, soak.

CHAPTER

41

Admitting and Transferring a Patient

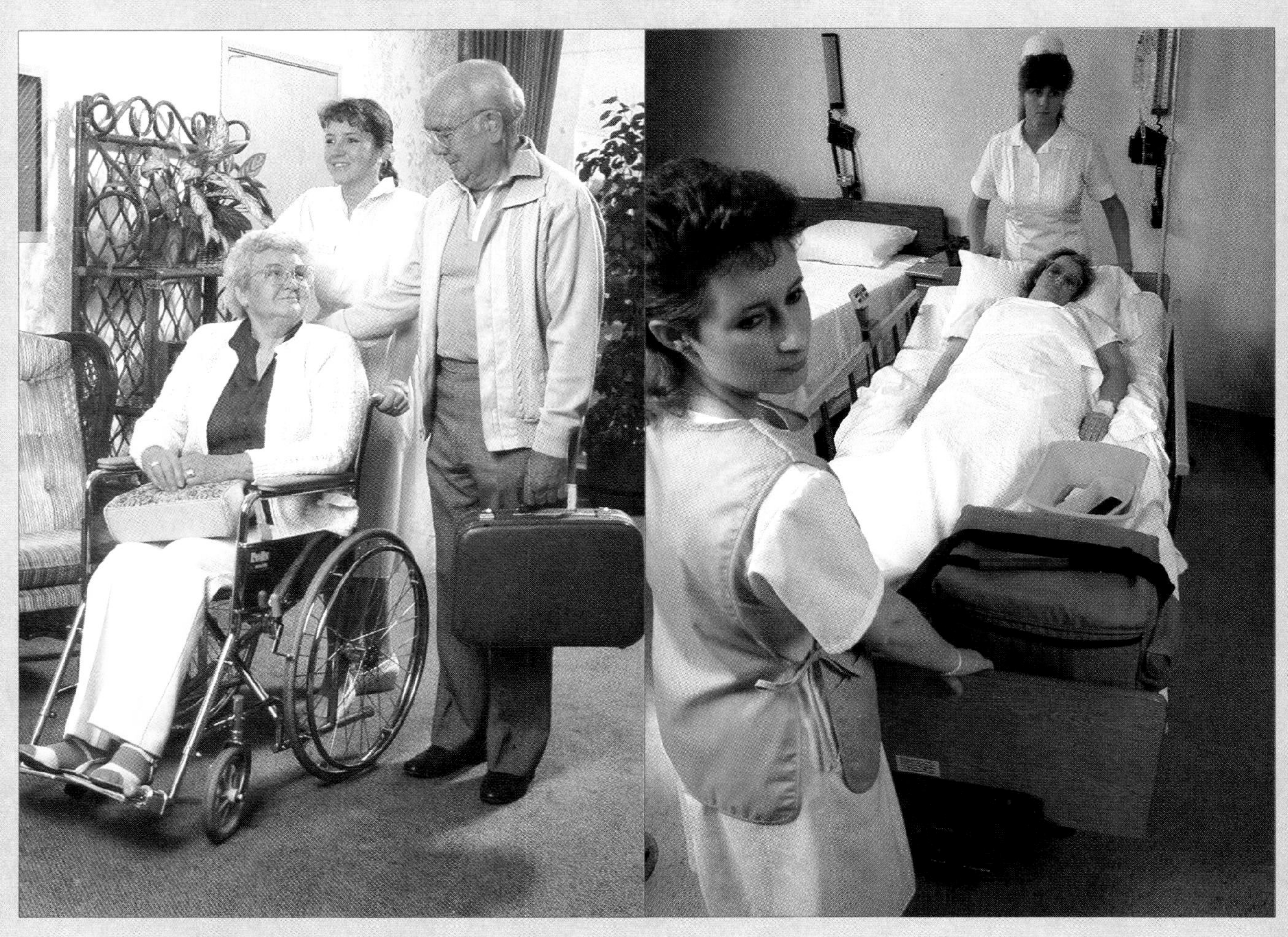

WARNING

For all patient contact, adhere to Universal Precautions. See page 91, 97, or the front cover flap. Wear protective equipment as indicated.

Objectives

What You Will Learn

When you have completed this chapter, you will be able to:

- Use the nursing care plan as a resource in providing quality patient care.
- Admit a patient to the nursing unit by following the correct procedure.
- Welcome the patient and his or her visitors in a pleasant and courteous manner.
- Make the patient feel comfortable and help him or her to adjust to the institutional environment.
- Fill in an admission checklist.
- Weigh and measure the height of a patient who is able to stand.
- Take care of the patient's valuables.
- Transfer a patient to another unit within the institution, following the correct procedure.
- Help the patient to stay calm and feel comfortable.
- Define: admission, assessing, evaluating, implementing, kilogram, nursing care plan, planning, transfer.

KEY IDEAS

Nursing Care Plans

Nursing Care Plan
A written plan stating the nursing diagnosis (the cause and nature of the patient's problems), the patient goals or expected outcomes (objectives), and the nursing orders, interventions, or actions (the procedures or activities that should be performed to obtain the desired results).

THE INDIVIDUALIZED NURSING CARE PLAN IS written by the registered nurse as a plan of action for assisting the patient to optimum wellness (Figure 41-1). Nursing care plans are one way for the nursing team to communicate. They provide a structure for **planning, assessing, implementing**, and **evaluating** individualized care. Each plan is written to meet the individual needs of the patient. One reason for the written care plan is to ensure that continuous and consistent care is provided for each patient.

NURSING CARE PLAN

DATE IDENTIFIED	NURSING DIAGNOSIS	DATE RESOLVED	PATIENT GOAL EXPECTED OUTCOME	NURSING ORDERS INTERVENTIONS/ ACTIONS

FIGURE 41-1 Nursing care plan.

Planning
Deciding what you are going to do and how you are going to do it; arranging in advance.

Assessing
Gathering facts to identify needs and problems.

Implementing
Carrying out or accomplishing a given plan.

Evaluating
Estimating or finding the value or worth of an action or an object.

The admitting registered nurse begins the plan by collecting information for a health history and completing a physical examination. Patient problems and nursing diagnoses are identified, long- and short-term goals are determined, and nursing interventions are planned to help the patient reach these goals. The registered nurse reevaluates the plan of care daily to meet the changing needs of the patient. This reevaluation is continued until discharge and includes patient health education and a discharge plan. All members of the multidisciplinary health care team collaborate on the nursing care plan and assist the patient to reach the goals by carrying out the interventions written into the plan.

The parts of the plan most directly involving the nursing assistant are the activities of daily living, direct bedside care, and making and reporting objective, factual observations. The nursing assistant must read the nursing plan of care for each of her or his assigned patients to ensure that the plan is followed. When the nursing plan of care is well developed and used appropriately, it is the single most important tool in providing quality patient care. (See Chapter 12 for a checklist of the activities of daily living.)

There are several ways that the nursing care plan can help the nursing assistant provide quality care on a daily basis. The plan of care provides:

- Specific instructions regarding care to be given
- Information needed prior to giving care
- Guidelines for continuity of care
- Information essential for organizing and planning work or special duties

You can see why this plan is the nursing assistant's most important resource in providing care. Each health care institution has its own policies and procedures related to the nursing care plans. Be sure you understand and follow your employer's policies.

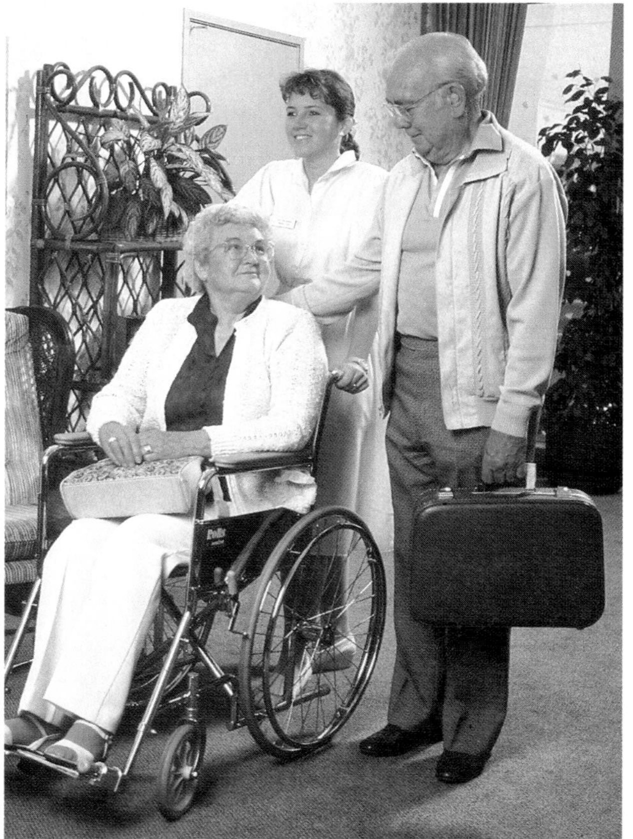

FIGURE 41-2 Help to make the admission of the patient as pleasant as possible.

KEY IDEAS

Admitting the Patient

Admission
The administrative procedures followed when a person enters the health care institution and becomes an inpatient; covers the period from the time the patient enters the door of the hospital until he is settled in his room.

A patient coming into a health care institution may be frightened and uncomfortable. He or she may or may not be seriously ill or in pain. This is a time when you, as a member of the nursing team, are very important to the patient. Being pleasant and courteous will make the patient's **admission** easier. A nice, relaxed environment and welcome will create a favorable first impression.

Introduce yourself (Figure 41-2). Learn the patient's name and use it often. Do not call an adult by his or her first name unless given permission to do so. Remember that the way you speak and behave will have a lot to do with the patient's impression of the institution. Smile, be friendly. Do not appear to be rushed or busy with other things. Do your work quietly and efficiently.

Procedure Admitting the Patient

1. Assemble your equipment on the bedside table:
   a) Admission checklist, if used in your institution
   b) Urine specimen container and laboratory requisition slip
   c) Institution gown or pajamas
   d) Clothing list
   e) Envelope for valuables
   f) Portable scale
   g) Blood pressure cuff and stethoscope
   h) Admission pack (contents vary in each health care institution)
   i) Thermometer
   j) Bedpan and/or urinal, emesis basin, and wash basin (may be in admission pack in some health care institutions)
2. Wash your hands.
3. Fan-fold the bed covers down to the foot of the bed to open the bed.
4. Place the hospital gown or pajamas at the foot of the bed.
5. Put the bedpan, urinal, emesis basin, wash basin, and admission pack in their proper place in the bedside table or stand.
6. When the patient arrives on the floor, introduce yourself to the patient and to his visitors. Smile, be friendly. Call the patient by his name. Shake hands and tell the patient your name and job title.
7. Escort the patient to his room. The patient may be brought to the room by an auxiliary worker. Introduce him to his roommates, if he has any.
8. Ask the visitors to leave the room while you finish admitting the patient, if this is your hospital's policy. At this time, follow the procedure for caring for the patient's valuables.
9. Close the door in a private room. Or draw the curtain around the bed for privacy.
10. Ask the patient to change into the hospital gown or his own pajamas. If necessary, help the patient get undressed and into the gown. Weigh the patient (see Procedure: Weighing and Measuring the Patient).
11. Help the patient to get into the bed. (If your immediate supervisor says the patient may sit in a chair, follow his or her orders.)
12. Raise the side rails on the bed, if necessary.
13. Complete the admission checklist of your institution (Figure 41-3).

FIGURE 41-3 A sample admission checklist.

ADMISSION CHECKLIST
(Fill in every statement and check every appropriate item)

Patient's name ________________ Room number ____
Time of admission ________ a.m./p.m. Date of admission ________
Admitted by stretcher ______ wheelchair ______ walking ______
Check identification bracelet? Yes ☐ No ☐ Bed tag in place? Yes ☐ No ☐
Side rails up? Yes ☐ No ☐
Bruises, marks, rashes, or broken skin noted? Yes ☐ No ☐
If yes, describe ________________
Weight ______ Height ______ Scale used? Yes ☐ No ☐
Temperature ____ Pulse ____ Respirations ____ Blood Pressure ____
Admission urine specimen collected? Yes ☐ No ☐ Sent to lab? Yes ☐ No ☐
Is the patient allergic to food? Yes ☐ No ☐ Allergic to drugs? Yes ☐ No ☐
Reason for admission ________________
Complaints ________________
Dentures? Yes ☐ No ☐ Partial? Yes ☐ No ☐ Full? Yes ☐ No ☐
Denture Cup? Yes ☐ No ☐
Vision problems? Yes ☐ No ☐ Does the patient wear glasses? Yes ☐ No ☐
Valuables: Money? Yes ☐ No ☐ Describe ________________
Jewelry? Yes ☐ No ☐ Describe ________________
Is the patient hard of hearing? Yes ☐ No ☐ Hearing aid? Yes ☐ No ☐
Artificial limb? Yes ☐ No ☐ Brace? Yes ☐ No ☐
Has the patient been admitted to this hospital before? Yes ☐ No ☐
Is the clothing list completed? Yes ☐ No ☐ Signed by ________________
Is the signal cord attached to the bed? Yes ☐ No ☐
Have drugs brought into hospital by the patient been given to the charge nurse? Yes ☐ No ☐
Name of the nurse drugs were given to ________________
Was the patient told not to eat or drink anything until the doctor's visit? Yes ☐ No ☐
Admitted by ________________

14. Have the patient put his toilet articles and small belongings into or on top of the bedside table. If the patient is unable to do this, do it for him.
15. Ask your immediate supervisor if the patient is NPO or is allowed to have drinking water. If he is allowed, fill the water pitcher.
16. To familiarize the patient with his new surroundings, show him where the signal cord or call bell is (Figure 41-4). Attach the signal cord to the bed where the patient can reach it easily. Test the signal cord, explaining how the intercom system works by showing and teaching. Permit the patient to work the signal cord light. Show him how to operate the remote-control TV, if there is one.
17. Explain the health care institution's policy on radios, television, newspapers, and mail. Tell the patient when his meals will be served. Help the patient to fill out the dietary slip for the next meal, if this is part of your institution's procedure.
18. Make the patient comfortable. Fix the lights the way he wants them. Be sure the top sheets and blankets are arranged properly.
19. If the patient is allowed to have the head of his bed elevated and the knee latch adjusted as high or low as is comfortable, adjust these to a position of comfort. If the bed is self-adjustable, explain how the bed works and show the patient how to adjust it. Lower the bed to a position of safety for the patient.
20. Pull the curtains back to the open position.
21. Raise the siderails where ordered, indicated, and appropriate for patient safety.
22. Wash your hands.
23. Report to your immediate supervisor:
    - That you have completed the admission
    - That the patient is in bed or sitting in a chair
    - That you have completed the admission checklist
    - That the side rails are in the up or down position
    - How the patient tolerated the procedure
    - Your observations of anything unusual

FIGURE 41-4

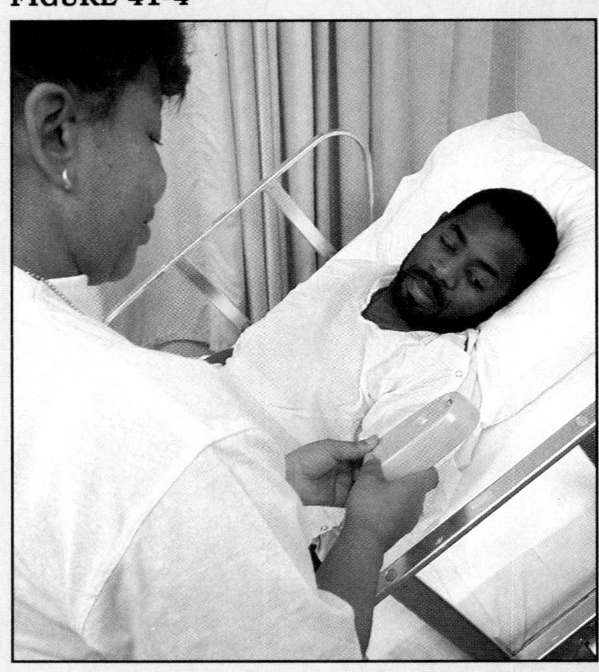

Procedure Weighing and Measuring the Height of a Patient Who Is Able to Stand

1. Assemble your equipment:
    a) Portable balance scale
    b) Paper towel
    c) Note paper
    d) Pen or pencil
2. Wash your hands.
3. Identify the patient by checking the identification bracelet.
4. Ask visitors to step out of the room, if this is your hospital's policy.
5. Tell the patient that you are going to weigh her.
6. Pull the curtain around the bed for privacy.
7. Balance the scale. To do this, make sure the scale is standing level. Both weights

(poises) must point to zero (0). If they do not, turn the balance screw until the pointer of the balance beam stays steadily in the middle of the balance area. The scale is now balanced.

8. Place a paper towel on the stand of the scale to protect the patient's feet.
9. Help the patient to stand with both feet firmly on the scale.
10. Ask the patient to place both hands at her side.
11. Adjust the weights (poises) until the balance pointer is again in the middle of the balance area.
12. Note the patient's weight by adding together the numbers on both the large balance and the small balance. Write it down on the note paper.
13. Raise the measuring rod above the patient's head.
14. Have the patient turn so that her back is against the measuring rod. Be sure she is standing very straight, with her heels touching the measuring bar.
15. Bring the measuring rod down so that it rests horizontally on the patient's head.
16. Note the patient's height. Write it down on the note paper.
17. Raise the measuring rod. Help the patient to step off the scale.
18. Assist the patient back into bed or help her to put on her robe and slippers.
19. Make the patient as comfortable as possible.
20. Lower the bed to a position of safety for the patient.
21. Pull the curtains back to the open position.
22. Raise the side rails where ordered, indicated, and appropriate for patient safety.
23. Place the call light within easy reach of the patient.
24. Wipe the entire scale with disinfectant solution.
25. Put the scale back where it belongs.
26. Wash your hands.
27. Report to your immediate supervisor:
    - That you have weighed and measured the height of the patient
    - Remind her or him if the patient has dressings (bandages) or braces, as this must be considered for the correct weight
    - The patient's weight and height
    - How the patient tolerated the procedure
    - Your observations of anything unusual

KEY IDEAS

Types of Scales

Many health care institutions have special equipment for weighing the patient who is unable to stand, such as the chair scale, bed scale, or wheelchair scale (Figure 41-5). Some institutions have special scales with bars on them to assist the patient in standing straight and to keep the patient from falling. For example, a bed scale is used for the patient on complete bedrest. Follow your institution's procedures for these different types of scales.

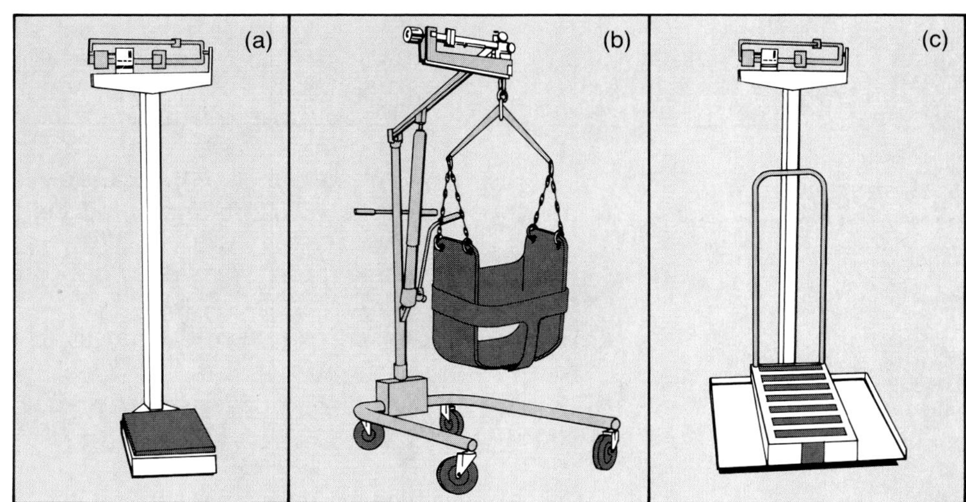

FIGURE 41-5 Types of scales: (1) standing scale; (b) scale with mechanical lift; (c) wheelchair scale.

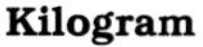

Kilogram
A unit for measuring weight in the metric system. One kilogram equals 1000 grams or 2.2 pounds.

KEY IDEAS

The Patient's Valuables

You may be responsible for taking care of the patient's jewelry, money, or other valuables at the time of admission. In some institutions the admitting office takes care of them; in other institutions a security officer takes care of them. If the family takes the valuables home, be sure to itemize them and have a family member sign that she or he is taking the valuables home. Follow the procedure used in your institution.

Procedure Caring for the Patient's Valuables

1. Assemble your equipment:
   a) Valuables envelope
   b) Pen or pencil
2. Wash your hands.
3. Identify the patient by checking the identification bracelet.
4. Ask visitors to step out of the room, unless they are needed as witnesses, if this is your hospital's policy.
5. Tell the patient that you are going to assist him with his valuables by making an accurate list of them.
6. Pull the curtain around the bed for privacy.
7. Itemize the valuables on the admission checklist or on the appropriate form.
8. When listing the valuables, be careful in describing each item. It is not the job of a nursing assistant to decide how much any article is worth. A good description might be: "gold-colored metal earrings," rather than "gold earrings"; a "silver-colored ring with a clear stone," rather than "diamond white gold ring"; a "fur coat," rather than a "mink coat." Never touch the patient's money. Let the patient count it in your presence. Record the amount on the admission checklist.
9. Ask the patient to place his valuables into the envelope that is clearly marked with his name, room number, doctor's name, and identification number.
10. Close the envelope while you are with the patient. Make sure he sees you do this.
11. Have the patient or relatives (if they are the witnesses) sign the itemized list of valuables.
12. Lower the bed to a position of safety for the patient.
13. Pull the curtains back to the open position.
14. Raise the side rails where ordered, indicated, and appropriate for patient safety.
15. Place the call light within easy reach of the patient.
16. Wash your hands.
17. Report to your immediate supervisor:
    - That you have itemized the patient's valuables and that the list is signed.
    - Give the valuables envelope to your immediate supervisor who will dispose of it in one of the proper ways:
      - The security officer will pick it up and take it to the vault.
      - A relative will take the envelope after he has signed the list that he is taking them home.
      - A bonded admissions clerk will come to the floor, take the valuables envelope to the safe, and give both the head nurse and the patient a receipt for the valuables.
    - How the patient tolerated the procedure
    - Your observations of anything unusual

KEY IDEAS

Transferring the Patient

Transfer
Moving a hospital patient from one unit or facility to another.

During his stay, a patient may be **transferred** from one unit or facility to another (Figure 41-6). This may be done for several reasons:

- He may have asked for a private room, but none was available when he was admitted.
- He may ask to be transferred from a private room to a semiprivate room.
- He may be moved to another unit because of a change in his medical condition.

Physiological
Referring to the study of the ways the body functions and responds.

Psychological
Referring to the study of the ways the mind functions and responds.

Sociocultural
Responses to methods of education, discipline, and training that are determined by the culture of the social group.

Spiritual
Referring to a person's responses to religious or inspirational ideas.

- **Physiological:** as seen in a person's biological response (physical changes) to alterations in the body's structures and functions.
- **Psychological:** as seen in a person's cognitive (level of knowledge) and emotional responses to himself and his environment.
- **Sociocultural:** as seen in a person's noninherited intra- and interpersonal responses to socialization practices learned and transmitted from families and communities.
- **Spiritual:** as seen in a person's personal response to inspirational forces.

Your immediate supervisor will include the following topics in the discharge and patient health education plan.

- *Explanation of the patient's disease/disorder:*
  - History and/or explanation of disease or disorder
  - Signs and symptoms expected and those not expected
  - What to report to the physician; his or her name, phone number, and address
- *Explanation of medications as ordered by the physician:*
  - Name of medication
  - Dose: how much he or she is to take
  - The correct times to take the medication
  - The purpose and expected effects of the medication
  - Signs and symptoms of side effects of the medication
  - What to report to the physician; his or her name, phone number, and address
- *Explanation of treatments ordered by the physician:*
  - Purpose of treatments
  - Time of treatments
  - How to perform treatments
  - Return demonstrations of treatments
  - What to report to the physician; his or her name, phone number, and address
- *Explanation of nutrition and diet:*
  - Type of diet ordered by physician
  - Foods allowed on this diet and foods not allowed
  - Amounts of food to be consumed
  - Available home health agencies for help; name, phone number, and address
- *Explanation of care in the home environment:*
  - Elimination of hazards in the home environment
  - Available transportation to the physician's office or clinic
  - Available housekeeping services
  - Available economic support agencies; name, phone number, and address
- *Explanation of progression of activities of daily living:*
  - Outline activities of daily living for the first two weeks following hospitalization, with progressive activities
  - Signs and symptoms of inability to perform activities
  - What to report to the physician; his or her name, phone number, and address
- *Explanation of future appointments that have been made with the physician or clinic:*
  - Time and date of appointment
  - Name of physician and/or clinic

- Phone number and address of physician or clinic
- The reason why these future appointments are necessary for follow-up care

- *Explanation of referral agencies:*
  - Names of agencies
  - Address of agencies
  - Phone number of agencies
  - Name of contact person at the agency

KEY IDEAS

Discharge Planning

Your immediate supervisor is responsible for the following discharge planning activities. You will be instructed on what you should do as your part of this discharge plan. Be sure to follow your immediate supervisor's instructions.

Your immediate supervisor will:

- Start discharge planning at the time of admission.
- Work with the physician, health care team members, social worker, dietitian, family, and significant others.
- Contact the necessary community agencies for referral, if necessary.
- Include the discharge plan in patient education with family members and/or significant others present when possible.
- Assess the patient's ability for self-care in the home setting.
- Give the patient and/or family members a written plan for all medications (stating time and amount), exercises, and any other pertinent data.
- Make future appointments in the physician's office, clinic, health agency, outpatient department, physical therapy, and social services, as indicated. Give the patient and/or family members a written schedule of appointments (date and time).
- Discuss activities of daily living with the patient and interested family members.
- Give the patient and family members a written outline for any exercises or special activities. Advise proper time for continuance of normal activities and life-style.
- Advise patient and/or family members to call, giving them phone number and extension, if they have any questions after they get home.
- Document the entire discharge plan on the permanent record and the patient's reaction to the plan.
- If permitted by your institution's policies, give the patient a copy of the discharge checklist.

Procedure Discharging the Patient

1. Assemble your equipment, according to the needs of the patient:
   a) Wheelchair
   b) Stretcher
   c) Discharge slip, if used in your institution
   d) Cart
2. Wash your hands.
3. Identify the patient by checking the identification bracelet.
4. Help the patient collect and pack personal possessions (Figure 42-1).
5. Be sure all valuables and medications are returned to the patient.
6. Help the patient get dressed, if necessary.
7. Check that the written instructions are given to the patient by your immediate supervisor, such as:
   a) Doctor's orders to follow at home

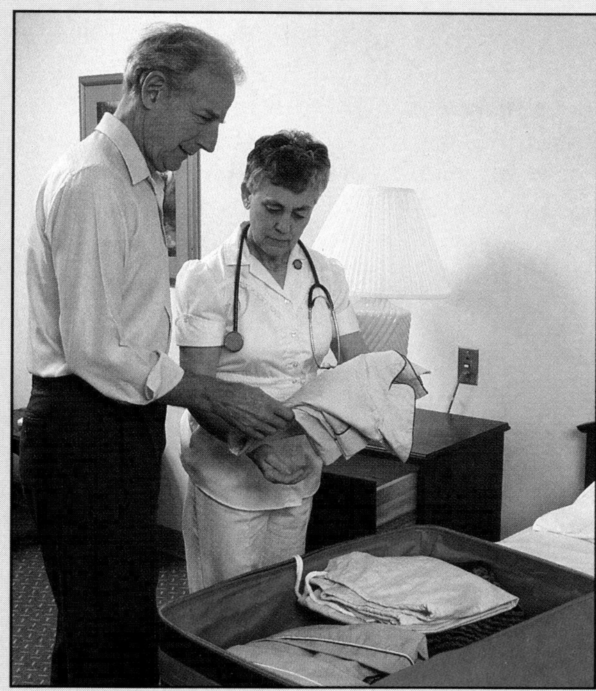

FIGURE 42-1

   b) Prescriptions
   c) Follow-up schedule of appointments with the doctor or clinic

8. Bring the wheelchair to the patient's bedside. Help the patient into it. (Figure 42-2.)

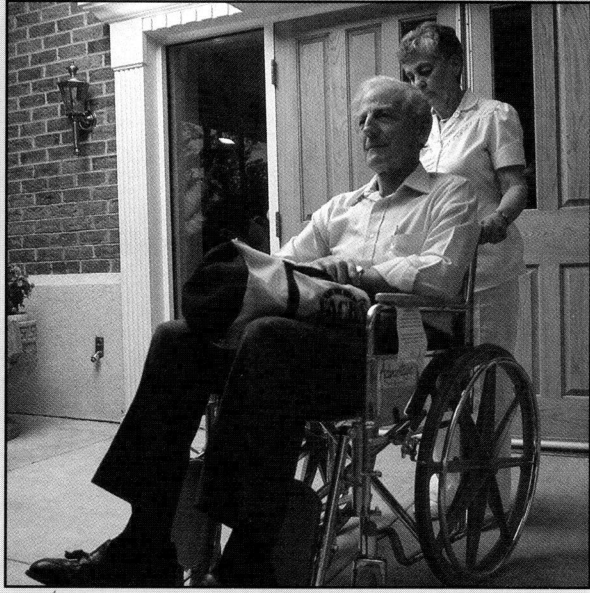

FIGURE 42-2

9. Before wheeling the patient off the floor, get the discharge slip from your immediate supervisor.
10. Take the patient in the wheelchair to the discharge desk, cashier, or business office, if her family has not already done this for her. Give the clerk the discharge slip. Get a release form in return.
11. Wheel the patient to the front door. Help her out of the wheelchair and into her car.
12. Say goodbye to the patient (Figure 42-3).

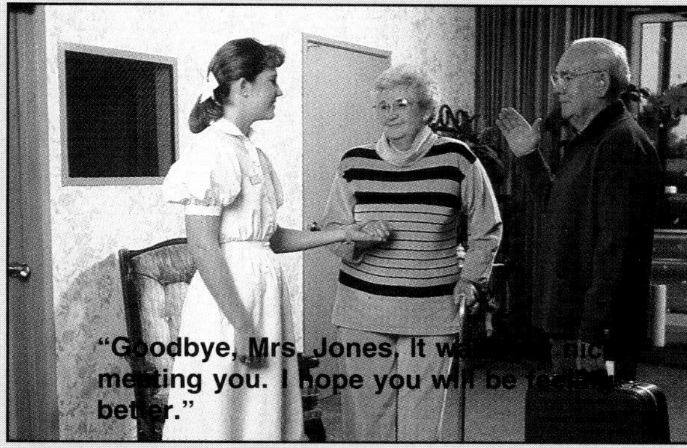
“Goodbye, Mrs. Jones. It w
meeting you. I hope you will be
better.”

FIGURE 42-3

13. Take the wheelchair and release form back to the floor.
14. Wipe the entire wheelchair with an antiseptic solution.
15. Strip the linen from the bed unless this is done by the environmental services department in your institution. Place it in the dirty linen hamper.
16. Notify the environmental service or housekeeping department that the discharge has taken place and the unit is ready to be cleaned.
17. Wash your hands.
18. Report to your immediate supervisor:
    - That the patient has been discharged
    - The time of the discharge
    - The type of transportation used for the discharge
    - Who accompanied the patient: husband, wife, daughter, friend
    - Give her or him the release form from the business office, cashier, or discharge desk
    - That patient was given a copy of the discharge
    - Patient's reaction to the discharge
    - That environmental service has been notified that the unit is ready to be cleaned
    - Your observations of anything unusual

KEY QUESTIONS

1. How can the holistic approach be applied to the discharge/health teaching plan?
2. Which topics should be included in the discharge plan?
3. List the discharge planning activities for which the discharge nurse, head nurse, or team leader is responsible.
4. Outline the discharge procedure.
5. Define: convalescence, discharge, holistic, physiological, psychological, sociocultural, spiritual.

CHAPTER 43

Preoperative Nursing Care

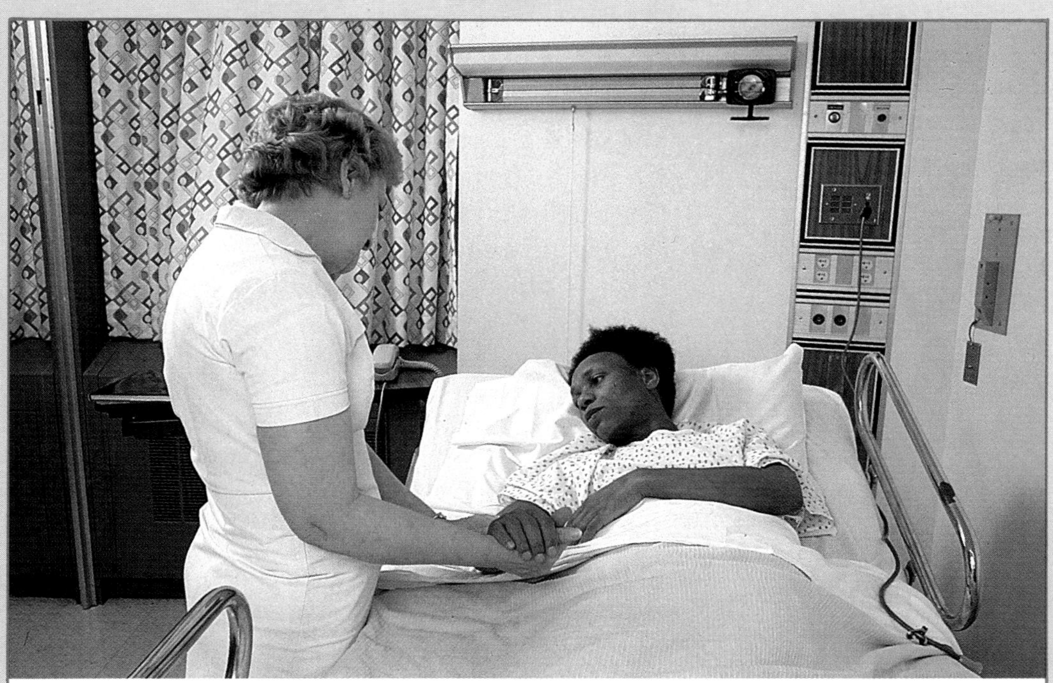

- To assist the nurse in performing certain functions for the physical care of the patients by completing the preoperative check list.
- To ease the patient's mind in anticipation of the surgery.

WARNING

For all patient contact, adhere to Universal Precautions. See page 91, 97, or the front cover flap. Wear protective equipment as indicated.

Objectives

What You Will Learn

When you have completed this chapter, you will be able to:

- Describe the purpose of preoperative education and list the topics included.
- Identify five things that might worry the preoperative patient.
- Complete a preoperative checklist accurately.
- Shave a patient in preparation for surgery.
- Name and describe the areas to be shaved in preparation for surgery.
- Describe the tasks you will perform the morning of surgery.
- Get the patient's unit ready for her or his return from the operating or recovery room.
- Define: abdominal prep, complication, NPO, postoperative, preoperative, scrotal prep, skin prep, vaginal prep.

KEY IDEAS

Preoperative Care

Preoperative
Before surgery.

Postoperative
After surgery.

TWO VERY IMPORTANT WORDS ARE USED often in this chapter. They are **preoperative** and **postoperative**.

- The word *operative* means an operation or surgery.
- *Pre* means before.
- *Post* means after.
- *Preoperative* means before surgery.
- *Postoperative* means after surgery.

Preoperative Patient Education

Preoperative patient education prepares the patient for surgery. Each step of the surgical experience is explained to eliminate fear of the unknown. Each member of the health care team is responsible for assisting with preoperative patient education. Your immediate supervisor will instruct you as to your part in this education. The patient will be instructed about the routine before surgery, the morning of surgery, what to expect upon arrival in the surgical suite, the recovery room, and postoperative care, including:

- Deep breathing and coughing exercises
- Turning from side to side
- Patient participation in self-care
- Leg and foot exercises
- Getting out of bed
- Pain or discomfort; how to ask for medication

- Safety: side rails in the up position
- Explanation of NPO

Psychological Aspects of Preoperative Care

Almost every patient who enters a hospital for surgery will be a little nervous and upset. Part of your job as a nursing assistant is to help the patient feel as calm and relaxed as possible.

Some things that might worry the preoperative patient are:

- Concern for the family
- Being away from work; financial fears
- A possible disability because of the operation
- The possibility of death or serious complications
- Fear of the unknown
- Concerns about scars or the loss of a body part.

Good physical and emotional preoperative care can help to reduce anxiety and fears. Give the patient all your attention. Make him feel that you care about him and how the operation comes out. Listen and show interest in what the patient says. Many frightened people relieve their tension by talking a lot and asking lots of questions. Others do not say anything. You can give support to your patient by being there when he needs assistance, by staying calm if he seems upset, and by being tactful. Alert your immediate supervisor if the patient appears abnormally upset or fearful.

Your immediate supervisor will give you the preoperative checklist (Figure 43-1) and instruct you as to:

- What each patient has been told about his operation
- What you are to tell the patient to prepare him for his surgery and postoperative care, including teaching deep breathing exercises
- How to handle and answer the patient's questions
- What care to give the patient the evening before surgery
- What care to give the patient the morning of surgery
- What portion, if any, of the preoperative checklist you are to complete

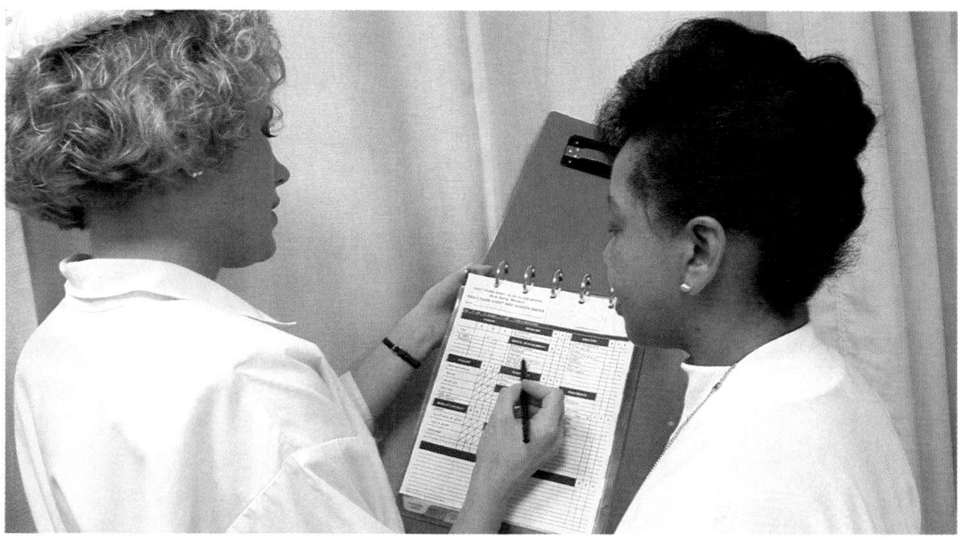

FIGURE 43-1 The immediate supervisor will give the nursing assistant the preoperative checklist.

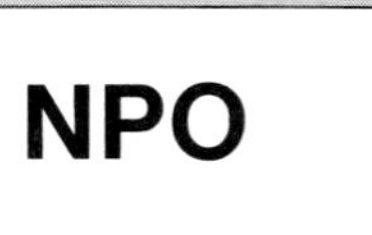

FIGURE 43-2 Nothing by mouth sign, usually placed at the head or foot of the patient's bed, if required.

NPO
Nothing by mouth.

You may be asked to take away the patient's water pitcher and glass at midnight and to post a sign saying **NPO** (Figure 43-2). NPO is taken from the Latin *nils per os*, which means "nothing by mouth." The sign is usually put at the head or foot of the bed; follow your immediate supervisor's instructions.

In most hospitals, you will be given a preoperative checklist along with your instructions (Figure 43-3). The checklist shown is a sample. By filling out this checklist, the nursing staff can be sure the patient has been prepared properly for surgery.

FIGURE 43-3 Sample preoperative checklist to be completed by the nursing assistant.

PREOPERATIVE CHECKLIST

EVENING BEFORE SURGERY

Patient's Name ______________________

Identify the patient by checking his identification bracelet Yes ____ No ____

Skin prep done by ______________________ at ____ p.m.

Skin prep checked by ______________________ at ____ p.m.

Food restrictions, if any, explained to patient . . . . Yes ____ No ____

"NPO AFTER MIDNIGHT" sign put on patient's bed
AND EXPLAINED TO THE PATIENT . . . . Yes ____ No ____

Enema administered by ______________________ at ____ p.m.

MORNING OF SURGERY

Bath . . . . Yes ____ No ____

Oral hygiene . . . . Yes ____ No ____

False teeth (dentures) & removable bridges removed . . . . Yes ____ No ____

Jewelry and pierced earrings removed . . . . Yes ____ No ____

Hairpiece, wig, hairpins removed . . . . Yes ____ No ____

Lipstick, makeup, and false eyelashes removed . . . . Yes ____ No ____

Nail polish removed . . . . Yes ____ No ____

Eyeglasses and contact lenses removed . . . . Yes ____ No ____

Prosthesis (artificial hearing aid, eye, leg, arm, and so forth)
removed . . . . Yes ____ No ____

All clothing removed except clean hospital gown . . . . Yes ____ No ____

Patient allergic or sensitive to drugs . . . . Yes ____ No ____

Pre-op urine specimen obtained and sent to lab . . . . Yes ____ No ____

Urinary drainage bag emptied . . . . Yes ____ No ____

Side rails in up position . . . . Yes ____ No ____

Temperature ________ Pulse ________ Respiration ________

Blood Pressure ____ Weight ____ lbs. Height ____ ft. ____ in.

Time patient leaves for the operating room ______________________

Observations ______________________

Signature and title ______________________

Preventing Chest Complications

Complication
An unexpected condition, such as the development of another illness in a patient who is already sick.

Preoperative patient education includes deep breathing exercises. To prevent chest **complications** following surgery, watch for these symptoms in preoperative patients:

- Signs of respiratory infection
- Sneezing, sniffling, or coughing
- Complaints or signs of chest pains
- Elevated temperature

Report any of these immediately to your immediate supervisor.

KEY IDEAS

Skin Preparation

Skin prep
Shaving the area of the body where an operation is going to be performed in preparation for surgery.

Before an operation, the patient's skin in the operative area must be free of hair and as clean as possible. Hair on the body is a breeding place for microorganisms. Because hair cannot be sterilized, it must be removed by shaving. The **skin prep** covers the area on the body where the operation is going to be done. When you are shaving a patient before an operation, watch for scratches, pimples, cuts, sores, or rashes on the skin. If you see anything on the skin that looks unusual, be sure to report this to your immediate supervisor. For some procedures, shaving is no longer performed. The nicks caused by shaving may actually harbor more microorganisms than the skin and hair.

In some hospitals, the patient is sent to the operating room suite one hour before he is scheduled for surgery. At that time, the nurses in the operating room will prep the patient (shave the skin in preparation for surgery). This is done in those hospitals that have holding areas in the operating room suite. In the holding area, each patient has his own cubicle (sometimes an anteroom) where preparation for surgery, including administration of medications, starting of intravenous infusions, and skin preps, are done.

In other hospitals, the staff does the prep the evening before surgery. The operating room staff does another complete prep after the patient is on the operating room table.

The prep is done with a special prep kit, which is obtained from the central supply room for each patient. After it is used, it is discarded in the dirty utility room. Each kit contains a safety razor and a sponge filled with soap. Most hospitals have a special place (usually a covered metal container) to dispose of razors in the dirty utility room. If your hospital does not supply a disposable prep kit, get the individual items from central supply.

Procedure Shaving a Patient in Preparation for Surgery

1. Assemble your equipment:
   a) Disposable prep kit (Figure 43-4) containing:
      - Razor and razor blades
      - Sponge filled with soap
      - Tissues

   b) Basin of water at 115°F (46.1°C)
   c) Bath blanket
   d) Towels
   Note: Some health care institutions do a "dry prep"; they shave the skin without soap. Follow the policies of your institution.

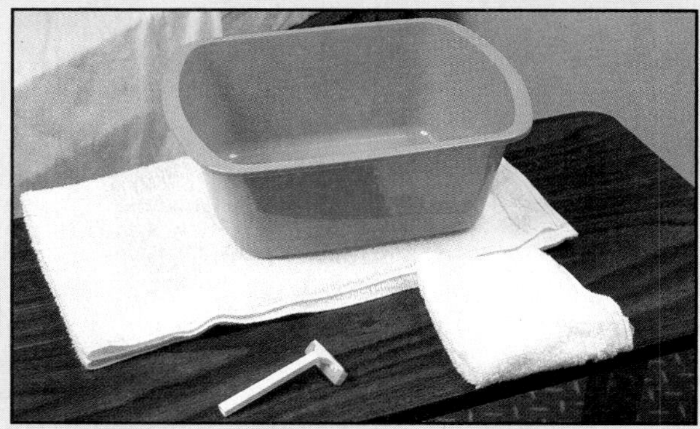

FIGURE 43-4 Disposable prep kit.

2. Wash your hands.
3. Identify the patient by checking his identification bracelet.
4. Ask visitors to step out of the room, if this is your hospital's policy.
5. Tell the patient that you are going to shave him.
6. Pull the curtains around the bed for privacy.
7. Raise the bed to a comfortable working position.
8. Place the bath blanket over the bedspread and top sheet. Ask the patient to hold the blanket in place. Fan-fold the top sheets to the foot of the bed. Do this from underneath the blanket without exposing the patient.
9. Adjust the bedside lamp so that the area is well lighted. There should be no shadows where you will be working.
10. Open the disposable prep kit.
11. Wet the soap sponge in the basin of water. Then soap the area to be shaved. Work up a good lather with the sponge.
12. Check to be sure the razor blade is in the correct position in the razor.
13. Hold the skin taut with a dry tissue. Shave in the direction the hair grows. Rinse the razor often. Keep the razor and the patient's skin wet and soapy throughout the procedure.
14. Clean the patient's umbilicus (navel) if it is in the area to be shaved.
15. Wash the soap off the patient's skin. Dry thoroughly with the towel.
16. Clean your equipment and put it in its proper place. Discard disposable equipment.
17. Cover the patient with the top sheet and bedspread. Ask him to hold them while you take the bath blanket from underneath without exposing the patient.
18. Make the patient comfortable.
19. Lower the bed to a position of safety for the patient.
20. Pull the curtains back to the open position.
21. Raise the side rails where ordered, indicated, and appropriate for patient safety.
22. Place the call light within easy reach of the patient.
23. Wash your hands.
24. Report to your immediate supervisor:
    - The time at which you shaved the patient
    - How the patient tolerated the procedure
    - Your observations of anything unusual

KEY IDEAS

Areas to Be Shaved in Preparation for Surgery

The areas to be shaved in preparation for various types of surgery are shown in Figures 43-5 through 43-11. The area not being operated on is called the *unaffected side.* The area where the operation will be done is called the *affected side.*

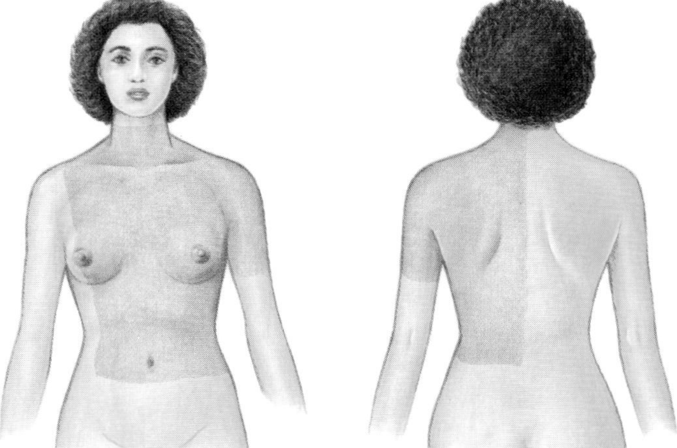

FIGURE 43-5 Prep for breast surgery. Shave from the nipple line of the unaffected side to the middle of the patient's back on the affected side. On the affected side, shave from the chin down to the umbilicus (navel), the axilla (armpit), and part of the upper arm.

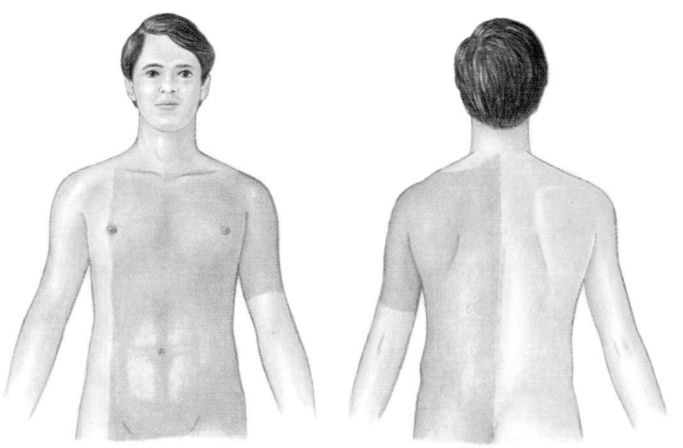

FIGURE 43-6 Chest prep for thoracic surgery. Shave the area extending from the nipple of the unaffected side, across the chest area of the affected side, and across the back, from the top of the shoulders down to the pubic hair.

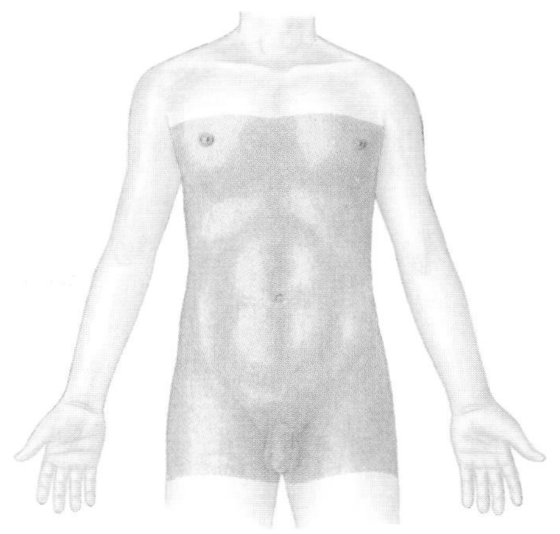

FIGURE 43-7 Abdominal prep. Shave from the nipple line on male patients and from below the breasts on female patients down to and including the pubic area. Shave the width of this area to each side of the body.

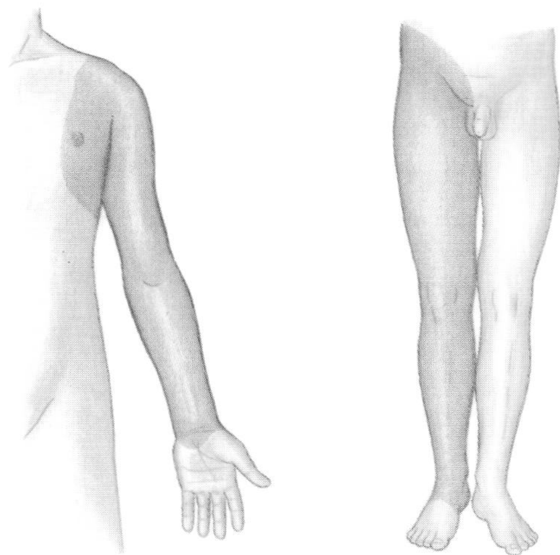

FIGURE 43-8 Prep for surgery of an extremity (arm or leg). If a joint such as an elbow or knee is going to be operated on, you will shave up to the next joint above and down to the next joint below. For example, if the patient's elbow is going to be operated on, you will shave the entire arm from the shoulder down to the wrist. If an area between joints is going to be operated on, you will shave the entire area, including the joints above and below. Shave all around an arm or a leg.

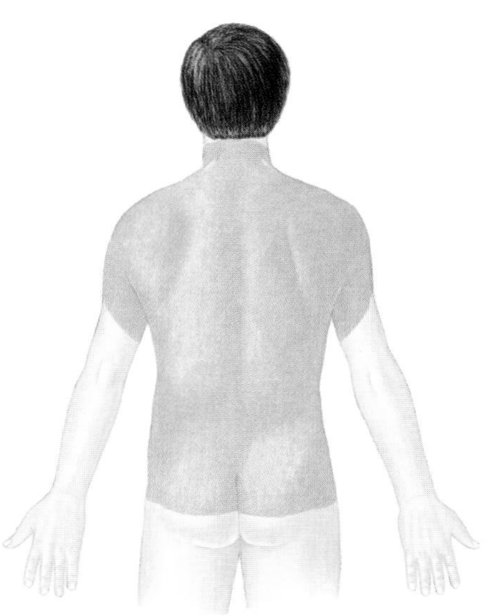

FIGURE 43-9 Back prep. Shave the patient's entire back from the hairline on the neck down to the middle of the buttocks, including the axillary area.

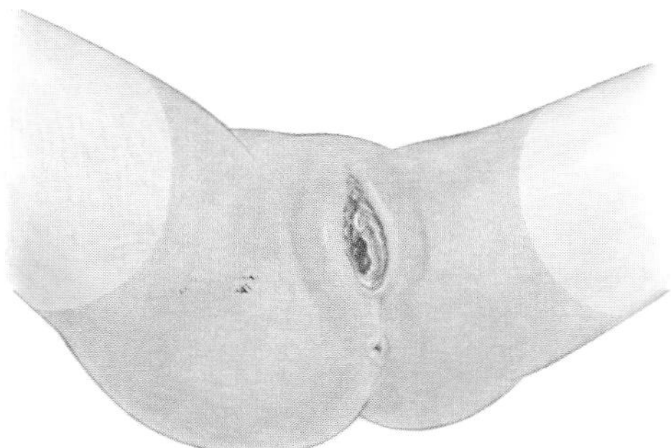

FIGURE 43-10 Vaginal prep, or the preparation of the genital area of female patients.

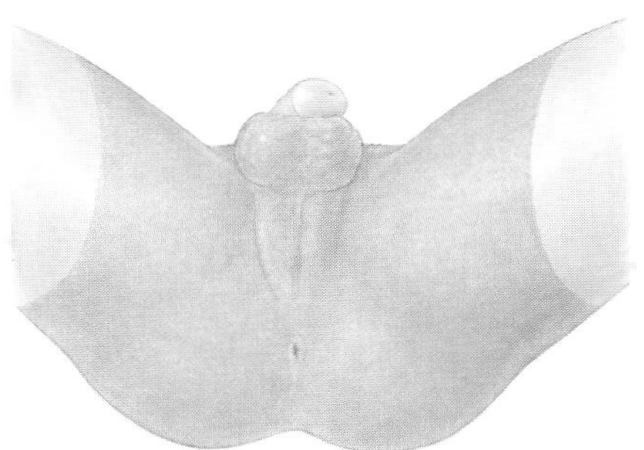

FIGURE 43-11 Scrotal prep, or the preparation of the genital area of male patients.

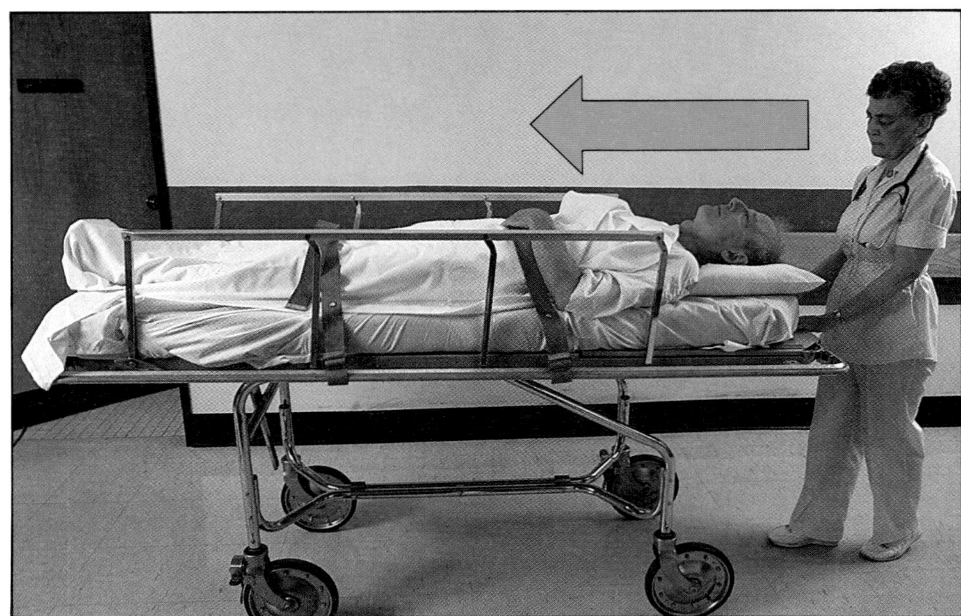

FIGURE 43-12 When transporting the patient to the operating room, cover the patient with a blanket or sheet, be sure the straps are secure, stand at the patient's head, and push the stretcher slowly.

KEY IDEAS

The Morning of Surgery

Abdominal Prep
The procedure for making the patient's abdomen ready for surgery; includes thorough cleansing of the skin and careful shaving of body hair in the abdominal area.

After the patient has been given his preoperative medications by the medication nurse:

- Keep the side rails in the up position.
- Remind the patient that he or she is not to smoke, eat, or get out of bed.

The transportation attendant or the operating room assistant will come to the floor at the proper time to take the patient to the operating room suite. Move the furniture out of the way. Make the room ready for the stretcher to be brought into the room. Assist with moving the patient from the bed to the stretcher. Tell the patient you or another nurse will see her in her room after the surgery.

The transportation assistant will then wheel the patient on the stretcher to the nurse's station (Figure 43-12). At this time, the nurse

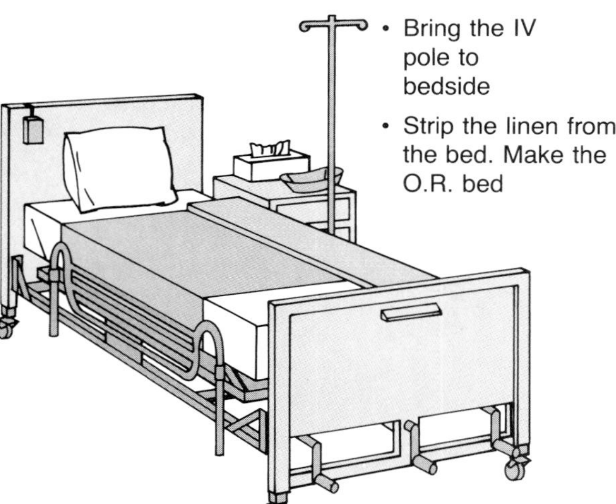

• Bring the IV pole to bedside
• Strip the linen from the bed. Make the O.R. bed

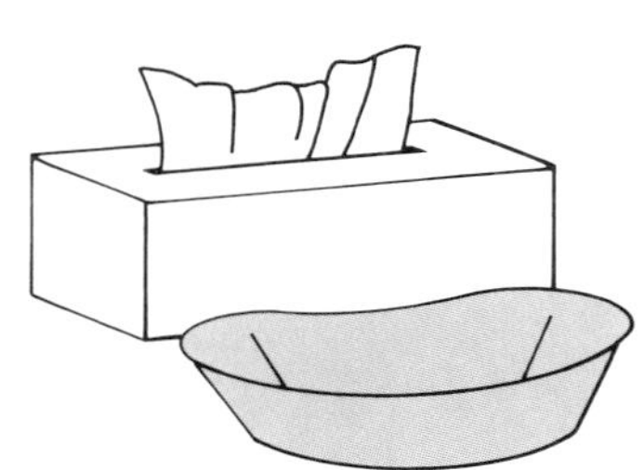

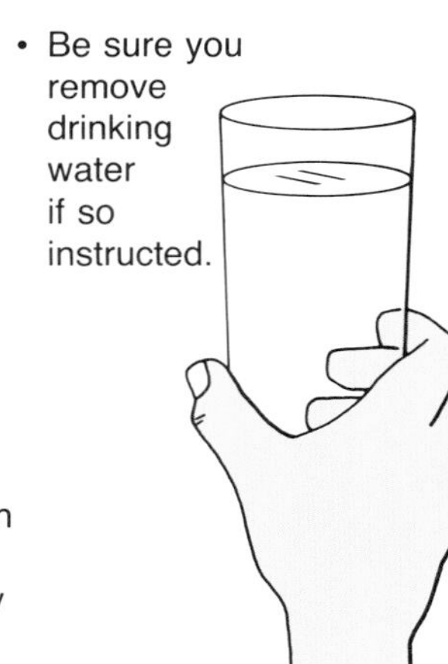

• Be sure you remove drinking water if so instructed.

FIGURE 43-13 Responsibility list for preparing for the return of the postoperative patient.

Vaginal Prep
The procedures for making the genital area of a female patient ready for surgery. The preparation includes thoroughly cleansing the skin and carefully shaving the pubic hair. It may also include a cleansing douche.

Scrotal Prep
The procedures for making the genital area of a male patient ready for surgery. The preparation includes thoroughly cleansing the skin and carefully shaving the hair in the area.

or unit clerk will give the attendant the patient's chart and will check the name on the identification bracelet against the name on the chart. The attendant then takes the patient and chart to the operating room.

Preparing the Patient's Unit to Receive the Patient after Surgery

Your next task is to strip the linen from the bed, make the operating room bed, and prepare the unit to receive the patient postoperatively (Figure 43-13).

KEY QUESTIONS

1. What is the purpose of preoperative education? What topics should be included in preoperative education?
2. What are five things that might worry the preoperative patient?
3. What will your immediate supervisor ask you to fill out on a preoperative checklist?
4. Why must the skin be shaved to remove hair before surgery?
5. Name and describe the areas to be shaved in preparation for surgery.
6. What are your responsibilities when preparing the patient's unit to receive the patient after surgery?
7. Define: abdominal prep, complication, NPO, postoperative, preoperative, scrotal prep, skin prep, vaginal prep.

CHAPTER

44

Postoperative Nursing Care

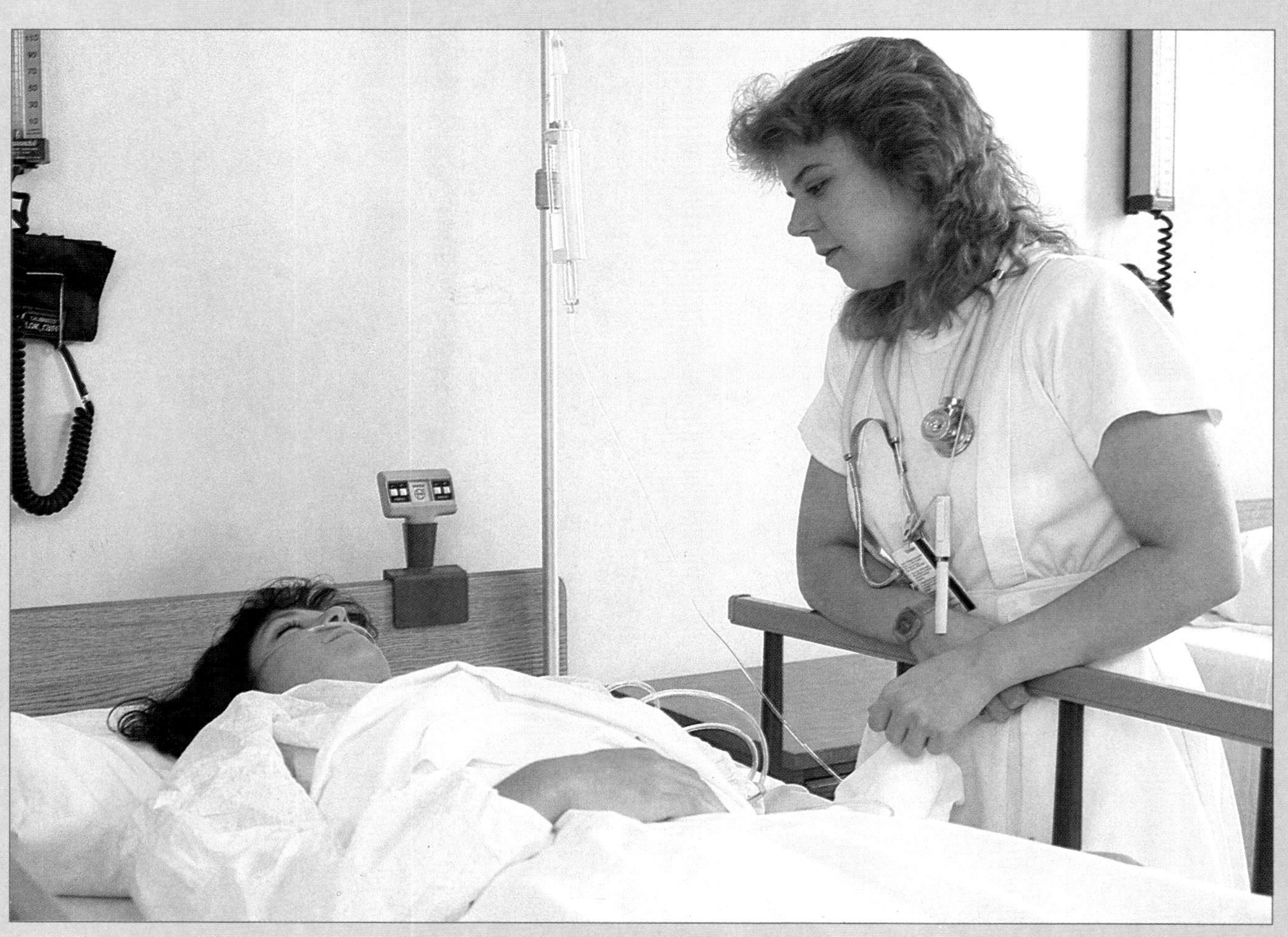

WARNING

For all patient contact, adhere to Universal Precautions. See page 91, 97, or the front cover flap. Wear protective equipment as indicated.

Objectives

What You Will Learn

When you have completed this chapter, you will be able to:

- Explain five reasons chest complications may occur following anesthesia.
- Assist with postoperative care when the patient returns to his room.
- Observe the patient for signs of postoperative problems.
- Care for the patient who is vomiting.
- Carry out your responsibilities concerning the patient's first voiding after surgery.
- Turn the postoperative patient.
- Assist the patient with deep breathing exercises.
- Define: anesthesia, anesthesiologist, anesthetic, anesthetist, aspirate, general anesthetics, local anesthetics, spinal anesthetics, unconscious, void.

KEY IDEAS

Postoperative Nursing Care

Anesthesia
Loss of feeling or sensation in a part or all of the body; local anesthesia is the loss of sensation in a part of the body; general anesthesia is complete loss of sensation in the entire body.

Anesthetic
A drug used to produce loss of feeling; can be given orally, rectally, by injection, or by inhalation. A person who has been given an anesthetic is anesthetized.

General Anesthetics
Anesthetics that cause a loss of sensation in the whole body.

Local Anesthetics
Anesthetics that cause numbness or a loss of sensation in only a part of the body.

Spinal Anesthetics
Anesthetics that cause a loss of feeling in a large area of the body, usually from the umbilicus down to and including the legs and feet.

POSTOPERATIVE CARE MEANS TAKING CARE OF a patient right after surgery. Most patients are taken to a surgical recovery room immediately following surgery. They remain in the recovery room until they begin to recover from the effects of anesthesia and vital signs have stabilized. When the patient returns to his or her room, you will begin assisting with postoperative nursing care.

Anesthesia

Before surgery, the patient is given special medications that cause a loss of feeling in all or part of the body, which means the patient feels no pain. When the patient is under the influence of these special medications, called **anesthetics**, he is in a state of **anesthesia**. Some anesthetics cause the loss of sensation in the whole body. These are called **general anesthetics**. Some anesthetics cause a numbness or loss of feeling in only a part of the body. These medications are called **local anesthetics**. A **spinal anesthetic** causes loss of feeling in a large area of the body, usually from the umbilicus down to and including the legs and feet.

The doctor who administers the anesthetic to the patient in the operating room is a medical doctor who is known as an **anesthesiologist**. The registered nurse who assists in administering the anesthetic to the patient in the operating room is known as an **anesthetist**.

Chest complications following anesthesia may happen for several reasons:

- The anesthetic may irritate the patient's respiratory passages (mouth, nose, trachea, lungs) and cause the secretions in these passages to

Anesthesiologist
The medical doctor who administers the anesthetic to the patient in the operating room.

Anesthetist
The registered nurse who assists the anesthesiologist.

Unconscious
Unaware of the environment; occurs during sleep and in temporary episodes, ranging from fainting or stupor to coma.

Aspirate
To remove material from a body cavity using a tube; also, to draw material such as saliva, mucus, or food particles into the lungs from the mouth.

increase. This might raise the chance of an infection in the lungs or other parts of the respiratory system.

- Smoking tends to irritate the whole respiratory system. Smoking may increase the secretion of mucus, which can also raise the chance of an infection.
- After surgery, many patients are so sore they cannot breathe deeply. They cannot cough up the increased amount of mucous material being secreted in the lungs. This can cause a respiratory infection, such as pneumonia.
- A patient might vomit while he is still **unconscious** after surgery. The vomitus (emesis, vomited material) might be **aspirated**, that is, drawn back into the lungs. This could very quickly cause an infection or even the patient's death. Saliva might also be drawn into the throat and block the air passages, which could cause an infection.
- Unconsciousness and inactivity during anesthesia allow mucus to accumulate in the patient's respiratory passages. If ordered by the physician, the head nurse or team leader will call the inhalation therapy department (pulmonary medicine). Staff persons from that department will treat the patient with chest complications.

When the Patient Comes Back from Surgery

The patient will be coming back to his or her unit on a stretcher. Move the furniture out of the way and make sure the bedside area is clear. The stretcher then can be brought easily and quickly to its place next to the bed.

When the patient is brought back to the unit, you will do the following things:

- Help move the patient safely from the stretcher to the bed.
- Be sure the patient is covered with blankets to keep warm.
- Be sure the bedside rails are raised after the patient is in bed.
- Measure the patient's vital signs (TPR and BP) as instructed by your immediate supervisor.
- Place the signal cord within the patient's reach (Figure 44-1).

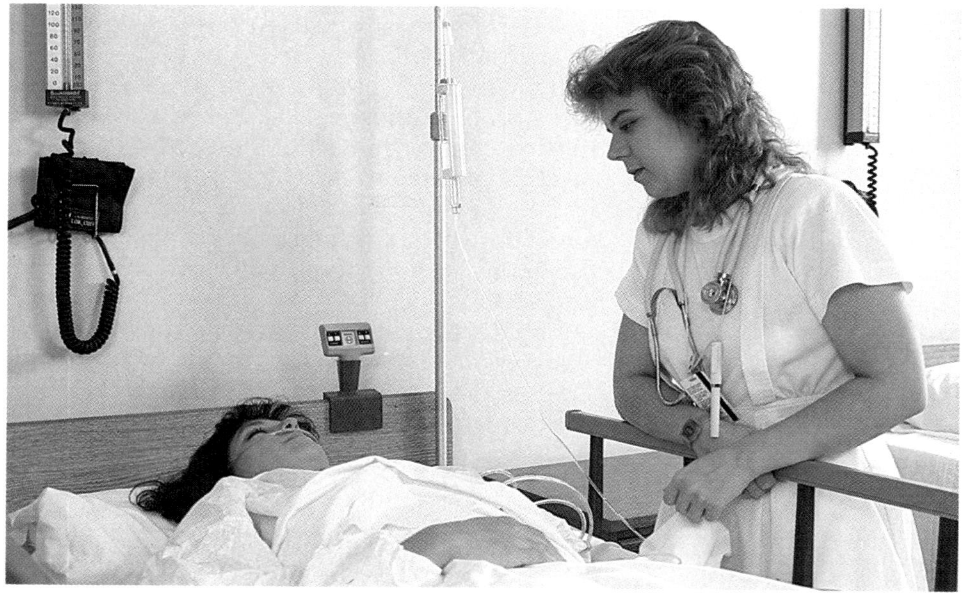

FIGURE 44-1 When the patient awakens from the anesthesia, call the patient by his preferred name. This reassures the patient that someone who knows him is present. Be sure the signal is within easy reach.

Signal your immediate supervisor immediately if you observe any of the following signs or symptoms:

- Rise or fall of blood pressure
- Choking
- Pulse: fast (above 100), slow (below 60), or an irregular pulse beat
- Respirations: rapid (above 30), labored, very slow or shallow
- Skin, lips, fingernails are very pale or turning blue (cyanosis)
- Thirst: patient asks for water often
- Unusual or extreme restlessness
- Moaning or complaining of pain
- Sudden, bright red bleeding
- Any other noticeable sudden changes

Figures 44-2 through 44-5 provide additional information on the techniques for postoperative care.

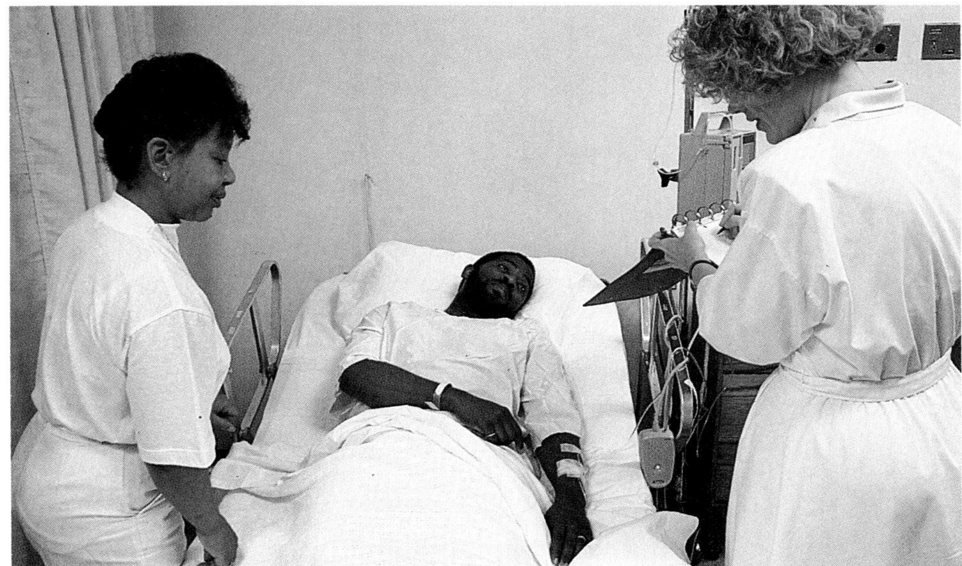

FIGURE 44-2 The postoperative patient may appear to be unconscious, but not really be. He may be able to hear you. Say only those things you would want the patient to hear if he were fully conscious. Speak normally. Always tell the patient who you are and what you are doing.

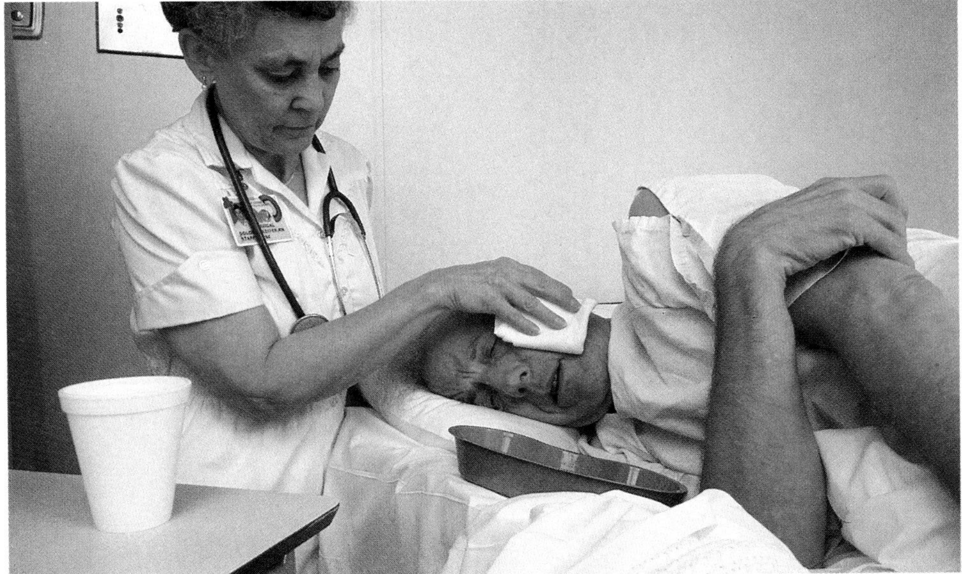

FIGURE 44-3 If the patient vomits, turn his head to one side to prevent vomitus from being drawn back into the lungs (aspiration). Wipe off the patient's mouth and chin. If the patient is conscious, rinse out his mouth with cold water. *Caution:* The patient is not to swallow the water.

Void
To urinate, pass water.

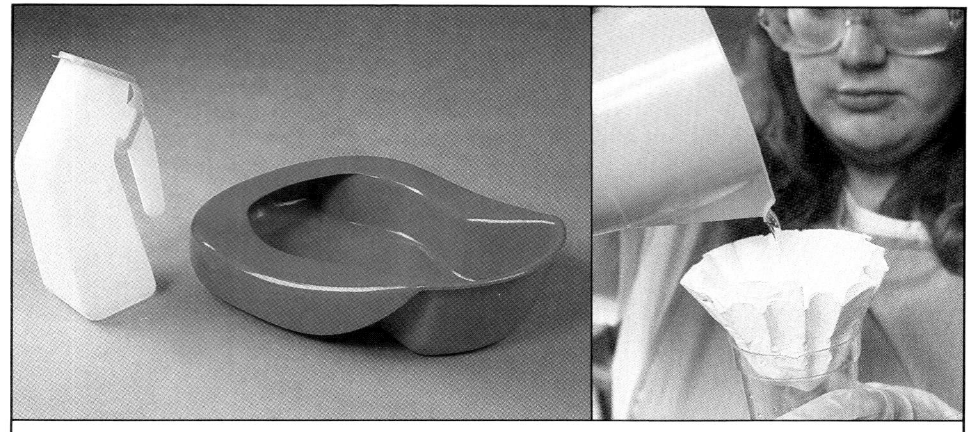

- Collect for a routine urine specimen
- Measure for amount
- Check for odor and color
- Record in proper place on output side of I and O sheet
- Report if the patient has not voided on your shift
- Report if the patient voids only a few drops of urine
- If an indwelling urinary catheter is present:
  Be sure it is unclamped and draining
  Observe amount and color in the drainage bag

FIGURE 44-4 The first voiding after surgery.

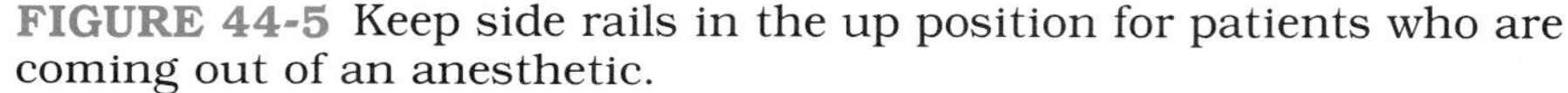

FIGURE 44-5 Keep side rails in the up position for patients who are coming out of an anesthetic.

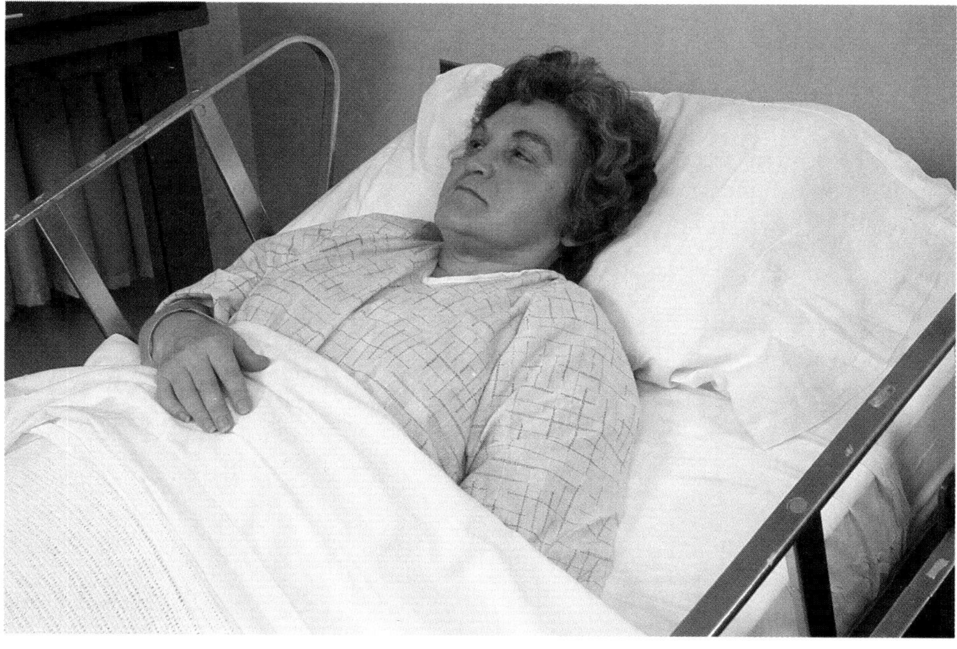

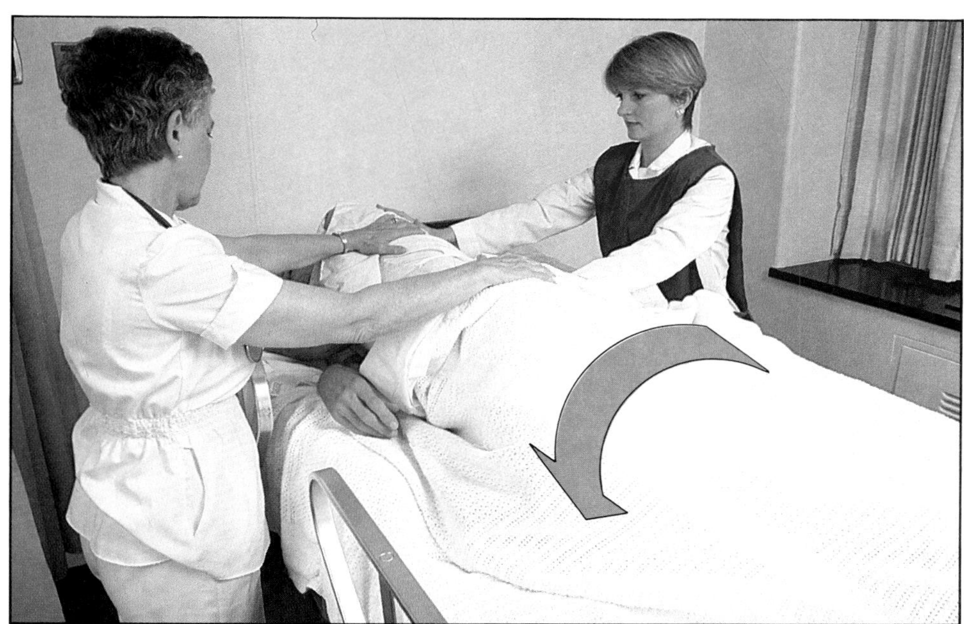

FIGURE 44-6 Turning the postoperative patient.

Turning the Postoperative Patient

Unless you are instructed not to, you should move a postoperative patient into a new position every 2 hours (q2h). This protects his skin, promotes healing, and helps prevent pneumonia. Each time the patient is moved, he should be turned onto his opposite side so that he faces the other side of the bed (Figure 44-6). Move the patient's legs at the same time.

If the patient's gown becomes wet, change it immediately. Change the bed linens whenever they become damp and soiled. Take the blankets off the bed if the patient complains of being too warm. Keep the side rails up at all times.

Check dressings when you turn patients. Report to your immediate supervisor if there is new drainage (clear or red), or if the dressing is soaked.

KEY IDEAS

Deep-Breathing Exercises

Deep-breathing exercises expand the lungs by increasing lung movement and assist in bringing up lung secretions. These exercises will help prevent postoperative pneumonia, or pneumonitis.

Procedure Assisting the Patient with Deep-breathing Exercises

1. Assemble your equipment:
   a) Pillow
   b) Specimen container, if a specimen is ordered
   c) Tissues
2. Report to the medication nurse that you are ready to start deep-breathing exercises.
3. Wash your hands.
4. Identify the patient by checking her identification bracelet.
5. Ask visitors to step out of the room, if this is your hospital's policy.
6. Tell the patient that you are going to help her with deep-breathing exercises.

7. Pull the curtain around the bed for privacy.
8. Raise the bed to a comfortable working position.
9. Offer the patient a bedpan or urinal.
10. Dangle the patient's legs over the side of the bed, if allowed. If not, place the patient in as much of a sitting position as possible.
11. If the patient had abdominal surgery, place the pillow on the patient's abdomen for support. Ask the patient to hold the pillow across the abdomen to splint the incision.
12. Ask her to breathe deeply 10 times.
13. Count the respirations out loud to the patient as she inhales and exhales. If the patient cannot breathe deeply, ask her to cough. Coughing is just another way of breathing deeply.
14. Ask the patient to feel her chest as she breathes to encourage deeper breathing.
15. Tell the patient to cough up all loose secretions into the tissues, if a specimen is not necessary, or into a specimen container, if you have been instructed to collect a specimen.
16. Assist the patient to a position of comfort and safety in bed.
17. If a specimen has been collected, label it and send it to the laboratory with a requisition slip.
18. Discard disposable equipment.
19. Replace the pillow under the patient's head.
20. Make the patient comfortable.
21. Lower the bed to a position of safety for the patient.
22. Pull the curtains back to the open position.
23. Raise the side rails where ordered, indicated, and appropriate for patient safety.
24. Place the call light within easy reach of the patient.
25. Wash your hands.
26. Report to your immediate supervisor:
    - That you have helped the patient with deep-breathing exercises
    - The number of breathing exercises
    - The color, amount, and consistency of the secretions the patient was able to cough up
    - That a specimen was collected and sent to the laboratory
    - How the patient tolerated the procedure
    - Your observations of anything unusual

KEY QUESTIONS

1. What are five reasons chest complications might occur following anesthesia?
2. How should you assist with postoperative care when the patient returns to his room?
3. List the signs of postoperative problems that should be reported immediately by signaling for your immediate supervisor.
4. What should you do if a postoperative patient vomits?
5. What should you do the first time a patient voids following surgery?
6. Why should you turn the postoperative patient?
7. Why should the patient do deep-breathing exercises?
8. Define: anesthesia, anesthesiologist, anesthetic, anesthetist, aspirate, general anesthetics, local anesthetics, spinal anesthetics, unconscious, void.

CHAPTER

45 Special Procedures

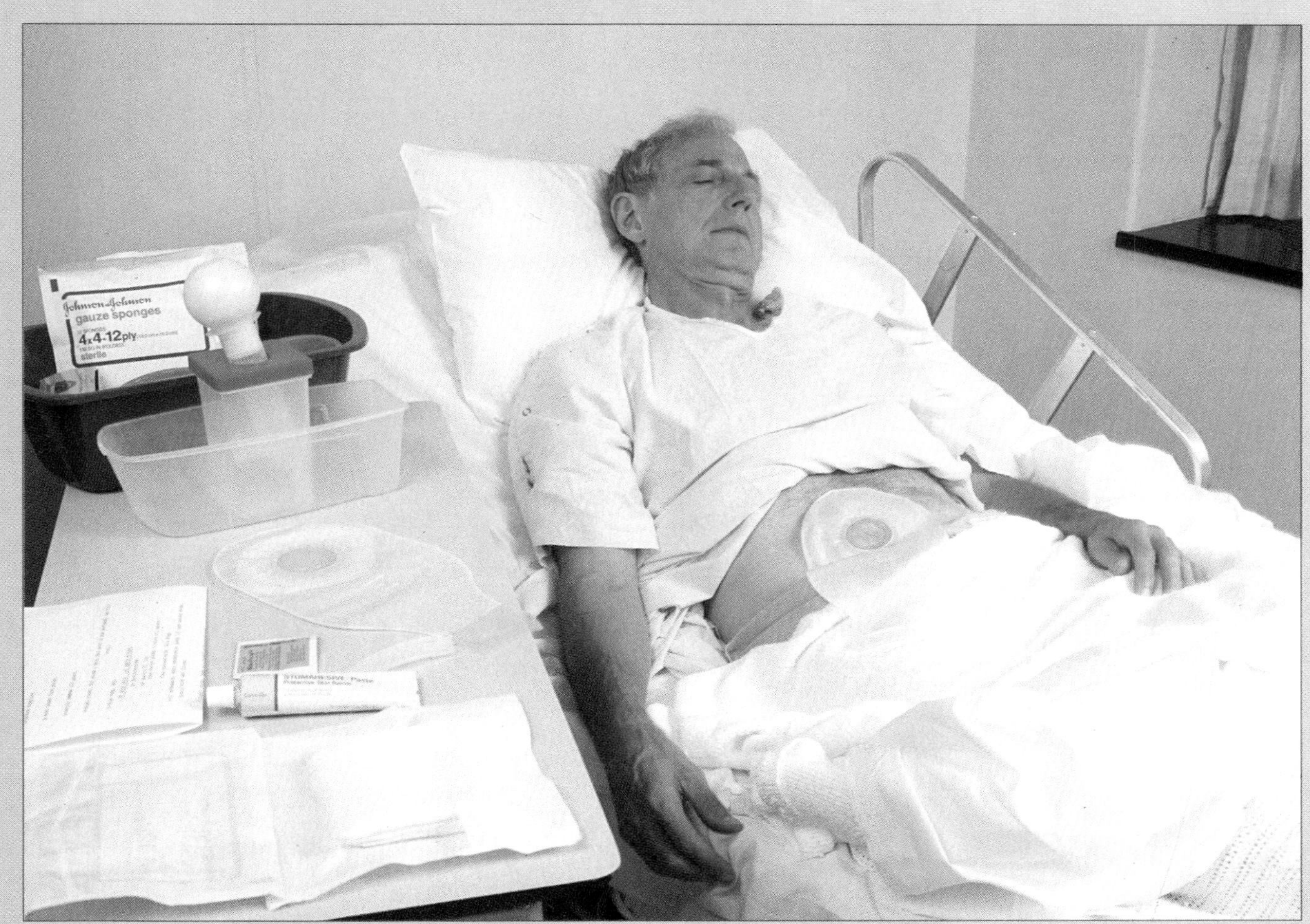

WARNING

For all patient contact, adhere to Universal Precautions. See page 91, 97, or the front cover flap. Wear protective equipment as indicated.

Objectives

What You Will Learn

When you have completed this chapter, you will be able to:

- Label the parts of the intravenous infusion equipment on a diagram.
- Change the gown of the patient with an intravenous infusion.
- Check the intravenous bottle, drip chamber, tubing, and the patient's arm so that you can promptly report anything unusual to your immediate supervisor.
- Describe the psychological aspects of caring for the ostomy patient.
- Give ostomy care.
- List three reasons for the use of binders.
- Apply the five types of binders.
- Explain the purpose of antiembolism elastic stockings and elastic bandages.
- Apply elastic bandages and antiembolism elastic stockings.
- Apply triangle sling bandages.
- Define: binder, infiltration, intravenous infusion, ostomy, phlebitis, stoma, thrombophlebitis.

KEY IDEAS

Intravenous Infusion (IV) Equipment

Intravenous Infusion
Refers to the injection of fluids into a vein. Foods in liquid form and medications can be put into the patient's body in this way.

AN INTRAVENOUS INFUSION IS OFTEN USED in the hospital to put fluids into the patient's body. A tube is connected to a bottle or plastic container. The container holds a fluid that could be a solution of salt or sugar, a prescribed medication, or blood (Figure 45-1).

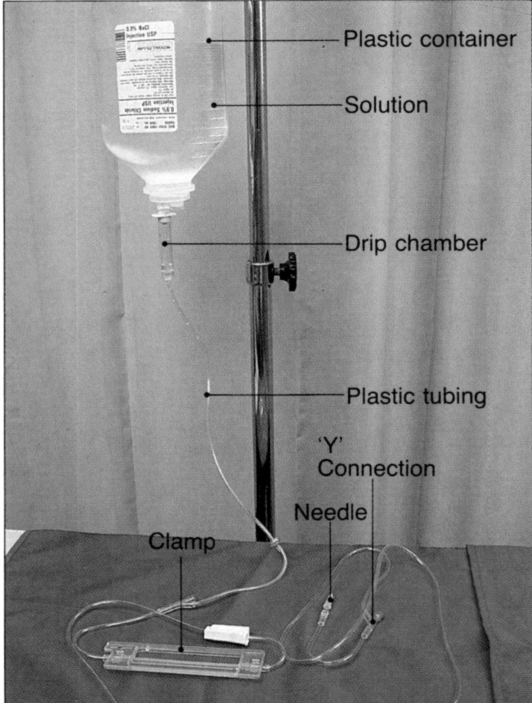

FIGURE 45-1 Intravenous (IV) infusion equipment.

The other end of the tube is connected to a needle. The needle is inserted by the doctor or the nurse into the patient's vein to give fluids, nourishment, or medications to the patient. It may be used to change the balance of certain chemicals in the patient's body. The solution flows from the container into the patient's vein and is circulated through the body.

The amount of fluid that can flow into the patient's body is controlled by a clamp on the tube. This clamp allows only a certain number of drops per minute to flow from the container. You, the nursing assistant, should never touch this clamp. Only a doctor or a nurse may change or regulate the amount of flow of a solution. You may have to move the patient in bed or change his position without interrupting the flow of the solution.

Procedure Changing the Gown of a Patient on IV (Intravenous Infusion)

☐ If the gowns used in your institution have Velcro® or snaps at the shoulders they can be placed directly on the patient. If the IV is on a pump you will not be able to run the gown around the pump. Follow the instructions of your immediate supervisor.

1. Assemble your equipment: Clean hospital gown.
2. Wash your hands.
3. Identify the patient by checking his identification bracelet.
4. Ask visitors to step out of the room, if this is your hospital's policy.
5. Tell the patient that you are going to change his gown.
6. Pull the curtain around the bed for privacy.
7. Raise the bed to a comfortable working position.
8. To remove the patient's soiled gown:
   a) Untie the gown.
   b) Remove the arm without the IV from the sleeve.
   c) Remove the gown from the arm with the IV carefully, considering the tube and the container of fluid as part of the arm. Move the sleeve down the arm, over the tubing, and up to the bottle or container.
   d) Remove the container or bottle from the hook, being careful not to lower the bottle below the area on the patient's arm where the needle is inserted.
   e) Slip the gown over the bottle and return the bottle or container to its hook.
   f) Place the soiled gown on a chair.
9. To put the clean gown on the patient, consider the bottle or container and tube as part of the patient's arm.
   a) Lift the bottle from the hook carefully. Do not put the bottle or container below the area on the patient's arm where the needle has been inserted.
   b) Then slip the sleeve of the gown over the bottle or container quickly.
   c) Replace the bottle on the hook.
   d) Slip the gown down the tube and then over the patient's arm.
   e) Then slip the gown over the other arm without the IV.
   f) Tie the back straps for the patient's comfort.
10. Make the patient comfortable.
11. Lower the bed to a position of safety for the patient.
12. Pull the curtains back to the open position.
13. Raise the side rails where ordered, indicated, and appropriate for patient safety.
14. Place the call light within easy reach of the patient.
15. If your immediate supervisor has instructed you to keep the patient's arm straight, encourage the patient to do so. If he bends his wrist or elbow, he may cut off the flow of solution.
16. Make sure the patient is not lying on top of the IV tubing. Watch for and straighten out any kinks that may form in the tubing. This may happen when the patient changes his position. Pressure or kinks might stop the flow of the solution.

17. Wash your hands.
18. Report to your immediate supervisor:

- That you have changed the patient's gown without disturbing the IV
- If there is still solution in the bottle but you cannot see the drops of solution passing from the bottle into the tubing
- If the plastic drop chamber is filled completely with the solution
- If you see blood in the tubing at the needle end
- If all the solution has run out of the bottle or that the bottle is almost empty
- If the needle has been removed from the patient's arm and whether this occurred deliberately or accidentally
- If the tubing has been disconnected and the bed is being saturated while the patient is bleeding freely from the connection
- If the patient complains of pain or tenderness at the site (place) where the needle is inserted
- If you notice a lumpy, raised, or inflamed (red) area on the patient's skin near the place where the needle is inserted. This might mean that the solution is not running into the vein but, instead, is running into the tissue nearby. This is called **infiltration** of an IV solution.
- How the patient tolerated the procedure
- Your observations of anything unusual

Infiltration
When an IV solution runs into nearby tissue instead of into a vein.

Caring for the Patient with an Intravenous Infusion

- Check the IV solution or blood transfusion to make sure it is flowing (Figure 45-2).

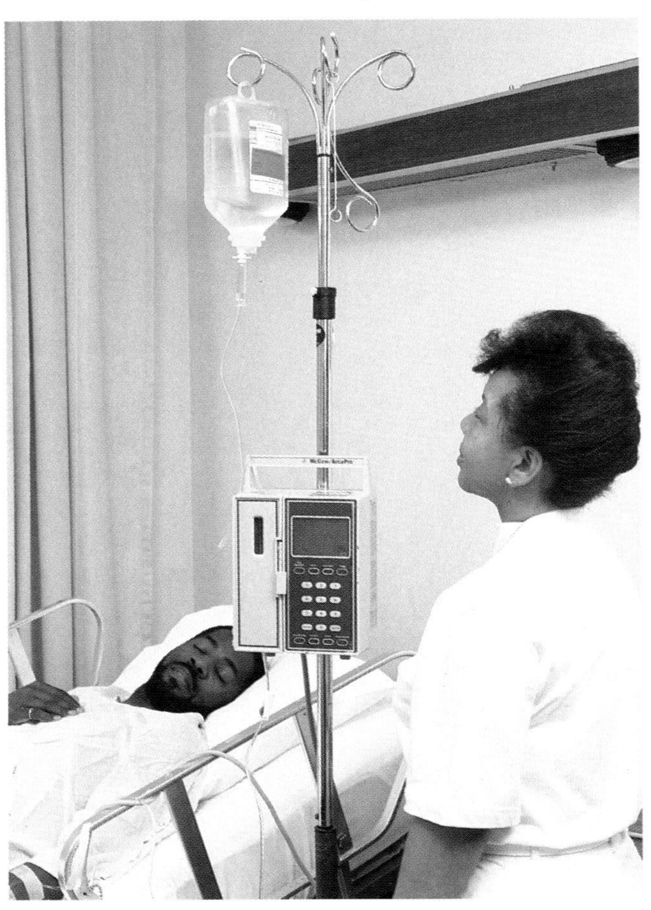

FIGURE 45-2 When a patient is receiving IV fluids, check the IV, drip chamber, and tubing.

- Make sure the tubing is not kinked and that the patient is not lying on the tubing.
- Check the skin for swelling, bleeding, or pain around the needle.
- Do not adjust the clamps or flow rate.
- Notify your supervisor immediately if the patient's skin around the needle is swollen or bleeding or if the fluid is not running properly.

KEY IDEAS

The Ostomy

Ostomy
A surgical procedure that provides the patient with an artificial opening, either temporary or permanent. The person's feces or urine then can leave the body through this opening. The opening is usually made through the abdominal wall into a part of the large intestine.

Stoma
An artificially made opening connecting a body passage with the outside, such as in a tracheotomy or colostomy.

An **ostomy** is a surgical procedure (operation) in which a new opening, called a **stoma**, is created in the abdomen, usually for the release of wastes (urine or feces) from the body. A stoma created surgically may be to divert the path of the patient's feces from the rectum. This is done when the colon is diseased or injured. The ostomy is most often performed when it is necessary to remove tumors. Sometimes the surgery is done to permit repair of bowel injuries.

A person with a stoma must wear an *ostomy appliance* to collect waste matter released through the stoma (Figure 45-3). This is a collecting bag usually held over the opening with a special adhesive paste.

Figures 45-4 through 45-8 describe types of ostomies and show the position of the stoma in each case.

As a nursing assistant, you will be taking care of the ostomy after the patient has been fitted with an ostomy appliance. This is sometimes referred to as an "old ostomy." A fresh surgical patient with a new ostomy is cared for by a registered nurse.

Sometimes the patient is able and wants to care for the ostomy himself. In this case, get permission from your immediate supervisor.

Psychological Aspects

The psychological reaction of the patient to an ostomy may be a feeling of loss of personal worth or dignity. The patient is faced with dealing with the ostomy and coping with life with an altered body image. The patient may become quiet and withdrawn. He may express feelings of loneliness or helplessness. Or he may become very angry, hostile, noisy,

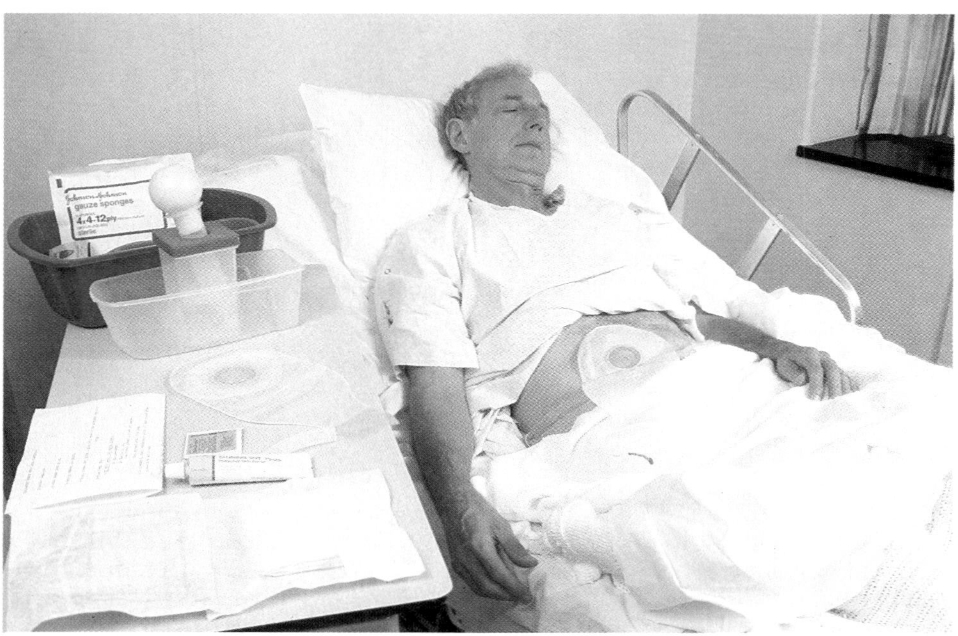

FIGURE 45-3 Ostomy appliance in place over the stoma.

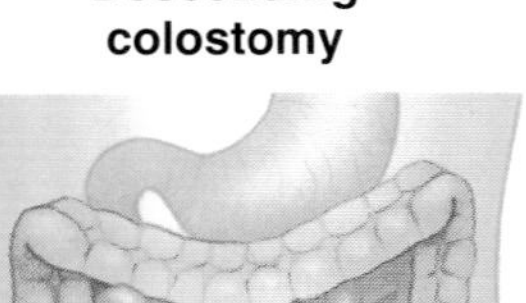

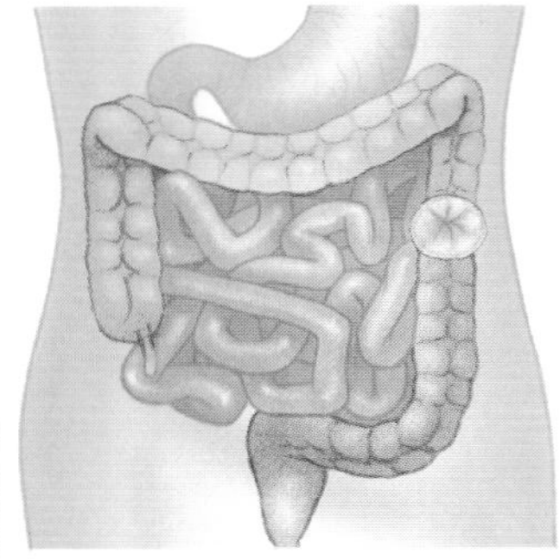

FIGURE 45-4 Following surgery, the type of discharge from a sigmoid or descending colostomy may be semiliquid until, through management of diet, the discharge begins to resemble a normal bowel movement.

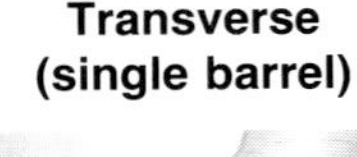

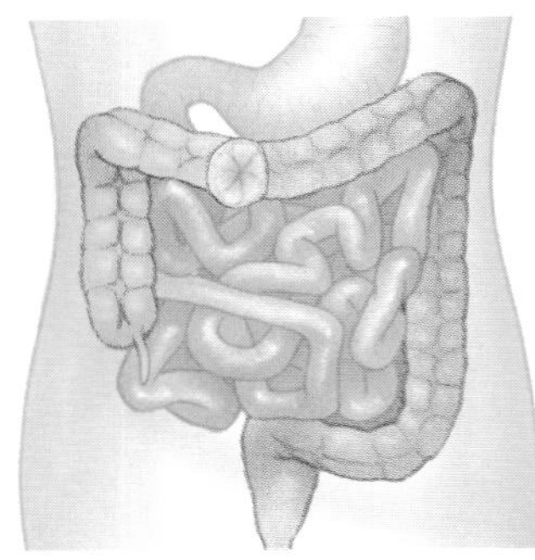

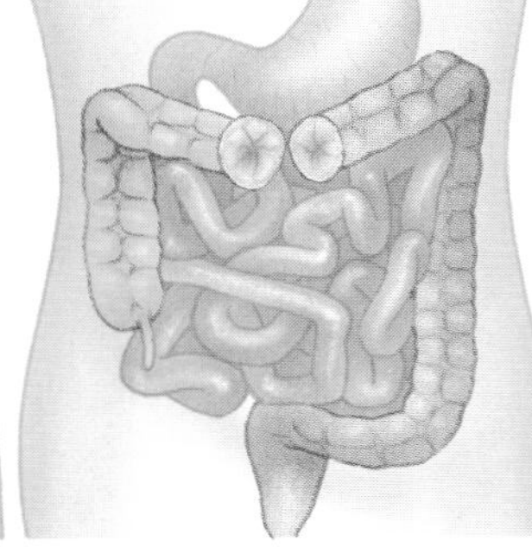

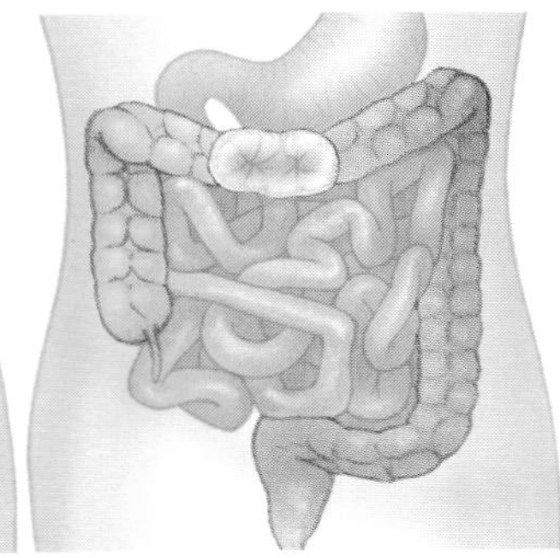

FIGURE 45-5 Frequently, the transverse single barrel, the transverse double barrel, and the transverse loop colostomy are temporary. Common patient problems with these types of ostomies include skin irritation, leakage from the appliance, and odor control.

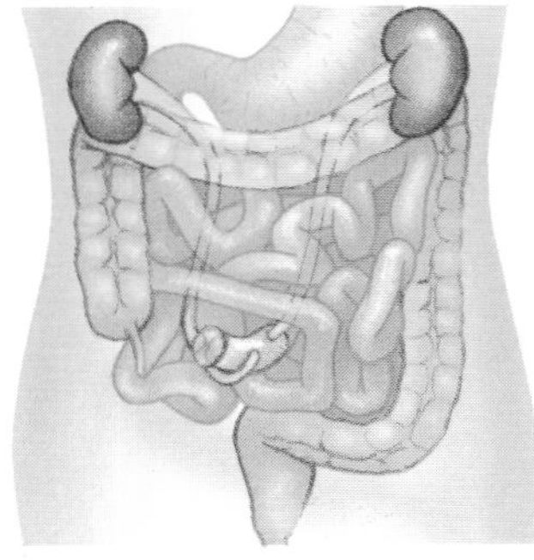

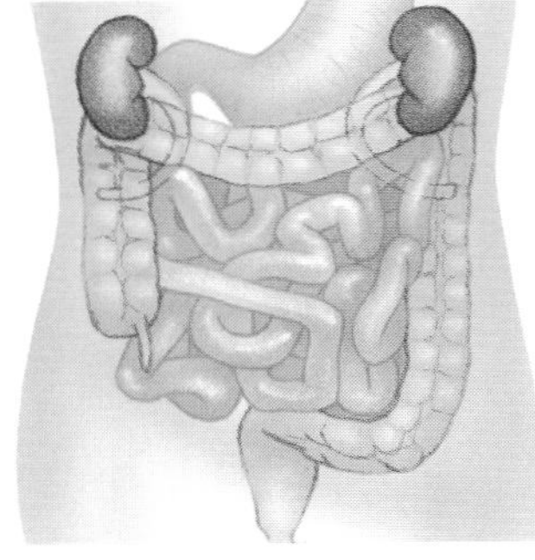

FIGURE 45-6 Urinary diversion (ureterostomy) is performed for malfunction of the urinary bladder. When the patient has a bilateral cutaneous ureterostomy or an ileal conduit, prevention of leakage and skin protection are of utmost importance.

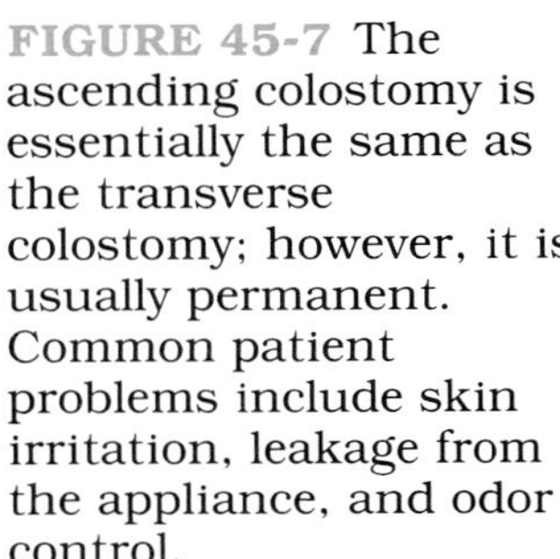

FIGURE 45-7 The ascending colostomy is essentially the same as the transverse colostomy; however, it is usually permanent. Common patient problems include skin irritation, leakage from the appliance, and odor control.

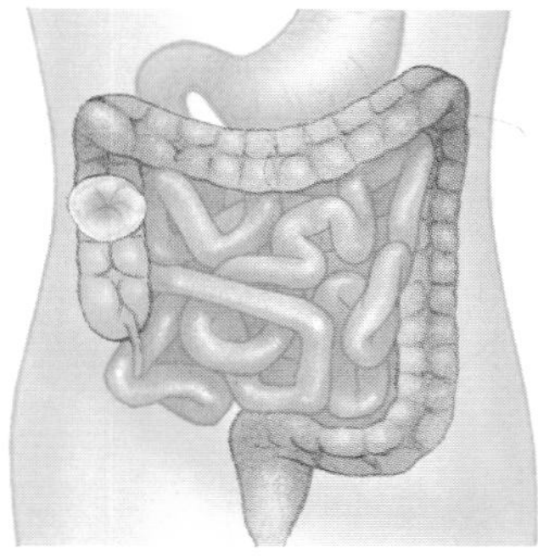

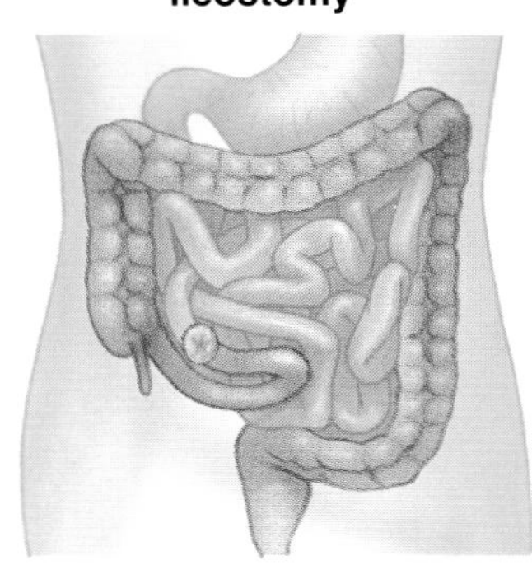

FIGURE 45-8 The ileostomy. Common patient problems with the ileostomy include skin irritation and odor control.

and disruptive. The patient may develop mood changes, appearing very anxious or depressed. Anxiety is a natural response felt by the patient. Fear is another emotion that causes the patient to develop feelings of doom or panic. When the patient does not adjust easily, all his emotions will get stronger. Family members and significant others who provide emotional support are very important. Report to your immediate supervisor any behavioral changes you observe in the patient.

Procedure Caring for an Ostomy

1. Assemble your equipment:
   a) Bedpan
   b) Disposable bed protector
   c) Bath blanket
   d) Large emesis basin
   e) Water with flange
   f) Clean stoma bag with stoma adhesive paste
   g) Toilet tissue
   h) Basin of water at 115°F (46.1°C)
   i) Soap or cleanser as ordered by your immediate supervisor
   j) Disposable washcloth
   k) Disposable gloves
   l) Towels
   m) Lubricant or skin cream as ordered
2. Wash your hands.
3. Identify the patient by checking the identification bracelet.
4. Ask visitors to step out of the room, if this is your hospital's policy.
5. Tell the patient that you will take care of and change his ostomy appliance.
6. Pull the curtain around the bed for privacy.
7. Raise the bed to a comfortable working position.
8. Cover the patient with the bath blanket. Ask the patient to hold the top edge of the blanket. Without exposing him, fanfold the top sheet and bedspread to the foot of the bed under the blanket.
9. Place the disposable bed protector under the patient's hips. This is to keep the bed from getting wet or dirty.
10. Place the bedpan and emesis basin within easy reach.
11. Fill the wash basin half full with water at 115°F (46.1°C). Have soap or cleanser as ordered, disposable washcloth, and bath towels on the bedside table.
12. Remove the soiled plastic stoma bag.
13. Put the soiled plastic bag into the bedpan. Wipe the area around the ostomy with toilet tissue. This is to remove any loose feces. Place the dirty tissue in the bedpan or emesis basin.
14. Wet and soap the washcloth. Wash the entire ostomy area with a gentle circular motion working from the stoma outward.
15. Rinse the entire area well. Be careful not to leave any soap on the skin. (Soap has a drying effect and may irritate the skin.)
16. Dry the area gently with a bath towel.
17. With clean scissors, cut the wafer in the center to fit over the stoma. (Follow the instructions of your immediate supervisor for cleaning the scissors.) Apply adhesive stoma paste to the skin around the stoma. Peel paper backing from the wafer. Place wafer, adhesive side down, over adhesive stoma paste. (Note that the wafer is *not* changed every time the stoma bag is changed.)
18. Place a clean stoma bag in place on the wafer. Seal tightly.
19. Remove the disposable bed protector. Change any damp linen.
20. Replace the top sheet and bedspread and remove the bath blanket.
21. Make the patient comfortable.
22. Lower the bed to a position of safety for the patient.
23. Pull the curtains back to the open position.
24. Raise the side rails where ordered, indicated, and appropriate for patient safety.
25. Place the call light within easy reach of the patient.
26. Remove all used equipment. Dispose of waste material in the large hopper or into the toilet.

27. Discard disposable equipment.
28. Clean the bedpan and put it where it belongs.
29. Empty the wash basin. Wash it thoroughly with soap and water.
30. Rinse and dry it and return it to its proper place.
31. Wash your hands.
32. Report to your immediate supervisor:

- That the ostomy was cleaned
- The amount of drainage
- The consistency of the excretions
- The color and appearance of the stoma and ostomy area
- How the patient tolerated the procedure
- Your observations of anything unusual

KEY IDEAS

Binders

Binder
A wide cloth bandage.

Binders are wide cloth bandages, usually made of cotton. They are applied mainly to the torso of the patient for several reasons. Binders can be used postoperatively, or after childbirth, or whenever it is desirable to:

- Give support to a weakened body part
- Hold dressing and bandages in place
- Put pressure on parts of the body to make the patient more comfortable

Your immediate supervisor will tell you if a particular patient is to have a binder applied and what kind of binder is to be used. Remember, unless the binder is put on properly, it can be more uncomfortable for the patient than if it had not been used at all. Binders are obtained from central supply.

Rules to Follow

BINDERS

- Keep the binder smooth and clean. Otherwise, it will be uncomfortable in the same way that crumbs or wrinkles in the patient's bed are uncomfortable. Bedsores (decubitus ulcers or pressure ulcers) can be caused by wrinkles or wetness of a binder.
- Watch for reddened areas on the patient's skin. Report these to your immediate supervisor.

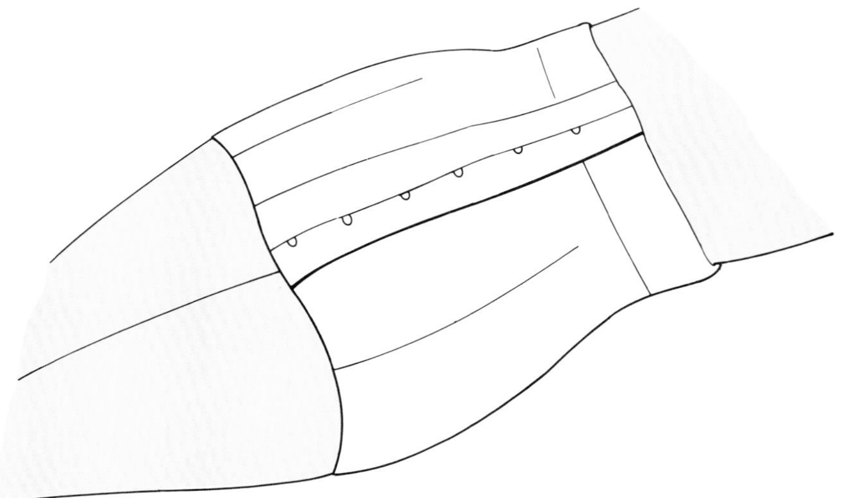

FIGURE 45-9 Straight abdominal binder.

- Use the correct type of binder. Be sure it is the correct size. Three different types of binders are commonly used:
  - Straight abdominal binder (Figure 45-9)
  - Scultetus (many tailed) binder (Figure 45-10)
  - T binder

The T binder is used to keep dressings in place on the perineal (genital) area and rectal area. This binder is often used after a hemorrhoidectomy (an operation to remove hemorrhoids) or after the delivery of a baby. The binder is first wrapped around the patient's waist. Part of the binder then goes between the patient's legs and is brought back up to be fastened at the waist.

FIGURE 45-10 Scultetus (many tailed) binder.

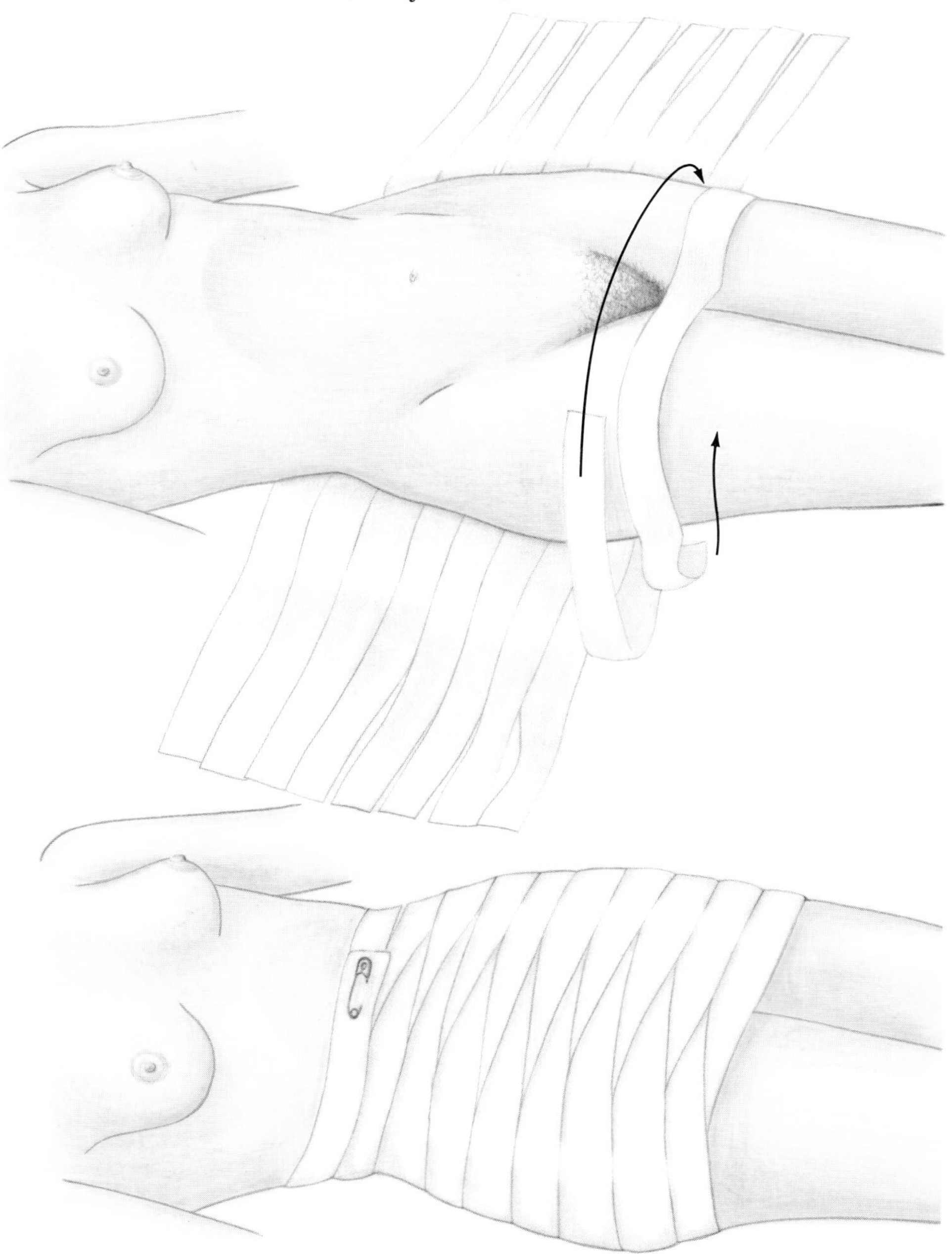

KEY IDEAS

Elastic Stockings and Elastic Bandages

Phlebitis
Inflammation of a vein.

Thrombophlebitis
Inflammation and blood clots in a vein.

Antiembolism elastic stockings and elastic bandages are applied to the body extremities (arms, hands, legs, feet). In postoperative care, they are most often used on the lower extremities or legs. They are used either as treatment for **thrombophlebitis** (blood clots in the veins) or for **phlebitis** (inflammation of the veins) or to prevent these conditions. The purpose of antiembolism elastic stockings and elastic bandages is to compress the veins and, therefore, improve the return of venous blood to the heart, which improves circulation.

In cases of sprain or strain at the joint, they are used to provide support and comfort.

Applying Antiembolism Elastic Stockings

Antiembolism elastic stockings can be either knee-length or full-length (Figure 45-11). Be careful to smooth out all the wrinkles. Be sure the stocking is pulled up firmly. Elastic stockings must be removed and reapplied at least once every 8 hours and more often if the doctor has so ordered. These stockings come in various sizes. Be sure they are the right size and fit the patient. They should be applied while the patient is lying down (not sitting in a chair) before getting out of bed. Elastic stockings should be applied only on the instructions of your immediate supervisor.

Elastic Bandages

Elastic bandages are long strips of elasticized cotton (Figure 45-12). They are wound neatly into rolls, with a metal clip or Velcro® to keep the end in place. They provide support, hold dressings in place, apply

FIGURE 45-11 Antiembolism stocking: (1) knee length; (b) full length.

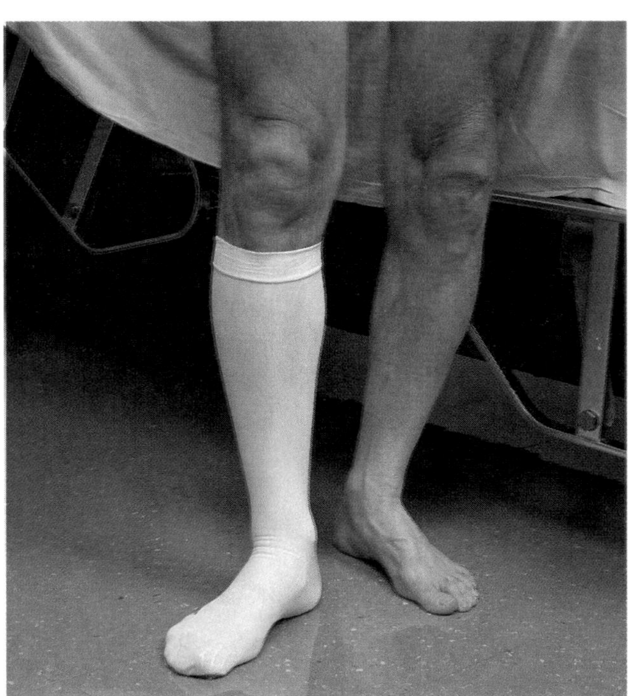

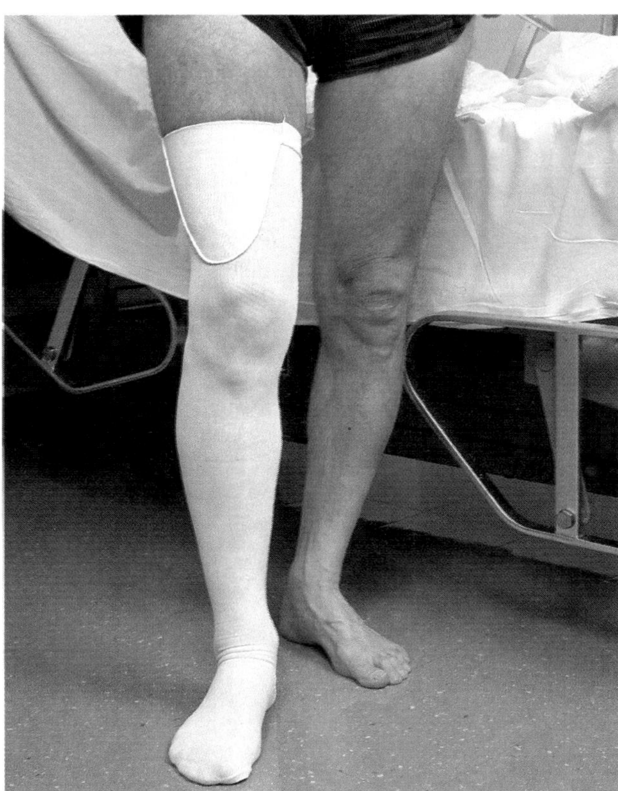

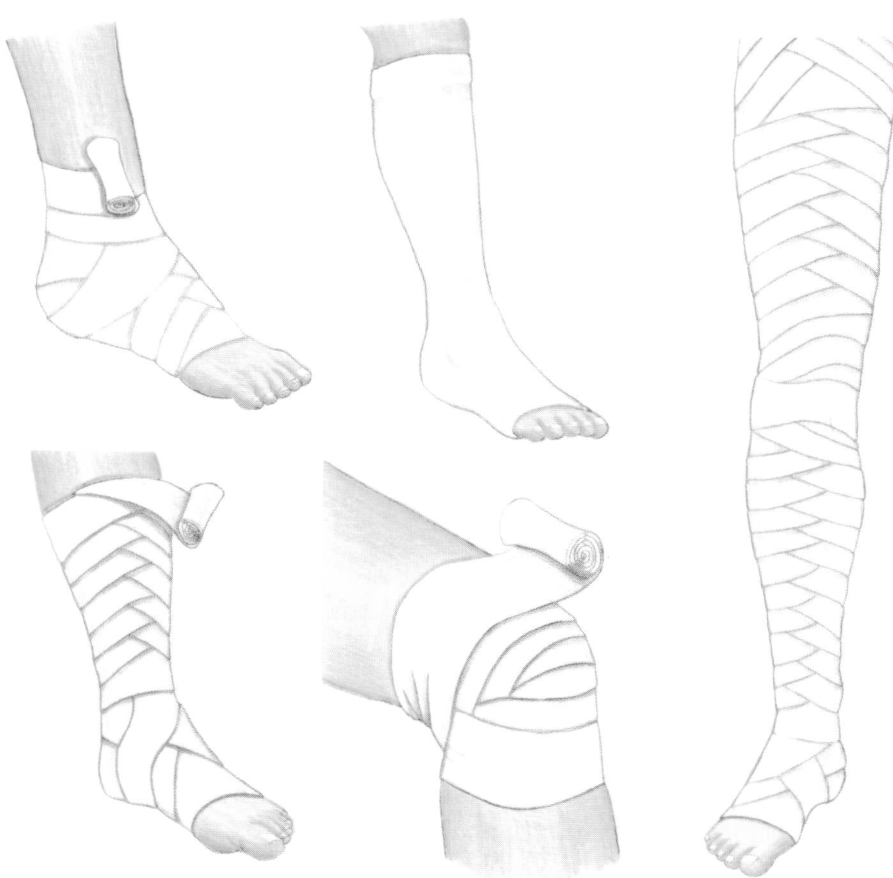

FIGURE 45-12 Elastic stockings and bandages.

pressure to a body part, and improve return circulation. Bandages may be ordered toes to knees, toes to mid-thighs, toes to groin, or heel-free (heel-free means heel uncovered). Follow the instructions given to you by your immediate supervisor. Use as many bandages as necessary to cover the area as ordered.

If the bandage has been wrapped too tightly, the patient's circulation may be impaired. She may develop such symptoms as paleness, coldness, blueness (cyanosis), pain, swelling, or numbness in the extremities. Be very careful to wrap these bandages firmly but not too tightly. Check the patient's condition frequently. Elastic bandages should be removed and reapplied once per shift. Observe the condition and color of the skin every hour (q.h.).

Procedure Applying Elastic Bandages

1. Assemble your equipment:
   a) Elastic bandages
   b) Clips or safety pins
2. Wash your hands.
3. Identify the patient by checking the identification bracelet.
4. Ask visitors to step out of the room, if this is your hospital's policy.
5. Tell the patient that you are going to wrap his leg or arm (or whatever area is to be wrapped) with an elastic bandage.
6. Pull the curtain around the bed for privacy.
7. Raise the bed to a comfortable working position.
8. Place the patient in a comfortable posi-

tion that is convenient for you to work. Expose the area to be wrapped.

9. Extend the part of the body to be bandaged. Support the patient's heel or wrist.
10. Stand directly in front of the patient or facing the part to be bandaged.
11. Hold the bandage with the loose end coming off the bottom of the roll.
12. Anchor the bandage by two circular turns around the body part at its smallest point. This usually is the ankle or the wrist.
13. Apply the bandage in the same direction as venous circulation, that is, toward the heart.
14. Roll the bandage smoothly and wrap it firmly but not too tightly.
15. Exert even pressure. Keep the bandage smooth. Be sure no skin areas show between the turns.
16. If possible, leave the toes or fingers exposed for observation of circulatory changes.
17. Continue wrapping upward with a spiral turn. Each turn should overlap the one before about one-half width of the bandage.
18. After applying the bandage, secure the terminal end by pinning it with a safety pin, by applying bandage clips, or with Velcro®.
19. If more than one bandage is used, overlap them to prevent the bandages from slipping.
20. To remove the bandage, unwind it gently. Gather it into a loose mass, passing the mass from hand to hand as the bandage is unwound. Then roll the bandage smoothly so it is ready for the next application.
21. Make the patient comfortable.
22. Lower the bed to a position of safety for the patient.
23. Pull the curtains back to the open position.
24. Raise the side rails where ordered, indicated, and appropriate for patient safety.
25. Place the call light within easy reach of the patient.
26. Wash your hands.
27. Report to your immediate supervisor:
    - That you have applied or removed the elastic bandages
    - The area of application
    - How the patient tolerated the procedure
    - Your observations of anything unusual

Procedure Applying a Triangle Sling Bandage

1. Assemble your equipment:
    a) Triangle of material or a square of cloth folded into a triangle
    b) Pin
    c) Small pieces of soft absorbent material
2. Wash your hands.
3. Identify the patient by checking her identification bracelet.
4. Ask visitors to step out of the room, if this is your hospital's policy.
5. Tell the patient that you are going to apply the sling bandage.
6. Pull the curtain around the bed for privacy.
7. Raise the bed to a comfortable working position.
8. Assist the patient to a comfortable position. If the patient is permitted to sit on the side of the bed (dangle), have her do so.
9. Place small pieces of soft, absorbent material wherever two areas of skin touch. This will prevent body parts from rubbing against each other, causing friction. Areas to place these absorbent pieces are the folds of the body where skin touches skin, such as under the breasts, between the arm and the chest, and in the axilla.
10. Place one end of the triangle over the shoulder on the uninjured side with the point of the triangle extending under the injured arm or shoulder.

11. Be gentle. Bring the other end of the triangle over the shoulder on the injured side, allowing enough of the bandage to reach around the back of the neck.
12. The patient's hand must be higher than the elbow and be supported to prevent "wrist drop."
13. To give desired support, adjust the sling to the patient size.
14. Tie the ends of the bandage at the side of the neck (Figure 45-13).

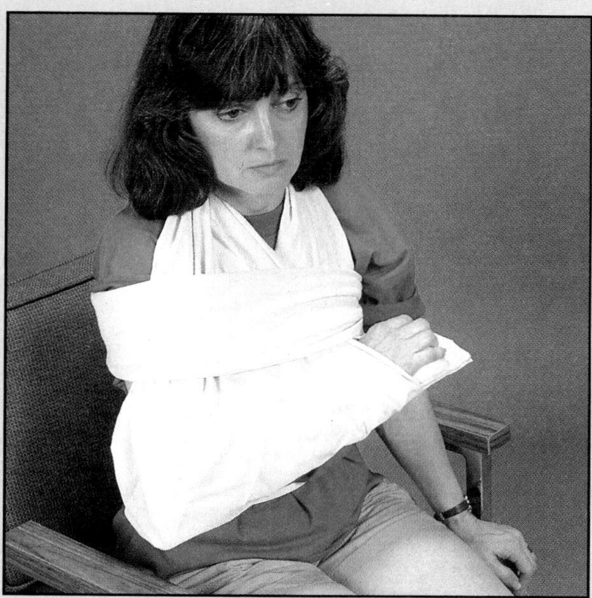

FIGURE 45-13 Triangle sling bandage.

15. To avoid a pressure point, use a square knot.
16. Tie a knot or fold the corner of the bandage at the elbow and pin it in place to keep the elbow from moving out of the support.
17. Check this patient every hour (q.h.) for skin color, positioning, circulation, and comfort.
18. Make the patient comfortable.
19. Lower the bed to a position of safety for the patient.
20. Pull the curtains back to the open position.
21. Raise the side rails where ordered, indicated, and appropriate for patient safety.
22. Place the call light within easy reach of the patient.
23. Wash your hands.
24. Report to your immediate supervisor:
    - That the triangle bandage has been applied
    - The time it was applied
    - The patient's comments as to the comfort of the bandage
    - How the patient tolerated the procedure
    - Your observations of anything unusual

KEY QUESTIONS

1. Name the parts of the intravenous infusion equipment.
2. How should you change the gown of a patient with an IV?
3. List the observations that should be reported after checking the intravenous equipment and the patient's arm, when the patient is receiving an intravenous infusion.
4. Discuss the psychological reactions of the ostomy patient.
5. What are your responsibilities when giving ostomy care?
6. Why are binders used?
7. List and describe the five types of binders.
8. Why are antiembolism elastic stockings and elastic bandages used?
9. In postoperative care, where are elastic stockings and bandages used?
10. When applying a triangle bandage, should the patient's hand be higher or lower than his elbow? Why?
11. Define: binder, infiltration, intravenous infusion, ostomy, phlebitis, stoma, thrombophlebitis.

CHAPTER

46

Geriatric Care

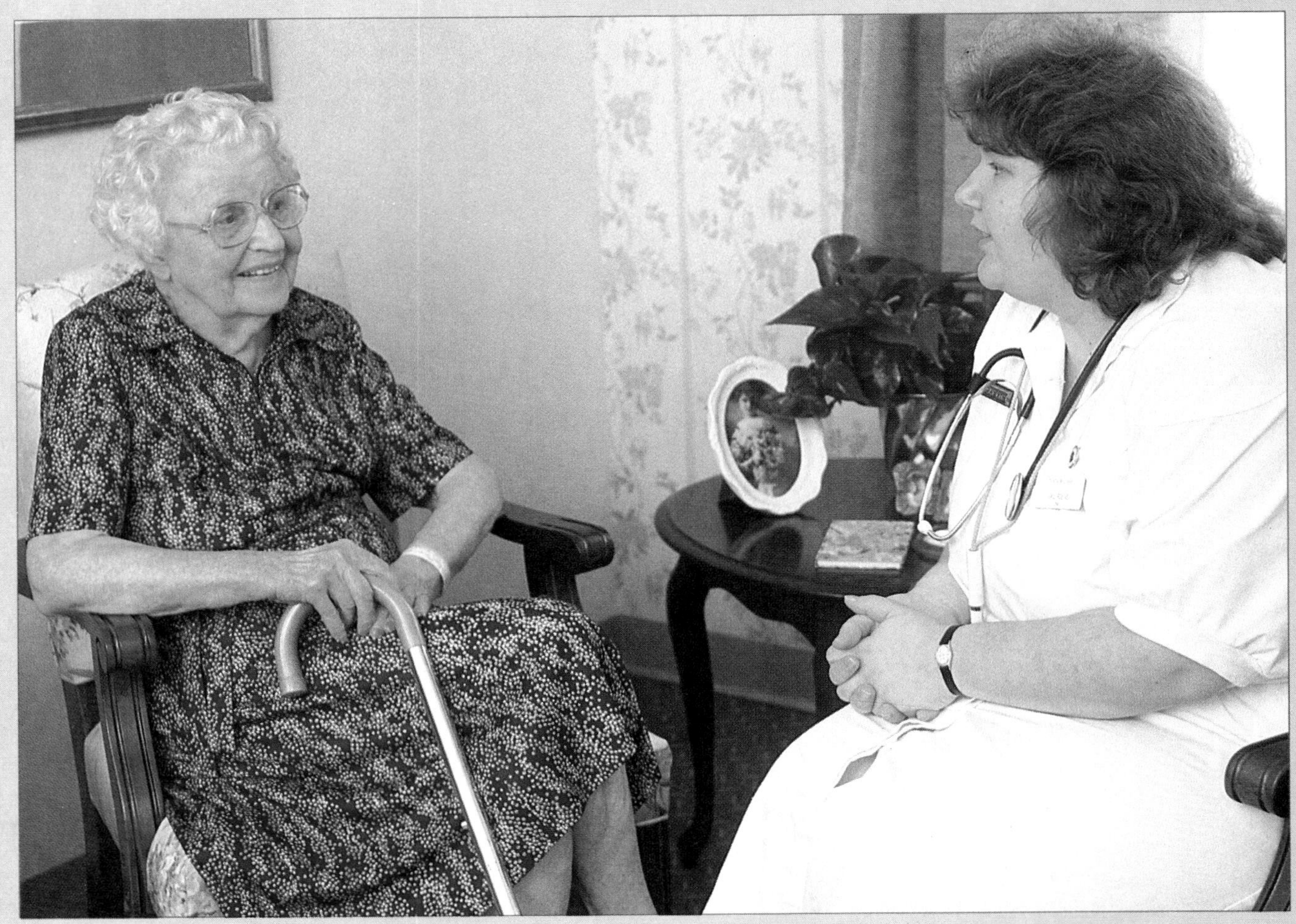

WARNING

For all patient contact, adhere to Universal Precautions. See page 91, 97, or the front cover flap. Wear protective equipment as indicated.

Objectives

What You Will Learn

When you have completed this chapter, you will be able to:

- Describe the geriatric patient physically and emotionally.
- Assist with reality orientation.
- Create a safe environment for the geriatric patient.
- Safely assist with ambulation.
- Give skin care.
- Assist the bed-bound patient.
- List and define common chronic conditions of the geriatric patient.
- Define: dangling position, dementia, deteriorate, disoriented, flammable, geriatric.

KEY IDEAS

Physical Changes of the Geriatric Patient

AS WE GROW OLDER, MANY PHYSICAL changes take place that make functioning independently more and more difficult. The body's central nervous system slows down. This can create problems in detecting heat, pain, and cold and slower reflexes. Thought processes may be slow and memory may become poor. All the senses (hearing, sight, taste, touch, and smell) may not be as sharp as they once were. Muscle tone may be poor due to lack of exercise. A disturbed sense of balance might make the patient unsteady on his feet or cause a change in his walking patterns. The bones tend to become brittle and break easily. Quick changes in position can cause the blood pressure to drop and, as a result, the patient will feel dizzy or faint. Posture may become more stooped. Circulation becomes less efficient and bodily processes slow down. The skin loses elasticity and some fat.

Geriatric
Aging; elderly; over 65 years of age.

Common Physical Changes in the Geriatric Person

The following changes may or may not occur in all patients.

Skeletal System

- Softening of the bones (osteoporosis)
- Decreased flexibility of joints (arthritis)
- Changes in vertebrae and feet (difficult ambulation)

Muscular System

- Decrease in muscle mass and muscle tone
- Decreased elasticity of tendons and ligaments

Cardiovascular System

- Decreased cardiac output
- Decreased elasticity of blood vessels (poor circulation; edema)

Respiratory System

- Reduced tone of respiratory muscles and diaphragm
- Decreased lung capacity
- Increased risk of upper respiratory disease

Endocrine System

- Increased incidence of metabolic disease (diabetes)
- Decreased hormonal functioning (menopause)
- Decreased ability to heal

Nervous System

- Decreased touch sensation (hot, cold, pain)
- Decreased equilibrium, or motor coordination
- Decreased reaction and response time
- Decreased taste perception
- Decreased sense of smell
- Decreased visual perception (night vision, depth and color perceptions, drying of cornea)
- Decreased elasticity of ear drum (alteration in hearing, delayed auditory impulse)

Integumentary System

- Decreased fat cells
- Decreased elasticity of skin
- Decreased sweat and sebaceous gland secretions (loss of ability to regulate body temperature)
- Increased pigmentation (aging spots)
- Thinning of skin layers

Urinary System

- Decreased kidney function (urinary output)
- Decreased bladder tone (incontinence)

Gastrointestinal System

- Alteration in metabolic rate
- Alteration in bowel habits

Mental Health

- Increased incidence of depression (loneliness, decrease in socialization)
- Changes in sleeping patterns

KEY IDEAS

Psychosocial and Psychological Aspects of Aging

- *Psycho:* mental or emotional processes
- *Social:* interactions and relations among people

Social changes may be caused by physical problems, life crises, or the pressure of society. These may include:

- Retirement
- Change in income

- Fear of illness
- Isolation from friends and family
- Death of a spouse or significant other
- Change in housing
- Increased dependence on others

To foster health and well-being provide opportunities for the patient to participate in a variety of activities that will be mentally stimulating and meaningful. Purposeful activity should be designed to involve the patient with other people. This will encourage geriatric patients to live their lives to the fullest. The feeling of being needed will stimulate feelings of self-accomplishment and satisfaction for the patient. By persuading the patient to participate and interact with others the nursing assistant can possibly decrease loneliness in the geriatric patient. Such rehabilitative measures help to eliminate the physical dependency and mental depression commonly seen in the geriatric patient.

Rules to Follow

MEETING THE PSYCHOSOCIAL NEEDS OF SOME GERIATRIC PATIENTS

- Maintain a safe environment.
- Help the patient to feel confident in the health care team.
- Pay attention to the patient and make him or her feel important.
- Encourage the patient to do as much as he or she is able to do.
- Show respect for the individual patient.
- Provide care with a gentle touch and in a kind and considerate manner.
- Be a good listener (pay attention to what the patient is saying).
- Provide for the patient's privacy.
- Accept the person as he or she is now, without passing judgment.
- Call the patient by the patient's preferred name at each contact.
- Touch the patient when you speak to him or her if acceptable to the patient.
- Talk directly to the patient.
- Keep the room well lighted.
- Have the patient's personal belongings where the patient wants them.
- Encourage the patient to interact with family, visitors, and other patients.
- Assist the patient to see himself or herself as a valuable, needed, and successful person.
- Provide opportunities for the patient to make decisions and to be independent.
- You may be one of the few your patient sees and talks to. Provide socialization by being friendly, understanding, and patient while completing your work with the patient.

Reality Orientation for the Confused Patient

Sometimes geriatric patients are confused for short or lengthy periods. The patient may not know where he is. He may be speaking to people who are not in the room. Report any new episodes of or changes in confusion to your supervisor. They may be caused by any number of things, many of which are reversible. Make an effort to orient this patient. Tell him the time of day and where he is. Tell him who you are and why you are there.

Patients who are **disoriented** may have difficulty remembering, recognizing, or describing people, places, or times. They may be unable to tell others who they are, where they are or the day, date, or time.

These patients benefit from a consistent calm environment and routine. Display a clock and a calendar in a prominent place. Repetition is important. Remind the patient frequently of who he is, where he is, and the date and time. For example:

- Include the time when talking to the patient, "Good morning, it's 8 o'clock and breakfast is ready."
- Introduce yourself repeatedly.

When the disoriented patient asks for or speaks to a person who is no longer living, gently remind him or her that this person has passed away. Going along with the patient would only increase the disorientation. However, do not pressure the disoriented person to respond correctly. This also may increase the disorientation and lower self-esteem.

KEY IDEAS

Safety for the Geriatric Patient

Creating a Safe Environment for the Geriatric Patient

Be diligent in your efforts to protect your patient from accidents. Every patient is an individual and has different needs. Some patients may need your assistance to get in and out of bed or to walk from room to room. If you notice that your patient is unsteady, report it to your supervisor. The unsteady patient may benefit from the use of a cane or a walker or regular exercise. A sturdy, hard chair, placed beside the patient's bed, will give her or him something to hold on to when getting out of bed. Be sure the patient's clothing is not so long that he or she is likely to trip over it. If the height of the bed is adjustable, make sure it is in the lowest position at all times and the wheels are locked.

To keep the geriatric patient safe, the nursing assistant must continually observe the patient and the environment. For example:

- Bed-bound geriatric patients should be protected by side rails that are kept in the up position on both sides of the bed at all times. If the bed is adjustable, keep it at its lowest level in a position of safety for the patient at all times.
- Before the patient moves out of bed, he or she should come to a full sitting **(dangling)** position before standing.
- When the patient gets out of bed, the nursing assistant must check to see that both of the patient's feet are firmly on the floor before the patient begins to stand. Assist the patient in securing shoes before walking whenever possible.
- The geriatric patient who is permitted to smoke alone should be checked frequently. Provide a large ash tray to prevent ashes from falling on the bed or on any **flammable** article.
- Remove harmful substances from the confused patient's reach, such as sharp equipment, Clinitest or Acetest supplies, matches, cigarette lighters, knives, and unauthorized medications.
- Monitor at all times patients who may wander away.

Dangling Position
Sitting up on the edge of the bed with the feet hanging down loosely.

Flammable
Something that can be easily set on fire and burns quickly.

- Offer assistance to the patient with meals as needed while fostering independence. For example, tell a patient with vision loss where food is on the plate.
- Protect the patient from overexposure to sunlight.
- Keep frequently used articles within reach of the patient.
- Wipe up spills immediately.
- Be alert at all times for any condition that might cause an accident or injury to the patient.
- Keep the patient's environment free from clutter. Keep the path from the bed and chair to the toilet clear.

Ambulation Safety with and without the Walker

- When patients who are unsteady are using a walker they should be accompanied by the nursing assistant.
- A walker provides support for the unsteady patient (Figure 46-1). Make sure there are rubber tips on the legs of the walker so that it cannot slide. The patient is supported on both sides as he or she holds on to the walker with both hands and lifts it slightly ahead.
- When assisting the patient use an ambulation belt on the patient and hold it lightly from behind (Figure 46.2).

FIGURE 46-1 Using a walker for support.

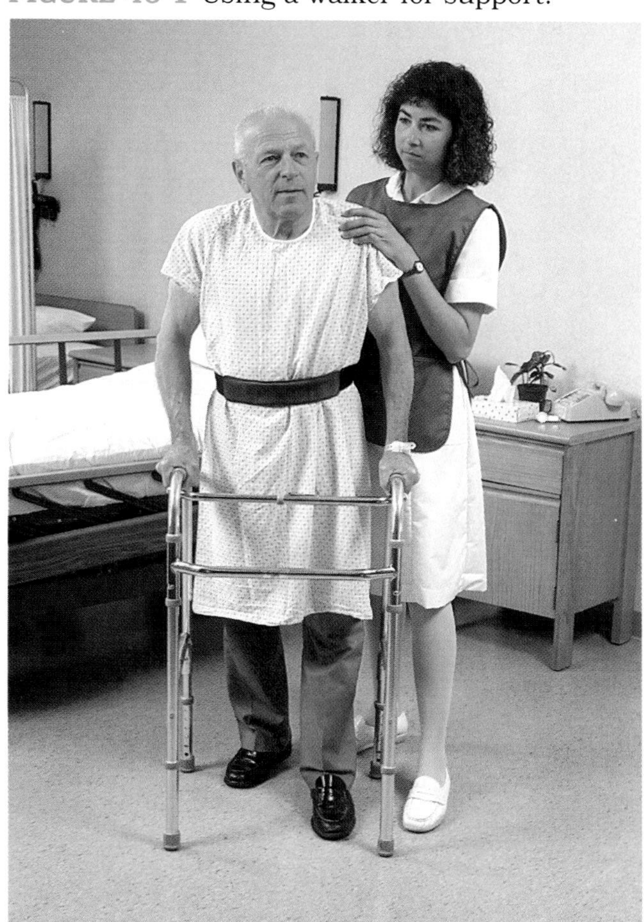

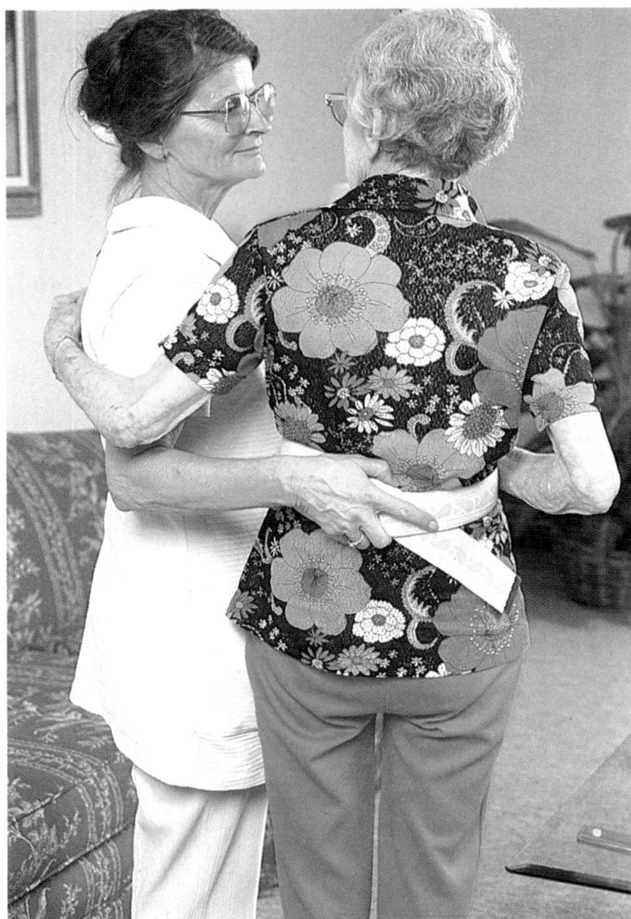

FIGURE 46-2 Steady the patient by holding the belt at the patient's back.

- Some walkers have wheels and are used with patients who cannot lift the walker.
- If the walker is being moved, the patient's feet should be stationary. If the walker is stationary, the patient may move his or her feet forward.

KEY IDEAS

Nursing Care for the Geriatric Patient

Skin Care

The patient's skin may be extremely dry, flaky, and wrinkled. This is due to the decreased amounts of oils being produced by the oil glands and poor circulation. Dry skin is less elastic and more sensitive than normal skin. Circulation tends to slow down in the older patient. Lack of frequent movement and exercise can contribute to problems. These problems of aging skin and circulation make the geriatric patient especially susceptible to pressure ulcers.

Give thorough skin care frequently and urge the patient to move about as often as he or she is able. Different patients will need varying amounts of assistance from you when changing position. If the patient is nonambulatory, you will need to turn him or her many times each day. Keep the principles of good body mechanics in mind and use a pull (turn) sheet to avoid friction. Sharpen your nursing skills concerning skin care by reviewing the section Pressure Ulcer Care (page 234).

The Bed-bound Geriatric Patient

When a patient is bed-bound, he or she has the same needs as an ambulatory patient, but will require more help in meeting these needs. Emotional support and encouragement can be very helpful. If family members are visiting the hospital often, involve them in the care of the patient by permitting them to suggest the patient's favorite foods, feed the patient, shave the patient, comb the patient's hair, or do simple tasks.

Proper positioning of the patient in bed will help make him or her comfortable. The back and joints should be supported to prevent unnecessary strain. Changing the patient's position at least every 2 hours will promote circulation and help in preventing pressure ulcers. Support the patient's arms and legs. Pillows can be used for support, but never put the support behind the knees, unless you have specific instructions to do so.

An air mattress or egg-crate mattress may promote comfort and prevent skin problems. At all times bed coverings should be smooth, clean, and dry.

Assist the bed-bound patient with the activities of daily living. A daily bed bath will not only keep the patient clean, but also will help him or her to feel relaxed and refreshed. Oral hygiene, back rubs, and care of the hair and nails all help the patient look and feel better. The bed-bound patient may need less food than before illness due to a lack of physical activity. Meals should be well balanced and served attractively. Constipation may be aggravated by the lack of exercise.

KEY IDEAS

Common Chronic Diseases and Conditions

Along with the normal body changes that occur as a person grows older, there are many chronic diseases or conditions that may result. The aging process is inevitable but it occurs at different rates in each person, as well as in each body system.

The following is a list of some common chronic diseases and conditions associated with the geriatric patient.

Common Chronic Diseases and Conditions	What Occurs as a Result of These Diseases and Conditions
Alzheimer's disease	Alzheimer's disease is a degenerative disorder that produces progressive dementia. Dementia is an irreversible deteriorative mental state. This disease is the most common cause of **dementia** in the geriatric patient. The **deterioration** in mental function causes the inability to perform the activities of daily living; a lack of orientation to time, place, and person and of memory, judgment, and understanding; mood changes; a general inability to care; and death. With today's increasing life-span, there is an increased incidence of this disease. Alzheimer's disease is divided into two classifications: (1) presenile dementia (before age 65), and (2) senile dementia (after age 65). The cause of Alzheimer's disease is not known. Nursing care of patients with this disease is based on the signs and symptoms they display. Contribute to the well-being of these patients by creating a safe environment, including careful observation to prevent the patients from harming themselves. Follow the principles of reality orientation and encourage these patients to do as much for themselves as possible.
Arteriosclerosis	A pathological condition in which there is a thickening, hardening, and loss of elasticity of the walls of the arteries. This results in

Dementia
An irreversible mental condition in which intellectual abilities are continuously reduced.

Deteriorate
To make or grow worse; degenerate.

altered function of the artery, that is, decreased flow of blood to parts of the body supplied by that artery.

Arthritis — Inflammation of the body joints causing pain, swelling, loss of movement, and changes in structure.

Atherosclerosis — A form of arteriosclerosis in which the arteries become clogged or blocked with various substances, such as plaque and deposits of calcium or fat.

Cataracts — Clouding of the lens of the eye, causing decreased vision.

Cerebral vascular accident (CVA) — Blood supply to the brain is reduced. This may be due to cerebral thrombosis, cerebral embolism, or intracerebral hemorrhage. Also called a *stroke.*

Congestive heart failure — The inability of the heart to pump out all the blood returned to it from the veins. The vital organs of the body do not receive an adequate supply of blood. Signs and symptoms of congestive heart failure are:

- Congestion in the lungs
- Difficulty breathing
- Restlessness, anxiety
- Edema of the legs, feet, hands, face
- Weight gain
- Weakness, fatigue
- Dizziness, confusion
- Chest pain
- Fall
- Confusion

Dementia and delerium — The terms dementia and delerium refer to a large group of acute and chronic mental disorders caused by or associated with brain damage or impaired cerebral function. The causes of dementia include multiple strokes, hardening of the arteries, and Alzheimer's disease. The patient suffering from delerium is often confused as a result of a temporary medical condition such as a fever, dehydration, or infection. Delerium is often misdiagnosed as dementia, but in many cases it is reversible. Signs and symptoms are:

- Loss or decrease in orientation
- Loss of memory
- Decrease in ability to do simple calculations
- Decrease in general information

When the acute condition is treated, the symptoms leave or are reversible. In the chronic stages there is a loss of cells in the cortex of the brain. One of the most common causes of irreversible mental impairment is Alzheimer's disease.

Diabetes mellitus — A disturbance of the carbohydrate metabolism because of an imbalance of the hormone insulin.

Emphysema — The tiny bronchioles of the lungs become plugged with mucus. The lungs becomes less elastic, and air inhaled is trapped in the lungs, making breathing difficult, especially during exhalation. Signs and symptoms of emphysema are:

- Persistent cough (moist cough and wheezing)
- Fatigue
- Loss of appetite
- Weight loss
- Anxiety due to difficult breathing
- Coughing up thick secretions
- Breathing with pursed lips

Fractures — Breaks in bone due to loss of mineralization or injury.

Gallstones	Crystals that settle out of the bile stored in the gallbladder. Stones often block the secretion of bile. This causes pain, nausea, and vomiting. Surgical or nonsurgical removal may be necessary.
Gastritis	Inflammation of the stomach caused by bacteria, viruses, vitamin deficiency, excessive eating, or overindulgence in alcoholic beverages.
Hemorrhoids	Engorged, blood-filled vessels that surround the area of the rectum. Hemorrhoids are painful and may bleed, causing the stool to become blood tinged.
Hypertension	High blood pressure. Signs and symptoms are: ■ Headache ■ Vision changes ■ Problems with urinary output Treatment may include medication, diet, and exercise.
Multiple sclerosis	Muscles lose tone due to damage to the nerves that control them.
Myocardial infarction (heart attack)	Arteries that supply the heart muscle become blocked; the heart muscle does not receive an adequate blood supply and parts of the heart muscle die or infarct.
Parkinson's disease	A chronic disease of the central nervous system, causing tremors in the body. Characterized by a peculiar gait or shuffling of the feet when walking and an expressionless face.
Pneumonia	Acute inflammation or infection in the lungs. Deep breathing and coughing are necessary to prevent the pooling of secretions (hypostatic pneumonia), which is a common condition occurring in geriatric patients who remain in the same position for long periods.
Stomach ulcer	An open sore or lesion that develops on the mucous membrane of the stomach. Ulcers are very painful and require special medications, diets, and occasionally surgical removal.
Urinary incontinence	Inability to control urination. This may be due to arteriosclerosis, which may affect the blood vessels that supply the urinary system. It may also be caused by inability to get to the toilet, or decreased muscle tone (stress, urge, or overflow incontinence).
Varicose veins	Type of vascular disease. The veins are distended or swollen, especially in the legs.

KEY QUESTIONS

1. What are the general physical and emotional characteristics of the geriatric patient?
2. How can you assist with reality orientation for the disoriented patient?
3. How can you create a safe environment for the geriatric patient?
4. How can you safely assist with ambulation?
5. Why is good skin care so essential for the geriatric patient?
6. What can you do to make the bed-bound patient comfortable?
7. What are the most common chronic conditions seen in the geriatric patient? Define each condition.
8. Define: dangling position, dementia, deteriorate, disoriented, flammable, geriatric.

CHAPTER

47

Holistic Approach to Rehabilitation

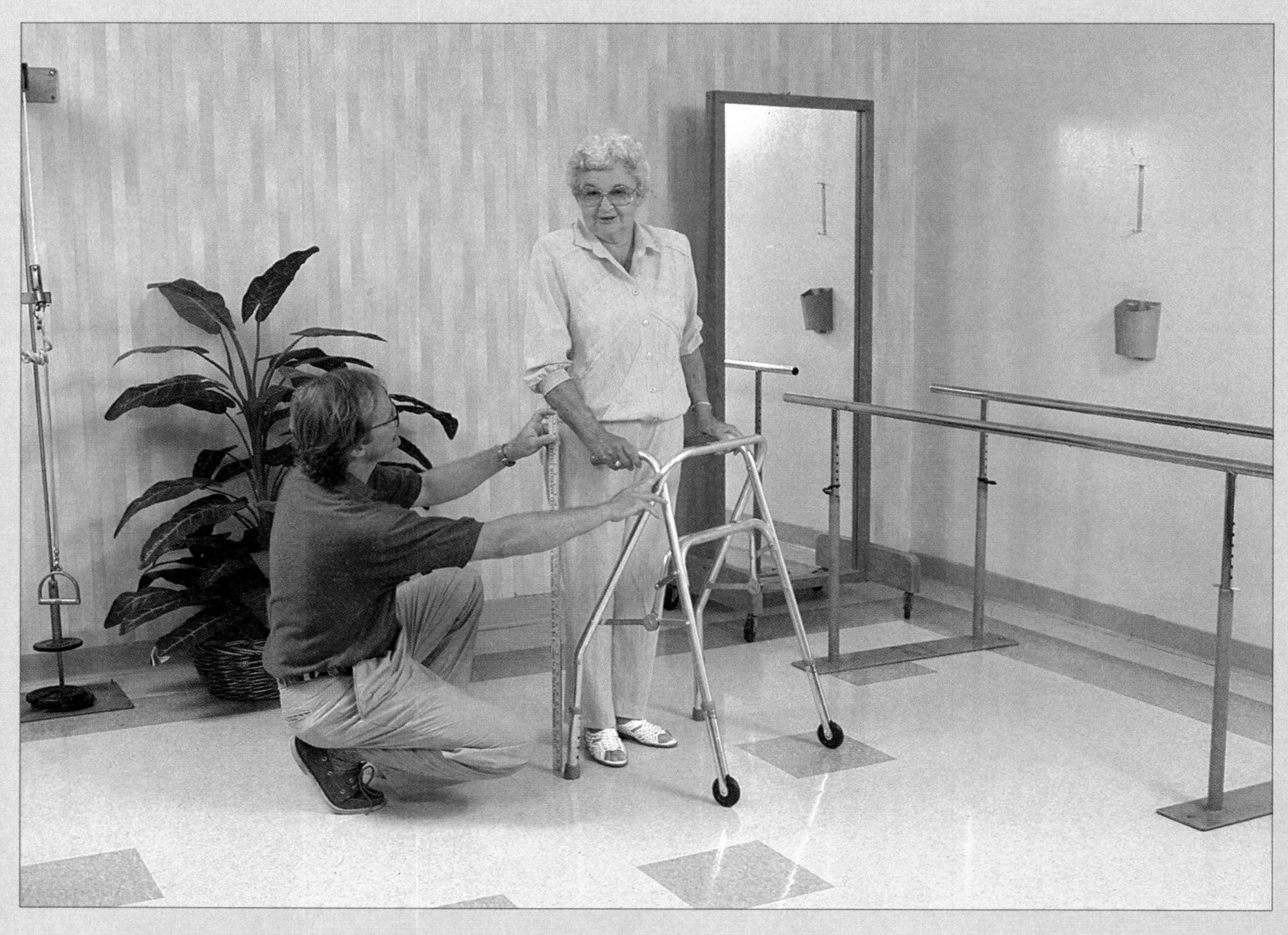

WARNING

For all patient contact, adhere to Universal Precautions. See page 91, 97, or the front cover flap. Wear protective equipment as indicated.

Objectives

What You Will Learn

When you have completed this chapter, you will be able to:

- Explain the goals of a holistic rehabilitation program.
- List the members of the rehabilitation team.
- List ten things the nursing assistant can do to assist the rehabilitation team.
- Describe the role of the nursing assistant in relation to the psychological aspects of rehabilitation.
- Define: depression, fatigue, holistic, motivation, occupational therapist, physical therapist, psychological, psychosocial, and rehabilitation.

KEY IDEAS

Rehabilitation

Rehabilitation
The process by which people who have been disabled by injury or sickness are helped to recover as much as possible of their original abilities for the activities of daily living.

Holistic
An approach to meeting the needs of the whole patient that comes from the belief that human beings function as complete units and cannot be treated part by part. Total of the interacting parts, more than the sum of the parts.

REHABILITATION MEANS HELPING THE PATIENT TO regain a state of health. In the **holistic** approach, the health care team is concerned with every aspect of the patient, not just the disease or ailment for which the patient was admitted to the health care institution. This is a comprehensive effort to restore patients to a medical, physical, psychological, psychosocial, and spiritual state of wellness. The goal is to help patients to do as much as they can, as well as they can, for as long as they can.

Assisting the patient in returning to the optimum level of wellness may require a rehabilitation program. This program is designed to offset the deteriorative effects of physical illness, trauma, and the consequences of:

- Surgery (for example, total hip replacement)
- Inactivity
- Poor positioning for long periods of time
- Lack of weight bearing
- Excessive stress
- Disuse of muscles
- Inability to perform activities of daily living

To restore or rehabilitate requires meeting the total needs of the patient including:

- Physical needs
- Emotional needs
- Social and economic needs
- Spiritual needs

Rehabilitation follows the stage of illness when short- and long-term realistic goals are set for the patient. Rehabilitation includes the patient's acceptance of learning to accomplish small goals. Sometimes a complete cure is not possible. However, the patient must come to enjoy the rewards from any small progress that is made. Skills are acquired or relearned through repetition and practice. As patients reach goals and become more independent, they will feel better about themselves and will attempt to reach additional goals. The nursing assistant should encourage patients, praise their accomplishments, remind them of what has been taught and accomplished, and report their reactions to the immediate supervisor.

KEY IDEAS

Pediatric Rehabilitation

Usually the process of rehabilitation in children is easier than in adults because of the child's age and their stage in growth and development. Learning the activities of daily living for children often requires a first learning, since they have not had the experience of being able to do many things for themselves yet. Because children are so adaptable, they can easily learn ways to compensate for their disabilities. For example, a child who was born with a certain kind of spinal defect may never be able to kick a football, but may learn to be an expert swimmer. A child who is born with a deformed limb learns to regard it as a natural part of his or her developing self-image.

The child's natural curiosity can be very helpful in the rehabilitation process. Where this curiosity may have caused an accident, as in the example of a child getting burned while playing with matches, this same curiosity can get the child interested in his or her treatment. A positive attitude on the part of the nursing assistant will encourage these same positive attitudes in the child and his or her family. Praise them for what they have done well and help them when they seem to need assistance. Always focus on the child's possibilities, not their disabilities.

KEY IDEAS

The Professional Rehabilitation Team

Physical Therapist
Trained person who assists the patient with activities related to motion.

Occupational Therapist
Trained person who assists the patient with performing activities of daily living.

- Rehabilitation nurse
- Rehabilitation psychologist
- Social worker
- Cardiac rehabilitation nurse
- Staff nurse
- Nursing assistant
- Speech therapist
- Recreational therapist
- Vocational counselor
- **Physical therapist**
- Physician that treats the acute condition (for example, cardiologist, orthopedist, neurologist, internist, or family practitioner)
- Individual professional personnel, where indicated
- Patient educator
- **Occupational therapist**
- Physiatrist or doctor of physical medicine and rehabilitation
- Spiritual counselor (priest, minister, or rabbi)

The nursing assistant will assist various members of the rehabilitation team when they work with the patient by:

- Repeating exercises with the patient to achieve the best result possible.
- Maintaining a safe environment
- Offering psychological support

- Contributing information about the patient's condition and progress
- Observing the patient
- Listening to the patient
- Establishing a relationship with the patient
- Maintaining a positive attitude
- Letting the patient know you expect her or him to regain some degree of independent activity within the limitations of the disease or injury.
- Motivating the patient to achieve the highest possible level of wellness

KEY IDEAS

Psychological Aspects

Psychological
All aspects of the mind, such as feelings and thoughts.

Depression
Low spirits that may or may not cause a change in activity.

Fatigue
A feeling of tiredness or weariness.

Depression

The nursing assistant must report signs of depression, which include:

- Pessimism
- Unhappiness
- Low self-esteem
- Withdrawal or personality changes
- Loss of interest
- Loss of appetite or excessive appetite.
- Constant **fatigue**
- Slow movement or constant movement
- Excessive irritability

Motivation
The reason, desire, need, or purpose that causes one to do something.

Motivation

The nursing assistant should try to:

- Involve the patient in recreational activities to provide a creative change of pace (Figure 47-1)
- Involve the patient in programs where the decisions are made by the patient

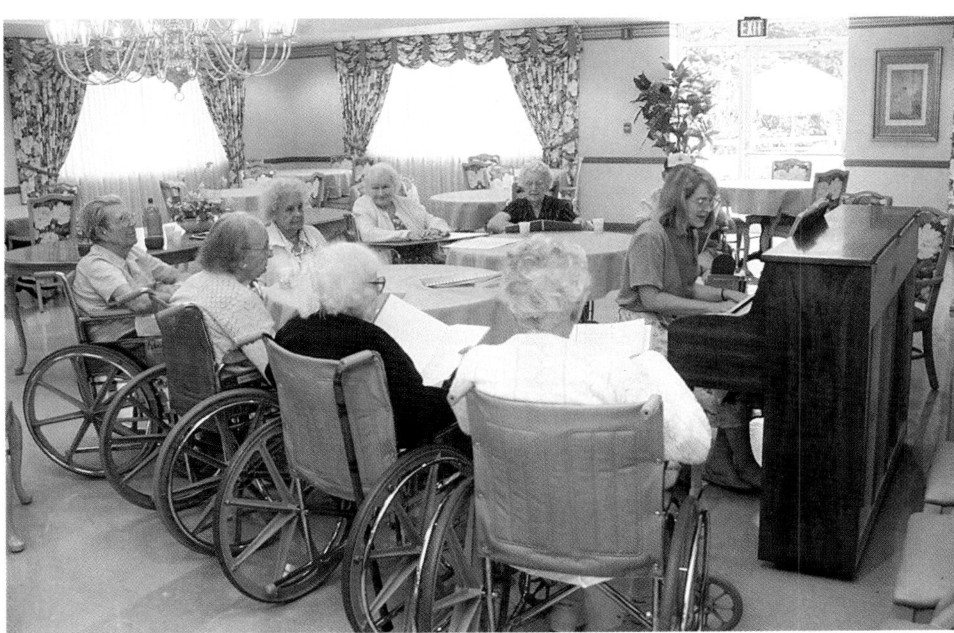

FIGURE 47-1 The nursing assistant should encourage the patient to participate in social activities.

- Constantly display a positive attitude toward rehabilitation and the patient's success
- Establish a genuine relationship with the patient by listening, understanding, and respecting the patient's individuality
- Report every change of condition and mental attitude to the immediate supervisor

Psychosocial
All aspects of living together in a group with other human beings.

Psychosocial Aspects of Rehabilitative Care

The nursing assistant will report the following signs and symptoms of potential **psychosocial** problems to the rehabilitation nurse or his or her immediate supervisor.

- Depression or discouragement
- Hopelessness or isolation
- Fear or distrustfulness
- Extreme hostility, anger, demanding behavior
- Total dependency without any effort toward self-care
- Apathy or hyperactivity

The rehabilitation team will write a plan of social activity for each patient individually. Under the team's directions, the nursing assistant's role will be outlined. To develop a good patient-nurse relationship, the nursing assistant will encourage the patient to:

- Actively participate in this plan of social therapy
- Participate in a variety of activities such as reading the daily newspaper, discussing the news, listening to the radio, or watching TV.
- Interact with the patient's support group (family, friends, and so on) through discussions, socialization, games, and so on
- Develop a feeling of belonging, self-respect, self-fulfillment, and responsibility for his or her own feelings and actions
- Tolerate stress in varying degrees and, in so doing, develop a stronger belief in his or her ability to regain functional independence

Rehabilitation services include:

- Medical care
- Surgical care
- Occupational therapy
- Rehabilitation nursing services
- Social services
- Speech therapy
- Prosthetic and orthotic services
- Psychological care
- Volunteer services
- Recreational activity
- Education, including both remedial and continuing
- Outpatient diagnostic and therapeutic services
- Inpatient diagnostic and therapeutic services
- Medical and paramedical services for acute and chronic rehabilitative care
- Vocational counseling

- Podiatry care
- Dental services
- Nutritional services
- Pastoral services
- Beautician services

KEY QUESTIONS

1. What are the goals of a holistic rehabilitation program?
2. Who are the members of the rehabilitation team?
3. What are ten things the nursing assistant can do to assist the rehabilitation team?
4. What is the role of the nursing assistant in relation to the psychological aspects of rehabilitation?
5. Define: depression, fatigue, holistic, motivation, occupational therapist, physical therapist, psychological, psychosocial, rehabilitation.

CHAPTER

48
Range of Motion

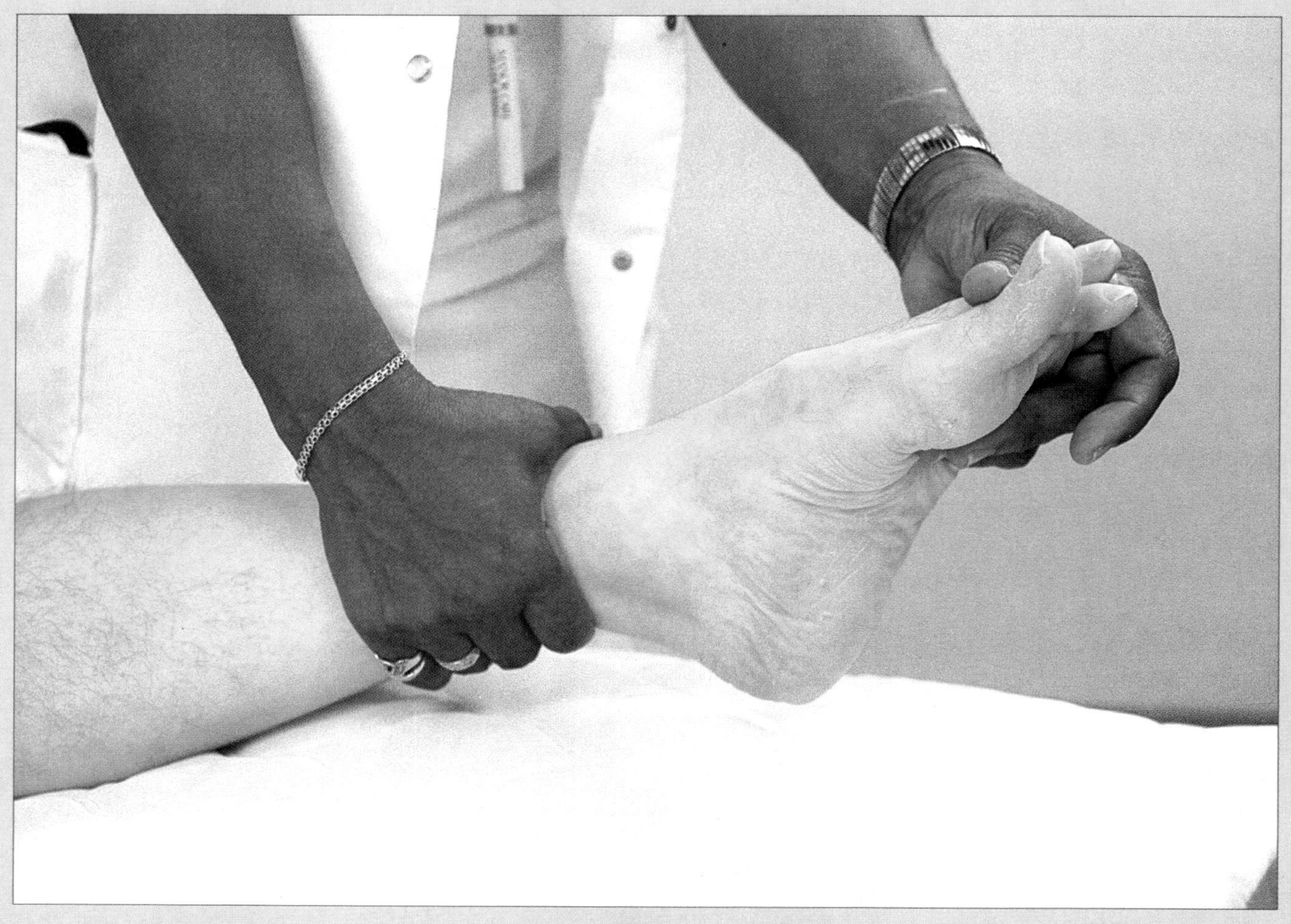

WARNING

For all patient contact, adhere to Universal Precautions. See page 91, 97, or the front cover flap. Wear protective equipment as indicated.

Objectives

What You Will Learn

When you have completed this chapter, you will be able to:

- Explain the principles and rules of range of motion exercises.
- Perform complete or partial range of motion exercises with a patient.
- Define: abduction, adduction, dorsal flexion, extension, flexion, hyperextension, pronation, range of motion, rotation, and supination.

KEY IDEAS

Range of Motion

Range of motion (ROM)
These exercises move each muscle and joint through its full range of motion and assist the patient who is confined to exercise her or his muscles and joints.

Pronation
To turn palm downward.

Supination
To turn palm upward.

Dorsal Flexion
To bend backward.

A PATIENT WHO IS CONFINED TO BED or is unable to get out of bed will not be getting the exercise she or he needs. Therefore, it may become necessary for the nursing assistant to help the patient exercise muscles and joints. This is accomplished through **range of motion** exercises (ROM). These exercises move each muscle and joint through its full range of motion using the basic movements of adduction, abduction, extension, hyperextension, **pronation**, **supination**, flexion, **dorsal flexion**, and rotation.

Your part in range of motion exercises will depend on the patient's level of ability and the physician's orders. According to these criteria range of motion exercises will be one of the following types:

- *Active Range of Motion (AROM):* The patient is able to move his limbs through their range of motion by himself.
- *Passive Range of Motion (PROM):* The nursing assistant moves the patient's limbs through the range of motion because the patient is unable, for whatever reason, to do it himself.
- *Active Assist Range of Motion (AAROM)*: The patient participates to the extent that he is able.

Rules to Follow

RANGE OF MOTION EXERCISES

- Do each exercise three times. (Follow the supervisor's instructions.)
- Follow a logical sequence so that each joint and muscle is exercised. For instance, start at the head and work your way down to the feet.
- If the patient is able to move parts of his body, encourage him to do as much as he can.
- Be gentle. Never bend or extend a body part farther than it can go.
- If a patient complains of unusual pain or discomfort in a particular body part, be sure to report this to your immediate supervisor.

Procedure Range of Motion Exercises

1. Assemble your equipment:
   a) Blanket
   b) Extra lighting, if necessary.
2. Wash your hands.
3. Identify the patient by checking the identification bracelet.
4. Ask visitors to step out of the room, if this is your hospital's policy.
5. Explain to the patient that you are going to help him exercise his muscles and joints while he is in bed.
6. Pull the curtain around the bed for privacy.
7. Raise the bed to a comfortable working position.
8. Place the patient in a supine position (on his back) with his knees extended and his arms at his side.
9. Loosen the top sheets, but don't expose the patient.
10. Raise the side rail on the far side of the bed.
11. Exercise the neck (Figures 48-1, 48-2, and 48-3).

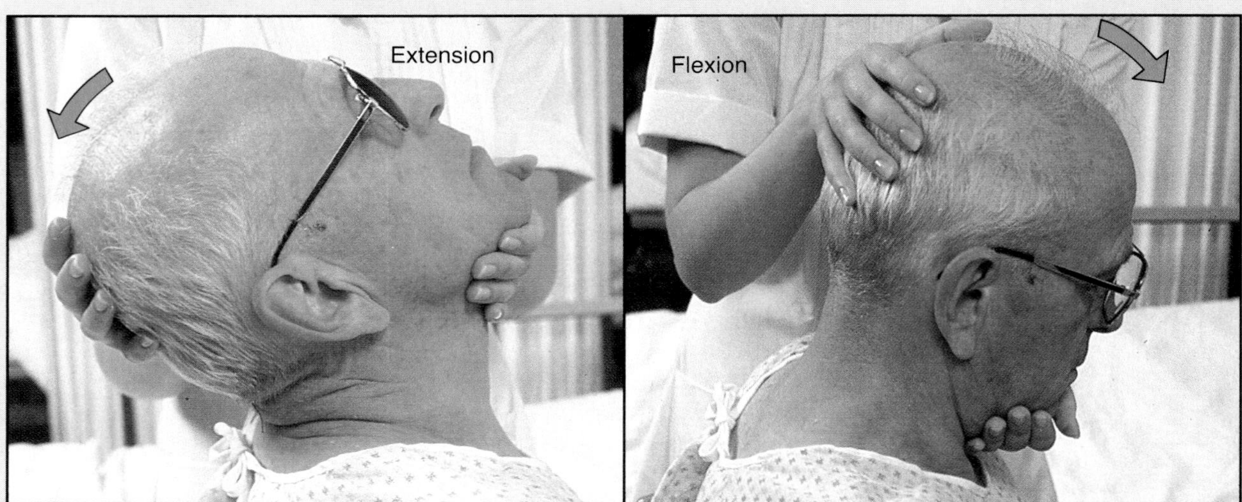

FIGURE 48-1

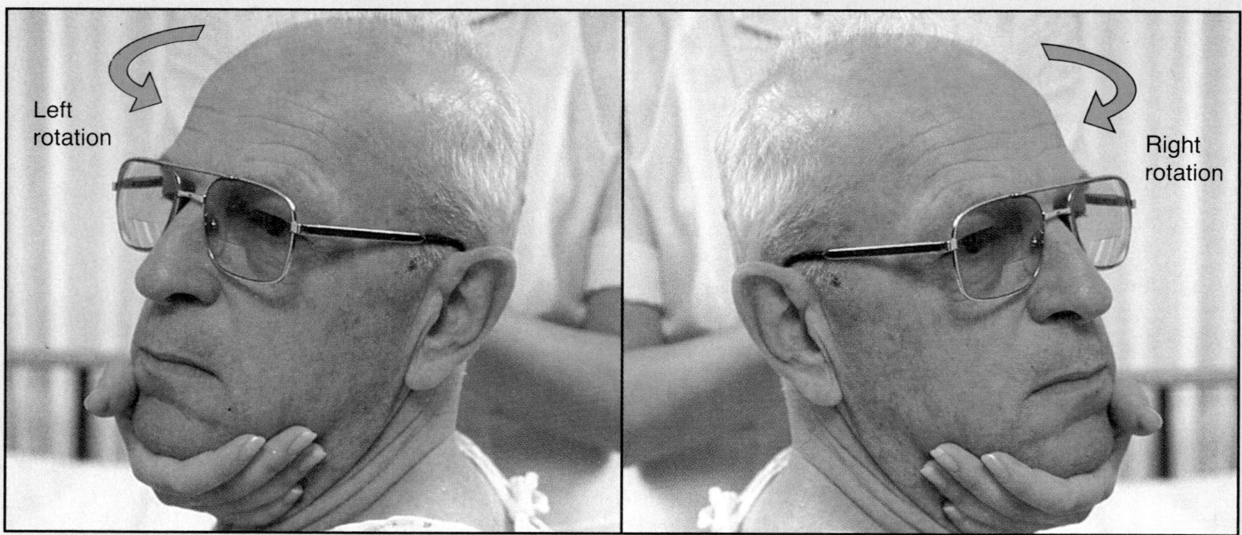

FIGURE 48-2

Extension
To straighten an arm or leg.

Flexion
To bend a joint (elbow, wrist, knee).

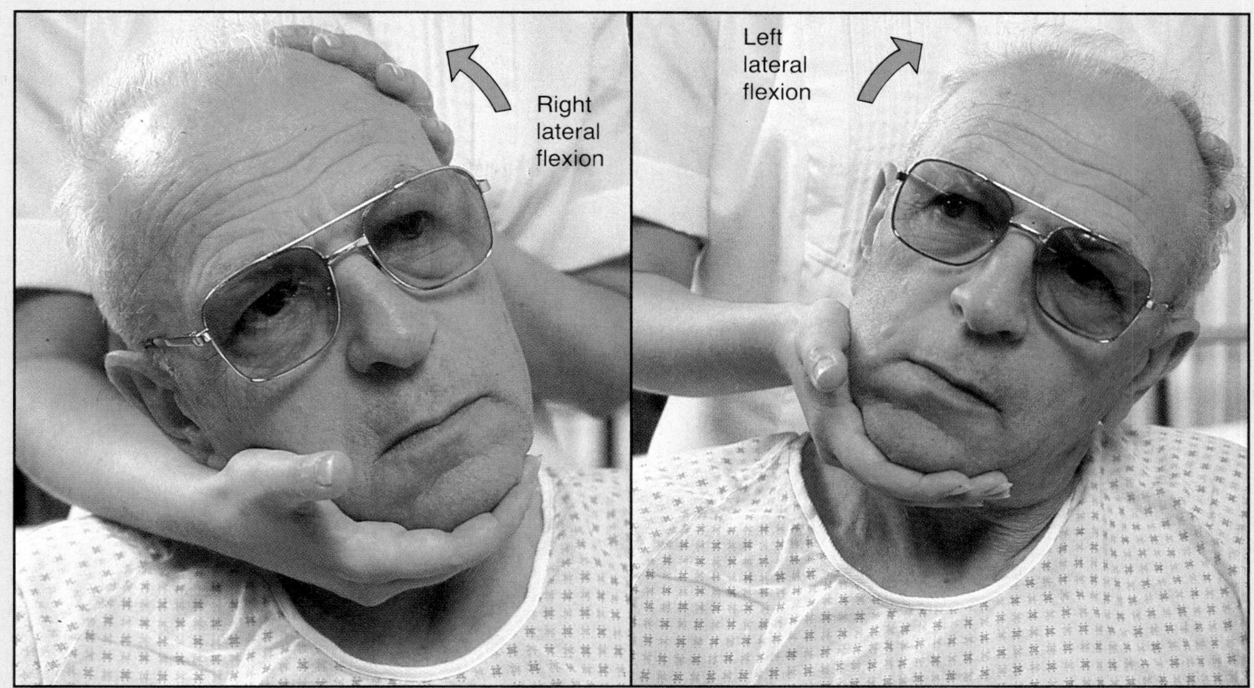

FIGURE 48-3

12. Hold the extremity to be exercised at the joint (for example, the knee, wrist, elbow).

13. Exercise each shoulder (Figures 48-4 and 48-5).

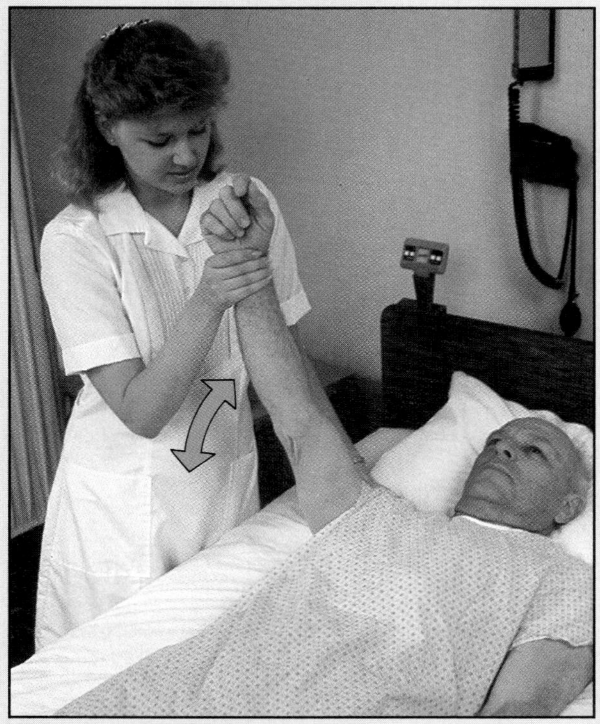

FIGURE 48-4

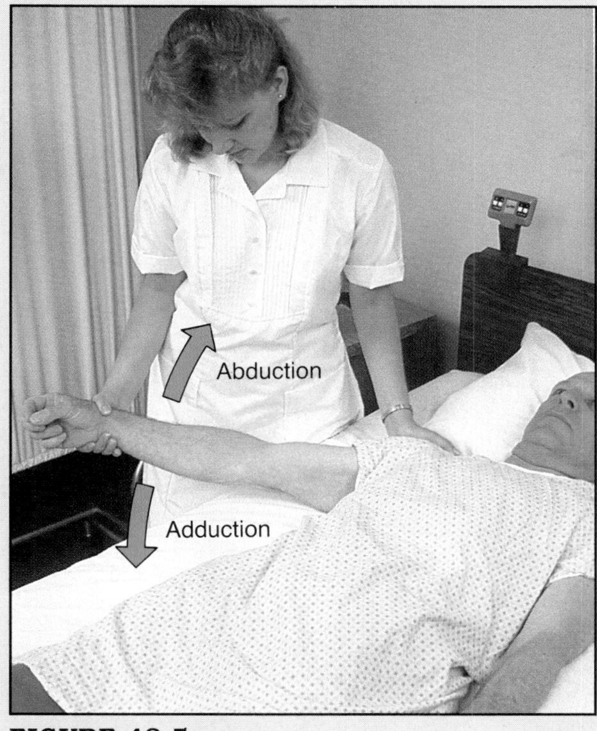

FIGURE 48-5

Rotation
To move a joint in a circular motion around its axis: internal, to turn in toward the center; external, to turn out away from the center.

14. Exercise each elbow (Figure 48-6).

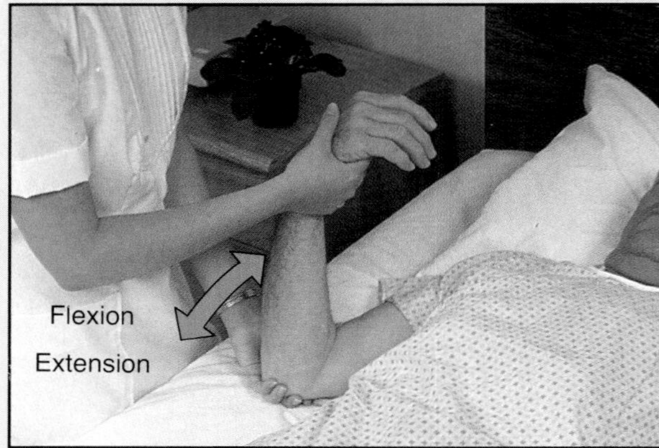

FIGURE 48-6

15. Exercise each wrist (Figures 48-7 and 48-8).

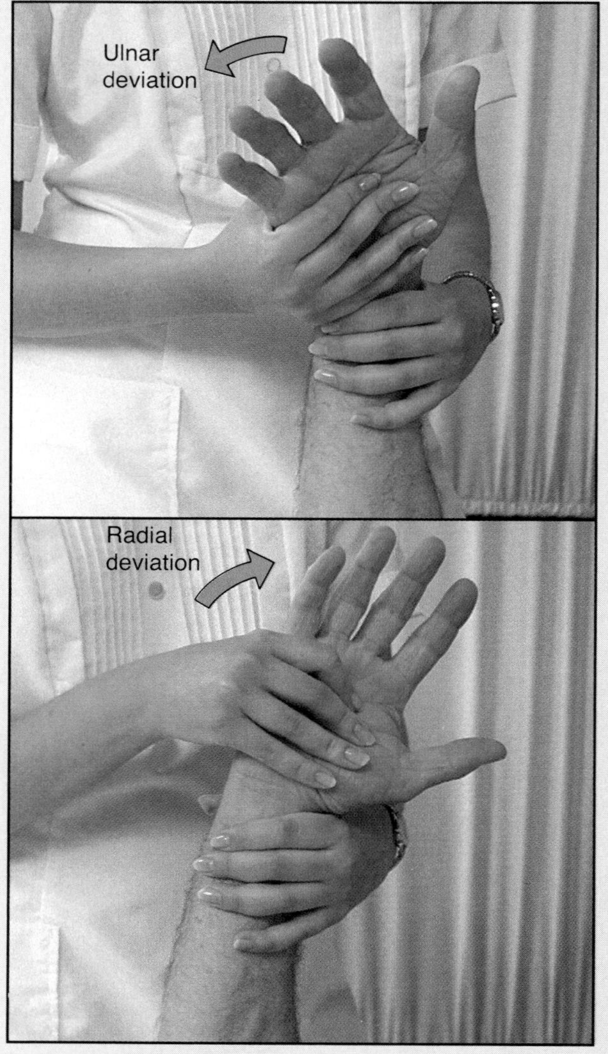

FIGURE 48-7

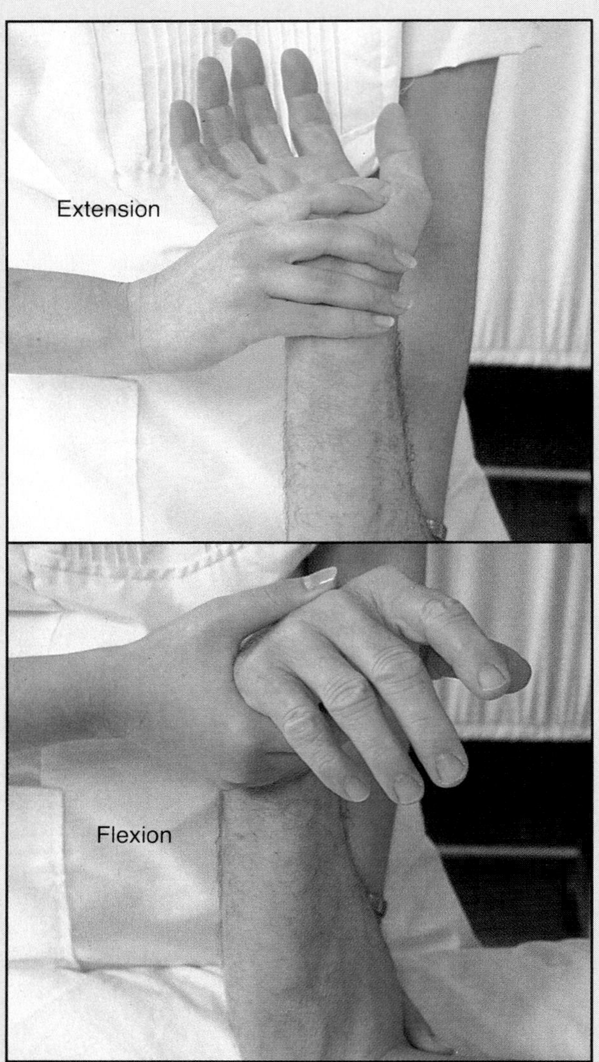

FIGURE 48-8

16. Exercise each finger (Figures 48-9, 48-10, and 48-11).

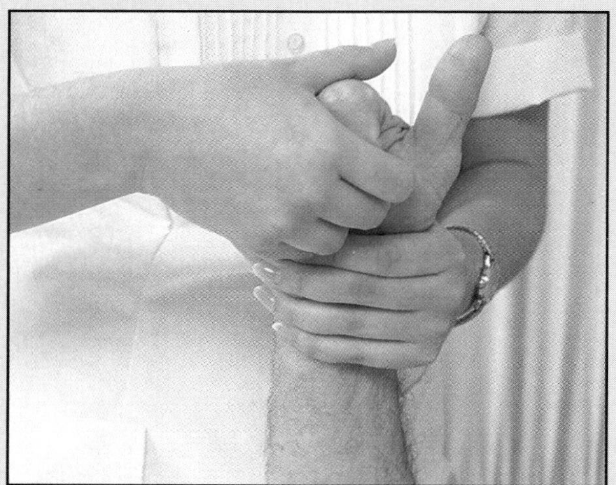

FIGURE 48-9

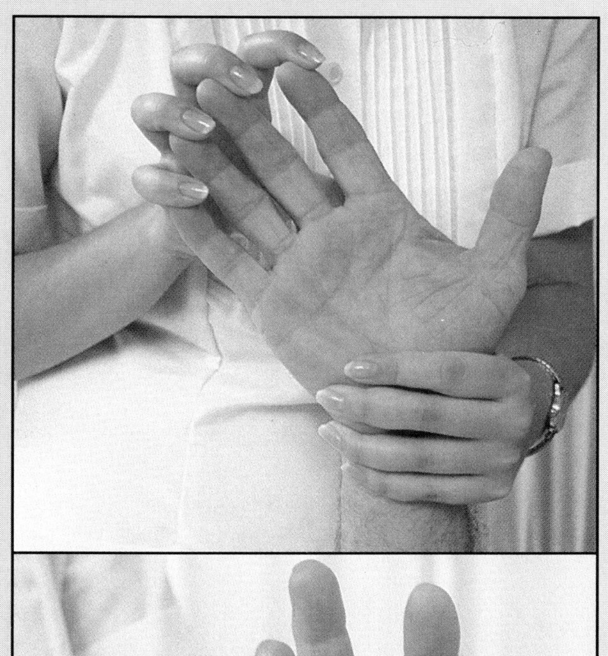

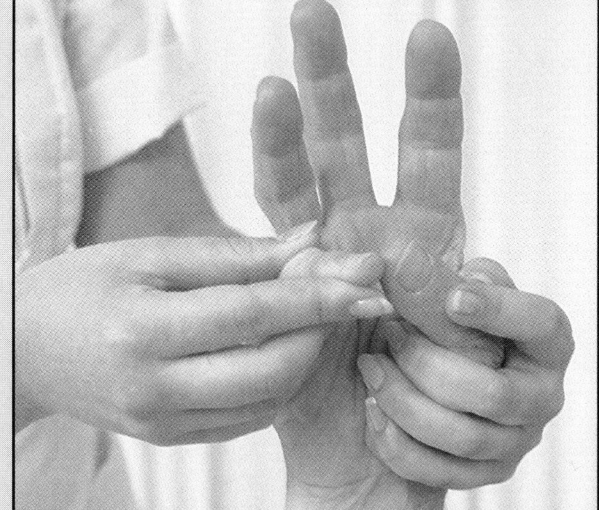

FIGURE 48-10

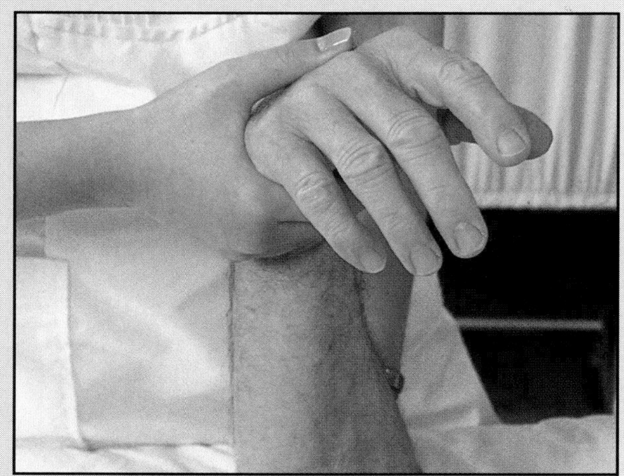

FIGURE 48-11

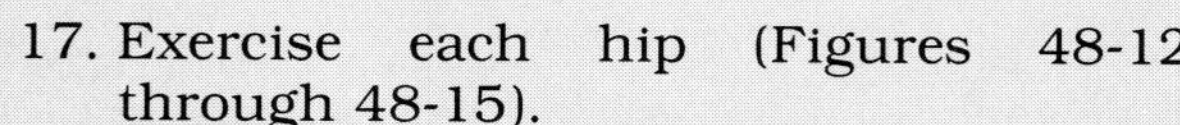

17. Exercise each hip (Figures 48-12 through 48-15).

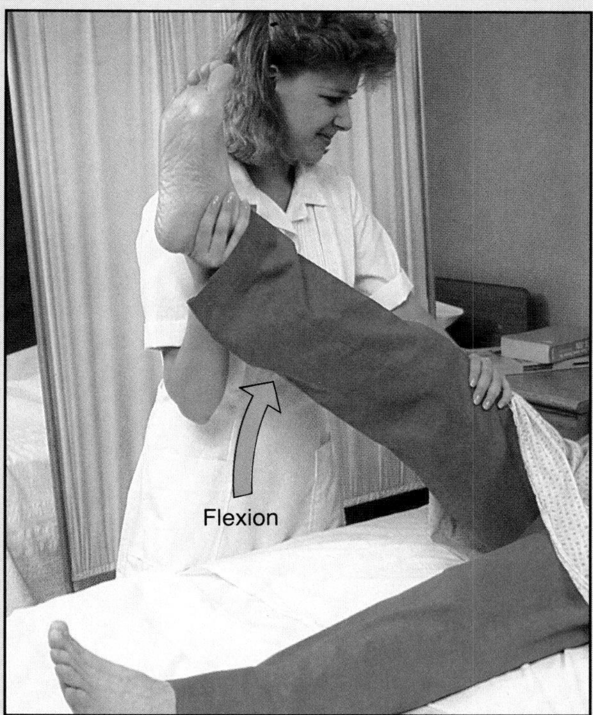

FIGURE 48-12

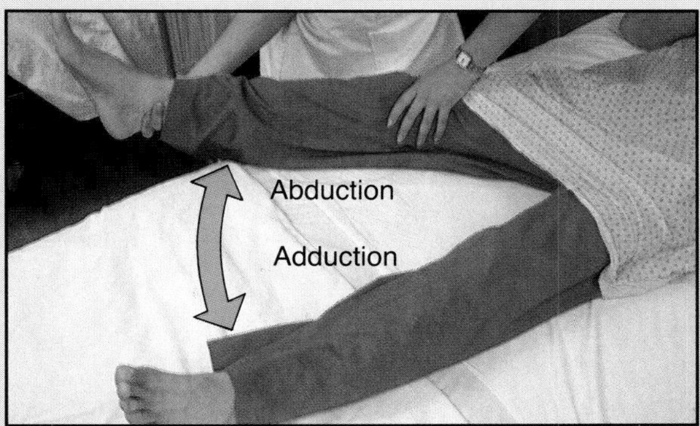

FIGURE 48-13

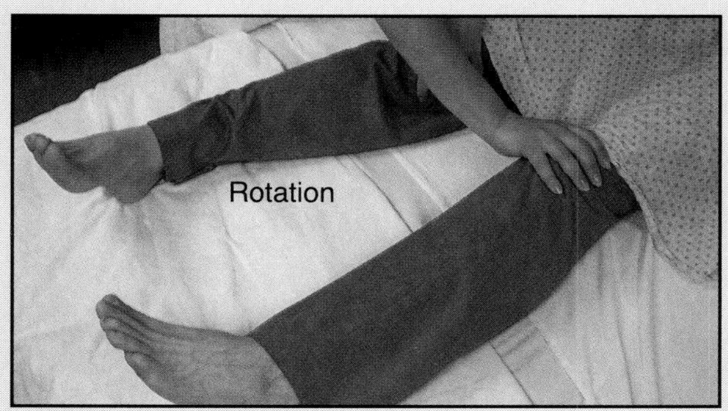

FIGURE 48-14

Abduction
To move an arm or leg away from the center of the body.

Adduction
To move an arm or leg toward the center of the body.

Hyperextension
Beyond the normal extension.

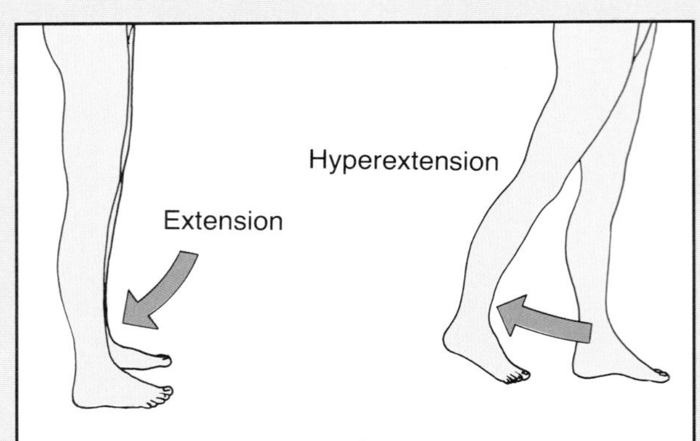

FIGURE 48-15

18. Exercise each knee (Figure 48-16).

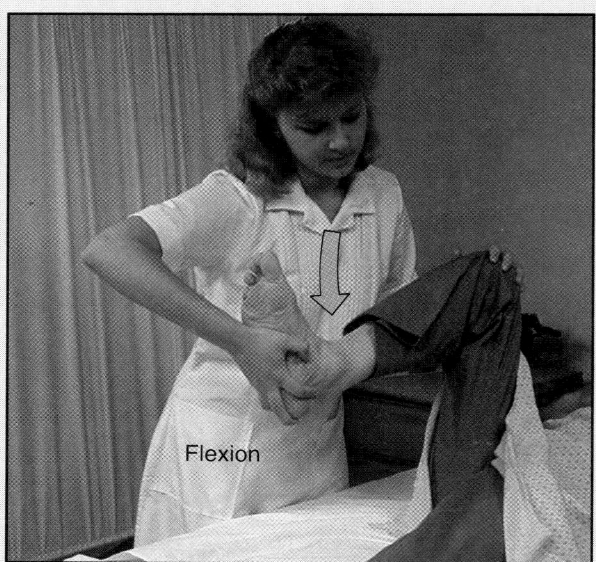

FIGURE 48-16

19. Exercise each ankle (Figures 48-17 and 48-18).

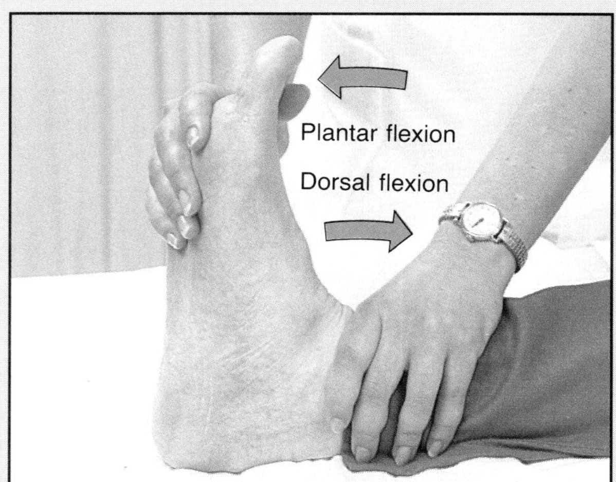

FIGURE 48-17

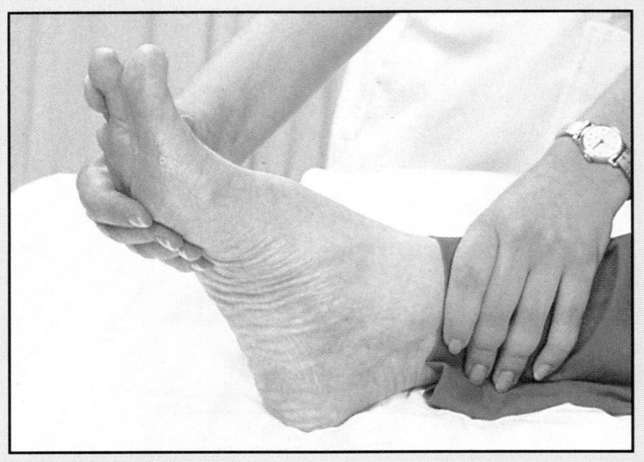

FIGURE 48-18

20. Exercise each toe (Figures 48-19 and 48-20).

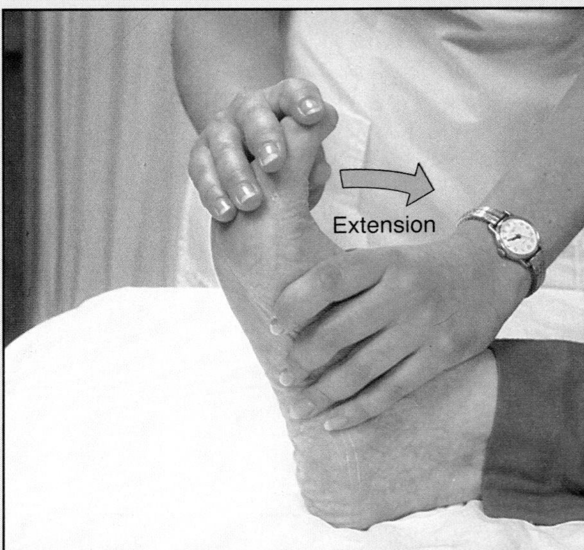

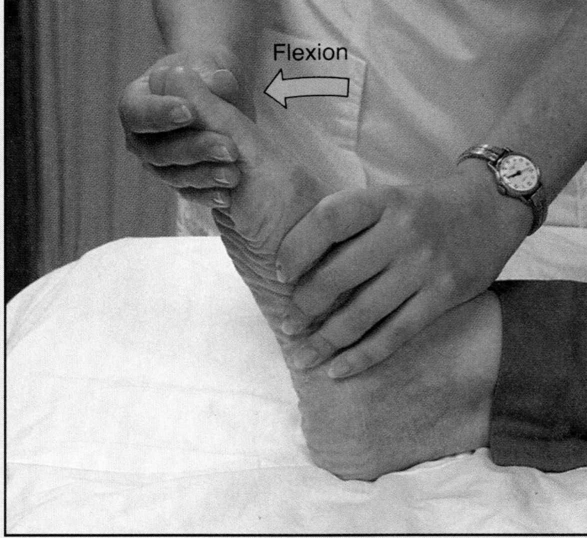

FIGURE 48-19

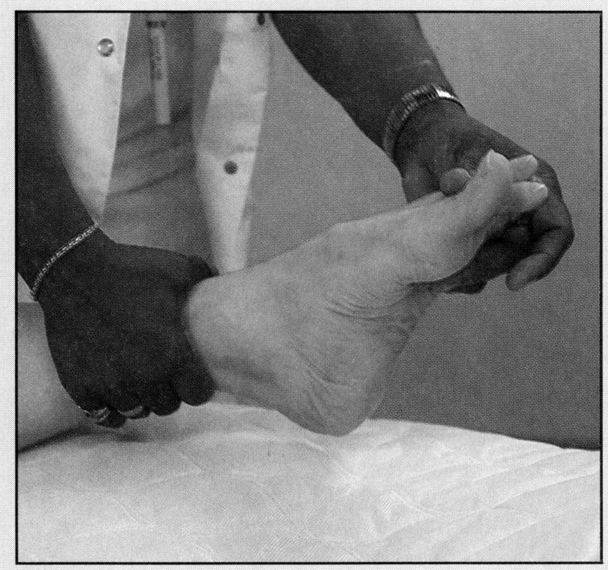

FIGURE 48-20

21. Make the patient comfortable.
22. Replace the sheets if a blanket was used. Fold and return the blanket to its proper place.
23. Lower the bed to a position of safety for the patient.
24. Pull the curtains back to the open position.
25. Raise the side rails where ordered, indicated, and appropriate for patient safety.
26. Place the call light within easy reach of the patient.
27. Be sure the signal cord is within the patient's easy reach.
28. Replace any extra lighting to its proper place after washing with an antiseptic or disinfectant solution.
29. Wash your hands.
30. Report to your immediate supervisor:
    - That you have completed range of motion exercises with the patient
    - The time the exercises were done
    - How the patient tolerated the exercises
    - Your observations of anything unusual

KEY QUESTIONS

1. What are the principles and rules of range of motion exercises?
2. How should range of motion exercises, both complete and partial, be performed?
3. Define: abduction, adduction, dorsal flexion, extension, flexion, hyperextension, pronation, range of motion, rotation, supination.

CHAPTER

49

Return to Self-care

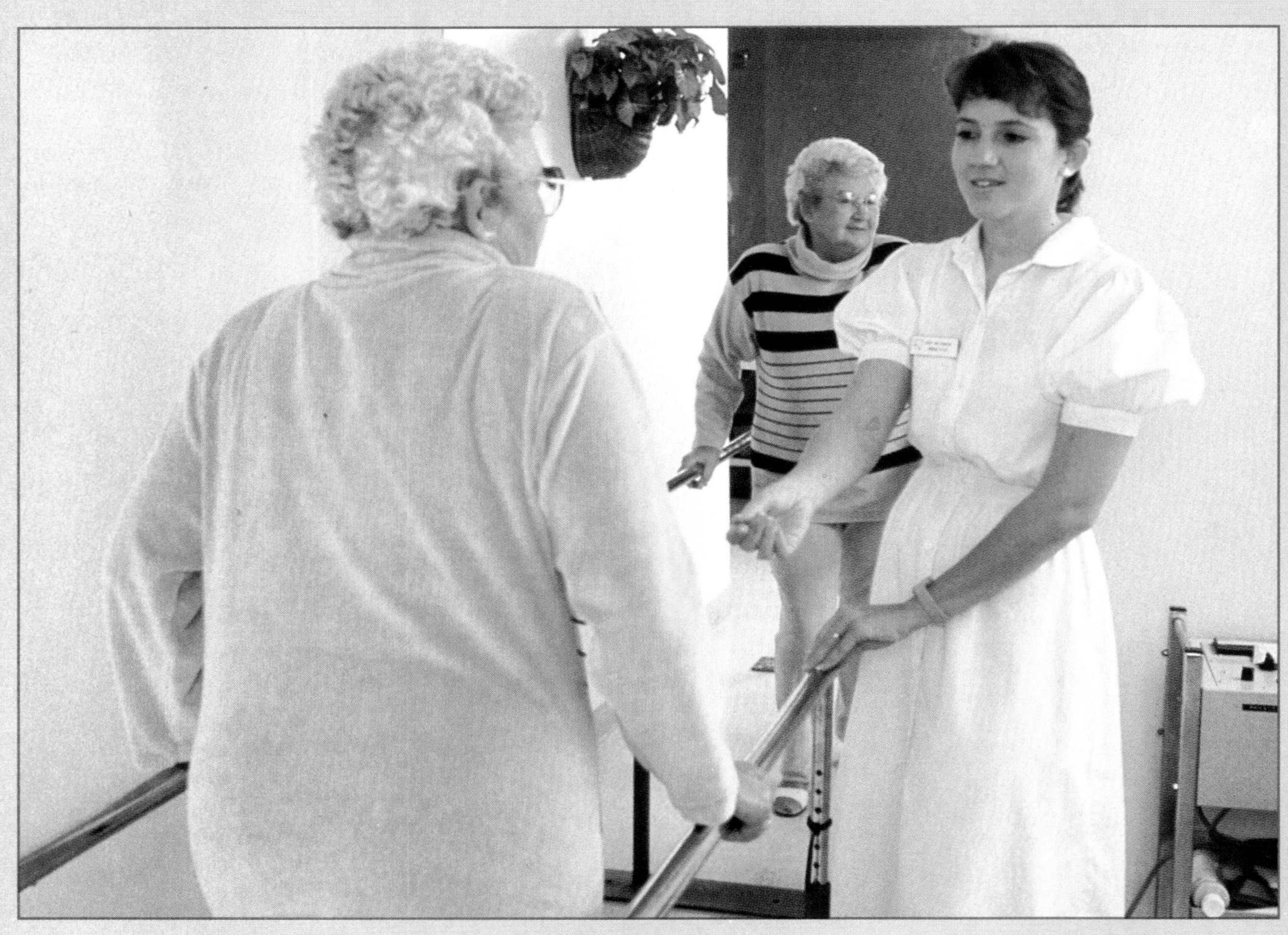

WARNING

For all patient contact, adhere to Universal Precautions. See page 91, 97, or the front cover flap. Wear protective equipment as indicated.

Objectives

What You Will Learn

When you have completed this chapter, you will be able to:

- Describe the roles of the rehabilitation nurse, the occupational therapist, the physical therapist, and the nursing assistant in helping the patient return to self-care.
- Assist the handicapped patient to bathe.
- Assist the handicapped patient with dressing and grooming.
- Assist the handicapped patient to eat.
- Assist with bowel and bladder rehabilitation and retraining for the incontinent patient.
- Insert rectal suppositories.
- Define: active, incontinence, mobilization, passive, suppository.

KEY IDEAS

The Role of the Rehabilitation Nurse

WHEN THE REHABILITATION NURSE ESTABLISHES A routine for the patient, the following patient needs will be taken into consideration:

- Physical
- Psychological
- Socioeconomic
- Spiritual
- Environmental

The rehabilitation nurse will then write a plan of care. This plan can measure and outline how long each step of rehabilitation will take. It will include all the members of the rehabilitation team, the patient, and the patient's family or significant order. Some factors taken into consideration during this planning session will be:

Active
Producing, involving, or participating in activity or movement.

Passive
Not active, but acted upon; enduring without effort or resistance.

- How much **active** or **passive** motion does the patient have
- The patient's sensory deficits in vision, hearing, speech, touch, and balance
- The patient's perception of his or her disability
- The patient's attitude, which will include:
  - Depression
  - Euphoria
  - Anger
  - Cooperation
  - Resentfulness
  - Frustration
  - Motivation
  - Acceptance of what has happened to him or her
- The patient's ability and what he will attempt to do for himself

- The patient's previous level of functioning prior to becoming disabled
- The patient's priorities
- The patient's barriers
- The available support system

KEY IDEAS

The Role of the Occupational Therapist and Activities of Daily Living

Mobilization
Making movable; putting into motion.

The occupational therapist focuses on increasing the functional ability of the patient within her or his environment. The therapist will teach the patient to work with and learn to adapt to new skills. The patient will be taught to take an active part in her or his daily care. The general areas in which the occupational therapist works are:

- **Mobilization:** Teaching the patient techniques to use to change position or to reach, grasp, or turn while sitting, or to maintain balance during an activity.
- **Activities of daily living tasks:** Teaching the patient tasks to be performed each day, such as toileting, bathing, dressing, feeding, grooming, homemaking, and leisure activities.
- **Coordination, strength, and activity tolerance:** Teaching the patient techniques to conserve his energy, to perform the task to meet his own satisfaction, and to use all his physical resources to the fullest without tiring quickly.

KEY IDEAS

The Nursing Assistant's Role in Assisting the Occupational Therapist

The nursing assistant will assist the occupational therapist by:

- Completely understanding what the patient is allowed to do
- Assisting the patient to perform activities of daily living as taught by the occupational therapist
- Assisting the patient to function independently following the occupational therapist's instructions
- Keeping the environment safe
- Discussing the outside world with the patient with regard to:
  - Change of seasons
  - What is happening in the community
  - Sports or other activity that the patient is interested in
- Involving the patient in the whole world
- Assisting the patient with daily needs by making them accessible
- Reporting observations of the patient to the occupational therapist:
  - Signs of pain
  - Signs of being tired
  - Signs of achievement of each task
  - Patient's tolerance of each procedure
  - Each time the patient attempts a newly taught procedure

Rules To Follow

BATHING THE HANDICAPPED PATIENT

- Do not attempt any technique that has not been taught or outlined to you or to the patient by the occupational therapist, head nurse, or team leader.
- Provide a safe environment.
- Assemble all equipment, placing it where the patient can reach it.
- Thin washcloths and small face towels may be easier for the patient to use.

- Place soap on a dampened sponge or face cloth where it will be less likely to slide.
- Assist the patient or permit the patient to undress following the instructions of the occupational therapist or your immediate supervisor.
- Always wash the involved arm first, reminding the patient to rinse off the soap and dry each part of the body, if he is washing in bed or at a sink.
- If the patient is learning to turn on the water faucets, be sure he turns the cold water on first to avoid burns.
- Wash the areas the patient cannot reach.

Rules To Follow

DRESSING AND GROOMING

People feel better about themselves when they are dressed. Even the wheelchair-bound or partially bed-bound patient should be encouraged to dress in street clothes. When the dependent person is up and dressed, it affects not only his feelings of self-esteem, but also his family's perceptions about his health. Let the patient select clothing and do as much of the dressing as is possible, no matter how long it takes. Always dress the weak or most involved extremity first and undress the weak or involved extremity last. Position the patient in front of a mirror and encourage a female patient to put on makeup. The occupational therapist may suggest certain tools to assist the patient to care for himself (Figures 49-1 and 49-2).

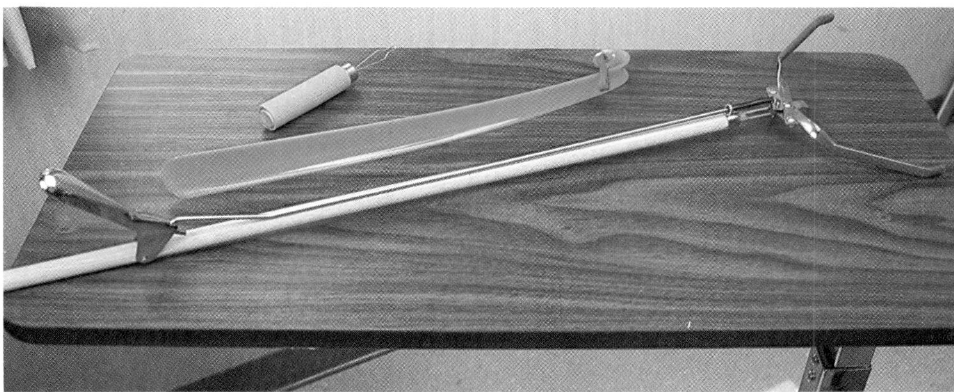

FIGURE 49-1 Tools to assist the patient in dressing himself.

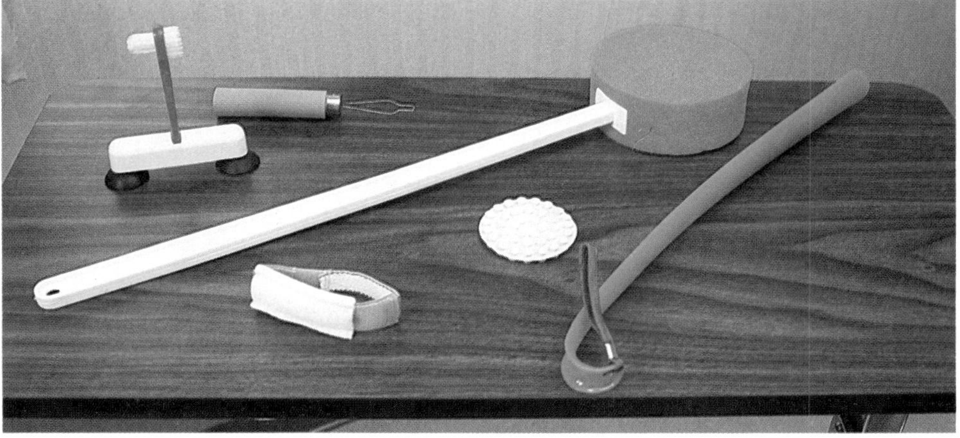

FIGURE 49-2 Tools to assist the patient in dressing, grooming, and bathing himself.

FIGURE 49-3
Equipment to aid the patient in feeding herself.

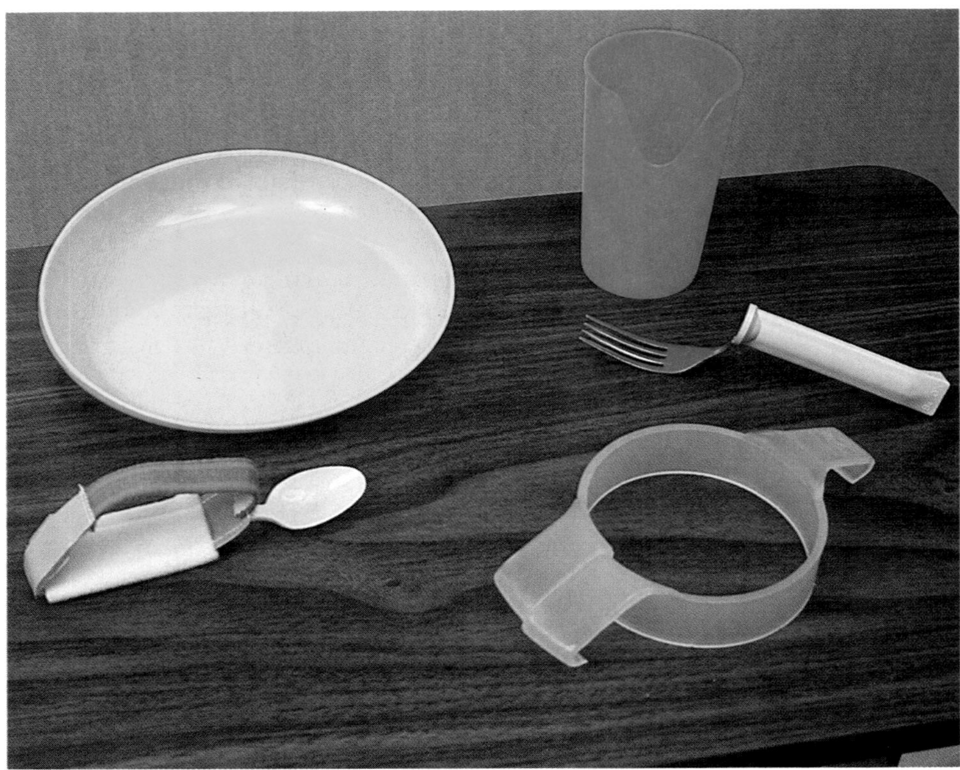

KEY IDEAS

Feeding the Handicapped Patient

- The nursing assistant should plan mealtimes so that the patient can use her available resources and feed herself partially or completely.
- The patient will eat more and feel better emotionally and physically when she can feed herself.
- The occupational therapist will assist the patient to gain many of the motor skills needed to perform this activity of daily living, which will motivate the patient to perform other activities of daily living skills.
- Set up the tray or table so tht it is convenient and attractive to the patient.
- The occupational therapist may suggest enlarging the gripping surface of the utensils so the patient can hold and lift the utensil. A plate guard, a plastic ring that slips over the edge of a plate and creates a bumper for the patient to push food against, may be one suggestion. This will make it easier for her to pick up her food (Figure 49-3).
- Use cups with handles to help the patient hold the cup to take a drink by herself.
- Food should be easy to chew and easy to swallow.
- Encourage family or friends to join the patient during a meal. This will help make the patient more independent when eating.
- Patients who have sensory deficits that affect eating may lack sensation if the facial muscles are weak on one side. This will affect the way they eat. If they cannot swallow easily, they may tend to pocket food between their cheeks and teeth on the involved side of their face. This can cause them to gag and choke as the food builds up. Place a mirror in front of the patient to enable her to use her eyes to make her aware of what occurs when she eats. The patient may begin to automatically wipe her mouth or to search with her tongue to dislodge stored food that remains on her lips.

KEY IDEAS

Bowel and Bladder Rehabilitation for the Incontinent Patient

Incontinence
The inability to control the bowels or bladder. An incontinent person cannot control urination or defecation.

Incontinent patients are those who have lost all or part of their control over their excretory functions. In some cases of **incontinence**, bladder or bowel training rehabilitation may be used to help the patient regain some or all of this control. Offering the patient the bedpan or urinal at regularly scheduled intervals may help the patient avoid incontinence.

If prescribed by the physician, a rectal **suppository** ordered on a regular schedule can help train the patient to empty his rectum while he is on the bedpan. Follow the instructions of your immediate supervisor for the time and type of suppository to be used. Follow the procedure for the insertion of the suppository.

Procedure Bowel and Bladder Rehabilitation and Training of the Incontinent Patient

1. Assemble your equipment:
   a) Urinal, if appropriate
   b) Bedpan or bedside commode
   c) Container of warm water at 105°F (40.5°C)
   d) Towel
   e) Suppositories, as ordered by the physician
2. Wash your hands.
3. Identify the patient by checking the identification bracelet.
4. Ask visitors to step out of the room, if this is your hospital's policy.
5. Tell the patient that you are going to assist him onto a bedpan, bedside commode, or toilet.
6. Pull the curtain for privacy.
7. Raise the bed to a comfortable working position.
8. Place the patient on a bedpan, on the bedside commode, or walk him to the bathroom every 2 hours to stimulate evacuation of the bowel and bladder.
9. Pour warm water at 105°F (40.5°C) over the genital area into the bedpan to stimulate elimination, if the patient has difficulty in voiding.
10. Insert a rectal suppository, using the approved procedure, as ordered by a physician.
11. Dry the patient with toilet tissue.
12. Remove the bedpan.
13. Help the patient back into bed from the bedside commode or toilet.
14. Wash the patient's hands.
15. Make the patient comfortable.
16. Lower the bed to a position of safety for the patient.
17. Pull the curtains back to the open position.
18. Raise the side rails where ordered, indicated, and appropriate for patient safety.
19. Place the call light within easy reach of the patient.
20. Wash your hands.
21. Report to your immediate supervisor:
    - That the patient was placed on the bedpan, commode, or toilet on a regular basis
    - The time this was done
    - If the patient urinated or moved his bowels into the bedpan, commode, or toilet
    - How the patient tolerated the procedure
    - Your observations of anything unusual

KEY IDEAS

Rectal Suppositories

Rectal suppositories are inserted into the rectum to aid in elimination, to assist in healing, to relieve pain, or to re-toilet train an incontinent patient (Figure 49-4). A single or double cone shape is used for adults; a long thin one is used for children. Simple, nonmedicinal suppositories are made of soap, glycerine, or cocoa butter. Medicinal suppositories that contain drugs are not administered by nursing assistants.

Suppository
A semisolid preparation (sometimes medicated) that is inserted into the vagina or rectum.

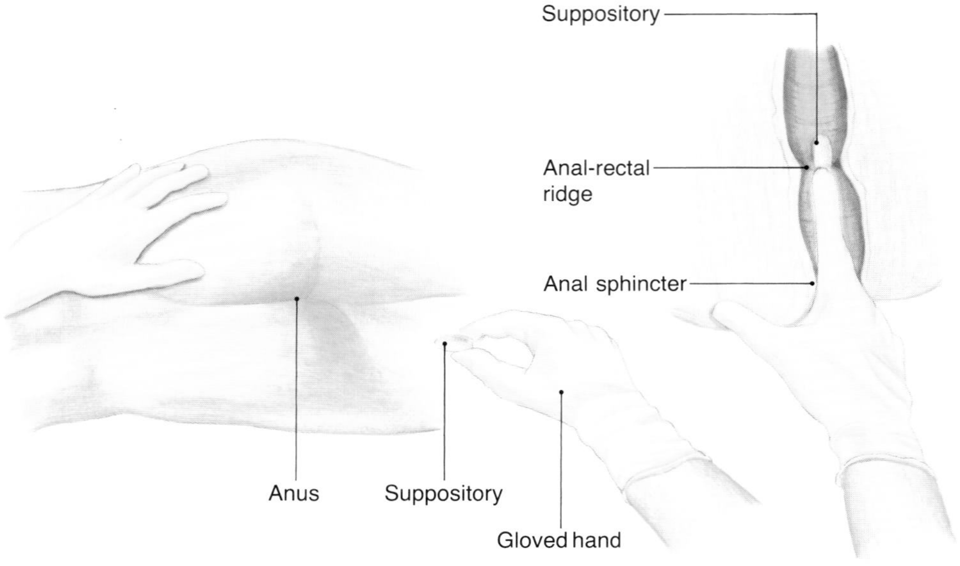

FIGURE 49-4 Inserting a rectal suppository.

Procedure Inserting a Rectal Suppository

1. Assemble your equipment:
   a) One small suppository as ordered
   b) Disposable gloves
   c) Lubricant
   d) Toilet tissue
   e) Bedpan and cover
2. Wash your hands.
3. Identify the patient by checking the identification bracelet.
4. Ask visitors to step out of the room, if this is your hospital's policy.
5. Tell the patient that you are going to insert a rectal suppository.
6. Pull the curtain around the bed for privacy.
7. Adjust the bed to the highest horizontal, comfortable, working position. Lock the bed in place.
8. Ask the patient to turn on his left side and raise his right knee toward his chest (left Sims's position). If he cannot do this, turn him and place the patient into position.
9. Expose the patient's buttocks by raising the blanket in a triangle over the anal area.
10. Put on the disposable gloves.
11. Put the lubricating jelly on a piece of toilet tissue and lubricate the suppository by gently rubbing the jelly on it with a tissue.
12. Raise the upper buttock so you can see the anal area.
13. Holding the suppository between the thumb and index finger, gently insert it through the anus into and along the wall of the rectum as far as the index finger will reach (2 inches).
14. Withdraw finger and press folded tissue against the anus briefly.
15. Remove the gloves, turning them inside out as you remove them and discard.
16. Replace the top sheets and turn the patient into a position of comfort.
17. Give the patient the signal cord and instruct him to signal you when he needs a bedpan.
18. If you are re-toilet training the patient, place him on a bedpan, commode, or toilet.
19. Raise the side rails and lock them in place when the patient is on the bedpan.
20. Check the patient every 5 minutes.
21. Make the patient comfortable.
22. Lower the bed to a position of safety for the patient.
23. Pull the curtains back to the open posi-

tion when you take the patient off the bedpan.

24. Raise the side rails where ordered, indicated, and appropriate for patient safety.
25. Place the call light within easy reach of the patient.
26. Wash your hands.
27. Report to your immediate supervisor:
    - That you have inserted the rectal suppository
    - The time you inserted it
    - The results obtained from inserting the suppository
    - How the patient tolerated the procedure
    - Your observations of anything unusual

KEY QUESTIONS

1. What are the roles of the rehabilitation nurse, the occupational therapist, the physical therapist, and the nursing assistant in helping the patient return to self-care?
2. How should the handicapped patient be helped to bathe?
3. How can the nursing assistant help the handicapped patient with dressing and grooming?
4. In what ways can the nursing assistant help the handicapped patient to eat?
5. How can the nursing assistant help with bowel and bladder rehabilitation and retraining for the incontinent patient?
6. How should rectal suppositories be inserted?
7. Define: active, incontinence, mobilization, passive, suppository.

CHAPTER

50

The Terminally Ill Patient

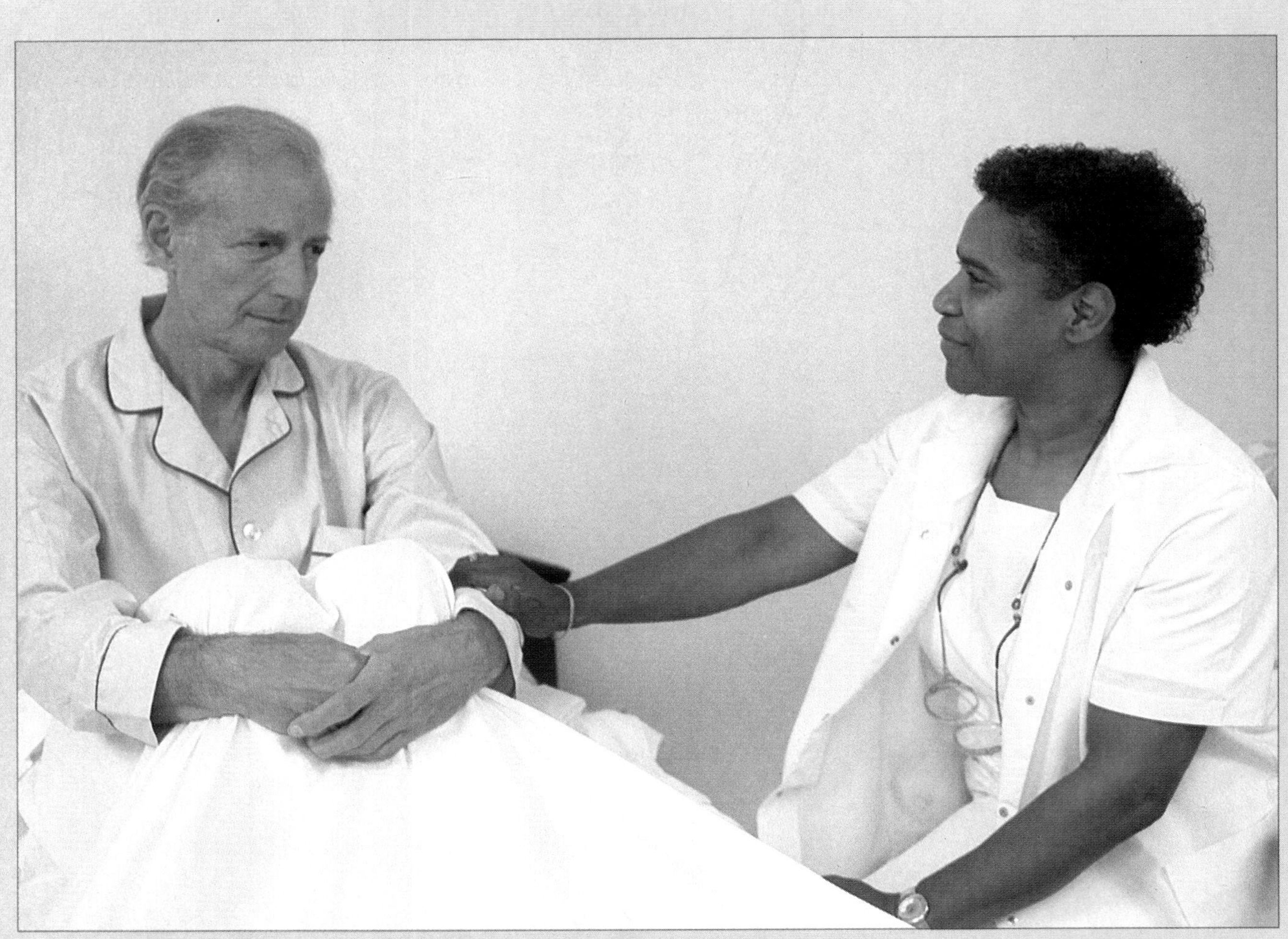

WARNING

For all patient contact, adhere to Universal Precautions. See page 91, 97, or the front cover flap. Wear protective equipment as indicated.

Objectives

What You Will Learn

When you have completed this chapter, you will be able to:

- Assist in meeting the psychological needs of the terminally ill patient.
- List common feelings of the patient who is dying.
- Assist in meeting the special care needs of the patient's family.
- Describe hospice care.
- Make the terminally ill patient comfortable.
- Identify the signs of approaching death.
- Describe *palliative care*, care designed to comfort the patient instead of curing him or her.
- Define: acceptance, anger, bargaining, denial, depression, hospice, terminally ill.
- Discuss advanced medical directives.

KEY IDEAS

Psychological Aspects of Caring for a Terminally Ill Patient

Terminally Ill
Having an illness that can be expected to cause death, usually within a known time.

SOME PATIENTS WHO ENTER A HEALTH care institution are **terminally ill**, that is, dying. Sometimes death is sudden or unexpected. More often it is not. Your first responsibility is to help make the patient as comfortable as possible. Your second responsibility is to assist in meeting the emotional needs of the patient and his or her family.

The most important single fact to remember when you are caring for a dying patient is that he or she is just as important as the patient who is going to recover. You will not have the satisfaction of contributing to recovery, but you will know that you have helped a human being to face the end of his or her life in peace, comfort, and dignity. Everyone must die. Surely we would all prefer to die in reassuring and comfortable surroundings.

Try to be very understanding. The patient may want to believe he will get well. He may want people around him to reassure him that he won't die. When a dying patient talks to you, listen. But don't give him false hopes. Don't tell him that he is getting better.

People have different ideas about death and the hereafter. These ideas depend on the patient's beliefs and background. You must show respect for the patient's beliefs. Be careful not to impose your own beliefs on him or his family.

When a patient suspects he is going to die, he may react in various ways:

- He may ask everyone about his chances for recovery.
- He may be afraid to be alone and want a lot of attention from you.
- He may ask a lot of questions.
- He may seem to complain constantly.
- He may often signal members of the staff.

- He may make many apparently unreasonable requests.
- He may rest and prefer to be left alone.

When a patient is told that he or she has a terminal disease or condition, the patient enters a very difficult time of life. Death may be frightening and the patient's reactions reflect the quality of emotional support provided by everyone interacting with him or her, as well as his or her culturally determined attitudes. Feelings of isolation, hopelessness, despair, sorrow and uselessness affect the coping mechanisms displayed by the patient and family members.

KEY IDEAS

Stages of Dying

Elizabeth Kübler-Ross describes five "stages" of dying in her book, *Death and Dying* (Figure 50-1). These are not intended to be stages that the patient must go through, however. Rather, they are emotional experiences that are common to terminally ill patients. This is especially true for the newly diagnosed patient and much less so for the patient who has been dying for a while. These "stages," or feelings common to terminally ill patients, are:

Denial
Refusal to admit the truth or face reality.

Anger
A strong emotional response of displeasure, irritation, and resentment.

Bargaining
Trying to make a deal to change the situation.

- **Denial:** This is a reaction to the shocking news. The patient may say, "No, this is not happening to me, this is something that happens to other people." This is sometimes the first reaction on the part of the patient.
- **Anger:** The patient resents that this has happened; all the unfinished plans, and the realization that they will be unable to finish or enjoy life's activities. It is at this point that the patient will begin to react to everything, making demands and asking for additional attention. The patient now is beginning to feel that soon he or she will be forgotten and that all is over.
- **Bargaining:** This is an attempt to make a bargain with God to postpone the inevitable. This bargaining may be connected with guilt for not having done what religious teachings tell us to do. It is here that the patient may request that a priest, minister, or rabbi be called.

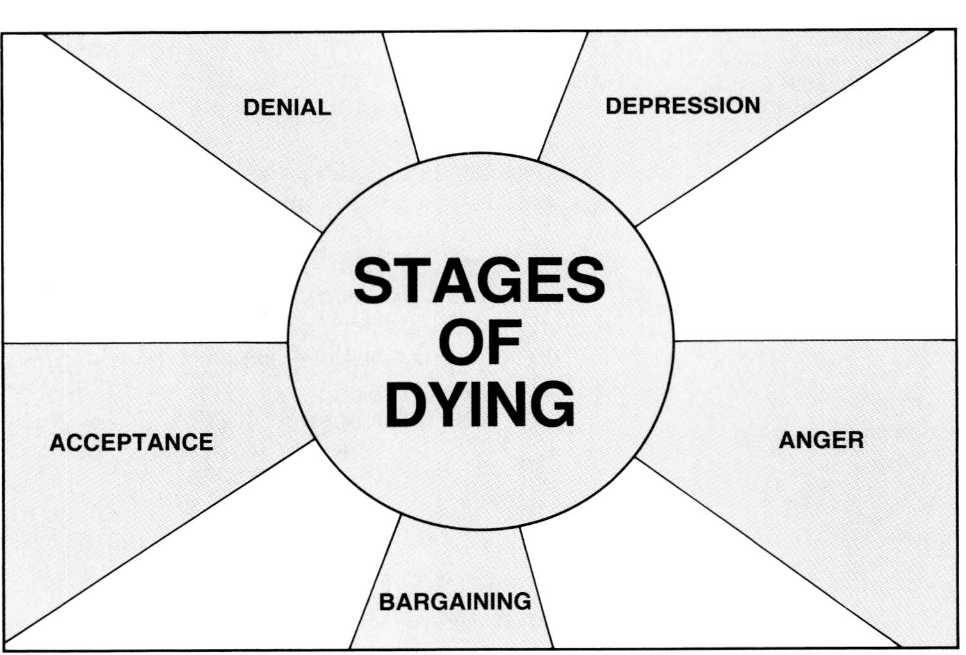

FIGURE 50-1 The five stages of dying.

Depression
A state of sadness, grief, or low spirits that may or may not cause change of activity.

Acceptance
Admitting, understanding, or facing the truth or reality of the situation.

- **Depression:** The patient reaches some acceptance of death. He or she may begin to grieve, to talk about innermost feelings, and may want you to listen. By being a good listener at this point, you can help the patient.
- **Acceptance:** Communication often becomes difficult. Some patients become quiet and withdrawn, while others may become more talkative after accepting the inevitable. The patient may communicate his or her needs to you through body language or gestures. Your job as a nursing assistant is to make the patient as comfortable as possible.

KEY IDEAS

The Terminally Ill Patient's Family

When it is known that death is approaching, the dying patient's family may want to spend a lot of time with the patient. This is usually permitted as much as possible.

Everyone on the staff should respect the family's need for privacy during their visits. If a private room is not available, the patient's area should be screened so that they will have the privacy they need. When the patient is visited by his pastor, priest, rabbi, or minister, assure them that they will not be disturbed.

Don't stop doing your work just because the patient's family is present. Carry out your job quickly, quietly, and efficiently (Figure 50-2). Don't wait until the family has gone before taking care of the patient. They might think that, because he is dying, he is being neglected by the hospital staff.

The patient's family may ask you many questions. Don't ignore their questions. Answer any you can. Also, do whatever is asked of you, if it is allowed.

There will be some questions that you can't answer. For example, you may be asked, "What did the doctor say today about his condition?" Refer the family to your immediate supervisor.

Even if the patient becomes unconscious, the family may want to stay with him. Family members may continue to hope for his recovery. They will watch you perform your patient care procedures. They will want you to make the patient comfortable, even if you cannot help him recover.

Unconscious patients require as thorough care as those who are conscious. Their needs must still be met. Sometimes you must ask the family to leave the bedside while you are giving care to the patient.

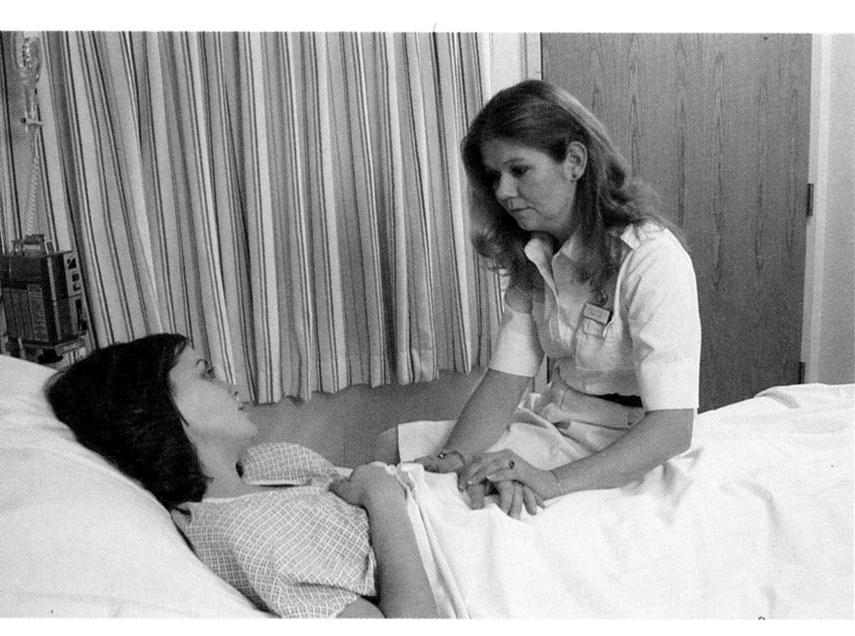

FIGURE 50-2 The nursing assistant should continue her regular care for the terminally ill patient even when family is present.

Explain this to the family. Tell them that you will let them know when you have finished.

Some visitors stay with the patient for many hours at a time. Be as helpful to them as you can. You might suggest that they have a cup of coffee. Tell them where the coffee shop is located. Also, learn the policy in your institution on serving meals to visitors. You may be able to arrange for trays to be delivered to the patient's family at mealtimes. If this is not allowed, tell the visitors where they can find the cafeteria or a nearby restaurant. Make sure the visitors know the location of the washroom, lounge, and telephones.

Remember at all times to be quietly courteous, understanding, sympathetic, and willing to help. These are the marks of a competent nursing assistant. Don't feel helpless or guilty because you can't improve the patient's condition. You can help the patient and his or her family most by maintaining a concerned and efficient approach to your work.

KEY IDEAS

Hospice Care

Hospice
Program that allows a dying patient to remain at home or in a nonhospital environment and die there while receiving professionally supervised care.

Hospice care is a method of health care delivery used to ensure individualized and humane care for the terminally ill. The philosophy of hospice stresses:

- Assisting with psychological, physiological, and spiritual problems.
- A family-oriented approach.
- Alleviating pain and other symptoms rather than effecting a cure in the advanced stage of disease.
- Offering professional and voluntary services to meet individual needs.
- Making the patient as comfortable as possible.

Principles of Hospice Care

- To provide physical comfort
- To provide psychological counseling
- To assist the patient to maintain her or his ability to participate in life
- To provide an environment that emphasizes the quality of life on a daily basis, rather than longevity
- To provide assurance that the patient and her or his family will not be alone in a moment of crisis
- To provide the patient with evidence that family, friends, and staff care about what the patient thinks and feels
- To provide an environment that permits the patient to return to her or his own schedule of activities of daily living
- To permit the patient to be surrounded by familiar belongings and people
- To provide assessment of changing needs
- To provide acceptance of the grieving patient's and family's behavior
- To provide the patient with the opportunity to die with dignity in familiar and caring surroundings

Characteristics of Hospice Programs

- Coordination of home and institutional care
- Patient and family regarded as one unit
- Physician and other health-care provider availability
- Care provided by an interdisciplinary team
- Control of symptoms

- Availability of care whenever needed, regardless of day or time
- Volunteer involvement
- Follow-up care for bereaved families
- System of open communication between staff, volunteers, patient, and family

KEY IDEAS

Making the Terminally Ill Patient Comfortable

Meeting Personal Needs

A patient approaching death continues to be given routine personal care, such as baths and mouth care. That is, he is given the same care he would receive if he were expected to recover. Members of the nursing staff should stay calm and sympathetic. This may help to relieve some of the patient's fears and make this time easier for him. As the patient becomes weaker, his condition may require more of your time. You may need to do many things for him that he had earlier taken care of himself.

Meeting Positioning Needs

The patient will tell you what position is most comfortable for him. However, it is important that the patient remain active for as long as possible, and his position in bed be changed regularly to protect the skin (Figure 50-3).

Meeting Communication Needs

Speak to the patient in your normal voice, even if he seems to be unconscious. You should still tell the patient who you are, what you are doing, and so on. The dying patient's hearing is usually one of the last senses to fail. We do not know how much an unconscious person hears or understands. It is guessed that this is a great deal. Encourage the family to continue to talk to the patient unless he is sleeping.

Meeting Visual Needs

Adjust the light in the room to suit the patient. For some, bright lights are irritating; for others, a dark room is frightening.

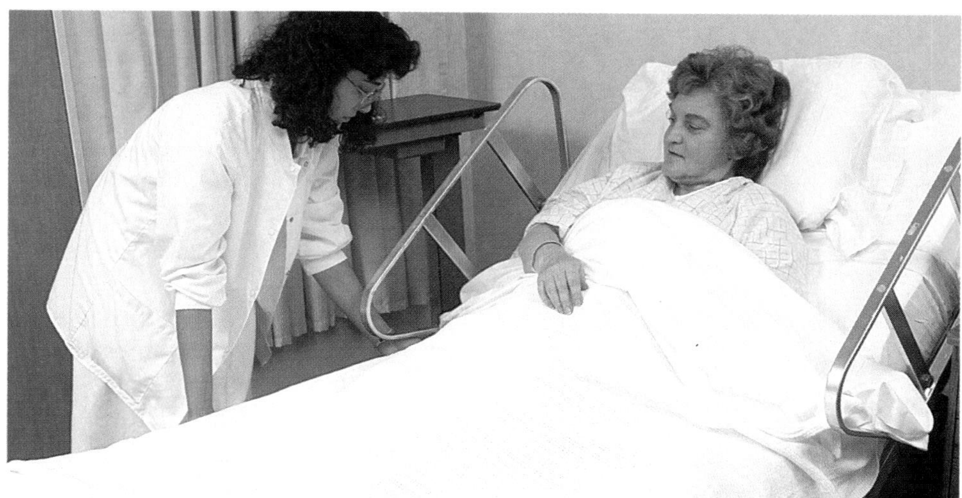

FIGURE 50-3 The nursing assistant should change the patient's position every 2 hours.

Meeting Elimination Needs

As death comes closer, the sphincters relax and the patient may lose control of the bowels and bladder. Your job is to keep the patient's body clean at all times. Change the bedding whenever necessary. This will keep the patient's skin from becoming irritated and will help to keep the patient comfortable. You may also be giving more back rubs than usual. The urine may become concentrated and strong smelling, and it is especially necessary to keep the skin clean. Foley catheters are rarely necessary with the use of incontinent pads and bed pads.

Meeting Nutritional Needs

Usually the patient is allowed whatever foods he or she desires. However there is often a decreased appetite. Semisoft foods or semi-frozen liquid may be easier to handle than liquids.

Meeting Oral Hygiene Needs

The patient approaching death needs special mouth care. His mouth may be dry because he is breathing through it. You might use an applicator with glycerine (or other lubricant) to swab the patient's mouth and lips. If the patient's mouth has a large amount of secretions in it, tell the nurse. She may use suction to remove the secreted material. If the patient has dentures, ask your immediate supervisor if you should leave them in the patient's mouth or take them out. If you remove the dentures, place them in a denture cup half filled with water, with the patient's name on the cover. A moist mouth will make it easier for the patient to eat. If the patient has cancer or AIDS, watch for and report sores in the mouth. Often persons near death have gums or lips that bleed. Using a dark-colored towel or washcloth may make this less frightening.

Meeting Oxygen Therapy Needs

A patient may be receiving oxygen through a nasal catheter or mask. If so, check his nostrils from time to time. Tell your immediate supervisor if the nostrils are dry and encrusted. Check the tops of the ears or any other place the tubing contacts. It can cause skin irritation.

A patient's nostrils also may become dry and encrusted because he has difficulty in breathing. If you notice dryness, with your immediate supervisor's permission, clean the nostrils with cotton swabs moistened slightly with glycerine (or other lubricant).

Meeting Spiritual Needs

Respect the patient's need for spiritual support. Learn the policy in your institution concerning religious observances and requirements at the time of death (Figure 50-4). If the patient has particular beliefs or practices relative to death, such as the care of the body, it is important to know these before death occurs.

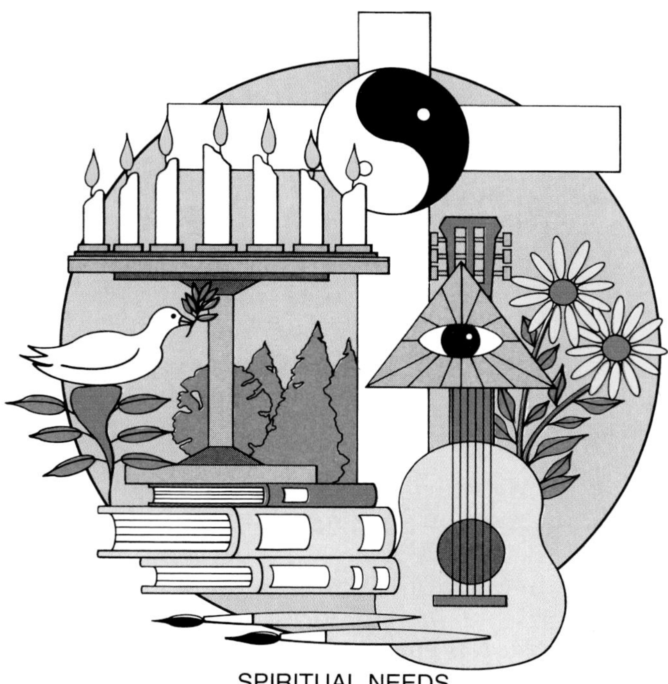

FIGURE 50-4 The patient's spiritual needs must be met.

KEY IDEAS
Signs of Approaching Death

Death comes in different ways. It may come quite suddenly. Or it may come after a long period during which there has been a steady decline of body functions. Death also may result from complications during convalescence. Here are some signs showing that death may be near:

- Blood circulation slows down. The patient's hands and feet are cold to the touch. If the patient is conscious, he may complain that he is cold. Keep him well covered.
- The patient's face may become pale because of decreased circulation.
- His eyes may be staring blankly into space. There may be no eye movement when you move your hand across his line of vision.
- The patient may perspire heavily, even though his body is cold.
- The patient loses muscle tone, and his body becomes limp. His jaw may drop and his mouth may stay partly open. Eyes may not close in sleep.
- Respirations may become slower and more difficult or faster, or there may be periods of no breathing.
- Mucus collecting in the patient's throat and bronchial tubes may cause a sound that is sometimes called the "death rattle."
- The pulse may be rapid or may become weak and irregular.
- Just before death, respiration stops and the pulse gets very faint. You may not be able to feel the patient's pulse at all.
- Contrary to popular belief, a dying person is rarely in great pain. As the patient's condition gets worse, less blood may be flowing to the brain. Therefore, the patient may feel little or no pain.
- The patient may talk to persons who have died.
- The patient's urine output may decrease.
- The patient's swallowing ability may decrease.
- The patient may have periods of confusion and/or agitation.

If you notice any of these signs or any changes in the patient's condition, report to your supervisor immediately. Find out what the patient would like you to do to help. Many want company. Others just want to know you're around.

Sometimes the patient requests, and the physician orders, that no resuscitative measures be taken when the patient's lungs and heart cease to function. This is referred to as *DNR* (Do Not Resuscitate) *status*. Your immediate supervisor will be aware of this and will not initiate resuscitative procedures. Follow his or her instructions.

KEY IDEAS

Advanced Medical Directives

An advanced directive can be a written or oral statement that has been witnessed in advance of serious illness or injury. There are two types of advanced directives. They are:

- Living will
- Health care surrogate designation

A living will is simply a statement of the patient's wishes regarding the use of life-support treatment in the event of serious illness or trauma. It is called a living will because it is prepared and executed while the patient is still alive.

A health care surrogate designation is a signed, dated, and witnessed document naming another individual to act as the patient's agent in making health care decisions for the patient should the patient become unable to make those decisions.

An individual may change his or her mind after making a living will or designating a surrogate.

KEY QUESTIONS

1. How can you assist in meeting the psychological needs of the terminally ill patient?
2. List common feelings of the patient who is dying.
3. How can you assist in meeting the special needs of the patient's family?
4. Describe hospice care.
5. List nine ways of making the terminally ill patient comfortable.
6. Identify the signs of approaching death.
7. Define: acceptance, anger, bargaining, denial, depression, hospice, terminally ill.
8. Discuss advanced medical directives.

CHAPTER

51

Postmortem Care

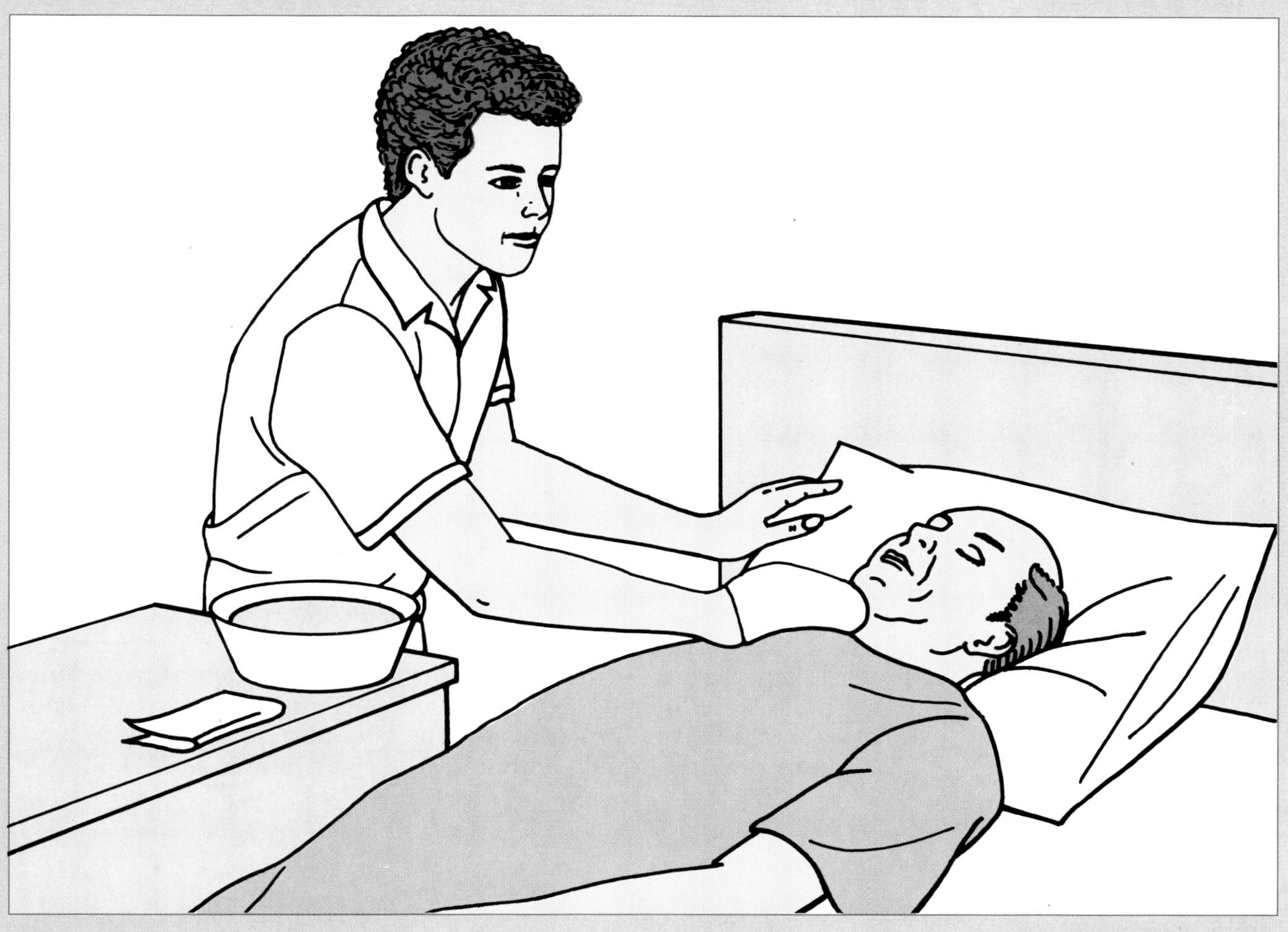

WARNING

For all patient contact, adhere to Universal Precautions. See page 91, 97, or the front cover flap. Wear protective equipment as indicated.

Objectives

What You Will Learn

When you have completed this chapter, you will be able to:

- Give postmortem care gently and respectfully.
- Protect the patient's valuables.
- Define: expired, morgue, postmortem, rigor mortis.

KEY IDEAS

Postmortem Care (PMC)

Postmortem
After death.

Expired
Died

Morgue
A place for storing dead bodies for identification and burial.

Rigor mortis
Stiffening of a person's body and limbs shortly after death.

IF YOU OBSERVE ANY SIGNS OF approaching death, tell the nurse immediately. The nurse will examine the patient and confirm what you have found. Until you have received direct instructions from your immediate supervisor, no **postmortem** care can be given to a patient.

In some health care institutions, a nurse confirms that a patient has no pulse or has stopped breathing and she calls a "code." Code Blue, Cardiac Arrest, or whatever name is used for the code in your institution is an emergency announcement to the entire staff. A preassigned team will come to help the patient and use every means available to keep the patient alive. Only when all efforts fail to keep the patient alive is the patient declared to be dead by a physician. In some cases, if it is known in advance that the patient may die, the physician may write a *Do Not Resuscitate* (DNR) order. In such cases the patient's death is not an emergency.

After a patient has **expired**, his or her body still must be treated with respect and must be given gentle care. If family members are present, they usually wait outside the room until the doctor has finished the examination. The patient's family will be allowed to view the body if they wish. Ask them if they would like to be alone with the body or if they would like you, or another member of the health care team, to stay with them.

Sometimes the family is not present when the patient dies. In this case, the nurse calls the doctor and tells him or her that the family is not there. Either the doctor or the nurse then notifies the family and finds out whether they wish to view the body before it is sent to the **morgue**. If so, the body usually stays in the room until the family arrives.

When the family is present, they are given the patient's personal belongings. These items are checked against the admission valuables list to be sure that everything is accounted for. You will learn the procedure in your health care institution for taking care of the deceased patient's clothes and belongings. If the members of the family do not wish to view the body, you will then proceed with the postmortem care.

Postmortem care should be done before **rigor mortis** sets in.

Rules to Follow
POSTMORTEM CARE

Each institution will have its own specific policies and procedures for postmortem care. You will need to learn and follow them, as well as the instructions of your immediate supervisor. Some general principles will apply in most institutions, however. For example, you may not remove tubes, bandages, and so on from the body.

- While you are preparing the body you may raise the bed to a comfortable working position. When you are finished, lower the bed to a low position.
- Lower the head of the bed so the patient is lying flat.
- If the body is soiled with urine or feces, clean gently to remove odor.
- Straighten the body in a dignified pose.
- Cover the body with clean bed linen, but do not cover the head.
- Straighten the room and remove any emergency equipment.
- Turn off oxygen, suction, or IVs at the nurse's or doctor's instructions.
- Turn off the bright light over the bed.
- Provide privacy and support for the family's visit.

Note: Many facilities no longer perform postmortem care. The funeral home comes to pick up the body, and the postmortem care is usually performed there.

KEY QUESTIONS

1. Describe postmortem care.
2. How should the patient's valuables and other belongings be cared for?
3. Define: expired, morgue, postmortem, rigor mortis.

CHAPTER

52

Introduction to Home Health Care

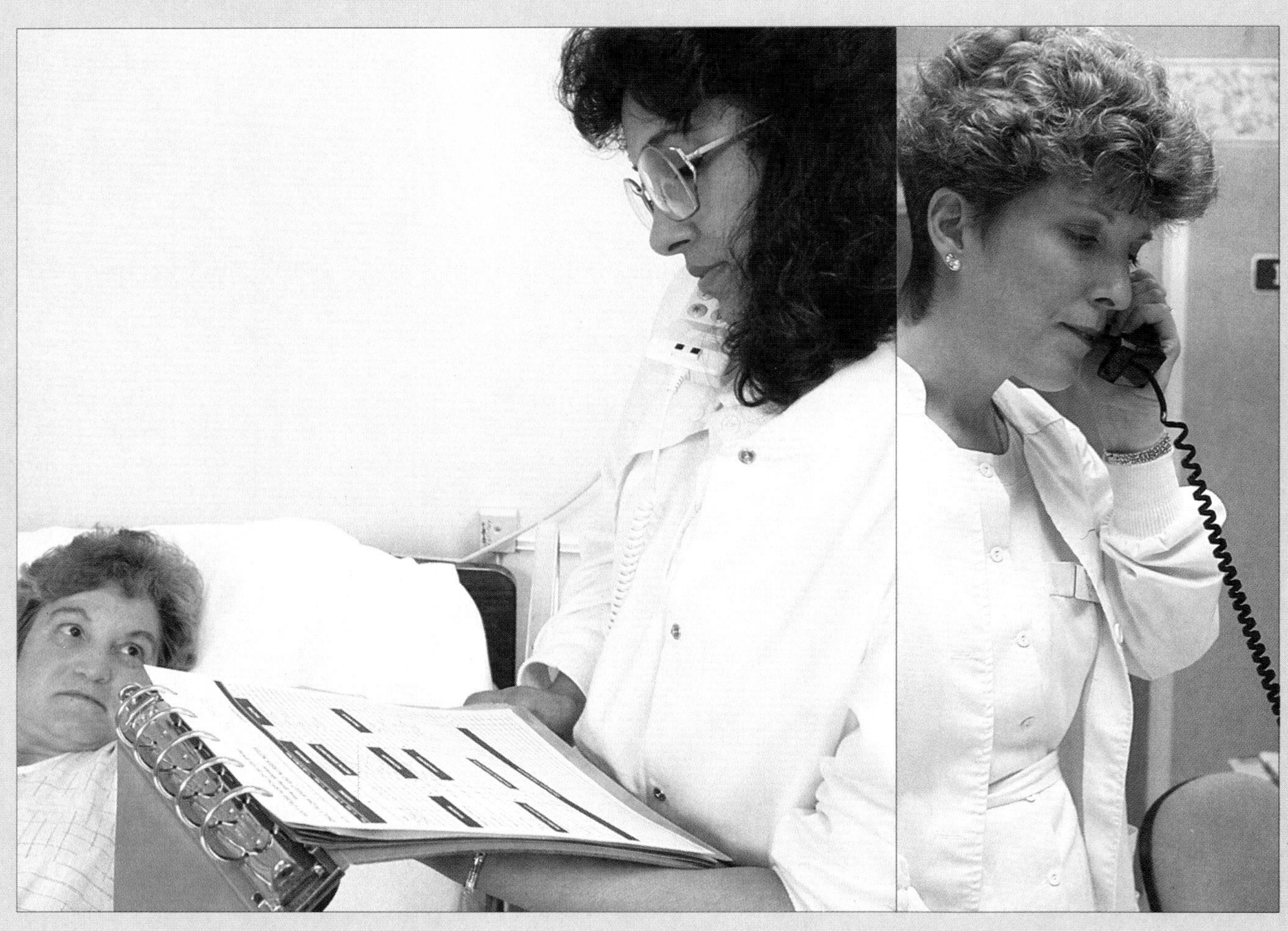

- Reporting to the home care supervisor your observations and anything unusual
- Recording all completed activities of daily living tasks

The reason the home health assistant may not perform the following tasks is that they are not licensed to do so.

Procedures Home Health Aide or Assistant May Not Do in the Home

The nursing tasks home health assistants are not permitted to do in the home vary from state to state. In most areas of this country, home health assistants may *not* do the following tasks:

- Change sterile dressings
- Irrigate body cavities (this includes administering enemas and irrigation of ostomies or wounds)
- Gastric lavage or gavage
- Catheterization
- Administer medications
- Apply heat by any method
- Care for a tracheostomy tube

In addition, do *not*:

- Disturb the patient's personal belongings, letters, pictures, and the like. You may suggest they be moved, however, to another place so that you can give better care.
- Perform heavy cleaning chores, such as moving heavy furniture, waxing floors, shampooing carpets, washing windows, and carrying firewood.

Helpful Personal Qualities of the Home Health Aide or Assistant

As a member of the health care team, you are expected to maintain a professional attitude in the home. The same qualities that will make you a successful nursing assistant in a health care institution will be necessary if you are to be successful as a home health assistant. The best home health assistants are those who are dependable, trustworthy, considerate, tactful, ethical, courteous, sympathetic, energetic, polite, careful, observant, and sensitive. Communication skills are an essential part of your job. You will be in close contact with the patient, family members, and visitors.

Behaving courteously means putting the needs of others before your own. It also means cooperating, sharing, and giving. Being polite and considerate of others shows that you care about them. Placing the needs of others first may mean quieting down your own feelings, such as cheerfulness around a person who is in pain, very ill, or depressed. Or it might mean the opposite, such as putting aside your own gloomy feelings to be more cheerful, positive, and receptive. You should never discuss your personal problems with the patient.

Having *empathy* is the ability to put yourself in someone else's place and to see things as they see them.

Respect
Recognition of the worth of another person.

Respect is recognition of the worth of another person. When you respect others, you recognize their right to make up their own minds and to make decisions.

Genuineness is simply being yourself. When your actions match what you say, you are genuine. Remember, "Actions speak louder than words."

Warmth is shown by demonstrating concern and affection. A nursing assistant shows warmth by the way care is delivered, by demonstrating kindness and patience, and by always using a gentle touch.

Compassion
Understanding the fears, problems, and distress of someone else, combined with a concern and desire to help.

Compassion or *caring* is understanding the fears, problems, and distress of someone else, combined with a concern and a desire to help. As a nursing assistant, you can demonstrate compassion in many ways through your actions. For example, answer the patient's call signal promptly, offer fluids to the patient, be sure the patient is clean and well groomed. Caring is doing, not just feeling.

Other personal qualities that enhance your relationship with the patient are courtesy, emotional control, tact, and ethical behavior. Demonstrate honesty and accuracy when handling the patient's money and valuables. Show respect by treating the patient's possessions carefully. Display dependability by never leaving before an assignment is completed. Because you are working alone, self-discipline, time management, and the motivation to do a good job are especially important qualities.

Transcultural Nursing in the Home

The atmosphere and life style will be different in every home in which you work. You must respect the rights of the patient and his or her family to have beliefs and opinions, culture, and customs that might be different from your own. People of different backgrounds may eat foods you have never seen or tasted; they may behave differently toward their family members than you would; their religious beliefs may seem unusual to you; and their standards of cleanliness or general life style may be different than yours. Accept these differences with respect and understanding, without judging or criticizing. Let the patient know it is your pleasure, not just your job, to assist him.

KEY IDEAS

The Family Unit

A *family* is a unit brought together by shared needs, interests, and mutual concern for the well-being of all its members.

An *extended family* typically has several generations living under the same roof. The family may consist of parents, children, and even friends living together with mutual needs.

Every family, regardless of its structure, has unique needs, rules, and customs. When you are working in the home setting, you must be aware and sensitive to the way this particular family functions.

The family may have values and behaviors that you are not familiar with or that you personally disapprove of. You may be sent to work in a home where you may feel uncomfortable or unsure of your actions.

You should discuss these feelings with your supervisor, who can help you understand what is happening. Being honest with yourself and, with the help of your supervisor, recognizing your feelings and reactions can help you provide the best care possible in a given situation. Don't let your feelings keep you from doing the best job you can.

KEY IDEAS

The Family and Family Reactions

Support systems
People or actions used to help a person adjust or live.

Caregiver
Refers to the family member who is taking the major responsibility for the patient.

Reactions of families to illness, disability, and crisis vary. How people and families deal with everyday life varies also. **Support systems** are people or actions used to help a person adjust to a new or difficult situation. Individuals who have strong support systems will be able to make the necessary adjustments in their functions and rally to the short- or long-term crisis of illness. Some families are unable to make any changes in their structure and will not be able to cope with crisis or illness. A sensitive home health aide or assistant can observe some of the problems within the family unit and discuss them with the home care supervisor. Often, when help is offered, a family in crisis can make the necessary changes to cope with illness. Remember, this is a family unit that has set up patterns of coping over a long period of time. You must work with these patterns. Crisis is not a good time to change coping mechanisms. The term **caregiver** refers to the family member who is taking the primary responsibility for the patient. Do not give advice, take sides, or make judgments about family conflicts. Offer sympathy with tact and do not get involved in family conflicts and problems.

It is important for you to have a good working relationship with the patient and the family. The patient's family may be unable or unwilling to provide daily health care because they:

- Work outside the home
- Care for small children or older parents or relatives
- Have physical limitations themselves
- Live far away from the patient and as a result they:
  - Cannot help with physical and personal care
  - Cannot provide a safe, clean environment
  - Cannot provide transportation
  - Cannot shop and prepare meals

KEY IDEAS

Safety in the Home

Patients are prone to having accidents in the home and may be unable to take care of themselves in case of an emergency. You, as the home health assistant, will be responsible for the patient's safety while you are present in the home. You can create a safe environment for your patient and yourself by eliminating, preventing, or correcting conditions that could cause accidents. Safety in the home includes proper infection control, electrical and fire safety, and accident prevention.

Safety Hazards

As you go about your work, be alert and look for the hazards listed below. Make a note of these things and bring them to the attention of the patient, family member responsible, and your supervisor. Some of the most common safety hazards in the home are:

Flammable
Capable of burning quickly and easily.

- Damaged electrical wiring on large and small appliances
- Faulty or uneven stairs
- Loose rugs that slip
- Poisons (highest incidence in children due to medication and cleaning solutions)
- **Flammable** cleaning rags, mops, and brooms (these should be cleaned after each use and stored in a well-ventilated place)
- Sharp objects such as knives, razors, and lawn tools
- Wet floor (spills should be wiped up immediately)
- Cluttered walkways
- Unstable furniture

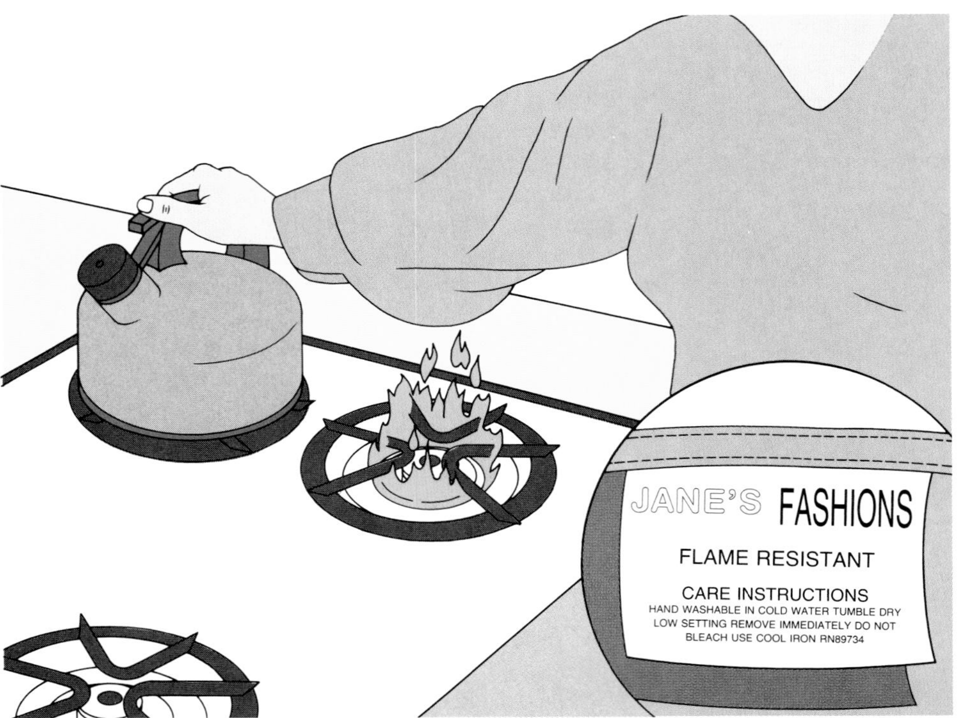

FIGURE 52-1 Many garment-related fires cause injuries when a loose-fitting portion of a garment, such as a sleeve or skirt hem, comes in contact with a stove burner, lighted candle, space heater, or fireplace fire. Flaming liquids also cause serious injuries when they splash onto a garment and ignite its fabric or when the textile is wet with a flammable liquid (such as lighter fluid), which is then ignited by a nearby spark or flame.

Fire Safety and Burn Prevention

- Avoid using flammable liquids.
- Use flame-resistant clothing for the patient and follow the washing instructions on the label inside the clothing to keep them flame resistant (Figure 52-1).
- Caution the patient against smoking while seated on upholstered furniture or the bed, especially when sleepy.
- If the patient is a smoker, use a deep, wide-rimmed ashtray and set it on a table. Extinguish smoldering butts when the patient is finished smoking.
- Do not use an extension cord or electric cord and plug unless it is in excellent condition.
- Arrange furniture with fire safety in mind. Place furniture well away from stoves, space heaters, and fireplaces.
- If a fire occurs, get the patient out of the house. Know the exit route. If the apartment is above the first floor, know where the stairs are.
- Have a fire extinguisher and smoke alarm in the home.
- Follow the safety rules of your local fire department.
- Keep matches away from children and confused adults.
- Check the temperature of water before using it on the patient.
- Check the temperature setting on the hot-water heater.

KEY IDEAS

Reporting an Accident or Emergency by Telephone

Phone Numbers to Keep Handy

If an accident or emergency does occur, you must be ready to handle the situation calmly and wisely. Report every accident to your supervisor immediately. It is important to have emergency phone numbers written next to the phone. The list should include:

- Emergency Medical Service (often *911*) if available
- Police department
- Fire department
- Responsible family member at work
- Your home care supervisor or agency
- Patient's physician
- Nearest hospital
- Ambulance service
- Poison control center
- If there is no phone in the home, arrange in advance to use a neighbor's phone in case of an emergency

Calling for Help

Many areas have a special phone number to call when an accident or emergency occurs in the home. You may call that number or the physician phone number that you have been given by the family or agency. No matter who you call, you must be clear in reporting the accident or emergency. Be sure to:

- Give your name and title.
- Give the name of the patient.
- Give the address and phone number of where you are.
- Clearly state the problem; objectively state exactly what has happened.
- Clearly state the condition of the patient or person who has had the accident or is in a crisis.
- If calling a city emergency number, give the phone number of the patient's physician to the person who answers the phone call.
- If you have a phone number for a member of the family, give that number to the emergency answering service.

KEY QUESTIONS

1. What are the differences between working in the home and the health care institution?
2. Where can you find the necessary instructions in order to assist the patient to follow his or her doctor's orders?
3. What are the responsibilities of the home health assistant?
4. What are the nine procedures a nursing assistant is *not* allowed to do in the home setting?
5. Give five examples of ways to behave on the job that display helpful personal qualities.

6. Discuss why it is important to show respect for the beliefs, opinions, culture, and customs of the patient and his family.
7. Describe possible family reactions to the illness of one of its members.
8. What should you do if you notice a safety hazard in the home?
9. Make a list of the emergency phone numbers for your city.
10. Define: care giver, compassion, flammable, respect, support systems.

CHAPTER

53

Household Management

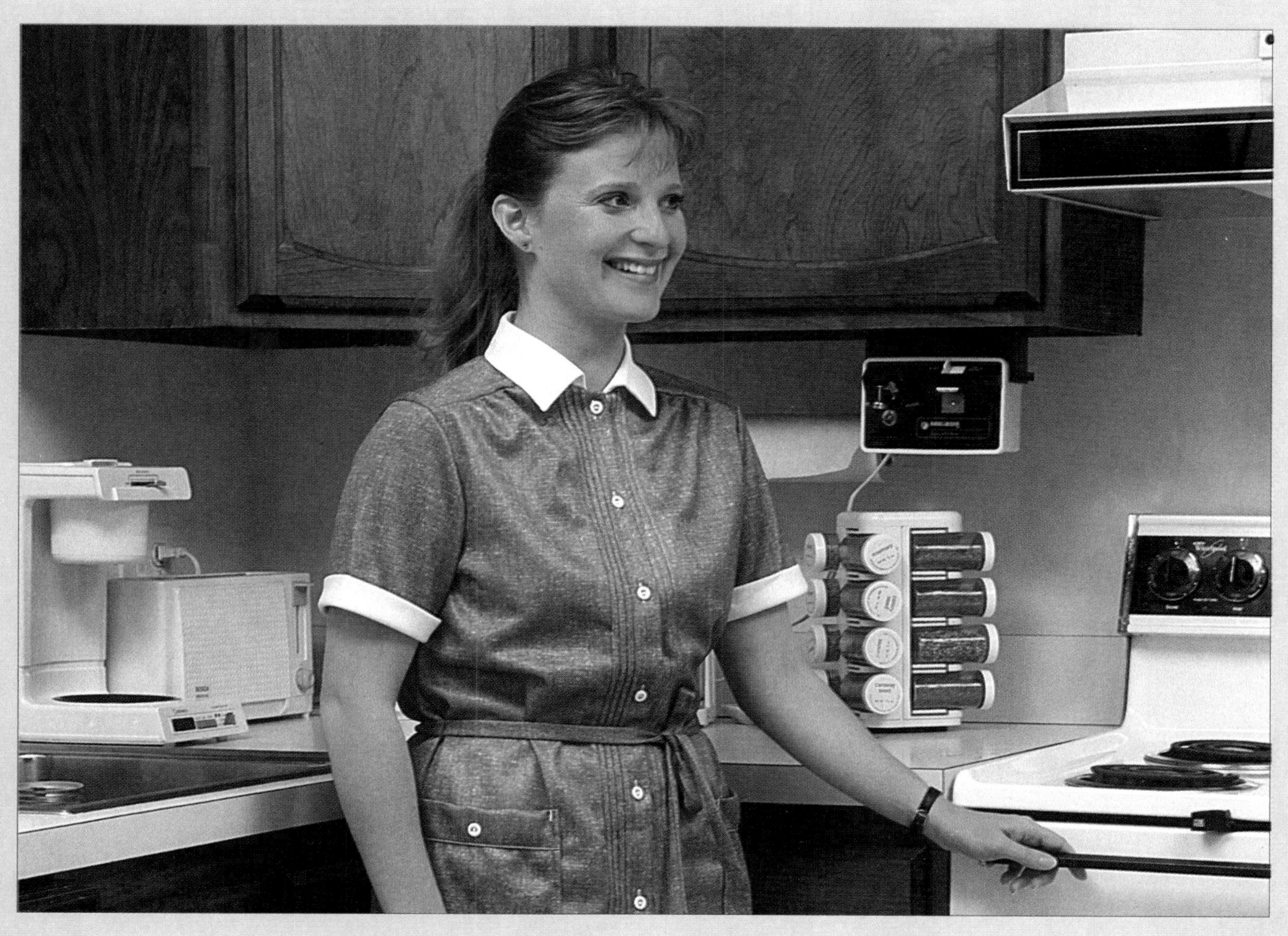

WARNING

For all patient contact, adhere to Universal Precautions. See page 91, 97, or the front cover flap. Wear protective equipment as indicated.

Objectives

What You Will Learn

When you have completed this chapter, you will be able to:

- Identify at least 15 housekeeping responsibilities of the home health aide or assistant.
- Discuss how to apply at least five principles of infection control to the home setting.
- Describe three ways to improvise when supplies are limited.
- Discuss nutrition and food service as it applies to the home setting.
- Record your activities and those of the patient every 15 minutes for an entire scheduled shift.
- Define: bed-bound, infection control, microorganism, responsibility.

KEY IDEAS

Household Management

PREPARING AND SERVING MEALS AND KEEPING the patient's home neat and clean are part of what is expected of you on the job. However, patient care and safety come first. Housekeeping tasks should be done between nursing tasks, which are your first priority. Convenient times occur when the patient is sleeping, reading, watching television, or conversing with visitors.

Planning Your Time

Planning your schedule for the day can help you to minimize the time necessary to complete your tasks. The easiest way for some to organize is to make a list of your tasks and carry this with you, checking off each task as it is completed. Plan the patient's care and your other tasks so that the patient will have periods of activity followed by periods of rest. Be sure your plan will allow you to complete all your assigned tasks in the allotted amount of time.

Housekeeping Responsibility List

The tasks expected of you will vary from home to home. In some homes a family member might buy the groceries, but in another home your employer (supervisor) will want you to do the shopping. When handling money for the patient, keep an accurate written account of the amount of money given to you by the patient. Be sure to save the register receipt for the total amount spent. Return the correct amount of change. Include this information in your written report with date and time.

It is best to ask the family members and your supervisor to list exactly what is expected of you before you start the job. This will avoid future misunderstandings. Housekeeping tasks for the home health assistant often include:

- Making the patient's bed
- Preparing, planning, and serving the patient's meals
- Washing linens and clothing used by the patient
- Sweeping floors or vacuuming the carpets in the rooms the patient uses
- Straightening up
- Dusting
- Cleaning the bathroom, including tub, toilet, sink, floor, and mirror
- Returning used items to their proper places
- Taking out the garbage
- Wiping kitchen counters, tables, sink, and floors
- Wiping spills and crumbs from the stove, counters, and floors
- Keeping the refrigerator and freezer clean and free of spoiled food
- Reporting broken windows or screens to avoid an insect problem
- Reporting safety hazards
- Writing a shopping list
- Shopping for groceries
- Washing the dishes

Infection Control
To restrain or curb the spread of microorganisms.

Responsibility
A duty or obligation; that for which one is accountable.

Microorganism
A living thing so small it cannot be seen with the naked eye but only through a microscope.

Infection Control in the Home

It is your **responsibility** to control the spread of **microorganisms** in the home by using proper handwashing technique and by doing sufficient housecleaning to maintain a clean environment for the patient. You should use hot water and ample amounts of detergent when washing dishes. Cleaning the bathroom frequently with a disinfectant will help to eliminate odors and will cut down on the growth of bacteria. If there is more than one person using the bathroom, encourage them to use their own towels. Laundry bleach is an inexpensive and effective disinfectant that can be found in most homes. If there are no supplies available, discuss this with your supervisor.

Remember that aseptic technique—including ***handwashing***—is part of everything you do. Review Chapter 5 for the procedure on handwashing technique. Other precautions to be taken are:

- Maintain general cleanliness
- Wash clothes and linens frequently
- Dispose of garbage promptly
- Dispose of soiled supplies
- Wash fruits and vegetables before cooking or serving
- Refrigerate or freeze all perishable foods as appropriate
- Sterilize infant bottles and nipples

Equipment and Supplies

Check to see what cleaning supplies are already in the home and make a list of supplies needed. Submit your list to your employer or supervisor. In some homes, cleaning supplies and even patient care supplies may be limited. You will have to be flexible and improvise with what is available.

- If there is no toothpaste, substitute baking soda on a wet toothbrush or a solution of mouthwash and water.

- If there is no disinfectant cleaning liquid or powder, you can use a solution of liquid laundry bleach and water.

Nutrition and Food Service

Try to involve the patient and the family in meal planning. Ask about the patient's favorite foods and how to prepare them. Ask for the times that the patient prefers to have his or her meals. Inquire about food allergies and dislikes. Be sure to check with your supervisor or patient's doctor to see if a special or therapeutic diet has been prescribed by the physician. If so, you must be sure the patient adheres to it strictly.

Make a list of needed foods and supplies as you plan the menus. If you are asked to buy the groceries, save all receipts to give to your employer. If a family member will be doing the marketing, you can show your menu plan and grocery list to him or her. After the food is purchased, it is your responsibility to see that it is stored promptly to avoid health hazards. Be sure dairy products, partly used items, and leftovers are kept in the refrigerator.

Bed-bound
Unable to get out of bed.

The **bed-bound** patient's appetite may be small. Even if the meals are small, they must be well balanced. Be sure the patient is taking enough fluids. Some patients have difficulty in chewing because dentures do not fit well, their own teeth are in poor condition, or because they have mouth sores. If you notice this, report it to your supervisor or to the patient's family, and try to provide softer, more easily chewed foods.

KEY IDEAS

Reading Food Product Labels

Read the labels. You've heard that before. How important is it to know exactly what you are buying? Some patients, due to their medical condition, are required to be on special diets. People on a salt-free (sodium free) diet need to know if salt was used in preparing the food product. The low-sodium diet is prescribed for the person who must restrict the amount of salt they take in. Usually, the diet is restricted to 200–500 mg of sodium. Foods restricted on a low-sodium diet include all table salt, salted nuts, bacon, ham, and other products of high sodium content.

By reading food labels, diabetic and other people who need to restrict sugar in their diet can find out which products they can safely consume. *Sugar* is the common name applied to a group of carbohydrates that includes glucose, fructose, sucrose, lactose, and maltose. Whole grains, vegetables, peas, beans, potatoes, fruits, honey, and refined sugar are all sources of carbohydrates. Reading food labels can help in planning diets for those people who have allergies or sensitivities to food additives.

Food labels can help you plan a calorie-restricted diet as well. Most labels provide information about the number of servings in the package and how many calories are contained in each serving.

Generally, ingredients are listed on the label according to the amount found in the product. The ingredient that is found in the greatest amount is listed first. The ingredient found in the smallest amount is listed last.

Reporting and Recording

A carefully written record of your activities and those of the patient must be kept. Any medications taken by the patient and any treatments given should be recorded. The doctor and your supervisor may want a record of the patient's food intake, activity, vital signs, and blood and urine sugar and acetone results.

FIGURE 53-1 The home health aide daily progress record.

HOME HEALTH AIDE
DAILY PROGRESS RECORD

Patient's Name: (print)	Medical Record Number:	Date of Visit:
Home Health Aide's Name: (print)	Employee's ID#:	Time In: ______ am/pm Time Out: ______ am/pm
Home Health Aide's Signature:	Patient's Signature:	Regular Visit: ______ Refused Visit: ______

PERSONAL CARE

SKIN CARE:	YES	NO	TUB BATH:	YES	NO
SHAVE:	YES	NO	BED BATH:	YES	NO
ORAL HYGIENE:	YES	NO	SHOWER:	YES	NO
SHAMPOO:	YES	NO	SPONGE BATH:	YES	NO

LIGHT HOUSEKEEPING PERFORMED BY AIDE

LINEN CHANGE:	YES	NO	DISHWASHING:	YES	NO
PERSONAL LAUNDRY:	YES	NO	MEAL PREPARATION:	YES	NO
DUSTING:	YES	NO	CLEAN BATHROOM:	YES	NO
VACUUM:	YES	NO	SHOPPING:	YES	NO

PATIENT AMBULATION ACTIVITY

ASSIST OF WALKER/CANE:	YES	NO	BEDBOUND:	YES	NO
ASSISTANCE OF AIDE:	YES	NO	TRANSFER ASSIST:	YES	NO
ASSIST OF WHEELCHAIR:	YES	NO	EXERCISES:	YES	NO

COMMENTS: ______________________________

Your supervisor may provide you with special forms for recording this information. If not, you may use a clean sheet of plain white paper. Be sure your handwriting is neat and legible. Write down each activity as soon as it is completed. Do *not* rely on your memory. If you are to report to your supervisor by phone, be sure this is done. If you consult the last step of every procedure in this book, it tells you exactly what to report or write down to tell your home care supervisor.

Figure 53-1 shows a sample of an activities of daily living report. To document the activities of daily living on a flow sheet, see Chapter 12 for an example.

KEY QUESTIONS

1. List the housekeeping responsibilities of the home health assistant.
2. How can the principles of infection control be applied to working in the home?
3. What are three ways to improvise when supplies are limited?
4. Discuss nutrition and food service as it applies to the home setting.
5. When should your activities and those of the patient be recorded?
6. Define: bed-bound, infection control, microorganism, responsibility.

CHAPTER

54

Newborn and Infant Care in the Home

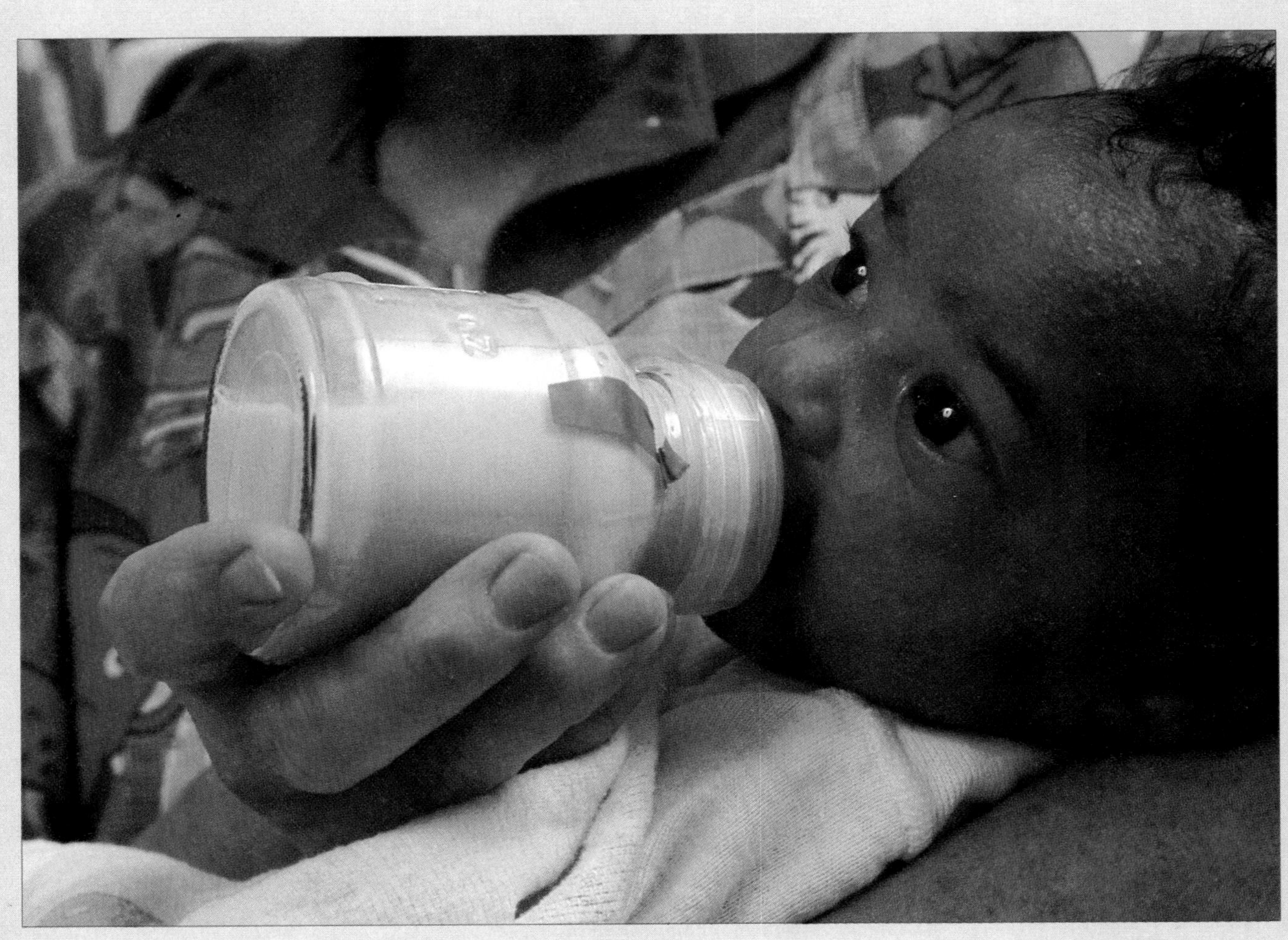

WARNING

For all patient contact, adhere to Universal Precautions. See page 91, 97, or the front cover flap. Wear protective equipment as indicated.

Objectives

What You Will Learn

When you have completed this chapter, you will be able to:

- List three rules to follow for storing infant formula.
- List three types of infant formula.
- Sterilize water, bottles, nipples, and caps.
- Feed and burp an infant.
- Recognize the difference between a normal and an abnormal infant bowel movement.
- Demonstrate umbilical cord care.
- Demonstrate an infant bath.
- List five safety precautions when caring for infants.
- Define: constipation, diarrhea, formula, infant, sterilizing, stool, umbilical cord.

KEY IDEAS

Care of the Infant in the Home

Formula
A liquid food prescribed for an infant containing most required nutrients.

MOST INFANTS ARE FED AT LEAST SIX TIMES a day, every 4 hours, but many infants need to be fed more often than that. If the mother is breast-feeding her baby, you may bring the baby to her when it is time for a feeding. If the baby is being bottle-fed, you may need to prepare the **formula**. Discuss the care of the newborn infant with the mother and your supervisor and follow their instructions.

Rules to Follow

STORING FORMULA

- Formula can be kept refrigerated for two days without spoiling.
- After two days, formula must be thrown away.
- If you are not sure how long formula has been in the refrigerator, discard it.
- Do not risk the baby's health by feeding him or her formula that might be spoiled.
- Formula will begin to spoil within 2 hours when it is left at room temperature.
- Keep the bottle refrigerated until 10 minutes before the feeding.

Different Types of Formula

- Ready to feed
- Powder
- Concentrated liquid

Ready-to-feed (prepared) Formula. *Before* opening the can or bottle the formula comes in from the store, it does not need to be refrigerated. Wash all cans and bottles before opening. This type of formula needs no preparation. Remember to shake it before opening. Open the can with a can opener that is clean (sterilized) and pour the contents into sterile (clean) bottles. Open bottles of ready-to-feed formula by unscrewing the cap. All you need to do now is screw a clean (sterilized) standard nipple right on the bottle the formula came in and feed the baby. Some ready-to-feed formulas come in disposable bottles, to which you attach a sterile nipple.

Powdered Formula. Powdered formula costs less per serving than ready-to-feed formula. Wash and dry all cans before opening. Use a clean can opener. Follow the instructions on the label carefully as to the amounts of powder and sterile water to mix together. Be sure to mix the powder with water that you have boiled and allowed to cool. Mix the powder and sterile water in sterile bottles. Once mixed, this formula must be kept refrigerated.

Concentrated Liquid Formula. Concentrated liquid is the least expensive type of formula. Shake and wash all cans before opening. Use a clean can opener. To prepare this formula, mix one part concentrate to one part boiled water (one can concentrate to one can boiled water). You must boil the water before you mix the formula. Be sure to mix the formula in sterile bottles or a sterile pitcher. Once mixed, this formula must be kept refrigerated.

Sterilizing
Destroying all microorganisms, including spores.

In certain areas, you will not be instructed to boil water to sterilize bottles and nipples. Ask your supervisor for instructions for your area.

Procedure Sterilizing Tap Water

1. Assemble your equipment:
   a) Saucepan
   b) Water
   c) Stove
   d) Timer, watch, or clock
2. Wash your hands.
3. Fill the saucepan two-thirds full with water.
4. Place the filled pan on the stove burner and turn on to high or full.
5. When the water comes to a full boil, begin timing. Allow the water to remain at a full boil for 20 minutes in covered pan.
6. Turn off the burner.
7. Allow the water to cool before using it to mix the formula.
8. Wash your hands.

Procedure Sterilizing Bottles

1. Assemble your equipment:
   a) Bottles
   b) Nipples, caps, and jar
   c) Bottle brush
   d) Dishwashing detergent
   e) Hot water from the tap
   f) Large pot with cover or a special sterilizing pot for baby bottles
   g) Small towel
   h) Tap water
   i) Stove
   j) Timer, watch, or clock
   k) Tongs
2. Wash your hands.
3. Scrub bottles, nipples, and caps with hot soapy water. Use the bottle brush to

clean inside the bottles. Always squirt hot, soapy water through the holes in the nipples to clean out any dried-on formula.

4. Rinse thoroughly with hot water.
5. Fold the small towel to fit the bottom of the pot and lay it there. This will prevent the bottles from breaking. (This is done when you do not have a bottle rack.)
6. Stand the washed bottles on the towel in a circle around the inside of the pot (Figure 54-1).

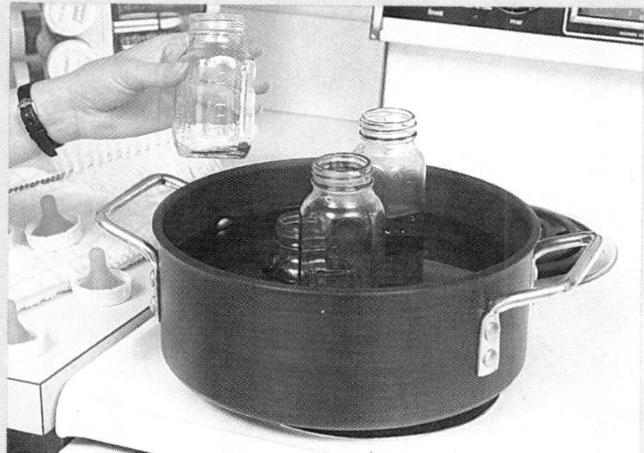

FIGURE 54-1 In certain areas, you will not be instructed to sterilize bottles and nipples. Ask your supervisor for instruction for your area.

7. Place the caps and nipples into the clean, empty jar. Place into the pot at the center of the bottles.
8. Pour water into and around the bottles and into the jar with the nipples until two-thirds of each bottle is under water. Place the tongs upright in the pot to sterilize them.
9. Cover the pot.
10. Place the pot on the stove burner and turn on the burner to the high or full setting.
11. When the water comes to a full boil, begin timing. Allow the water to remain at a full boil for 25 minutes.
12. Using the sterile tongs, remove the nipples and caps in the jar 10 to 15 minutes after the full boil began. With the nipples still inside the jar, stand the jar on the table to cool.
13. Turn off the burner.
14. Take the cover off the pot and allow it to cool.
15. Remove the sterile bottles from the pot with sterile tongs.
16. Empty the water out of the pot. The pot is now sterilized, so you can use it for mixing the formula, if needed.
17. Wash your hands.

KEY IDEAS

Feeding the Baby from a Bottle

Figures 54-2 through 54-5 provide guidance for feeding a baby from a bottle.

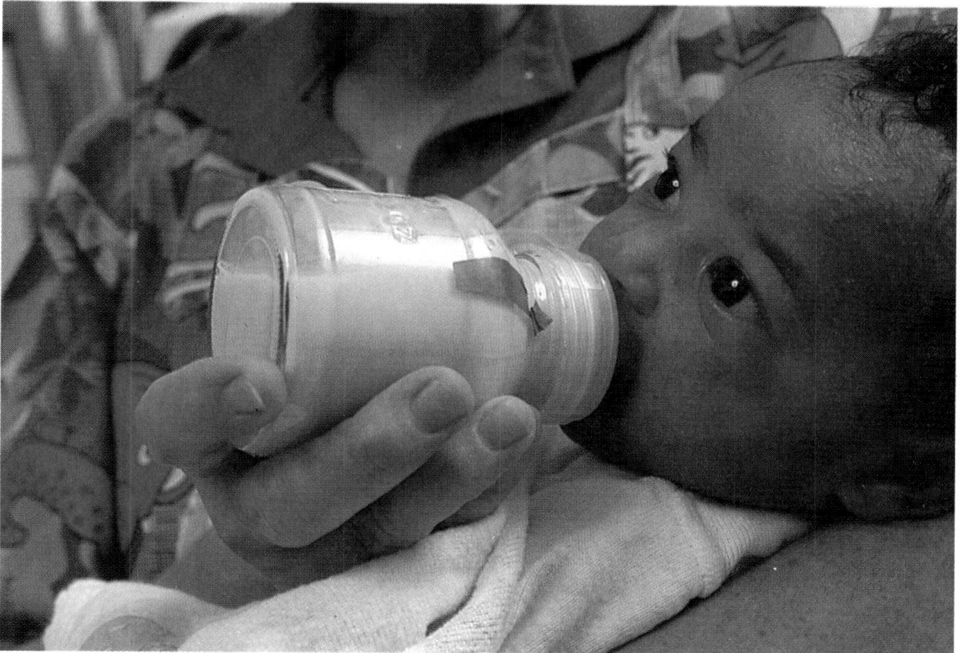

FIGURE 54-2 Tilt the bottle so the nipple is always full of milk and the air in the bottle rises.

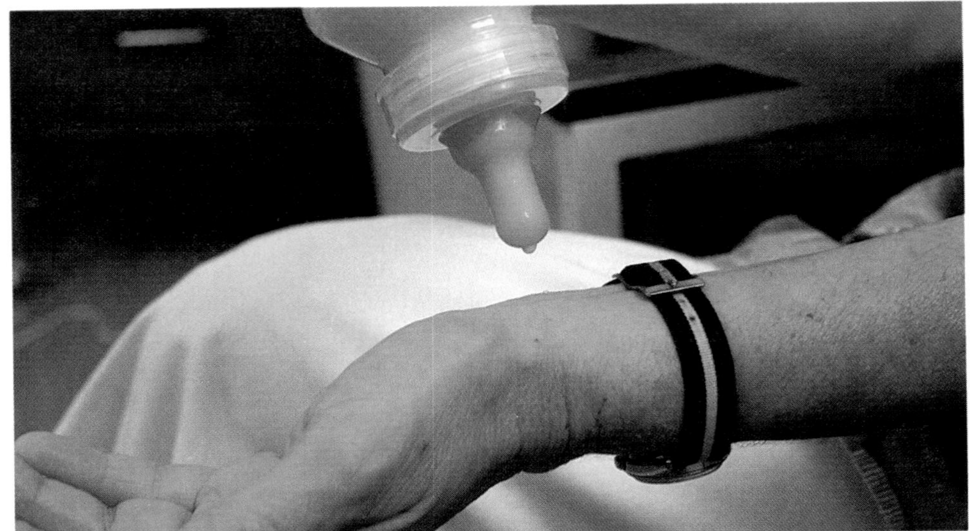

FIGURE 54-3 Check the temperature of the formula.

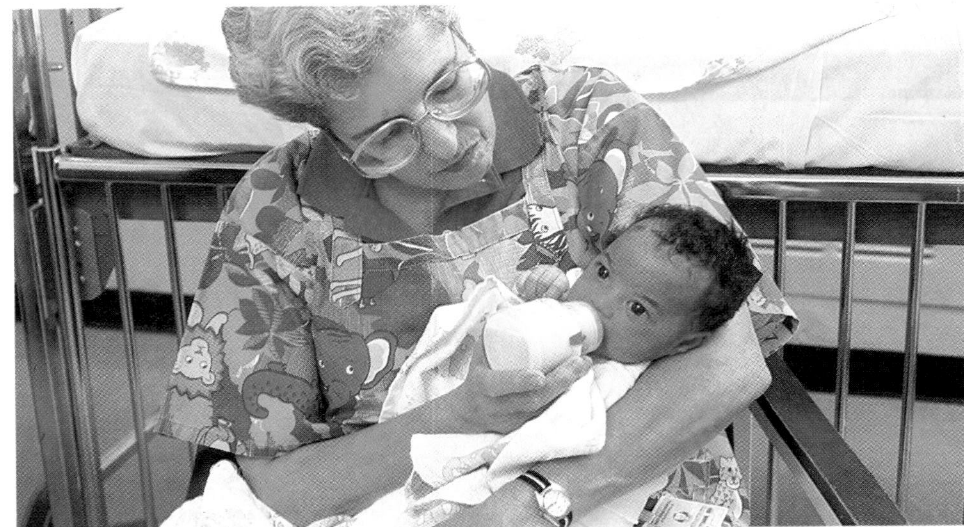

FIGURE 54-4 The infant should be held during feeding. Do not prop the bottle and leave the baby.

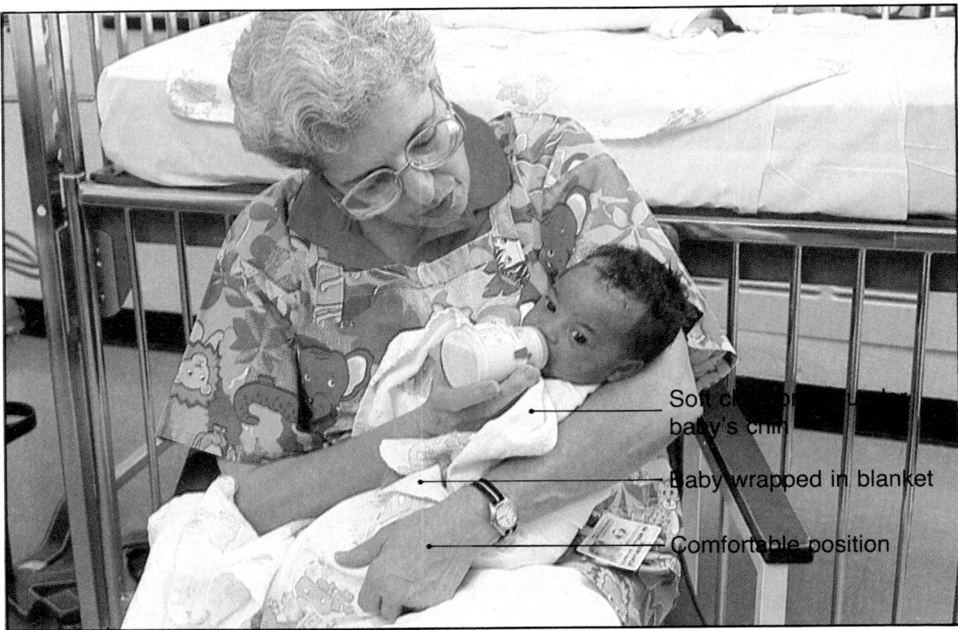

FIGURE 54-5 The infant should be made comfortable while being fed.

KEY IDEAS

Burping the Infant

Most infants, especially those who are bottle-fed, swallow some air while drinking. Air in the gastrointestinal tract can cause vomiting and abdominal pain. You can prevent a buildup of the air by feeding the infant slowly, stopping after every 1–2 ounces (30–60 cc) to burp the baby.

There are two methods for burping the baby:

Method A. Cover your shoulder with a clean cloth (a small towel or a cloth diaper). Hold the baby in a vertical position, so his head is resting on your shoulder (Figure 54-6). Gently rub and/or pat the infant's back until you hear the burp.

Method B. Sit the infant on your leg so his feet are dangling on your side. Put one of your hands on the infant's chest and lean the baby over so your hand is supporting him (Figure 54-7). Gently rub and pat the baby's back with your other hand until you hear the burp.

FIGURE 54-6 Method A for burping a baby. Use a diaper or towel over your shoulder. Press the baby against your shoulder. Pat the baby gently on the back.

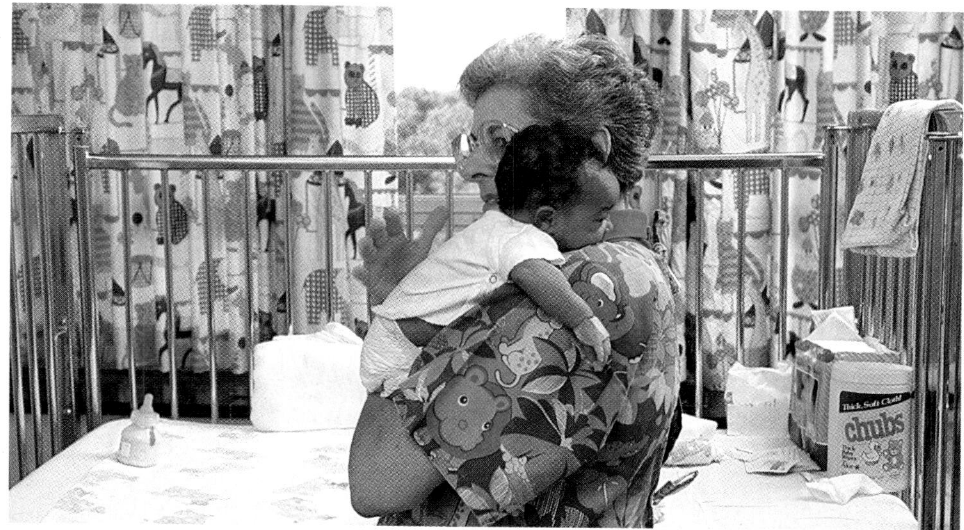

FIGURE 54-7 Method B for burping the baby.

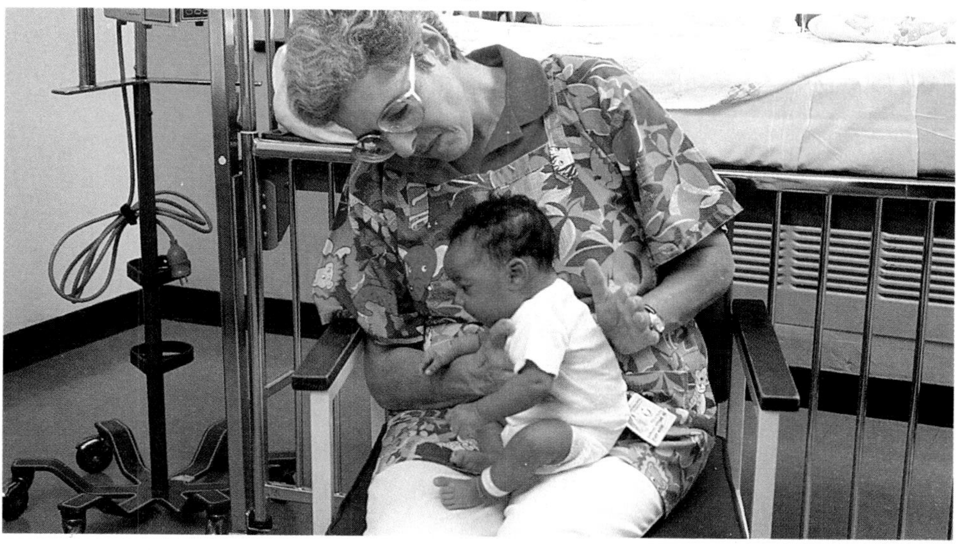

KEY IDEAS

Observing the Infant's Stool

Stool
Solid waste material discharged from the body throughout the rectum and anus. Other names includes feces, excreta, excrement, bowel movement, and fecal matter.

Constipation
Difficult, infrequent defecation with passage of unduly hard and dry, fecal material.

Diarrhea
An abnormally frequent discharge of fluid fecal material from the bowel.

You will need to observe the infant's **stool** at each diaper change in order to detect **constipation** or **diarrhea**. When you observe a change from what has been normal for your patient, report your observations to the nurse.

The bottle-fed infant will have stools that are yellowish or mustard color. They will be lumpy but soft. One to three bowel movements each day is normal for an infant that is bottle-fed every 3 to 4 hours.

The breast-fed infant will have stools that are yellowish or mustard color, but the color may change slightly and may appear to have a greenish tint, depending on the mother's diet. The stools will be looser and smoother than the stools of a bottle-fed infant. It is not unusual for the stools to look like there are tiny seeds in them. A bowel movement after every feeding or only once or twice a day is normal for an infant that is breast-fed every 2 to 3 hours. Check with your supervisor if you suspect that the infant is constipated. An infant whose bowel movement is dry and formed is considered to be constipated. Often, all that is necessary to correct this situation is to offer the infant some plain sterile water between each formula feeding. Usually the infant will drink ½ to 1½ ounces (15–45 cc) of water. If the constipation persists, report this to the nurse.

Diarrhea in Infants

Diarrhea in infants can be a very serious problem and requires immediate attention. Infants can lose all their body fluids and chemicals very quickly. An infant with diarrhea can become dehydrated within two days. You will be able to see a noticeable change in the infant's elimination pattern and in the actual color and consistency of the stools when an infant has diarrhea. The stools may appear green and watery, running right out of the diaper. There may be a distinct odor. The frequency of the stools may increase to two or three times within just a few hours. At the first sign of diarrhea, report to your immediate supervisor.

There are many causes for diarrhea in infants. It may be caused by equipment that was not sterilized (cleansed) properly, by carelessly prepared or spoiled formula, or by allergies. Much diarrhea is caused by passing bacteria to the infant from the hands of those who handle him or her. This is the reason proper handwashing is so essential when caring for an infant. Encourage everyone who handles the infant to wash their hands frequently and certainly before handling the baby or equipment used in its care. Be sure to explain why you are asking them to do this, to avoid offending anyone. Frequent handwashing can prevent and limit unnecessary diarrhea.

Umbilical Cord
A rather long, flexible, rough organ that carries nourishment from the mother to the baby. It connects the umbilicus of the unborn baby in the mother's uterus to the placenta.

KEY IDEAS

Care of the Umbilical Cord

Before birth, the **umbilical cord** serves as a lifeline, connecting the fetus with the mother's placenta. All nourishment is passed from mother to fetus through the umbilical cord. At the time of delivery, the cord is clamped and cut, and the healing process of the umbilicus begins. Within 5 to 10 days the cord will dry, turn black, and eventually fall off.

Rules to Follow

CARE OF THE UMBILICAL CORD

- Keep the diaper folded down away from the cord. A wet diaper on top of the cord could cause an infection.

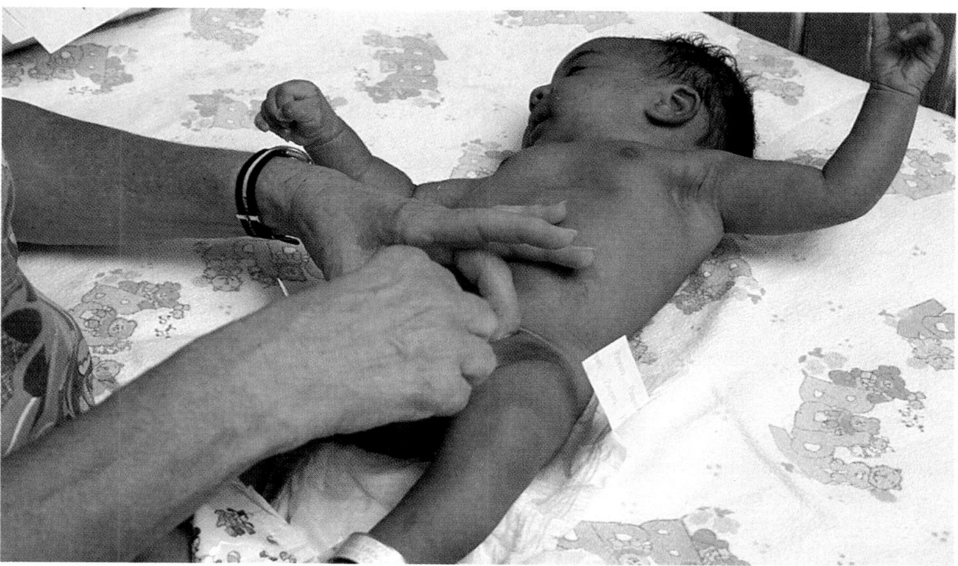

FIGURE 54-8 Checking the baby's umbilical cord. Report anything unusual, such as oozing and bleeding.

- At every diaper change, check the baby's cord (Figure 54-8). Wash the cord with plain rubbing alcohol on a cotton ball or according to your institution's policy. The alcohol will help speed up the drying process and will keep the cord clean.
- Ask your supervisor if you may use the alcohol. Follow his or her instructions.
- Never pull on the cord. Let it fall off by itself. Laying the infant on his abdomen will not hurt the cord. Binders or belly bands are not advised.

KEY IDEAS

Bathing the Infant

Sponge Bathing

While the umbilical cord is still attached to the baby, he or she can be washed using a sponge bath. A tub bath is not permitted until the cord has fallen off. The infant should receive a sponge bath at least once a day.

Sponge bathing an infant means gently washing each part of the baby's body with mild soap and warm water, but not submerging the infant in water. Safety and the infant is very important. Whenever in doubt about anything, ask the nurse. A safe table or counter is a convenient place to give a sponge bath. Clear off the counter and wash it well. Spread a towel on the counter to make a soft and warm place on which to place the baby. Prepare warm water, mild soap, washcloth, blankets, and towels before bringing the baby to the counter. Only one part of the body is washed at a time. Wash, rinse, and dry each body part or area very well. Then cover the body part right away with the bath blanket. If you do not have a bath blanket, use a towel.

Tub Bathing

After the cord has fallen off, the infant can be given a tub bath. You can use a large sink or a baby bath tub. If you are using a sink, be sure to clean the sink and counter. Scrub the sink with a cleanser and rinse it thoroughly. Assemble your equipment before you begin so you will not need to leave the room to get something that you may have forgotten. Do not leave the infant in the tub or on the counter to answer the phone or the doorbell.

Bath time should be a pleasant and enjoyable time for mother and baby. Try to involve the mother as much as she is able and take the opportunity to teach her how to care for the baby. The infant's safety is your first responsibility. Keep your hands and eyes on the baby throughout the bath.

Procedure Giving the Infant a Tub Bath

1. Assemble your equipment:
   a) Infant tub or sink
   b) Two bath towels (soft)
   c) Cotton balls
   d) Wash cloth
   e) Warm water 100°F (37.8°C) (warm to the touch of the elbow)
   f) Baby soap
   g) Baby shampoo (optional)
   h) Baby powder, lotion, or cream
   i) Diaper
   j) Clean clothes
2. Wash your hands.
3. Wash the sink or tub with a disinfectant cleanser and rinse thoroughly.
4. Line the sink or tub with a bath towel.
5. Place a towel on the counter next to the sink or tub as you may want to lay the infant down to dry him.
6. Fill the tub or sink with 1 to 2 inches of warm water 100°F (37.8°C). This will be warm to the touch of the elbow.
7. Undress the infant, wrap him in a towel or blanket, and bring him to the tub or sink (Figure 54-9).

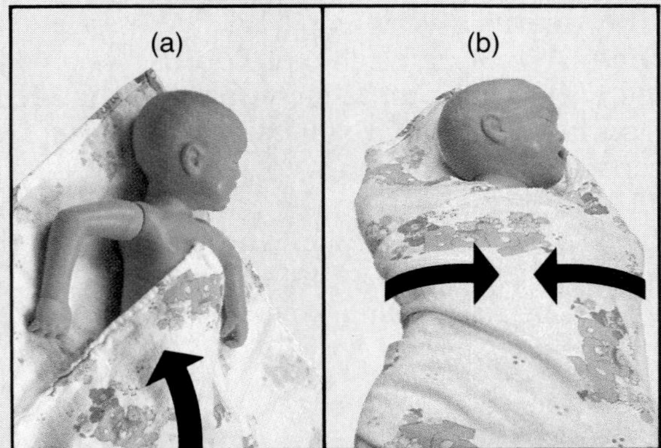

FIGURE 54-9 Wrapping the baby. (a) Fold the lower corner of the blanket over the legs and feet. (b) Fold the two side corners under the arms and over the chest.

8. Using a cotton ball moistened with warm water and squeezed out, gently wipe the infant's eyes from the nose toward the ears. *Use a clean cotton ball for each eye* (Figure 54-10).

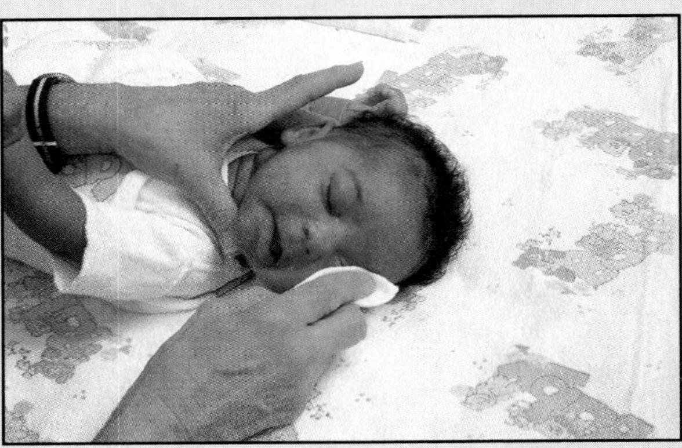

FIGURE 54-10

9. To wash the hair, hold the infant in the football hold, with the baby's head over the sink or tub (FIgure 54-11). This will

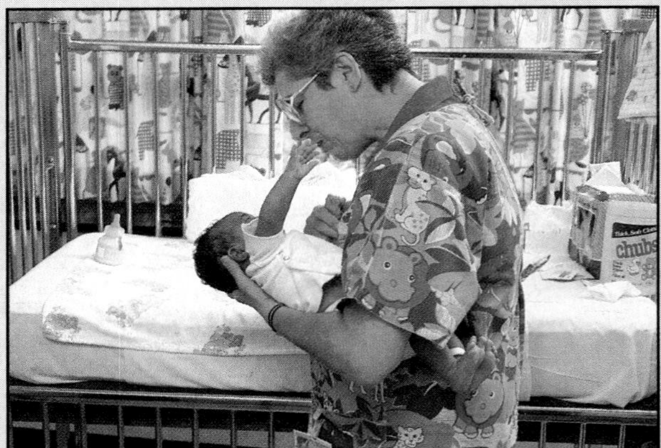

FIGURE 54-11 The football hold. Support the baby's head in the palm of your left hand. The baby's back will be supported along your left forearm. His hips will be pressed against your waist by your left elbow, holding him securely in place. You may use either arm for this hold, as long as you support his head and neck.

free your other arm to wet the hair, apply a small amount of shampoo, and rinse the hair.

10. Dry the infant's head with a towel.
11. Unwrap the infant and gently place him on the towel in the sink or tub. One of your hands should always be holding the baby. Never let go, not even for a second.
12. Wash the infant's body with the soap and the washcloth, being careful to wash between the folds (creases) of the skin (Figure 54-12).

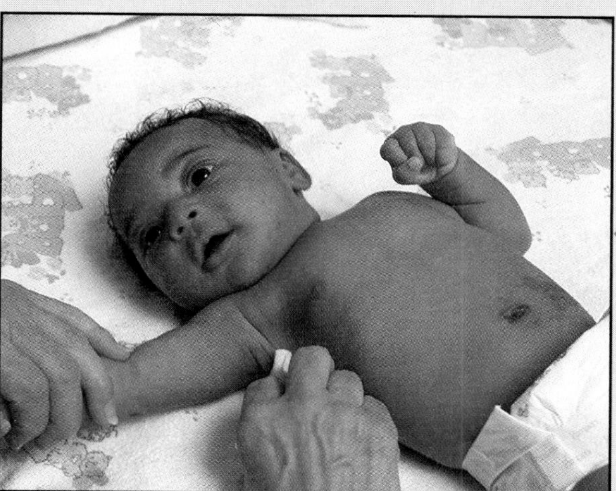

FIGURE 54-12 Cleaning creases.

13. If the infant is female, always wash the perineal area from front to back (Figure 54-13).

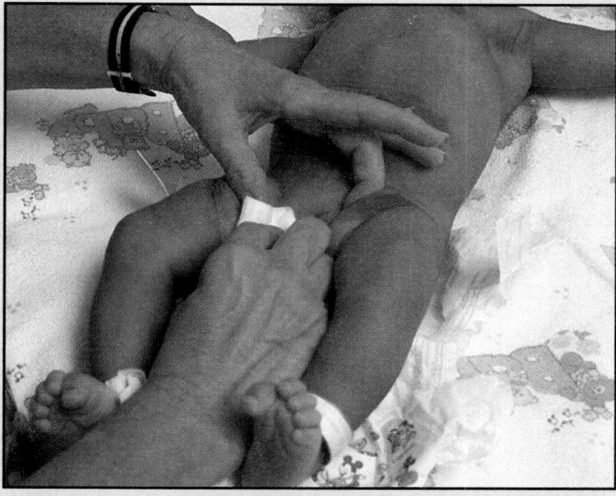

FIGURE 54-13 Cleaning the genital area.

14. Rinse the infant thoroughly with warm water.
15. Lift the infant out of the water and onto the towel you laid out on the counter.
16. Dry the infant well, being careful to dry between the folds of skin.
17. Now you can apply powder, lotion, or cream to the infant, whichever the mother prefers or as instructed by the nurse.
18. Diaper and dress the infant (Figures 54-14 and 54-15).

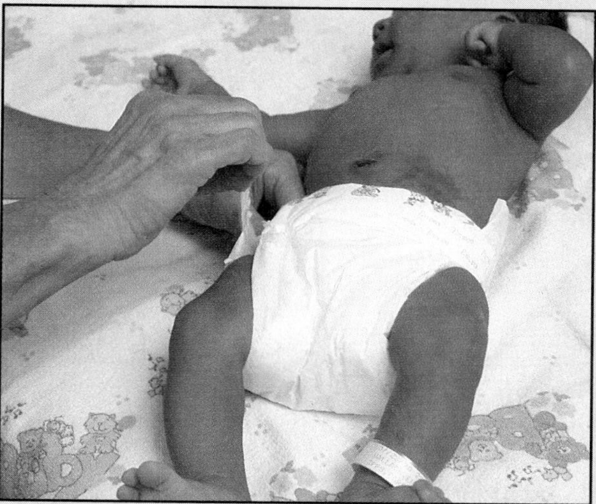

FIGURE 54-14

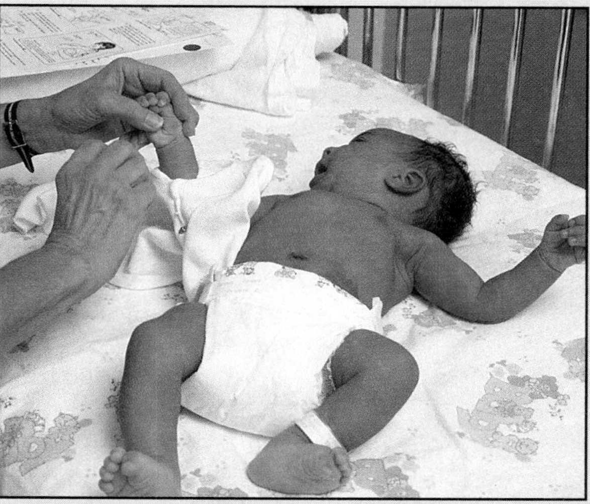

FIGURE 54-15 Slip the fingers of one hand inside the sleeve of the shirt. With that hand, take the baby's hand. With your other hand, pull the sleeve up over the baby's arm. Turn the baby gently on her side. Slip the shirt down over her back. Turn her gently back, and draw the shirt to the other side. Put the baby's other arm into its sleeve in the same way. Fasten the ties or snaps.

19. Place the infant in his crib and raise the crib side rails or allow the mother to hold him. Show the mother how to hold the

infant in either the upright position (Figure 54-16) or the cradle position (Figure 54-17).

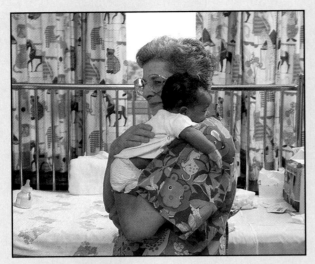

FIGURE 54-16 To hold an infant in the upright position, your left forearm should be under the baby's buttocks. His body is pressed against your shoulder and chest. The infant's cheek rests on your left shoulder. Use your right hand to support his head and back.

20. Clean and return the equipment and supplies to their proper place.

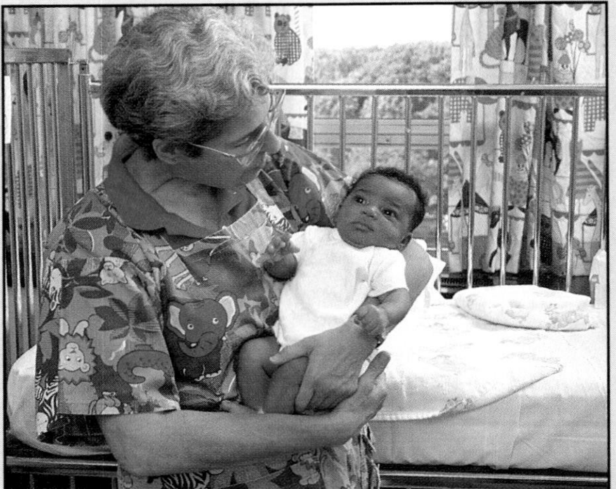

FIGURE 54-17 To lift and carry an infant in the cradle position, slide your left hand and arm under the baby's back. Use your left arm to support his head, back, and buttocks. Put your right hand under the baby's buttocks. Then move your left arm and hand up toward the infant's head before picking him up. You use your left arm and hand to give more support to the back, shoulders, and head while your right hand and arm support his buttocks, legs, and feet. Pick up the baby by cradling him in your arms, with his body against your chest.

21. Clean the area where the bath was given.
22. Wash your hands.

KEY IDEAS

Infant Safety

Infant
A child not over two years of age; a baby.

When the patient is an **infant**, you must take special precautions to protect the baby from preventable accidents. Even if an infant has not yet learned to roll over, he can wiggle and kick until he falls off beds, chairs, tables, or counters. Never leave an infant unattended on any of these surfaces. If you are far from the infant's crib and you must leave him unattended for a few seconds, put him on the floor. The safest place for an infant is in his crib, with the side rails up. Some people keep babies in a carriage or a drawer because they do not have a crib. Other things you can do to prevent accidents when caring for an infant include:

- Washing your hands before handling the infant or her supplies
- Placing the infant on her side or belly after eating to prevent aspiration
- Keeping the crib rails in the up position when the infant is sleeping or playing
- Using only 1 to 2 inches of bath water and never leaving the infant alone in the water.
- Never placing the infant who is in an infant seat on tables, chairs, beds, or counters
- Keeping all medications and cleaning solutions out of the reach of all children (Figure 54-18).

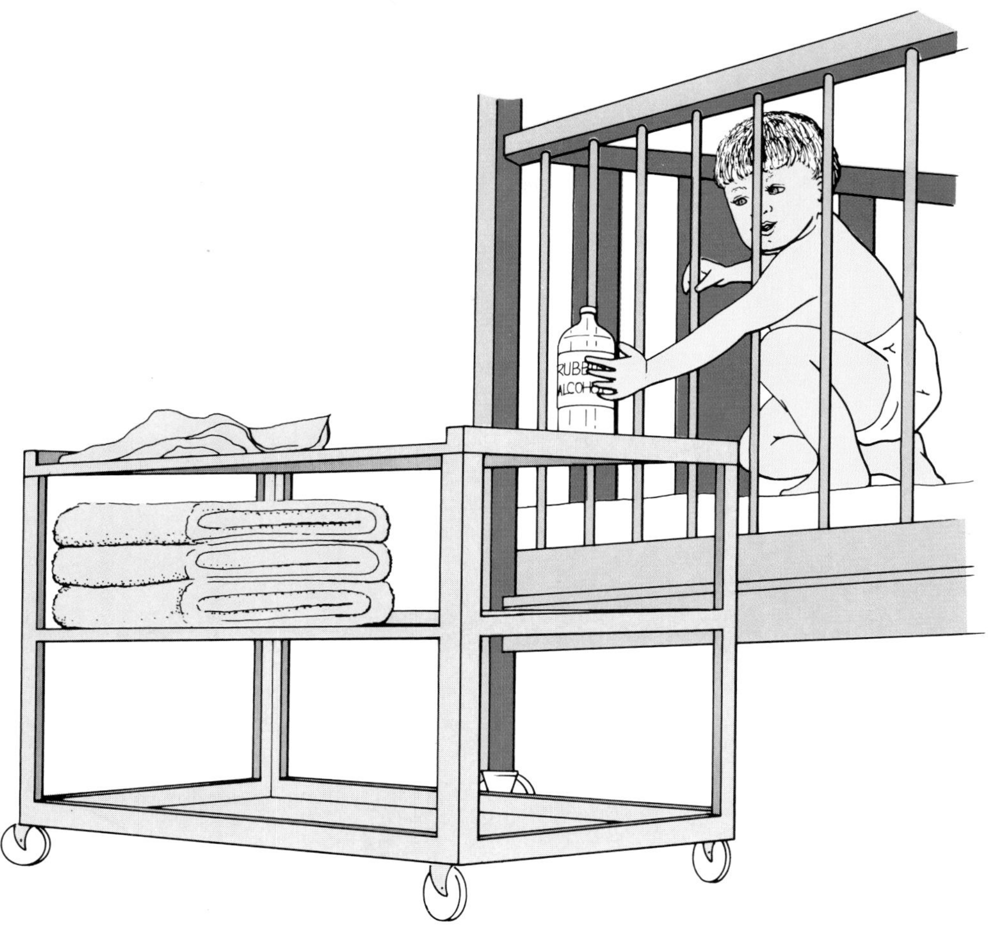

FIGURE 54-18 Keep hazards out of reach of all children.

KEY QUESTIONS

1. What are three rules you should follow when storing infant formula?
2. Describe three types of infant formula.
3. Your employer, a new mother, asks you to teach her how to sterilize water, bottles, nipples, and caps. Explain these procedures to her.
4. There are two methods of burping a baby. What is the difference between them?
5. What are the first signs of diarrhea in infants, and why is it dangerous?
6. List three rules to follow when caring for the umbilical cord.
7. When bathing the infant, what is your first responsibility and how can you do this?
8. List five safety precautions to follow when caring for infants.
9. Define: constipation, diarrhea, formula, infant, sterilizing, stool, umbilical cord.

Glossary

Abbreviation A shortened form of a word or phrase used to represent the complete form.

Abdomen The region of the body between the chest and the pelvis.

Abdominal prep The procedure for making the patient's abdomen ready for surgery; includes thorough cleansing of the skin and careful shaving of body hair in the abdominal area.

Abdominal respiration Breathing in which the patient uses mostly the abdominal muscles.

Abduction To move an arm or leg away from the center of the body.

Absorb To take or soak in, up, or through.

Absorption The process of the end products of digestion entering the bloodstream.

Acceptance Admitting, understanding, or facing the truth or reality of the situation.

Accountable To be answerable for one's behavior; legally or ethically responsible for the care of another.

Accuracy The quality of being exact or correct; exact conformity to truth and rules; free from errors or defects.

Acetest® A test used to measure the amount of acetone in the patient's urine.

Acetone A chemical compound found in the blood and urine of diabetic patients.

Active Producing, involving, or participating in activity or movement.

Activities of daily living The activities or tasks usually performed every day, such as toileting, washing, eating, or dressing.

Acute Illness that comes on suddenly.

Adduction To move an arm or leg toward the center of the body.

Adhere Stick to.

Admission The administrative procedures followed when a person enters the health care institution and becomes an inpatient; covers the period from the time the patient enters the door of the hospital until he is settled in his room.

Adrenal glands Two glands in the upper posterior dorsal area of the abdomen, near the kidneys.

Aging process Changes in the body caused by growing older.

AIDS (acquired immune deficiency syndrome) A viral infection characterized by decreased immunity to opportunistic infections. It is a group of signs and symptoms that characterize a lethal disorder in T-cell immunity.

Allotted Given or assigned.

Alternating-pressure air mattress A pad similar to an air mattress that can be placed beneath the patient to reduce pressure on the shoulders, back, heels, and elbows.

Alveoli A microscopic air sac in the lung where oxygen passes into the blood.

Ambulate To walk or move about.

Ambulation Walking or moving about in an upright position.

Ambulatory Able to walk about; not bedridden.

Amputation The cutting off of a body part by accident or through surgery.

Anal Pertaining to the anus.

Anatomical position A person standing facing you, feet together, palms forward, head up.

Anatomy The study of the structure of an organism.

Aneroid sphygmomanometer Dial-type blood pressure equipment.

Anesthesia Loss of feeling or sensation in a part or all of the body; *local* anesthesia is the loss of sensation in a part of the body; *general* anesthesia is complete loss of sensation in the entire body.

Anesthesiologist The medical doctor who administers the anesthetic to the patient in the operating room.

Anesthetic A drug used to produce loss of feeling; can be given orally, rectally, by injection, or by inhalation. A person who has been given an anesthetic is anesthetized.

Anesthetist The registered nurse who assists the anesthetist.

Anger A strong emotional response of displeasure, irritation, and resentment.

Anterior Located in the front; opposite of posterior.

Anus The posterior opening in the body through which feces are excreted.

Aorta The name for the major artery that carries blood away from the heart.

Aphasia Loss of language or speech.

Apical pulse A measurement of the heartbeats at the apex of the heart, located just under the left breast.

Appetite Desire for food or drink.

Artery A blood vessel that carries blood away from the heart.

Aseptis The condition of being free of disease-causing organisms.

Aspirate To remove material from a body cavity by using a tube; also, to draw material such as saliva, mucus, or food particles into the lungs from the mouth.

Atrophy Muscles wasting away or decreasing in size.

Auricles/atria The two upper chambers of the heart, which are side by side. Each is known as an *atrium*, the left atrium or the right atrium.

Autoclave Equipment used to sterilize instruments and other articles in the health care institution.

Autonomic nervous system The part of the nervous system that carries messages without conscious thought.

Axillary The area under the arms; the armpits.

Bacteria Sometimes called germs; one kind of microorganism; many bacteria cause disease.

Bargaining Trying to make a deal to change the situation.

Bed-bound Unable to get out of bed.

Bed cradle A frame shaped like a barrel cut in half lengthwise used to keep bed linens off a part of the patient's body.

Bedpan A pan used by patients who must defecate or urinate while in bed.

Bedridden (bed-bound) Unable to get out of bed.

Benign A tumor or neoplasm that stays at its site of origin and does not usually regrow once removed.

Binder A wide cloth bandage.

Bladder A membranous sac that serves as a container within the body, such as the urinary bladder, which holds urine.

Blood The fluid that circulates through the heart, arteries, veins, and capillaries; it carries nourishment and oxygen to the tissues and takes away waste matter and carbon dioxide.

Blood and lymph tissue Tissue composed of singular cells that move within a fluid to every part of the body circulating nutrients, oxygen, and antibodies and removing waste products.

Blood pressure The force of the blood exerted on the inner walls of the arteries, veins, and chambers of the heart as it flows or circulates through them.

Body alignment Refers to the arrangement of the body in a straight line; the placing of portions of the body in correct anatomical position.

Body language Communication through hand movements (gestures), facial expressions, body movements, and touch.

Body mechanics Special ways of standing and moving one's body to make the best use of strength and avoid fatigue.

Brain The main organ of the central nervous system; the center of thought, movement, emotion, and speech; controls coordination of the nerves and responses from the sense organs.

Bronchial tubes Branches of the trachea that lead into the lungs.

Bursa A sac found within a joint capsule; filled with synovial fluid, which helps to buffer the movement of the bones against one another.

Calibrated Marked with lines and numbers for measuring.

Calories Units for measuring the energy produced when food is oxidized in the body.

Cancer Refers to malignant neoplasms. Cancer cells interfere with normal body function, grow and spread between cells, invade surrounding tissue, and sometimes cause death.

Cannula A flexible tube that can be inserted into one of the body cavities. A cannula may be used to draw fluids out or to give oxygen or fluids.

Capillaries The very small blood vessels that carry blood to all parts of the body and the skin; a link between the ends of the arteries and the beginning of the veins.

Carbohydrate One of the basic food elements used by the body; composed of carbon, hydrogen, and oxygen (includes sugars and starches).

Cardiac Pertaining to the heart.

Cardiac arrest The unexpected stopping of the heartbeat and circulation.

Cardiac muscle tissue Involuntary muscle tissue found only in the heart.

Cardiopulmonary resuscitation (CPR) An emergency procedure used to reestablish effective circulation and respiration in order to prevent irreversible brain damage.

Cardiovascular system Circulatory system.

Caregiver Refers to the family member who is taking the major responsibility for the patient.

Cartilage A tough connective tissue that holds bones together.

Catheter A tube inserted into a body opening or cavity.

Catheterization Inserting a catheter into a body opening or cavity.

Cell The basic unit of living matter.

Centigrade A system for measurement of temperature using a scale divided into 100 units or degrees. In this system, the freezing temperature of water is 0°C. Water boils at 100°C. Often referred to as Celsius.

Central nervous system The part of the nervous system made up of the brain, nerves, and spinal cord.

Central supply A central place for storing supplies and equipment; also called Central Supply Room, Special Purchasing Department, or Central Supply Department.

Cerebral Pertaining to the cerebrum, a part of the brain.

Cerebrovascular accident Stroke or CVA; blood vessels in the brain become blocked or bleed, interrupting the blood supply to that part of the brain and damaging the surrounding area of the brain.

Channel Path.

Check and balance A safeguard for health in which the systems of the body have built-in mechanisms that keep their activity in a state of balance.

Cheyne-Stokes respiration One kind of irregular breathing. At first the breathing is slow and shallow; then the respiration becomes faster and deeper until it reaches a kind of peak. The respiration then slows down and becomes shallow again. The breathing may then stop completely for 10 seconds, and then begin the pattern again. This type of respiration may be caused by certain cerebral (brain), cardiac (heart), or pulmonary (lung) diseases or conditions.

Chronic Illness continues over many years or a lifetime.

Circulation The continuous movement of blood through the heart and blood vessels to all parts of the body.

Circulatory system The heart, blood vessels, blood, and all the organs that pump and carry blood and other fluids throughout the body.

Clean A term used in health care institutions to refer to an object or area that is uncontaminated by harmful microorganisms.

Clean catch Refers to the fact that the urine for this specimen is not contaminated by anything outside the patient's body.

Clinitest® A test used to measure the amount of glucose in the patient's urine.

Colon The large bowel; extends from the large intestine to the anus.

Coma A state of deep unconsciousness, often caused by disease, injury, or drugs.

Commode A movable chair enclosing a bedpan or with an opening that can fit over a toilet.

Communicable disease A disease that is easily spread from one person to another; also called infectious disease.

Communication The exchange of thoughts, messages, or ideas by speech, signals, gestures, or writing.

Compassion Understanding the fears, problems, and distress of someone else, combined with a concern and a desire to help.

Complication An unexpected condition, such as the development of another illness in a patient who is already sick.

Compress Folded piece of cloth used to apply pressure, moisture, heat, cold, or medication to a specific part of the body.

Congenital Born with, or from birth; refers to a physical or mental characteristic present in a baby at birth. Sometimes referred to as a birth defect.

Connective tissue Tissue that connects, supports, covers, ensheathes, lines, pads, or protects.

Constipation Difficult, infrequent defecation with passage of unduly hard and dry fecal material.

Continuous Uninterrupted, without a stop.

Contract Get smaller.

Contracture When muscle tissue becomes drawn together, bunched up, or shortened because of spasm or paralysis, either permanently or temporarily.

Convalescence The period of time when a person is getting well or recovering after an illness or surgery.

Convert Change.

Cooperate To work or act together; to unite in producing an effect or to share an activity for mutual benefit.

Courtesy Being polite and considerate.

Cubic centimeter Having a volume equal to a cube whose edges are 1 centimeter long.

Cyanosis When the skin looks blue or gray, especially on the lips, nailbeds, and under the fingernails. In a black patient, it may appear as a darkening of color. This occurs when there is not enough oxygen in the blood.

Dangling position Sitting up on the edge of the bed with the feet hanging down loosely.

Deceased Another word for dead.

Deep Distant from the surface of the body.

Defecate To have a bowel movement; to excrete waste matter from the bowels.

Dehydration A condition in which the body has less than the normal amount of fluid.

Dementia An irreversible mental condition in which intellectual abilities are continuously reduced.

Denial Refusal to admit the truth or face reality.

Dentures Artificial teeth. Dentures may replace some or all of a person's teeth; they are described as being partial or complete and upper or lower.

Dependability A quality shown by coming to work every day on time and doing what is asked at the proper time and in the proper way.

Depression A state of sadness, grief, or low spirits that may or may not cause change of activity.

Dermis The inner layer of skin.

Deteriorate To make or grow worse; degenerate.

Development An increase in the ability to do things.

Deviate To differ from the normal.

Diabetes mellitus A disorder of carbohydrate metabolism that develops when the body cannot change sugar into energy, due to inadequate production or utilization of insulin. When this sugar collects in the blood, the patient needs a special diet and may have to be given medications.

Diabetic coma A coma (abnormal deep stupor), which can occur in a diabetic patient from lack of insulin.

Diagnosis Finding out what kind of disease or medical condition a patient has. A medical diagnosis is always made by a physician.

Diarrhea An abnormally frequent discharge of fluid fecal material from the bowel.

Diastolic blood pressure In taking a patient's blood pressure, one records the bottom number as the reading for the diastolic pressure. This is the relaxing phase of the heartbeat.

Died Expired.

Dietitian An individual who plans well-balanced nourishing diets, designed to meet the needs of individual patients.

Digestion The process in the body in which food is broken down mechanically and chemically and is changed into forms that can enter the bloodstream and be used by the body.

Dilate Get bigger; expand.

Dirty A term used in the health care institution to refer to an object or area as being contaminated by harmful microorganisms.

Disability Loss of the ability to use a part or parts of the body in a normal way.

Discard To throw away or get rid of something.

Discharge (1) The procedure for helping patients to leave the health care institution, including teaching them how to care for themselves at home. (2) Flowing out of material (secretion or excretion) from any part of the body, such as pus, feces, urine, or drainage from a wound.

Discoloration Change in color.

Disinfection The process of destroying most disease-causing pathogenic organisms or rendering them inert.

Disoriented Unaware of or unable to remember, recognize, or describe people, places, or times; confused perception of reality.

Disposable equipment Equipment that is used one time only or for one patient only and then thrown away.

Dorsal Refers to the back or to the back part of an organ.

Dorsal flexion To bend backward.

Dorsal recumbent position Refers to the back or to the back part of an organ; the posterior part; lying down or reclining.

Douche A stream of water or air applied to a part or cavity of the body for cleansing or for the treatment of a localized condition.

Drape A covering used to provide privacy during an examination or an operation.

Draping Covering a patient or parts of the patient's body with a sheet, blanket, bath blanket, or other material. Draping is usually done during the physical examination of the patient and during surgery.

Draw sheet A small sheet made of plastic, rubber, or cotton placed crosswise on the middle of the bed over the bottom sheet to help protect the bedding from a patient's discharges, and/or to tighten the foundation.

DRGs Diagnosis-related groups of patients. A DRG classifies patients by diagnosis or surgical procedure to determine payment for hospital costs.

Dry application An application of warmth or cold in which no water touches the skin.

Edema Abnormal swelling of a part of the body caused by fluid collecting in that area. Usually the swelling is in the ankles, legs, hands, or abdomen.

Egg-crate mattress A foam pad shaped like an egg carton with many depressions and fingerlike projections used in addition to a mattress pad to reduce pressure on the back, shoulders, heels, elbows, and bony prominences.

Eliminate To rid the body of waste products; to excrete, expel, remove, put out.

Embolus A blood clot or mass of other undissolved matter that travels through the circulatory system from its place of formation to another site, lodges in a small blood vessel, and causes an obstruction.

Emergency Event that calls for immediate action.

Emesis Stomach material brought up (vomited) from the stomach.

Emesis basin A pan used for catching material that a patient spits out, vomits, or expectorates.

Empathy The ability to put yourself in another's place and to see things as they see them.

Endocrine gland Ductless glands that produce hormones and secrete them directly into the blood or lymph.

Endocrine system The system composed of the endocrine glands that regulates body function by secreting hormones into the blood or lymph to be circulated to all parts of the body.

Enema A liquid that flows through a tube into the rectum to wash out its contents.

Environment All the surrounding conditions and influences affecting the life and development of an organism.

Enzyme A substance manufactured by living tissue that stimulates certain chemical changes in the body. For example, pancreatic enzymes cause complex food proteins to break down into simpler structures that can be absorbed by the intestines.

Epidermis The outer layer or surface of the skin.

Epithelial tissue Tissue that protects, secretes, absorbs, and receives sensations.

Equipment Materials, tools, devices, supplies, furnishings, necessary things used to perform a task.

Esophagus A muscular tube for the passage of food, which extends from the back of the throat (pharynx), down through the chest and diaphragm into the stomach.

Estrogen A female hormone produced by the ovaries that causes a buildup of the lining of the uterus. It prepares the uterus for possible pregnancy, and is responsible for the development of secondary sexual characteristics, for example, pubic hair.

Ethical behavior To keep promises and do what you should do; to act in accordance with the rules or standards for right conduct or practice.

Evacuation Emptying out.

Evaporate To pass off as vapor, as water evaporating into the air.

Excreta Urine and feces; waste matter from the body.

Excrete To eliminate or expel waste matter from the body.

Excretory system (urinary system) The group of body organs, including the kidneys, ureters, bladder, and urethra, that removes wastes from the blood and produces and eliminates urine.

Exhaling The process of breathing out air in respiration.

Exocrine glands Glands that produce hormones and secrete them either directly or through a duct to epithelial tissue such as a body cavity or the skin surface.

Expectorate To cough up matter from the lungs, trachea, or bronchial tubes and spit it out.

Expired Dead.

Extension To straighten.

Extra nourishment Snacks.

Fahrenheit A system for measuring temperature. In the Fahrenheit system, the temperature of water at boiling is 212°. At freezing, it is 32°. These temperatures are usually written 212°F and 32°F.

Fan-fold A method of arranging bed linens so that the covers and spread are folded back out of the way but still are on the bed and within easy reach.

Fatigue A feeling of tiredness or weariness.

Feces Solid waste material discharged from the body through the rectum and anus. Other names for feces are stool, excreta, excrement, BM, bowel movement, and fecal matter.

Fertile Capable of reproduction.

Fertilization When the sperm and ovum join to form a new cell.

Fever The term for a person's condition when the body temperature is above normal.

First aid The first action taken to help a person who is in crisis.

Flammable Capable of burning quickly and easily.

Flatus Intestinal gas.

Flex To bend.

Flexion To bend a joint (elbow, wrist, knee).

Flow sheet A checklist or chart for recording the activities of daily living.

Fluid Applies to both liquid and gaseous substances.

Fluid balance The same amount of fluid that is taken in by the body is given out by the body.

Fluid imbalance When too much fluid is kept in the body or when too much fluid is lost.

Fluid intake The fluid taken into the body, from whatever source.

Fluid output The fluid passed or excreted out of the body, no matter how.

Fluid retention Intake of fluids exceeds amounts of fluid output causing edema.

Force Strength or power; used to describe the beat of the pulse.

Force fluids (FF) Extra fluids to be taken in by a patient according to the doctor's orders.

Formula A liquid food prescribed for an infant containing most required nutrients.

Fowler's position The patient's position when the head of the bed is at a 45 degree angle.

Fracture A break in the bone.

Fresh urine Urine that has accumulated recently in the patient's urinary bladder.

Friction The rubbing of one surface against another. Friction between the patient's body and the bedclothes often produces bedsores (pressure ulcers).

Functional nursing A method of organizing the health care team in which the head nurse assigns and directs all patient care responsibilities for the nursing staff. This is sometimes called direct assignment.

Gait training Rehabilitative exercise to help the patient improve his ability walking.

Gastrointestinal system The group of body organs that carries out digestion; the digestive system. Sometimes called the GI system; an abbreviation for gastro (stomach) and intestinal.

Gatch handle A handle used on manually operated hospital beds to raise or lower the backrest and kneerest.

Gavage Feeding a patient by putting a tube into the stomach. In nasogastric gavage, the tube is passed through the patient's nostril and then through the esophagus into the stomach.

General anesthetics Anesthetics that cause a loss of sensation in the whole body.

Generalized Affecting, involving, or pertaining to the whole body.

Generalized application One in which warmth or cold is applied to the entire body.

Genital Refers to the external reproductive organs.

Geriatric Aging, elderly; over 65 years of age.

Germicide A chemical compound used to destroy bacteria.

Gland An organ that is able to manufacture and discharge a chemical that will be used elsewhere in the body.

Glucose A sugar formed during metabolism of carbohydrates; blood sugar.

Graduate A measuring cup marked along its side to show various amounts so that the material placed in the cup can be measured accurately. The marks are called calibrations.

Growth An increase in physical size.

Gynecological patient Patients being treated for diseases or conditions of the female reproductive organs, including the breasts.

Hazard A source of danger; a possible cause of an accident.

Health care institution Hospital, extended care facility, nursing home, convalescent home, or clinic where health care services are provided both on an inpatient and outpatient basis.

Heart A four-chambered, hollow, muscular organ that lies in the chest cavity, pointing slightly to the left. It is the pump that circulates the blood through the lungs and into all parts of the body.

Heart attack Interruption of or damage to the blood supply to the heart muscle; myocardial infarction.

Heat cradle A combination of a bed cradle and a heat lamp used for dry heat applications or to maintain the temperature of a warm compress.

Hemiplegia Paralysis of only one-half of the body.

Hemisphere Half of a sphere. In the nervous system it refers to one half of the brain.

Hemorrhage Excessive bleeding; extreme or unexpected loss of blood; bleeding.

Hepatitis B A blood-borne pathogen that can be life-threatening. This infection is transmitted by exposure to blood and other infectious body fluids and tissues.

Hereditary Characteristics passed down from parent to a child. An example is eye color. Some diseases apparently are hereditary. An example is diabetes.

Holistic An approach to meeting the needs of the whole patient that comes from the belief that human beings function as complete units and cannot be treated part by part. Total of the interacting parts, more than the sum of the parts.

Homeostasis Stability of all body functions at normal levels.

Hormones Protein substances secreted by endocrine glands directly into the blood to be circulated to another part of the body, where they stimulate increased activity by chemical action.

Hospice Program that allows a dying patient to remain at home or in a nonhospital environment and die there while receiving professionally supervised care.

Hygiene The science that deals with the preservation of health. When used to describe an object or a person, it means clean and sanitary.

Hyperextension Beyond the normal extension.

Hyperglycemia Abnormally high blood sugar.

Hypertension High blood pressure.

Hypoglycemia Abnormally low blood sugar.

Hypotension Low blood pressure.

Hypothalamus A tiny structure at the base of the brain that has great influence over all body activities, especially the activity of the pituitary gland.

Immobile Unable to move.

Improvise To create from available materials.

Impulse An electrical or chemical change transmitted through certain tissues, especially nerve fibers and muscles.

Incident Any unusual event or occurrence, such as an accident or a condition that is likely to cause an accident.

Incontinence The inability to control the bowels or bladder.

Incontinent Unable to control the bowels or bladder.

Indwelling urinary catheter A bladder drainage tube that is allowed to remain in place within the bladder.

Infant A child not over 2 years of age; a baby.

Infection A condition in body tissue in which germs or pathogens have multiplied.

Infection control To restrain or curb the spread of microorganisms.

Inferior Refers to the lower portion of the body.

Infiltration When an IV solution runs into nearby tissue instead of into a vein.

Inflammation A reaction of the tissues to disease or injury. There is usually pain, heat, redness, and swelling of the body part.

Inhaling The process of taking in air in respiration.

Insensible fluid loss Fluid that is lost from the body without being noticed, such as in perspiration or in air breathed out.

Insulin A hormone produced naturally by the pancreas that helps the body change sugar into energy. Insulin can be produced from an animal pancreas for use in the treatment of diabetes.

Insulin shock A condition that can occur in a diabetic patient with too much insulin, which results in very low blood sugar.

Integumentary system The group of body organs, including the skin, hair, nails, sweat, and oil glands, that provides the first line of defense against infection, maintains body temperature, provides fluids, and eliminates wastes.

Intermittent Alternating; stopping and beginning again.

Intravenous infusion Refers to the injection of fluids into a vein. Foods in liquid form and medications can be put into the patient's body in this way.

Intravenous pole Also called IV pole. A tall poll on rollers or casters used to hold the containers or tubes needed, for example, during a blood transfusion.

Involuntary Without conscious will, control, or decision.

Irregular respiration The depth of breathing changes, and the rate of the rise and fall of the chest is not steady.

Isolation gown A special gown worn over a uniform when coming in contact with a patient with a communicable infectious disease. The gown protects the uniform from being contaminated by harmful bacteria.

Isolation techniques and protective care Special procedures used in caring for patients with infectious communicable diseases, to prevent infection or disease from spreading to other persons, as well as to keep other types of infections or diseases from coming in contact with the patient.

Job description The fundamental nursing tasks and procedures you will be accountable for in your work will be found in the job description given to you by your employing health care institution or agency.

Joint Body part where two bones come together.

Ketones Organic chemical substances that are produced when fatty acids combine with oxygen.

Kidney The organ lying in the upper posterior portion of the abdomen. It removes waste products and water from the bloodstream and excretes them as urine.

Kilogram A unit for measuring weight in the metric system. One kilogram equals 1000 grams. One kilogram equals 2.2046 pounds.

Knee-chest position A bent posture with the knees and chest touching the examining table. This position is sometimes used for examining the rectum. It is also used for women who have recently given birth to get the uterus to fall forward into its normal position.

Labored respiration Working hard to breathe.

Lamb's wool A wide strip of lamb's hide with the fleece attached or a man-made imitation used to relieve pressure in the treatment or prevention of bed sores.

Lavage Refers to the washing out of the stomach when drawing a specimen or draining fluids through a nasogastric tube.

Licensed practical nurse (LPN) or licensed vocational nurse (LVN) A member of the nursing health care team who is educated in a one-year course and licensed to give bedside nursing care and treatments. In some states, with additional training the LPN is permitted to dispense medications.

Ligament A tough, white, fibrous cord that connects bone to bone.

Liquid Flowing freely, like water.

Lithotomy (dorsal) position The patient lies on her back with her legs spread apart and her knees bent. The position is used for performing a pelvic (vaginal) examination.

Liver The body's largest gland, located in the abdominal cavity. The liver has many functions in the chemistry and metabolism of the body and is essential to life.

Local anesthetics Anesthetics that cause numbness or a loss of sensation in only a part of the body.

Localized Limited to one place or part; affecting, involving, or pertaining to a definite area.

Localized application One in which warmth or coldness is applied to a specific area or small part of the body.

Lubricant A substance such as petroleum jelly, glycerine, or cold cream that is used to make a surface smooth or moist.

Lungs The primary organs of breathing.

Malignant A tumor or neoplasm that grows, spreads, invades, and destroys organs.

Malpractice Negligence when applied to the performance of a professional.

Medical asepsis Special practices and procedures for cleanliness to decrease the chances for disease-causing bacteria to live and spread.

Medical terminology The special vocabulary of words used in the health care professions.

Membrane A thin layer of tissue. An example is the mucous membrane, as in the lining of the nose and throat.

Menstruation The periodic (monthly) loss of some blood and a small part of the lining of the uterus.

Mercury sphygmomanometer Blood pressure equipment containing a column of mercury.

Metabolism The total of all the physical and chemical changes that take place in living organisms and cells, including all the processes involved in the use of substances taken into the body.

Metastasis The spreading of cancer cells through the body systems.

Metric system A system of measurement based on the decimal system. Units are 10s, 100s, and so forth.

Microorganism A living thing so small that it cannot be seen with the naked eye but only through a microscope.

Midstream Catching the urine specimen between the time the patient begins to void and the time he stops.

Mitered corner A special way to fold the bedding at the corners when making a hospital bed. The mitered corner keeps the bedding neat and stretched tightly so that wrinkles are avoided. It is sometimes called a square corner or hospital corner.

Mobilization Making movable; putting into motion.

Modified Changed.

Moist application An application of warmth or cold in which water touches the skin.

Morgue A place for storing dead bodies for identification and burial.

Motivation The reason, desire, need, or purpose that causes one to do something.

Mucus A sticky substance secreted by mucous membranes, mainly in the lungs, nose, and parts of the rectal and genital areas.

Muscle Tissue composed of fibers with the ability to elongate and shorten, causing bones and joints to move. Voluntary muscles are in body parts such as the neck, arms, fingers, and legs. Involuntary muscles are in organs such as the heart and intestines.

Muscle tissue Tissue that ensures movement; it is capable of stretching and contracting.

Muscular system The group of body organs that makes it possible for the body and its parts to move.

Nasal Pertaining to the nose and the nasal cavity.

Nasogastric tube Levine tube, n/g tube, stomach tube.

Negligence The commission of an act or failure to perform an act, where the respective performance or nonperformance deviates from the act that should have been done by a reasonably prudent person under the same or similar conditions.

Neoplasm New growth in which the cells grow without any control, organization or purpose.

Nephron The functional unit of the kidney that filters out those substances the body does not need, reabsorbing those it does need, and secreting those products that are harmful to the body. The result of this process is urine.

Nerves Bundles of neurons held together with connective tissue. Nerves are spread throughout all areas of the body in an orderly way and send messages to and from the brain through the spinal cord.

Nerve tissue Tissue that carries nervous impulses between the brain, the spinal cord, and all parts of the body.

Nervous system The group of body organs, consisting of the brain, spinal cord, and nerves, that controls and regulates the activities of the body and the function of the other body systems.

Neuron A nerve cell that moves nerve impulses.

Nonambulatory Not able to walk.

Nosocomial infection Hospital-acquired infections.

Nothing by mouth (NPO) Cannot eat or drink anything at all.

Nourishment The process of taking food into the body to maintain life.

Nurse A person educated and trained to care for sick people and to help physicians and surgeons. Nurses are licensed as registered nurses (RNs) and licensed practical nurses (LPNs).

Nursing assistant A person who helps the registered nurse to care for patients. Nursing assistants usually work in hospitals, in other health care institutions, or in the patient's home.

Nursing care plan A written plan stating the nursing diagnosis, (the cause and nature of the patient's problems), the patient goals or expected outcomes (objectives), and the nursing orders, interventions, or actions (the procedures or activities that should be performed to obtain the desired results).

Nutrients Chemical substances found in food. Some 50 individual nutrients are needed to build the body. They work better together than alone. There are six classes of nutrients: carbohydrates, fats, minerals, proteins, vitamins, and water.

Nutrition The process by which the body takes in and uses food.

Obese Very fat.

Objective observations Symptoms that can be observed and reported exactly as they are seen.

Objective reporting Reporting exactly what you observe.

Observation Gathering information about the patient by noticing any change.

Occupational therapist Trained person who assists the patient with performing the activities of daily living.

Omit Leave out.

Oral Anything to do with the mouth.

Oral hygiene Cleanliness of the mouth.

Orders A command, direction, or instruction given by a superior requiring obedient execution of a task.

Organ A part of the body made of several types of tissue grouped together to perform a certain function. Examples are the heart, stomach, and lungs.

Organism A living thing.

Orthopedics (orthopaedics) The medical specialty that covers the treatment of broken bones, deformities, or diseases that attack the bones, joints, and muscles.

Ostomy A surgical procedure that provides the patient with an artificial opening, either temporary or permanent. The person's feces or urine then can leave the body through this opening. The opening is usually made through the abdominal wall into a part of the large intestine.

Ovulation The process whereby an ovum is released from one ovary into the opening of the Fallopian tube and moves to the uterus.

Ovum The female reproductive cell produced in the ovaries, which is capable of uniting with a sperm cell and developing into a new organism.

Oxygen A colorless, odorless, tasteless gaseous element that is essential for respiration. Air is 21% oxygen.

Oxygen tent Equipment used in the health care institution to provide large amounts of extra oxygen for a patient.

Pancreas A large gland, 6 to 8 inches long, that secretes enzymes into the intestines for digestion of foods. It also manufactures insulin, which is secreted into the bloodstream.

Paralysis Loss of the ability to move a part or all of the body.

Paraplegia Paralysis of the legs and lower part of the body.

Parenteral intake Fluids taken in intravenously.

Passive Not active, but acted upon; enduring without effort or resistance.

Pathogens Disease-causing microorganisms.

Patient lift A mechanical device with a sling seat used for lifting a patient into and out of such equipment as the hospital bed, bathtub, or wheelchair.

Patient oriented Nursing care that is arranged according to the total needs of the individual patient.

Patient unit The space for one patient, including the hospital bed, bedside table, chair, and other equipment.

Pediatric patient Any patient under the age of 16 years.

Perineum (perineal area) The body area between the thighs. It includes the area of the anus and the external genital organs.

Peristalsis Movement of the intestines that pushes the food along to the next part of the digestive system.

Perspiration Sweat.

Phlebitis Inflammation of a vein.

Physical therapist Trained person who assists the patient with activities related to motion.

Physician A doctor; a person who is licensed to practice medicine.

Physiological Referring to the study of the ways the body functions and responds.

Physiology The study of the functions of the body.

Pituitary gland Sometimes called the master gland. It is attached to the base of the brain and directs the flow of all hormones in the body.

Plaque Fatty deposits within blood vessels attached to vessel walls.

Pleural cavity The chest cavity containing the lungs. The pleura is the membrane lining the chest cavity and covering the lungs.

Poison Any substance ingested, inhaled, injected, or absorbed into the body that will interfere with normal physiological functions.

Posterior Located in the back or toward the rear.

Postmortem After death.

Postoperative After surgery.

Postoperative bed A standard hospital bed made up in a special way for a patient who is coming back to his or her unit after an operation. Sometimes called recovery bed, stretcher bed, or operating room bed.

Postpartum Following childbirth.

Prefix A word element added to the beginning of a root.

Preoperative Before surgery.

Pressure ulcers Also called skin breakdown ulcers; areas of the skin that become broken; caused by continuous pressure on a body part.

Prevent To keep from happening.

Primary nursing A patient-oriented method of organizing the health care team in which the professional registered nurses are responsible for the total nursing care of the patient.

Professional registered nurse A member of the nursing health care team who is educated for from two to four years and licensed to plan and carry out total patient care. The duties of the registered nurse may include dispensing medication, administering treatments, assisting physicians, and supervising other members of the nursing health care team. The job of head nurse or team leader is an example of one important role filled by a registered nurse.

Prominences Places where bones are close to the surface of the body.

Pronation Rolling the palm downward.

Prone Lying on one's stomach.

Prosthesis An artificial body part. There are prostheses (plural) for legs, arms, hands, feet, breasts, eyes, and teeth.

Protective device A type of restraint that keeps the patient from harming himself and, therefore, creates a safe environment for the patient.

Psychological Referring to the study of the ways the mind functions and responds, including feelings and thoughts.

Psychosocial All aspects of living together in a group with other human beings.

Pulmonary Refers to the lungs.

Pulse The rhythmic expansion and contraction of the arteries caused by the beating of the heart. The expansion and contraction show how fast, how regular, and with what force the heart is beating.

Pulse deficit A difference between the apical heartbeat and the radial pulse rate.

Quadriplegia Paralysis of both the upper and lower parts of the body.

Radial pulse The pulse felt at a person's wrist at the radial artery.

Range of motion (ROM) These exercises move each muscle and joint through its full range of motion and assist the patient who is confined to exercise his or her muscles and joints.

Rate Used to describe the number of pulse beats per minute.

Reagent A substance that detects the presence of another substance in a chemical reaction.

Rectal Pertaining to the rectum.

Rectal irrigation Washing out the rectum by injecting a stream of water; giving an enema.

Rectum The lower 8 to 10 inches of the colon. The anus is the body opening from the rectum.

Recumbent position Lying down or reclining.

Rehabilitation The process by which people who have been disabled by injury or sickness are helped to recover as much as possible of their original abilities for the activities of daily living.

Relax In a resting position; the time following contraction of a muscle in which tension decreases, fibers lengthen, and the muscle returns to a resting position.

Reproductive system The group of body organs that makes possible the creation of a new human life.

Respect Recognition of the worth of another person.

Respiration The body process of breathing; inhaling and exhaling air.

Respiratory system The group of body organs that carries on the body function of respiration. The system brings oxygen into the body and eliminates carbon dioxide.

Respond To react; to begin, end, or change activity in reaction to stimulation.

Responsibility A duty or obligation; that for which one is accountable.

Restraint Equipment used to protect, support, or hold a patient in a particular position.

Restrict fluids Fluids that are limited to certain amounts.

Restricted Not permitted.

Restrictions Limits on the amounts allowed; being limited or confined.

Retain To keep or hold in.

Retention To hold in; retain.

Reticuloendothelial system The body system primarily responsible for our resistance to disease. The tissue is made up of cells from various systems, all of which are capable of either producing antibodies or the process of phagocytosis.

Reverse isolation Procedures used to prevent harmful organisms from coming into contact with the patient. See isolation procedure.

Rhythm Used to describe the regularity of the pulse beats.

Rigor mortis Stiffening of a body and limbs shortly after death.

Roman numerals The letters used to represent numbers in the ancient Roman system.

Root The body or main part of the word.

Rotation To move a joint in a circular motion around its axis: internal, to turn in toward the center; external, to turn away from the center.

Rupture Break open.

Saliva The secretion of the salivary glands into the mouth. Saliva moistens food and helps in swallowing. It also contains an enzyme (chemical) that helps digest starches.

Scrotal prep The procedures for making the genital area of a male patient ready for surgery. The preparation includes thoroughly cleansing the skin and carefully shaving the hair in the area.

Secrete To produce a special substance and expel or discharge it. The salivary glands secrete saliva. The pancreas secretes insulin.

Secretions The substances that flow out of or are produced by glandular organs; the process of producing this substance; for example, sweat, bile, lymph, saliva, or urine.

Seizure An episode, either partial or generalized, which may include altered consciousness, motor activity, or sensory phenomena and convulsions.

Self-care Activities or care tasks performed by the patient.

Sexually Transmitted Diseases Diseases acquired as a result of sexual intercourse with a person who is infected.

Shallow respiration Breathing with only the upper part of the lungs.

Shock The failure of the cardiovascular system to provide sufficient blood circulation to every part of the body.

Shroud A cloth or sheet in which a body is wrapped for burial.

Side lying Lying on one's side.

Signs Objective evidence of disease. Signs can be observed by a trained person such as a doctor or nurse. Vital signs are special signals that doctors and nurses always look for. These are the patient's temperature, pulse, respiration, and blood pressure.

Sim's position The patient lies on the left side with the right knee and thigh drawn up. This position permits a satisfactory rectal examination.

Sitz bath A bath in which the patient sits in a specially designed chairtub or a regular bathtub with the hips and buttocks in water.

Skeleton The bony support of the body.

Skin prep Shaving the area of the body where an operation is going to be performed in preparation for surgery.

Soak Immerse the body or body part completely in water.

Social Refers to interactions and relations among people.

Sociocultural Responses to methods of education, discipline, and training that are determined by the culture of the social group.

Solution Liquid containing dissolved substances.

Spasm An involuntary sudden movement or convulsive muscular contraction.

Specialty bed A bed that constantly changes pressure under the patient. Used to minimize pressure points in the treatment or prevention of bedsores.

Specimen A sample of material taken from the patient's body. Examples are urine specimens, feces specimens, and sputum specimens.

Sperm The male reproductive cell produced in the testes, which is capable of uniting with an ovum and developing into a new organism.

Sphincter A ringlike muscle that controls the opening and closing of a body opening. An example is the anal sphincter.

Sphygmomanometer An apparatus for measuring blood pressure.

Spinal anesthetics Anesthetics that cause a loss of feeling in a large area of the body, usually from the umbilicus down to and including the legs and feet.

Spinal cord One of the main organs of the nervous system. The spine is another name for the human backbone. The spinal cord carries messages from the brain to other parts of the body and from parts of the body back to the brain. The spinal cord is inside the spine (backbone).

Spiritual Referring to a person's responses to religious or inspirational ideas.

Spleen An abdominal organ that manufactures blood cells during the life of the embryo.

Splint A thin piece of wood or other rigid material used to keep an injured part, such as a broken bone, in place.

Spores Bacteria that have formed hard shells around themselves for protection. Spores can be destroyed only by sterilization.

Sputum Waste material coughed up from the lungs or trachea.

Staphylococcus One type of bacteria that causes infection found in health care institutions. Antibiotic drugs are used to fight staphylococcus infections.

Sterilization (sterilizing) The process of destroying all microorganisms, including spores.

Stertorous respiration The patient makes abnormal noises like snoring sounds when he or she is breathing.

Stethoscope An instrument that allows one to listen to various sounds in the patient's body, such as the heartbeat or breathing sounds.

Stimuli Changes in the external or internal environment strong enough to set up a nervous impulse or other responses in an organism.

Stoma An artificially made opening connecting a body passage with the outside, such as in a tracheotomy or colostomy.

Stool Solid waste material discharged from the body through the rectum and anus. Other names include feces, excreta, excrement, bowel movement, and fecal matter.

Stretcher A narrow, rolling table with or without a mattress or simply a canvas stretched over a frame used to transport patients. This may also be called a litter or a gurney.

Stroke Interruption of or damage to the blood supply to the brain; a cerebrovascular accident.

Subjective Observations Signs and symptoms that can be felt and described only by the patient himself, such as pain, nausea, dizziness, ringing in the ears, and headache.

Subjective reporting Giving your opinion about what you have observed. The nursing assistant should never use subjective reporting.

Suction The action of, or capacity for, vacuuming up. This is accomplished by reducing the air pressure over part of the surface of a substance.

Suffix A word element used to change or add to the meaning of a root. It is always added to the end of a root.

Superficial On or near the surface of the body.

Superior The upper portion of the body.

Supervision Direction and inspection of the performance of workers.

Supination Rolling the palm upward.

Supine Lying on one's back.

Support systems People or actions used to help a person adjust or live.

Suppository A semisolid preparation (sometimes medicated) that is inserted into the vagina or the rectum.

Surgical asepsis When an area is made totally free of microorganisms. The area may be called surgically clean.

Surgical procedure The repair of an injury or a disease condition. In a surgical procedure, the surgeon usually makes an incision; that is, he or she cuts through the skin into the body.

Symptom Evidence of a disease, disorder, or condition.

System A group of organs acting together to carry out one or more body functions.

Systolic blood pressure The force with which blood is pumped when the heart muscle is contracting. When taking a patient's blood pressure, the systolic blood pressure is recorded as the top number.

Tact Doing or saying the right things at the right time.

Task oriented Nursing care that is arranged according to what must be done.

Taut Pulled or drawn tight; not slack.

Team nursing A task-oriented method of organizing the health care team in which the team leader gives patient care assignments to each team member.

Temperature A measurement of the amount of heat in the body at a given time. The normal body temperature is 98.6°F (37°C).

Terminally ill Having an illness that can be expected to cause death, usually within a known time.

Testosterone The primary male sex hormone manufactured in the testes; it is essential for normal sexual behavior and the development of secondary sexual characteristics.

Therapeutic Refers mainly to the treatment of disease. Something that helps heal.

Therapeutic diet A diet designed to meet a patient's special nutritional needs; also called special diet, restricted diet, modified diet.

Thermometer An instrument used for measuring temperature.

Thrombophlebitis Inflammation and blood clots in a vein.

Thrombus A blood clot that remains at its site of formation.

Thyroid An endocrine gland, located in the front of the neck. It regulates body metabolism and secretes a hormone known as thyroxine.

Tissue A group of cells of the same type.

Tissue fluid A watery environment around each cell that acts as a place of exchange for gases, food, and waste products between the cells and the blood.

Toxins Poisonous substances of plant or animal origin.

Trachea An organ of the respiratory system located in the throat area. The trachea is commonly called the *windpipe*.

Tracheotomy A surgical procedure to make an artificial opening in a person's neck connecting his or her trachea with the outside. This surgery may be necessary when the trachea above the opening is blocked and the person cannot breathe.

Traction device Equipment for pulling and stretching parts of the patient's body by using pulleys and weights. Traction is used to keep broken bones in proper alignment while healing.

Transfer Moving a hospital patient from one unit to another, or from one facility to another.

Transporting Moving from one place to another.

Trapeze A metal bar suspended over the bed. It is used by a patient to help him or her raise or move the body more easily.

Traumatic Refers to damage to the body caused by injury, wound, or shock. Sometimes used to refer to mental disturbances caused by emotional shock.

Trendelenburg's position The bed or operating table is tilted so that the patient's head is about one foot below the level of the knees. This position is used to get more blood to the head and prevent shock. Also called the shock position.

Tumor A growth in or on the body. There are two kinds: (1) benign tumors, and (2) malignant tumors.

Ulcer A local destruction of the epidermis and dermis.

Umbilical cord A rather long, flexible, rough organ that carries nourishment from the mother to the baby. It connects the umbilicus of the unborn baby in the mother's uterus to the placenta.

Umbilicus A small depression on the abdomen that marks the place where the umbilical cord was originally attached to the fetus. Another name for the umbilicus is the *navel*.

Unconscious Unaware of the environment; occurs during sleep and in temporary episodes ranging from fainting or stupor to coma.

Ureters The tubes leading from the kidneys to the urinary bladder.

Urethra Tube leading from the urinary bladder to the outside of the body.

Urinal A portable pan given to male patients in bed so they can urinate without getting out of bed.

Urinalysis A laboratory test of the patient's urine done for diagnostic purposes.

Urinate To discharge urine from the body. Other words for this function are void, micturate, and pass water.

Urine The fluid secreted by the kidneys, stored in the bladder, and excreted through the urethra.

Vagina In the female, the birth canal leading from the vulva to the cervix of the uterus (vaginal canal, vaginal tract).

Vaginal irrigation or douche A procedure by which a stream of water is sent into the patient's vaginal opening. The water may be plain or it may contain medication.

Vaginal prep The procedures for making the genital area of a female patient ready for surgery. The preparation includes thoroughly cleansing the skin and carefully shaving the pubic hair. It may also include a cleansing douche.

Vascular Pertaining to blood vessels.

Vein A blood vessel that carries blood from parts of the body back to the heart.

Ventral On the abdominal, anterior, or front side of the body.

Ventricles The lower two chambers of the heart. They are side by side.

Villus A tiny, fingerlike projection in the lining of the small intestine into which the end products of digestion are absorbed and carried to the bloodstream and then to the individual cells.

Virus A microscopic living parasitic agent that can cause infectious disease.

Viscera Refers to the organs within the abdominal body cavity.

Vital signs Temperature, pulse, respiration, and blood pressure.

Void To urinate, pass water.

Voluntary Under control of the will; with conscious decision.

Vomiting Throwing up; the contents of the stomach are cast up and out of the mouth.

Vomitus Vomited material; emesis.

Walker A stable frame made of metal tubing used to support the unsteady patient while walking. The patient holds the walker while taking a step, moves it forward, and takes another step.

Well-balanced diet A diet containing a variety of foods from each of the basic food groups.

Wheelchair A chair on wheels used to transport patients.

Index

B

C

D

E

F

G

H

I

J

K

L

M

N

O

S

T